BMA

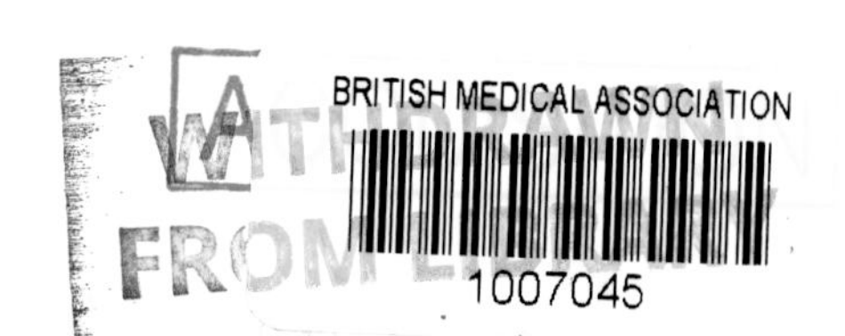

# PRACTICAL STATISTICS FOR MEDICAL RESEARCH

OTHER STATISTICS TEXTS FROM
CHAPMAN AND HALL

**The Analysis of Time Series**
C. Chatfield
**Problem Solving: A Statistician's Guide**
C. Chatfield
**Statistics for Technology**
C. Chatfield
**Introduction to Multivariate Analysis**
C. Chatfield and A. J. Collins
**Applied Statistics**
D. R. Cox and E. J. Snell
**An Introduction to Statistical Modelling**
A. J. Dobson
**Introduction to Optimization Methods and their Application in Statistics**
B. S. Everitt
**Multivariate Statistics – A Practical Approach**
B. Flury and H. Riedwyl
**Readings in Decision Analysis**
S. French
**Multivariate Analysis of Variance and Repeated Measures**
D. J. Hand and C. C. Taylor
**Multivariate Statistical Methods – A Primer**
Bryan F. Manley
**Statistical Methods in Agriculture and Experimental Biology**
R. Mead and R. N. Curnow
**Elements of Simulation**
B. J. T. Morgan
**Probability: Methods and Measurement**
A. O'Hagan
**Essential Statistics**
D. G. Rees
**Foundations of Statistics**
D. G. Rees
**Decision Analysis: A Bayesian Approach**
J. Q. Smith
**Applied Statistics: A Handbook of BMDP Analyses**
E. J. Snell
**Elementary Applications of Probability Theory**
H. C. Tuckwell
**Intermediate Statistical Methods**
G. B. Wetherill

*Further information of the complete range of* Chapman and Hall *statistics books is available from the publishers.*

# PRACTICAL STATISTICS FOR MEDICAL RESEARCH

Douglas G. Altman

*Head of Medical Statistical Laboratory*
*Imperial Cancer Research Fund*
*London*



CHAPMAN & HALL/CRC

**Boca Raton London New York Washington, D.C.**

**Library of Congress Cataloging-in-Publication Data**

Altman, Douglas G.
Practical statistics for medical research / Douglas G. Altman.
p. cm.
Originally published: London : Chapman & Hall, 1991.
Includes bibliographical references and index.
ISBN 0-412-27630-5
1. Medicine—Research—Stastical methods. I. Title.
R853.S7A48 1999
610'.7'27—dc21 99-15186
CIP



Direct all inquiries to CRC Press LLC, 2000 N.W. Corporate Blvd., Boca Raton, Florida 33431.



**Visit the CRC Press Web site at www.crcpress.com**

First edition 1991
Reprinted 1992 (twice), 1993, 1994, 1995, 1996, 1997
First CRC Press Reprint 1999
Originally published by Chapman & Hall


International Standard Book Number 0-412-27630-5
Library of Congress Card Number 99-15186
Printed and bound by CPI Group (UK) Ltd, Croydon, CR0 4YY
Printed on acid-free paper

To my parents

# Contents

# Preface

The difficulties many intelligent people have with 'sums' are infinite
Greenwood (1948)

This book on statistics is primarily aimed at medical researchers. Whether clinical or non-clinical, most will have received some statistics teaching as undergraduates, but it will have been fairly brief, a long time ago, and largely forgotten by the time it is needed. The book should also be useful to medical students, to clinicians who wish to understand the principles of the design and analysis of research, and to those attending postgraduate courses in medical statistics.

I have been motivated to write this book by the belief that most introductory texts do not explain adequately the concepts that underlie the whole subject of statistics, and in many cases they are divorced from the reality of carrying out and assessing medical research. This book should provide an understanding of the basic principles that underlie research design, data analysis and the interpretation of results, and enable the reader to carry out a wide range of statistical analyses. The emphasis is firmly on practical aspects of the design and analysis of medical research and I have paid special attention to the interpretation and presentation of results. By discussing both the use and misuse of statistics the book should also give the reader the material to be able to judge the appropriateness of the methods and interpretation in papers published in medical journals.

I have assumed that most researchers now have access to a computer so that the mathematical details are generally confined to self-contained sections that may be omitted. I have used real data throughout, mostly from published papers, and I have tried to find data that are interesting in their own right. In most cases all the raw data are given, so that the analyses can be reproduced either by computer or by hand calculation. This feature will assist in the evaluation of a statistical computer program.

Many data sets have been taken from published papers, not always used for the authors' original purpose. Some data sets have been reconstructed from graphs or summary statistics and others have come from my own collaborative studies. I thank everyone whose data I have used. I have tried to represent these studies fairly, and apologise if I have failed at all in this respect. I am grateful to the *British Medical Journal* and the *British*

*Journal of Obstetrics and Gynaecology* for permission to reproduce figures and Ciba-Geigy Ltd, the Biometrika Trustees and Oliver and Boyd for permission to reproduce statistical tables. Almost all of the figures were produced using STATA and STAGE (Computing Resource Center, Los Angeles).

I wish to thank everyone who has helped me to write this book. The whole book was read in draft by Martin Bland, Caroline Doré, Sheila Gore and Richard Wootton to whom I am especially grateful, and I also thank Peter Clark, Bianca De Stavola, David Hill and Patrick Royston for reading certain chapters. Their comments and suggestions have been enormously valuable, but I must take the blame for any remaining infelicities or errors. I especially thank Judy MacDonald for typing the manuscript, and dealing with numerous revisions; thanks too to Olive Waldron and Clare Wood who typed early drafts. Lastly I thank Sue for her encouragement and support.

Douglas Altman
1990

# 1

# Statistics in medical research

> At the thought of statistics, the Collector, walking through the chaotic Residency garden, felt his heart quicken with joy. . . . For what were statistics but the ordering of a chaotic universe? Statistics were the leg-irons to be clapped on the *thugs* of ignorance and superstition which strangled Truth in lonely byways.
>
> J. G. Farrell, *The Siege of Krishnapur*

## 1.1 STATISTICS AT LARGE

We are bombarded with statistics to an unprecedented degree. Newspapers contain a wealth of statistical information, relating to trade and industry, finance, (un)employment, road accident figures and the like, and there are frequent results of opinion polls and surveys. Statistics presented in this way are of varying reliability. While political opinion polls are performed with reasonably reliable methods, most surveys are based on asking questions of some convenient group of people, with no concern for their representativeness. They may even be based on volunteered information, as in phone-in polls.

It is also common to see reports of medical research in the media. Research findings are usually based on sound methodology, but as the results may be presented in a like manner the distinction in reliability is not widely perceived. For example, newspapers will report in similar terms the findings of a poll about attitudes to consumption of eggs in the light of worries about salmonella and also the results of an epidemiological study investigating the relation between use of the contraceptive pill and risk of breast cancer. Many medical issues are really too complex to be dealt with adequately in a short item in a newspaper or on television. Topics such as the possibility of raised rates of childhood leukaemia around nuclear power stations or the carcinogenic effect of adding fluoride to drinking water require an in-depth consideration of many complicated issues. The complexity of the fluoride debate may be judged by the fact that a court case lasted 201 days, with much of the evidence being statistical (Oldham, 1985).

The word 'research' has powerful connotations, with reliability being implicit. Few people outside the relevant field are concerned about *how* the research was done, only about what was found. One recent advertisement I have seen makes use of this weakness. The company supports its promotion of desk top binding systems with the opening comment that 'Research shows that a well presented document stands a 95% better chance of being properly read and well received'. I doubt whether any such research had been carried out, or even if it could be, but the power of research is successfully invoked.

At the other extreme from this piece of nonsense is the following excerpt from a newspaper report (*Guardian*, 23 August 1986) of a paper in a medical journal:

**Score system for heart risk**
A cheap 'ready reckoner' for identifying men at high risk of a heart attack has been devised by doctors it was announced yesterday. Expensive electrocardiograph tests and measurements of blood cholesterol levels can be supplanted by a simple scoring system. The system can identify more than half of the men likely to have a heart attack over the next five years, who can then be advised to adopt a healthier lifestyle or offered treatment. . . . The system requires measurement of blood pressure, an estimate of the number of years of cigarette smoking, knowledge of previous angina, heart attack or diabetes, and whether either parent died of heart trouble.

Clearly this study is potentially valuable to thousands of men. Are these results reliable and how was the 'ready reckoner' devised? Of course we would not expect to obtain this information from a short newspaper article, but the fact that no information is given about how the study was performed may put it in no better light than any other statistics reported in the same newspaper.

Another example is given by a newspaper article (*Guardian*, 19 May 1988) reporting a study of the relation between longevity and left-handedness:

**Not many old hands left, says scientist**
If you're over 80 and left-handed, you're in a class of your own. Nearly all the other left-handers have passed on. . . . It was, said Dr Halpern last night, a small sample. Generally the scientists found that there was no difference in death rates up till the age of 33; from then the left-handers slowly fade away.

She offered several reasons. One might be that low-weight babies tended to be left-handed, and low birthweight might mean reduced chances of survival. The other was that it was a right-handed world. The left-handed were simply at a disadvantage with automobiles and power tools, suffered from greater stress and had more accidents.

I shall explain in Chapter 5 why the interpretation of the results from this study is not valid. For the moment I shall just note that the study findings are reported uncritically, and the last paragraph contains unsupported speculations which do not even appear in the publication (Halpern and Coren, 1988). There is no way that readers of the newspaper could distinguish the reliability of the information in the two newspaper reports. Yet it is variation in scientific standards, and hence the validity of research findings, that fuels controversies in medical research. These often impinge on daily life, such that the public becomes confused about possible adverse health effects of numerous foods and drugs (Feinstein, 1988).

In general the emphasis is on results (which are presented as facts), with little or no regard to the manner in which they were obtained, which is probably why the subject of statistics is widely seen as relating solely to the analysis of data and the presentation of numerical results. While these are important parts of statistics, there is much else besides. In particular, how and why the data were collected are supremely important.

There is a wide perception of statistics (and perhaps statisticians too) as untrustworthy, as embodied in the idea that 'you can prove anything with statistics'. This saying, if it means anything, suggests that figures can be presented in a variety of ways, and that it is common for the most favourable view to be selected. While there is justification for this belief, it is not true that you can *prove* anything with statistics; the opposite is true, at least with regard to statistical methods used in research. Statistical analysis allows us to put limits on our uncertainty, but not to *prove* anything. Despite considerable mistrust of statistics, there is a tendency towards uncritical acceptance by the public of research findings, which may be attributed to the power of the printed word.

## 1.2 STATISTICS IN MEDICINE

Statistics are increasingly prevalent in medical practice. Nowadays much concern is devoted to hospital utility statistics, audit, resource allocation, vaccination uptake, numbers of new cases of AIDS, and so on. Journals and magazines for doctors are full of statistical material of this sort, as well as the findings of individual research studies. Statistical issues are implicit in all clinical practice when making diagnoses and choosing an appropriate treatment.

It is increasingly common to see statistical results from research papers quoted in promotional materials for drugs (especially) and other medical therapies. As an example, the following text is from an advertisement for a treatment for leukaemia appearing in a clinical oncology journal in 1989 (I have only changed the names of the drugs):

**Significantly more first-course responders with NOVORAN**

- 63% of all adults with ANLL treated with NOVORAN had a complete remission, compared with 53% of all patients treated with orsoran ($P = 0.15$)
- 56% of patients had a complete remission after one induction course with NOVORAN, compared with 36% of patients treated with orsoran ($P < 0.01$)*
- 89% of complete responders to NOVORAN responded after a single induction course, compared with only 68% of complete responders to orsoran.

* Single df $\chi^2$

To understand this passage it is necessary to know the meaning of expressions like '$P = 0.15$', and perhaps also the curious footnote. More importantly, however, we should wish to know how large the study was and what the design was. An appreciation of the methods by which these percentages were obtained and how to interpret them is thus at least useful and arguably essential for all those who treat patients. (We cannot obtain the information in this case as the results of this study were reported as being 'on file', i.e. unpublished.)

For those doing research statistical issues are fundamental, and so it is extremely important to understand basic statistical ideas relating to research design and data analysis, and to be familiar with the most common methods of statistical analysis.

## 1.3 STATISTICS IN MEDICAL RESEARCH

Colton (1974, p. 1) observed that 'statistics pervades the medical literature'. Since then the huge influx of statistics into medical research has continued. The aim is to improve the reliability and credibility of the findings from medical research, but there is no guarantee that the statistical aspects have been handled well or even validly. As I shall show in the final chapter, there is considerable evidence that many published papers contain statistical errors.

There are many reasons why errors in statistics are a matter for concern. Put most simply, if there are statistical errors the conclusions of the study may be incorrect. Readers of the paper may not detect the error and may be misled either with respect to clinical practice or further research. While this argument may overestimate the influence of a single published paper, there is much evidence that readers of medical journals accept uncritically the printed word, as does the general public.

There is also a similar belief that statistics is about data analysis, perhaps because this is the most visible part of the statistical contribution. Data analysis is certainly an important part of statistics, but this narrow view excludes in particular vital aspects relating to the design of research. Without the solid foundations of a good design the edifice of analysis is unsafe. Reliable results depend upon an appropriate research design: 'The justification for the analysis lies not in the data collected but in the *manner* in which the data were collected' (Schoolman *et al.*, 1968). Many controversies in medicine are traceable to varying quality of the design of the research.

## 1.4 WHAT DOES STATISTICS COVER?

Figure 1.1 shows the general sequence of steps in a research project. Statistical thinking can contribute to every stage, although the major steps of design, analysis and interpretation will be the prime focus of this book.

The key difference between medical research and clinical practice is their scope. In each, data are collected from individual subjects, but in medical research the aim is to be able to make some general statements about a wider set of subjects, and we are not usually especially interested in the particular subjects that have been studied. We thus use information from a **sample** of individuals to make some **inference** about the wider **population** of like individuals. The three words in bold are formal statistical terms that will be explained fully in later chapters. The important point here is that the subjects who are studied act as a proxy for the total group of interest.

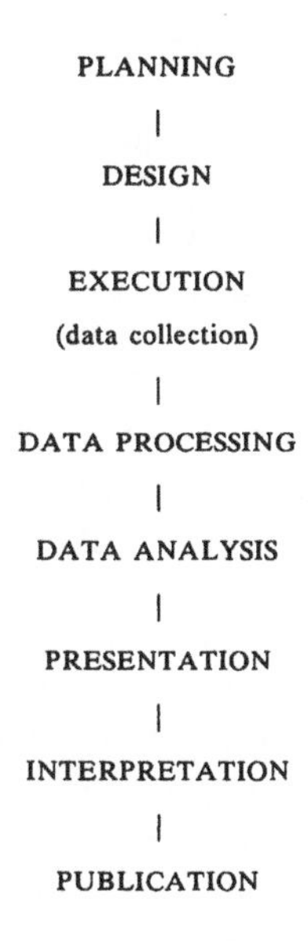


**Figure 1.1** General sequence of steps in a research project.

### 1.4.1 Research design

We can never study all diabetics, all pregnant women, or all people living in a geographical area. If we wish to investigate, for example, the relation between maternal weight gain in pregnancy and baby's birth weight we must study a sample of pregnant women. The aim of this research would be to extrapolate the findings from this sample to all pregnancies. For this inference to be reasonable, it is necessary for the sample of women to be representative of all pregnant women. In theory we can obtain a truly representative sample only by choosing women **at random** (a concept explained in Chapter 5) but even then the sample would be specific to a time period and geographical area. In practice, samples are nearly always chosen systematically and the subjects' characteristics are described so that their representativeness can be judged. The study just proposed would probably be carried out by taking all women registering at one or more specific hospitals in a set time period. In most studies it is necessary to exclude some people. Here women registering late in pregnancy would have to be excluded because they would not provide sufficient weight data. It is well known that this group is untypical in many respects. We might also wish to exclude premature births (< 37 weeks) and there would probably be some other minor reasons for exclusion, such as diabetes and twins.

It is customary for the report of such a study to list the criteria for including or excluding subjects in the study, and to describe important characteristics of the sample at the start of the study; in this case these would include age, parity (number of previous children), height and weight. It is then a subjective matter to decide whether or not it is reasonable to take the findings from the study sample as being representative of all pregnant women.

A comparative study would involve the same considerations as the observational study just described. For example, we might wish to compare groups of women given different dietary advice. Here we have the additional issue of how to decide which women get which advice. We would like a method that would result in the women in the two groups being of similar age, parity and pre-pregnancy weight. Further, we want a method that excludes the possibility of subjective influence on who receives which advice.

All the issues just described come under the broad heading of design, and are thus part of the statistical contribution to research. Another aspect is determination of a suitable sample size for the study. I hope that this example has illustrated some of the reasons why a correct design is an essential part of good research, and thus the importance of good statistical input at this early stage. Different problems arise in each study, but there are many general principles for good design, which are discussed in

Chapter 5. Clinical trials are considered in detail in Chapter 15.

A consequence of the fundamental role of study design is that the most important part of a research paper is the Methods section. It is here that we learn what was done and if the results will be useful. A study of maternal weight gain carried out only on women of above average weight or restricted to pregnancies ending with low birth weight babies might be of no interest, regardless of the findings, and a study carried out in Britain may be of little relevance to the situation in Africa or Asia. Put more generally, we cannot make valid generalizations from unrepresentative or **biased** samples. The avoidance of bias is one of the main aims of sound research design.

The report of the aforementioned study of men at high risk of heart attacks was published in the *British Medical Journal* (Shaper *et al.*, 1986). The 'Subjects and Methods' section of their paper (slightly shortened here) described exactly how the study was carried out:

The data used were derived from the British Regional Heart Study, which examined 7735 men aged 40–59 randomly selected from the age–sex registers of representative group general practices in 24 towns in England, Wales and Scotland. The 24 towns were selected from those with populations of 50 000–100 000; they represented the full range of cardiovascular disease mortality and included towns in all the major standard regions. The general practice selected in each town had a social class distribution representative of the town. The men were selected at random from age–sex registers; no attempt was made to exclude subjects with cardiovascular disease, and there was a 78% response rate.

Research nurses administered a questionnaire to and completed an examination of each man. In this study exposure to cigarette smoking was expressed as the number of years a man had smoked, irrespective of the quantity, as this was most strongly related to risk of ischaemic heart disease. Subjects were regarded as having angina if they indicated on the questionnaire that chest pain was present on exertion (walking uphill or hurrying). This included definite and possible angina. Results in this paper are confined to the 7506 men (97%) with complete data on all the above risk factors.

Only when armed with this information and details of the methods of analysis, can we make a proper assessment of the appropriateness of the authors' conclusions to all men aged 40–59. Extrapolation outside this age range is unwise.

If, however, important information is omitted from a paper, then we must reserve judgement on the findings. I consider this and other issues regarding reading medical papers in the final chapter.

### 1.4.2 Analysis and interpretation

Despite the preceding comments the analysis of data is the major part of learning about statistics. There are dozens of different methods of analysis, which makes difficult the choice of the correct method for a particular case. Before worrying about particular methods, however, it is necessary to consider the philosophy that underlies all methods of analysis. We will see that statistical methods of analysis are based on the same key idea that we use data from a sample to draw inferences about a wider population. Of course particular methods are important, but the general principles need to be absorbed first. The main general approaches to the statistical analysis of data are considered in Chapter 8, before particular methods are introduced.

The interpretation of results of statistical analysis is not always straightforward, but is simpler when the study has a clear aim and when there is an appreciation of the general principles that underlie the analysis. Indeed, if the study has been well designed and correctly analysed the interpretation of results can be fairly simple.

## 1.5 THE SCOPE OF THIS BOOK

In this book I have tried to give prominence to the concepts and principles of statistical design and analysis before considering specific methods of analysing data. Thus it is not until Chapter 9 that I start to describe the more familiar methods of analysis. The earlier chapters cover basic material including, as well as the main ideas of design and analysis, consideration of different types of data that may be encountered and advice on how to use a computer for statistical analysis. Chapters 9 to 12 describe the main methods of statistical analysis, while Chapters 13 to 15 consider specific medical topics. In Chapter 16 I look at the way statistics is used in the medical literature, and give advice on reading and writing medical papers with respect to the statistical content.

Medical research falls into the broad areas of clinical research, laboratory research and epidemiology, which may be regarded as relating to people, samples from people or populations of people. In each case the individuals studied may be a mixture of healthy and ill people. I use the term 'clinical' to include research in surgery, dentistry, nursing, psychology and so on.

The statistical methods described in this book apply to all of these areas, although the specific problems may vary. Epidemiology, however, has many special features and statistical methods, which are covered comprehensively in specialized texts.

One problem when writing a statistics textbook is the likely variation among readers in their familiarity with mathematical methods. I have adopted two devices to assist those who are less than comfortable with mathematics. Firstly, I have included an Appendix on mathematical notation (Appendix A), which includes brief explanations of all the terms used. Secondly, in most chapters I have put the mathematical formulae in self-contained sections, so that it is possible to read about a particular method without being confused or distracted by sometimes formidable looking equations. Although the formulae are not needed when using a computer, they do show the way in which the analysis works, and except in cases of extreme hypersensitivity I recommend that they should be examined. For the more advanced methods in later chapters I have not included the mathematical formulae as these are very complicated and the analyses are always done on a computer.

It is not necessary to be able to remember formulae – these can be looked up. What is important is to understand the general principles of the research process, from formulating an objective through all the steps shown in Figure 1.1, and to be aware of the limitations of what may or may not be deduced.

I do not pretend that statistics is easy to learn. On the contrary, I think it is rather difficult. Statistics is a curious amalgam of mathematics, logic and judgement. Although many are put off by the mathematics, it is often the logical processes that cause more difficulty – the principles of good design, and the concepts underlying data analysis and interpretation. If statistics were what many people expect, namely an extension of simple mathematics, it would be more straightforward. The mismatch between expectation and reality leads to many problems, a dislike of the subject, frustration and maybe even tears. In the past it has led to remarks such as the following: 'The truth of the matter is that most of us detest statistical analysis and welcome any excuse to dispense with it' (Seddon, 1937). Fortunately this is not an inevitable pathway. I hope that the approach that I have adopted in this book leads to a relatively painless acquisition of an understanding of statistics.

# 2

# Types of data

## 2.1 INTRODUCTION

There is a lot more to statistics than the analysis of data, and in later chapters I shall consider aspects such as the design of good experiments and the interpretation of results. Nevertheless statistics as a subject is very largely about data so it is sensible to start with a brief discussion of various types of data that may be encountered in medical work. The nature of the observations is of major importance in relation to the choice of correct statistical methods of analysis.

Data can be either **categorical** or **numerical** (otherwise known as **qualitative** and **quantitative**), but within these broad classifications there are various different types of data.

## 2.2 CATEGORICAL DATA

### 2.2.1 Two categories

The simplest type of observation on an individual is the allocation of that individual to one of only two possible categories. Often these relate to the presence or absence of some attribute. Examples of such categorizations for patients include:

1. male/female
2. pregnant/not pregnant
3. married/single
4. diabetic/non-diabetic
5. smoker/non-smoker
6. hypertensive/normotensive

Such data have numerous other names such as binary data, dichotomous data, attribute data, yes/no data, and 0–1 data. We will see later that there are some advantages in giving the numerical values 0 and 1 to the two categories.

Notice that whereas (1) and (2) above definitely split subjects into two groups the other examples are all simplifications of more complex data.

For example, without further information it is not clear how to categorize people who have been divorced in (3) or ex-smokers in (5). The classification of patients as hypertensive or not (6) imposes a cut-off point on values of a measurement (here blood pressure). In general this is an undesirable practice, not always just from the statistical viewpoint.

### 2.2.2 More than two categories

Clearly many classifications require more than two categories, such as country of birth or blood group. Examples (3) and (4) in the previous section might be expanded into several categories as follows:

married/single/divorced/separated/widowed

juvenile-onset diabetes/maturity-onset diabetes/non-diabetic

Another example is blood group: A/B/AB/O. Data of this type are also called **nominal** data.

In the above examples there is no obvious ordering of the categories, but often there is a natural order, as with the various staging systems for cancers (and other diseases) and social class. Returning to the example of cigarette consumption, it is common to classify subjects as

non-smokers/ex-smokers/light smokers/heavy smokers

where the degree of smoking could be subdivided further. Data of this type are also called **ordinal** data.

Another type of ordered categorical data arises with subjective assessment of something that cannot be measured. For example, a patient may classify their degree of pain as

minimal/moderate/severe/unbearable

(but see section 2.4.5).

Ordinal data are often reduced to two categories to simplify analysis and presentation, which may result in a considerable loss of information.

## 2.3 NUMERICAL DATA

### 2.3.1 Discrete data

**Discrete** numerical data arise when the observations in question can only take certain numerical values. Virtually all examples are counts of events, such as number of children, number of visits to the GP in a year, number of ectopic heart beats in 24 hours, etc.

The difference between such data as these and the ordered categorical data described earlier can be seen by considering an example of each:

*Ordered categorical:*

Stage of breast cancer: I II III IV

*Discrete numerical:*

Number of children: 0 1 2 3 4 5+

We cannot say that stage IV is twice as bad as stage II nor that the difference between stages I and II is equivalent to that between stages III and IV. In contrast, three children are three times as many as one (although not necessarily three times as bad!), and a difference of one means the same throughout the range of values.

In practice discrete data are often treated in statistical analyses as if they were ordered categories. This is not wrong, but it may not be getting the most out of the data. Conversely, where ordered categories are numbered, as with stage of disease or social class, the temptation to treat these numbers as statistically meaningful must be resisted. For example, it is not sensible to calculate the average social class or stage of cancer. The only information the numbers contain is in the ordering, which would be conveyed equally by calling them A, B, C, D and so on.

### 2.3.2 Continuous data

**Continuous** data are usually obtained by some form of measurement. Common examples include height, weight, age, body temperature, blood pressure and serum cholesterol. Such observations are not restricted to certain values except insofar as this is restricted by the accuracy of the measuring instrument.

It will not be necessary to record the data to numerous decimal places, but the fact that in principle it could be done is the distinguishing property of continuous measurements. Thus blood pressure is often recorded to the nearest 2 or perhaps 5 mm Hg, and body weight of adults to the nearest 100 g.

Sometimes it is reasonable to treat discrete data as if they were continuous, at least as far as statistical analysis goes. While age is a continuous measurement, age at last birthday is discrete. In studies of adults with ages ranging from, say, 16 to 80, no harm is done in considering age in years as a continuous measurement (and this is standard practice), but for studies of pre-school children it would be better to use age in months. Heart rate (in beats per minute) is another discrete measurement that is usually regarded as continuous. Although the essential requirement for this change of status is that there should be a large number of different possible values, in practice we do not worry too much about analysing discrete measurements as if they were continuous.

Conversely, continuous data are often reduced to several categories.

Where the variable is known to be imprecise, such as reported number of cigarettes smoked per day, it may be sensible to have categories such as

0/1–10/11–20/21 or more.

Otherwise, it is best to record the actual value of blood pressure, haemoglobin, etc. It is easy to convert to categories in the analysis, but the raw data cannot be retrieved later if only categories are recorded. Information is lost with no compensatory gain. Indeed, the statistical analysis of continuous data is more powerful, and often simpler.

When some calculation is necessary to derive the observation of interest this should be done by the computer. Thus it is much better to record date of birth and date of examination for subsequent calculation of age rather than to rely on mental arithmetic.

The degree of measurement accuracy and the type of data are both important in relation to carrying out a proper statistical analysis.

## 2.4 OTHER TYPES OF DATA

The preceding sections have covered the most common types of data likely to be encountered in medical research. In this section some miscellaneous other types of data are described.

### 2.4.1 Ranks

Occasionally the data in question are the relative positions of the members of a group in some respect. The most obvious (although non-medical) example is in sporting competitions or examinations. Sometimes there is a clear underlying measurement, such as time to run 400 metres, but in other cases there is not, for example when expressing preferences between different treatments.

Patients are sometimes given two or more treatments and asked to express a preference. Such rankings are rare in medical work, but the idea is important. As we shall see in later chapters, in some circumstances it is a good idea to convert the measurements on a group of individuals into a rank ordering before analysing the data.

### 2.4.2 Percentages

Percentages arise when one takes the ratio of two quantities. Examples are the left ventricular ejection fraction, which measures the percentage of blood ejected from the left ventricle when the heart beats, and the relative body weight (observed body weight divided by ‘desirable’ body weight). In the first example the ratio is of two quantities both of which have been measured, while in the second a single measurement is divided by a pre-existing (constant) value usually taken from published tables.

Although it is reasonable to use these calculated percentages for well-established measurements, it is in general desirable to retain the information regarding both quantities used in the calculation. It would not, for example, be a good idea to record for each individual just the percentage reduction in blood pressure achieved following treatment. There is no particular reason to consider the effectiveness of a drug in terms of percentage reduction.

Although percentages may usually be regarded as continuous measurements they can cause problems in analysis, especially where there can be values either side of 100% (e.g. relative weight), or where there can be negative values as when calculating the percentage change in some measurement. If your systolic blood pressure is 150 mm Hg then a 20% rise will increase it to 180 mm Hg, but a subsequent fall of 20% will take it back down to 144 mm Hg. Considerable care is necessary when considering such data.

### 2.4.3 Rates and ratios

A similar approach is used to convert an observed frequency to a **rate**. For example, the number of perinatal deaths is usually related to the total number of births by calculating the perinatal mortality rate per 1000 births.

Sometimes the frequency of events of a specific kind is compared with the expected number of events. For example, the expected number of new cases of leukaemia in an area in a given time period can be calculated by applying national age and sex specific rates to the numbers of people in the area in each age sex group. The ratio of the observed ($O$) to expected ($E$) frequencies yields the standardized mortality ratio as $100 \times O/E$.

### 2.4.4 Scores

When it is not possible to take direct measurements it is often possible to grade individuals in some way. In its simplest form, such a system may involve classifying a skin rash, for example, as mild, moderate or severe. More generally clinicians often use systems such as 0,+,++,+++. Although the meaning of such symbols is pretty obvious, the classes are usually undefined and will not be comparable from one doctor to another. Clearly, such simple scales are further examples of ordered categorical data.

Often, however, it is possible to classify patients in several ways, perhaps in relation to various symptoms and signs. For each symptom the different codings can be given numerical values and the various values added up to give a total score. This score is then the observation.

**Table 2.1** Apgar system of scoring newborn babies

| Sign | Score<br>0 | 1 | 2 |
|---|---|---|---|
| Heart rate | Absent | Slow (< 100) | > 100 |
| Respiratory effort | Absent | Weak cry; hypoventilation | Good strong cry |
| Muscle tone | Limp | Some flexion of extremities | Well flexed |
| Reflex irritability (response to skin stimulation to feet) | No response | Some motion | Cry |
| Colour | Blue; pale | Body pink; extremities blue | Completely pink |

A well-known example is the Apgar score for evaluating the well-being of newborn babies (Apgar, 1953). Table 2.1 (from Apgar *et al.*, 1958) shows how the 'Apgar score' is obtained. Infants are classified into one of three categories scored 0, 1 or 2 for each of five variables, and thus receive a total score of between 0 and 10. It is standard practice to calculate Apgar scores in all newborn babies at both one and five minutes after birth. At one minute a score of 7 or more is good, whereas a score of less than 3 is very bad.

This is not the place to discuss the usefulness or validity of this particular scoring system, but three aspects of the system, which is typical of such schemes, should be noted. Firstly, for most of the signs some subjectivity is involved. Secondly, the numerical coding implies that any difference from 0 to 1 or from 1 to 2 is equally important. Thirdly, the five signs are considered equally important. Composite scores thus incorporate considerable subjectivity, some inherent in the combination procedure and some in the assessment of individuals.

In a non-medical field there has been considerable controversy over the relative weights given to the different events in ice-skating championships, and the scoring system for the decathlon is being changed because advances in achievement in some events have tended to undervalue other events. The same problem occurs in combining marks from different exams. The weighting of constituent elements of a composite score does not have to be equal, although it usually is in clinical practice.

### 2.4.5 Visual analogue scales

Patients may be asked to assess their degree of something unmeasureable like pain, mobility or hunger. A technique for improving on ordered categories (illustrated in section 2.2.2) is the **visual analogue scale** (VAS) or **linear analogue scale**. The patient is shown a straight line (often 10 cm long) the ends of which are labelled with extreme states. They are asked to mark the point on the line which represents their perception of their current state. A VAS for post-operative pain might look like

no pain|------------X-------------------|unbearable pain
patient's mark

where X indicates the place on the scale where the patient judges himself to be. As such assessments are clearly highly subjective, these scales are of most value when looking at changes within individuals. We cannot put any absolute meaning on a score of, say, 2.2 (measured from the leftmost end of the scale), but a reduction to 1.4 in the same patient is interpretable. Caution is required in handling such data. We might, for example, prefer a method of analysis that is based on the rank ordering of scores rather than their exact values.

## 2.5 CENSORED DATA

An observation is called censored if we cannot measure it precisely but know that it is beyond some limit. Common situations often producing censored data are:

1. When measuring some trace constituent of blood the actual level may be below the lowest level that the machine or test can detect, even though it is known that the value should be greater than zero. Such values are termed non-detectable but are said to be censored at the limit of detectability. Because the convention is to plot data with low values to the left of a horizontal scale, this is also known as **left censoring**.
2. In some experiments, often with animals, there is a fixed length follow-up period. During this period the investigators may be looking for the appearance or perhaps disappearance of some specific condition, where the observation of interest is the time taken from the start of the experiment. Where nothing has happened by the end of the experiment, those observations are (right) censored at that time. Likewise, in long-term clinical trials the outcome of interest is often length of survival. Here the trial will usually stop at a fixed time after recruitment to the trial began, so that patients still alive at the end of the trial all have censored survival times, with the censoring being after different times of observation depending on how long the patient had been in the trial.

Special techniques for analysing censored survival data will be described in Chapter 13.

## 2.6 VARIABILITY

Statistics is largely about variability; in medical research this is often the variability between people. Sometimes it is the variability itself that is of prime interest, such as when describing the likely values of some measurement in a group of healthy subjects. Often, however, we are more interested in detecting underlying trends which may be obscured by variability. For example, when comparing two treatments on different groups of patients there may be considerable variation in the way patients respond to a particular treatment. The concept of variability is fundamental in statistics, and will recur throughout this book.

We use the term **variable** to denote anything that varies within a set of data. Although many variables relate to human subjects (or perhaps animals), the same considerations apply if one is studying variation from country to country (for example in perinatal mortality rates), comparing characteristics of small groups of individuals, or looking at variability in measurements of the same subject under different conditions.

All the examples of data given earlier in this chapter are called variables.

## 2.7 IMPORTANCE OF THE TYPE OF DATA

The many types of data just introduced can all be analysed by statistical methods, but the type of data can be critically important in determining which methods of analysis will be appropriate (and valid). In many medical studies variables of several types are collected, so that several different analytic methods may be needed. In Chapter 6 I shall give advice on how to record data for subsequent analysis.

Most statistical methods are specific to a certain type of data, with alternative techniques needed for different data types. The major distinction, however, is that between continuous and categorical variables. Further, for continuous or ordered categorical variables there is also the possibility of using alternative **rank** methods which are of much wider applicability.

These aspects of analysis will feature throughout this book. It is essential to use a method of analysis that is appropriate for the type of data.

## 2.8 DEALING WITH NUMBERS

### 2.8.1 Statistical analysis

When analysing data the rule is to use the full precision of the recorded data. There should not be any 'rounding' of intermediate results (see below). If you carry out your analysis on a computer the procedure just described will happen automatically. On a calculator it will happen only if intermediate calculations are stored in memory.

### 2.8.2 Presenting results

Advice on presentation of results appears in many later chapters, but some general introductory comments on presenting numbers may be helpful.

Analysis of categorical data often leads to counts of occurrences, such as the numbers of subjects in different blood groups, together with the corresponding percentages. If, as is usually desirable, the counts are given the percentages do not need to be given very precisely. Thus, for example, it is not necessary to express 17 out of 45 as 37.78% or even 37.8 – 38% is sufficient if the raw numbers are given too. Numbers with many digits are much harder to assimilate. Percentages may mislead in very small samples – saying that 25% of patients responded well to the treatment is not recommended when you mean one out of four patients.

The analysis of continuous data will lead to results that have many decimal places, such as an average diastolic blood pressure of 85.348074 mm Hg. Results like this clearly should be shortened by rounding (see next section), bearing in mind the accuracy of the original data. In this example no important information would be lost if the average blood pressure was reported as 85.3 mm Hg.

For numbers less than 1.0 a zero before the decimal point is preferable – thus 0.729 rather than .729.

It is usually best to quote all comparable results to the same number of decimal places.

### 2.8.3 Rounding numbers

If we wish to report a number such as 85.348074 to fewer decimal places, we use a simple rule for **rounding**. The rule is that excess digits are simply discarded if the first of them is less than five. Otherwise the last retained digit is increased by one. So rounding 85.348074 to three decimal places gives 85.348, while rounding to two decimal places gives 85.35. If the discarded information is a solitary 5 or a 5 followed by zeros some people recommend rounding to the nearest even digit, while others always round upwards. Thus rounding 17.75 to one decimal place gives 17.8, but 16.85 will give 16.8 or 16.9 depending upon your preference. Zeros on the end of a number should be retained. Thus if we round 28.402 or 28.399 to two decimal places we get 28.40.

Beware of rounding the same number twice, which can lead to errors. If 85.348074 is rounded to two decimal places we get 85.35. If we then decide to round this value to one decimal place we get 85.4 rather than the correct value of 85.3.

Rounding should not be used until the final presentation – full precision should be retained during the analysis.

# 3

# Describing Data

## 3.1 INTRODUCTION

If there is one key concept underlying the subject of statistics, it is that of variability. In medicine we can see this most obviously in the way people differ in their physiological, biochemical and other characteristics and also in their variable responses to disease and to therapy. We also often encounter variability between machines that are supposed to be identical, and between different observers. There are sometimes many sources of variability present at once. For example, if I have my blood pressure measured the value recorded by my GP will depend greatly on some unknown underlying 'true' value, but it will also relate to the time of day, whether I was late and had to run to the surgery, the type of sphygmomanometer being used, whether I was anxious about the outcome, and so on. When many people have their blood pressure measured other factors will affect between-subject variability, such as age, sex and race.

In general we can divide variability into that due to known causes and that which is unexplained. Thus, for example, in a study of men aged 25 to 65 part of the variability in their blood pressures may be ascribed to their age, but most of the rest is unexplained. We often refer to this unexplained variability as **random variation**.

In any study we will usually want to summarize some of the data in a simple way. Sometimes this will be as far as the statistical analysis goes, but often it is a first step. For categorical variables, such as sex and blood group, it is straightforward to present the number in each category, usually indicating the frequency or percentage of the total number of patients. When shown graphically this is called a **bar diagram**. Figure 3.1 shows a bar diagram of general aviation accident rates in 1974 by occupation (Booze, 1977). A similar diagram can also be used to relate frequencies (or rates) to values of another variable. For example, Figure 3.2 shows perinatal mortality per 1000 births in England and Wales in 1979 by day of the week. The higher mortality rates at the weekend are clearly seen. It is very important that the vertical axis of a bar diagram starts at zero, otherwise the visual impression is misleading, with the differences between groups being exaggerated.

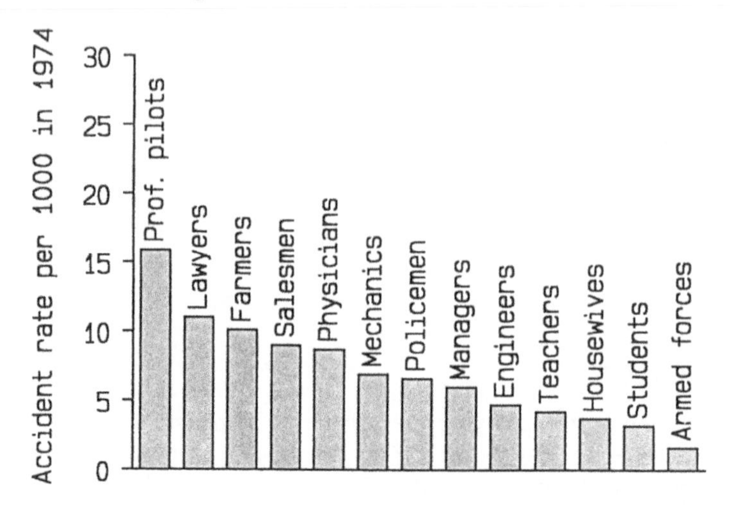


**Figure 3.1** Bar diagram showing general aviation accident rates (per 1000) in 1974 by occupation (Booze, 1977).

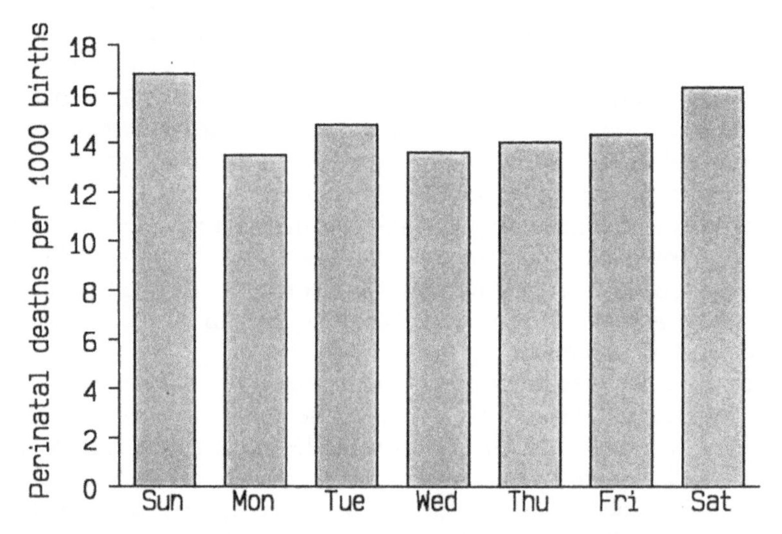


**Figure 3.2** Perinatal mortality in England and Wales in 1979 by day of the week (Macfarlane and Mugford, 1984).

For continuous variables, such as age and serum bilirubin, there will be a large number of different observed values, so an alternative approach is needed. The remainder of this chapter concentrates on ways of describing and summarizing such data both numerically and graphically.

In this chapter I shall introduce some mathematical notation for the first time. Further explanation of this notation can be found in Appendix A at the end of the book.

## 3.2 AVERAGES

The obvious first step when describing a set of observations of a continuous variable is to calculate the average value. In colloquial use the word 'average' does not have a precise meaning, but in statistics there are several so-called 'measures of central tendency' that are precisely defined and which can be taken as the average or typical value.

The most common of these is the **arithmetic mean**, usually just called the **mean**, which is the sum of all the observations divided by the number of observations. Table 3.1 shows age and lung function data for 25 patients with cystic fibrosis. The variable shown is the maximal static inspiratory

**Table 3.1** Age and PImax in 25 patients with cystic fibrosis (O'Neill *et al.*, 1983)

| Subject | Age (years) | PImax (cm $H_2O$) |
|---|---|---|
| 1 | 7 | 80 |
| 2 | 7 | 85 |
| 3 | 8 | 110 |
| 4 | 8 | 95 |
| 5 | 8 | 95 |
| 6 | 9 | 100 |
| 7 | 11 | 45 |
| 8 | 12 | 95 |
| 9 | 12 | 130 |
| 10 | 13 | 75 |
| 11 | 13 | 80 |
| 12 | 14 | 70 |
| 13 | 14 | 80 |
| 14 | 15 | 100 |
| 15 | 16 | 120 |
| 16 | 17 | 110 |
| 17 | 17 | 125 |
| 18 | 17 | 75 |
| 19 | 17 | 100 |
| 20 | 19 | 40 |
| 21 | 19 | 75 |
| 22 | 20 | 110 |
| 23 | 23 | 150 |
| 24 | 23 | 75 |
| 25 | 23 | 95 |

pressure (PImax) and is an index of respiratory muscle strength. The sum of the PImax values is 2315, so the mean is 2315/25 = 92.6 cm $H_2O$. The mean is the value usually meant when talking about 'the average'. The mean is sometimes indicated by $\bar{x}$ (pronounced 'x bar'), but this shorthand notation is best avoided other than in equations.

The other frequently used measure is the **median**. This is the value that comes half-way when the data are ranked in order. For the PImax data in Table 3.1 there are 25 observations, so the median is the 13th value in order. If we rank the PImax values in ascending order we get

| Rank | 1 | 2 | 3 | 4 | 5 | 6 | 7 | 8 | 9 | 10 | 11 | 12 | 13 |
|---|---|---|---|---|---|---|---|---|---|---|---|---|---|
| PImax | 40 | 45 | 70 | 75 | 75 | 75 | 75 | 80 | 80 | 80 | 85 | 95 | **95** |

| Rank | 14 | 15 | 16 | 17 | 18 | 19 | 20 | 21 | 22 | 23 | 24 | 25 |
|---|---|---|---|---|---|---|---|---|---|---|---|---|
| PImax | 95 | 95 | 100 | 100 | 100 | 110 | 110 | 110 | 120 | 125 | 130 | 150 |

and we can see that the median is 95 cm $H_2O$. More easily, we can see immediately from Table 3.1 that the median age of these patients was 14 years. When there is an even number of observations the median is defined as the average of the two central values: if we had 24 observations the median would be the average of the 12th and 13th values in an ordered listing of the observations. There are usually equal numbers of observations above and below the median. However, when there is more than one observation equal to the median, as for the PImax data, this may not be exactly true.

The median is especially useful when some extreme data values are censored. If observations are not recorded precisely when they are above a certain level or below a level of detection, we cannot calculate the mean, but we can calculate the median if we have definite values for over half the subjects. The median is also valuable in the analysis of survival times, which is considered in Chapter 13.

The mean and the median are both widely used to describe the average or typical value of a set of data. The mean is much more frequently used because this ties in well with the most common types of statistical analysis, but the median is in no way inferior as a descriptive statistic and in some circumstances it is much more useful than the mean, as we shall see later. In some situations we calculate another measure known as the **geometric mean**, which is usually close to the median. Its use is described in section 3.4.4.

A final indicator of the centre of a set of data is the **mode** which is simply the most common value observed. The mode is rarely of any practical use for continuous data.

## 3.3 DESCRIBING VARIABILITY

The second aspect of describing a set of observations of a continuous variable is to assess the variability of the observations in some way. Any set of data will contain many different values, for example the PImax data shown above. We are interested in the way these values are distributed – are they all similar or do they vary a lot? There are several ways of tackling this problem. I shall look first at graphical methods, and then consider numerical methods.

### 3.3.1 Histogram

A simple graphical way of depicting a complete set of observations is by means of the **histogram** in which the number (or frequency) of observations is plotted for different values or groups of values. Table 3.2 shows the **frequency distribution** of the immunoglobulin IgM in 298 healthy children aged 6 months to 6 years, and Figure 3.3 shows a histogram of

**Table 3.2** Concentrations of serum IgM in 298 children aged 6 months to 6 years (Isaacs *et al.*, 1983)

| IgM (g/l) | Number of Children |
|---|---|
| 0.1 | 3 |
| 0.2 | 7 |
| 0.3 | 19 |
| 0.4 | 27 |
| 0.5 | 32 |
| 0.6 | 35 |
| 0.7 | 38 |
| 0.8 | 38 |
| 0.9 | 22 |
| 1.0 | 16 |
| 1.1 | 16 |
| 1.2 | 6 |
| 1.3 | 7 |
| 1.4 | 9 |
| 1.5 | 6 |
| 1.6 | 2 |
| 1.7 | 3 |
| 1.8 | 3 |
| 2.0 | 3 |
| 2.1 | 2 |
| 2.2 | 1 |
| 2.5 | 1 |
| 2.7 | 1 |
| 4.5 | 1 |

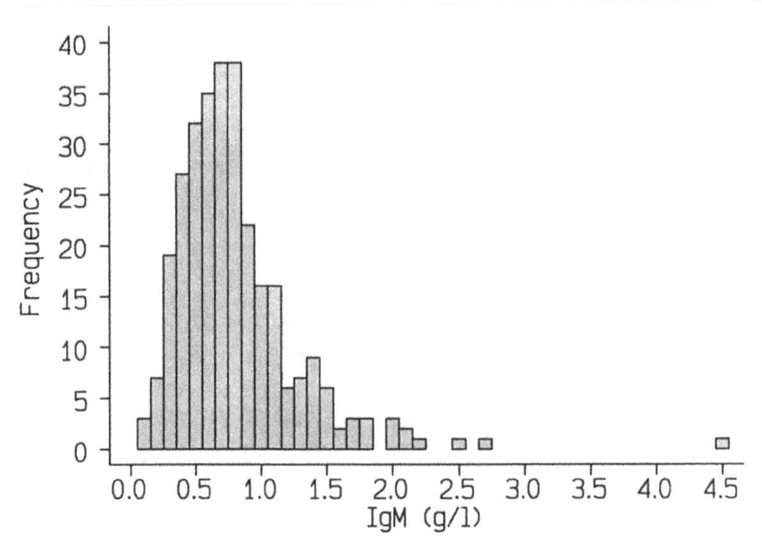


**Figure 3.3** Frequency histogram of IgM concentrations in 298 children aged 6 months to 6 years (Isaacs *et al.*, 1983).

these values. If there are many different values it is often desirable to group observations before constructing a histogram in order to get a better visual impression. Unless the sample is very large somewhere around 8 to 15 groups will usually suffice for a satisfactory display. This will depend upon the actual data, for it is desirable to keep the groupings simple. Although we could group the IgM data in intervals of, say, 0.25, this goes beyond the precision of the data. Better is the grouping in intervals of 0.2 shown in Figure 3.4. Note that the width of each vertical bar covers the range of values that have been grouped. So, for example, when we group 0.1 and 0.2 we are actually including values between 0.05 and 0.25 even though the data were not recorded that accurately. A histogram is similar to a bar diagram, but because the frequencies relate to a continuous variable adjacent bars of a histogram should touch.

The bars in histograms are usually all the same width, because the groupings are the same size. If the groups are not the same size this should be allowed for by remembering that it is the *area* of each bar that is proportional to the frequency, not its height. This principle is illustrated on data showing the age distribution of road accident casualties in the London borough of Harrow in 1985. Table 3.3 shows the data as presented. Most of the casualties were adults, with the greatest number in the age range 25 to 59. Clearly the widths of the groupings vary considerably, from 1 to 35 years in fact, and this must be taken account of in a histogram of the data. Note that in order to include the 60+ age group in a histogram we have to assume a reasonable upper age limit – here it will be taken as 80.

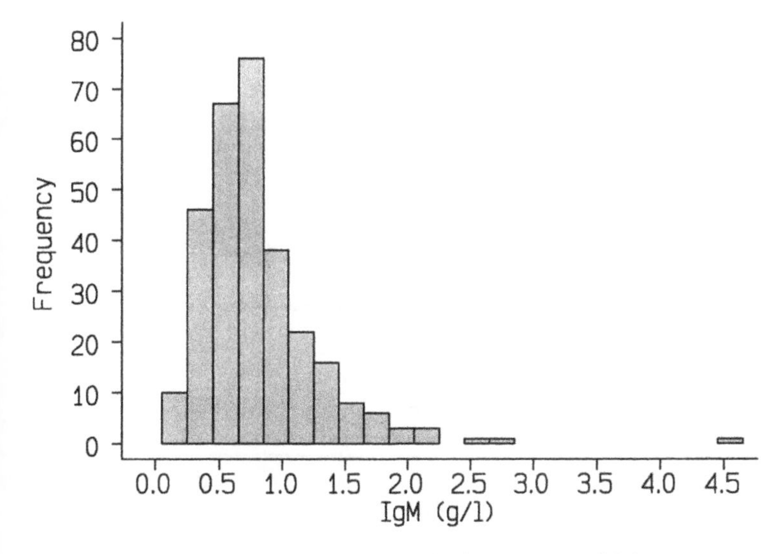


**Figure 3.4** As Figure 3.3 but data grouped in intervals of 0.2 g/l.

**Table 3.3** Road accident casualties in the London Borough of Harrow in 1985 (excluding 65 with unknown age)

| Age | Frequency |
|---|---|
| 0– 4 | 28 |
| 5– 9 | 46 |
| 10–15 | 58 |
| 16 | 20 |
| 17 | 31 |
| 18–19 | 64 |
| 20–24 | 149 |
| 25–59 | 316 |
| 60+ | 103 |
| Total | 815 |

First, consider what happens if we ignore the above warning and draw a histogram where, for each age group, the height indicates the frequency shown in Table 3.3 and the width shows the age range – this is shown in Figure 3.5. This histogram suggests that accident victims are much less likely to be 16 and 17 year olds than adults, whereas we would probably expect the opposite to be true. We get the correct picture by making the frequencies correspond to the area of each bar rather than its height, as is shown in Figure 3.6. What we have done is consider the number of casualties *per year of age* – where we don't have this explicitly we take the

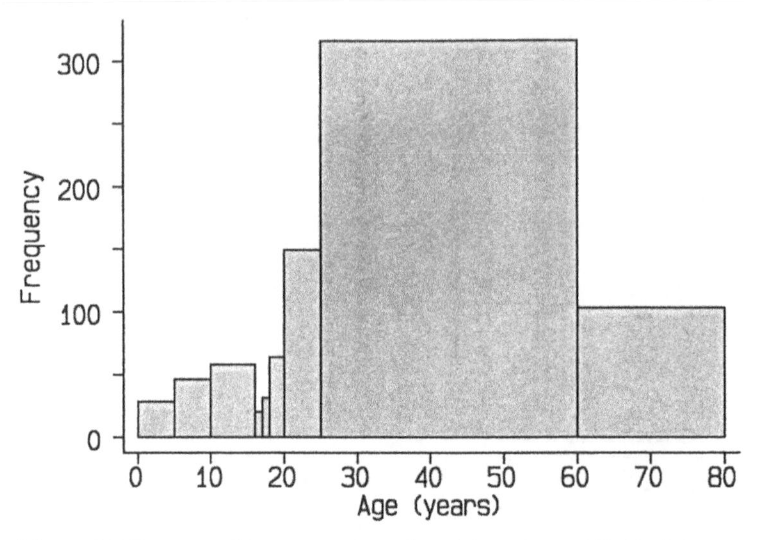


**Figure 3.5** Incorrect histogram of road accident data of Table 3.3.

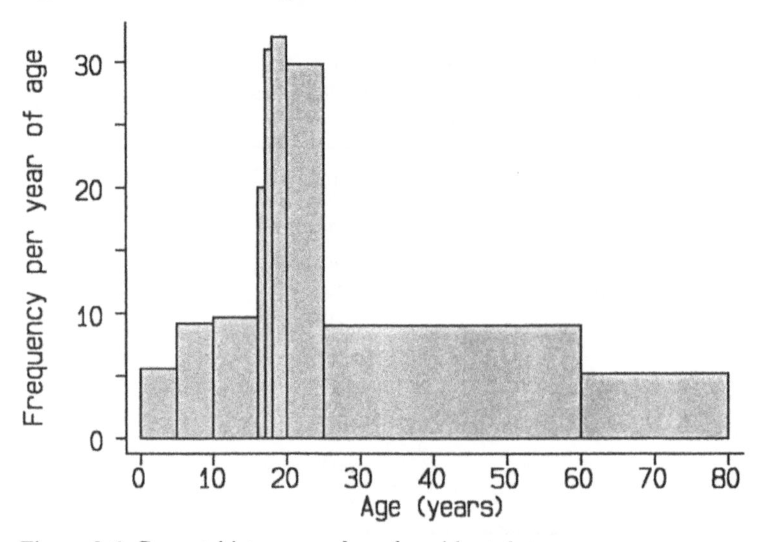


**Figure 3.6** Correct histogram of road accident data.

average value in that age group. Figure 3.6 shows a true impression of the data, from which we can see that road accident casualties are more likely to be aged 16 to 24 than any other age group.

Note that this histogram just shows the observed numbers of casualties. It does not indicate the *risk* of a road accident for people of varying age – for this we would also need to know the age distribution of the population, and would need to assume that all casualties lived in Harrow and that no Harrow residents had accidents elsewhere.

It is sometimes more useful to show the proportion of the sample in each interval. All the frequencies are converted into percentages by dividing by the sample size and multiplying by 100. Figure 3.7(a) shows the resulting **relative frequency histogram** for the IgM data, which differs from Figure 3.3 only in the way the vertical axis is labelled. An alternative way of plotting the data is to join the mid-points of the tops of all the vertical bars of the histogram; this is called a **frequency polygon**. Figure 3.7(b) shows such a plot for the same data.

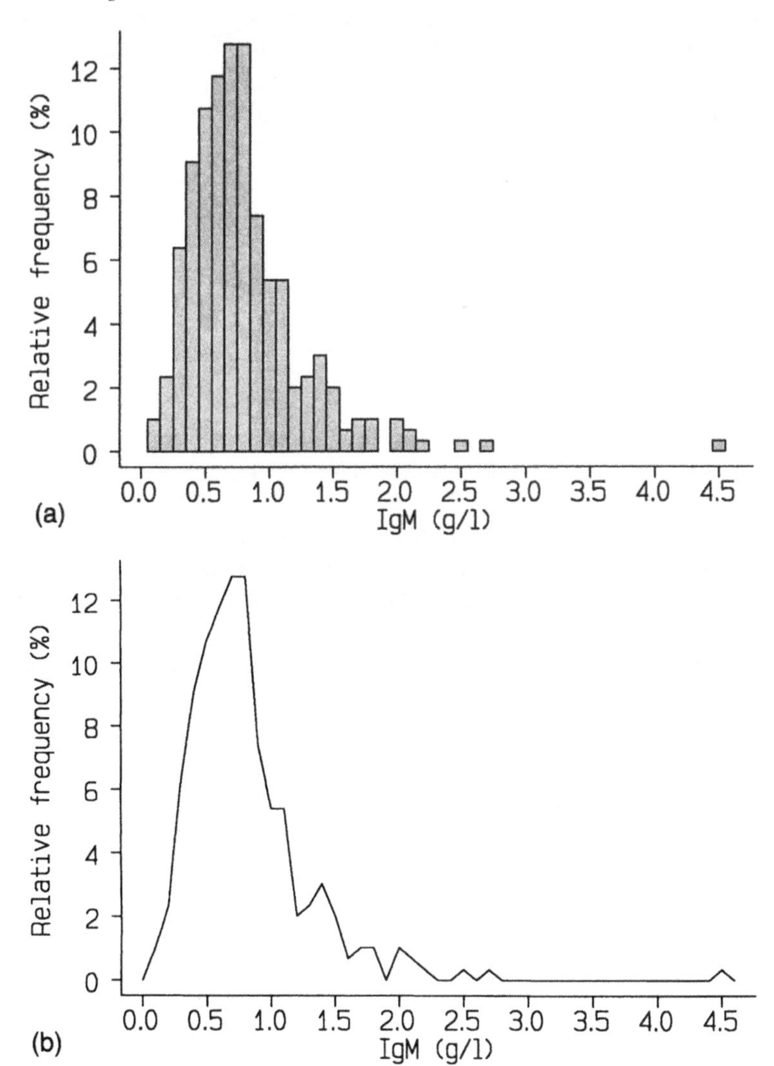


**Figure 3.7** IgM data in Figure 3.3 shown as (a) Relative frequency histogram, (b) Relative frequency polygon.

The vertical axis of a histogram must start at zero, and there should not be any breaks in the scale. Otherwise the visual impression will be misleading. Likewise three-dimensional effects should not be used.

### 3.3.2 Stem-and-leaf diagram

A clever modification of the histogram called a **stem-and-leaf** diagram allows all the actual observations to be shown too. Figure 3.8 shows the PImax data from Table 3.1 redrawn as a stem-and-leaf diagram. The raw data can be reconstructed by joining the numbers on the left (the stems) to each of the numbers on the right (the leaves) on the same row. This is a very economical way of reproducing the raw data, and is more useful than a simple list of the data.

```
 4  05
 5
 6
 7  05555
 8  0005
 9  5555
10  000
11  000
12  05
13  0
14
15  0
```

**Figure 3.8** Stem-and-leaf diagram of PImax data in Table 3.1.

The stem-and-leaf diagram works well in many circumstances, especially where there are many different values, but the best format depends on the nature of the data and the sample size. The IgM data in Table 3.2 cannot be made into a successful stem-and-leaf diagram using five 'stems' (0, 1, 2, 3, 4), but we can split each group to get a useful diagram, as in Figure 3.9.

```
0  111
0  22222223333333333333333333
0  444444444444444444444444444555555555555555555555555555555555
0  66666666666666666666666666666666666677777777777777777777777777777777777777777
0  888888888888888888888888888888888888888899999999999999999
1  00000000000000000000001111111111111111
1  2222223333333
1  444444444555555
1  66777
1  888
2  00011
2  2
2  5
2  7
2
3
3
3
3
3
4
4
4  5
```

**Figure 3.9** Stem-and-leaf diagram of IgM data in Table 3.2.

### 3.3.3 Cumulative frequencies

We saw earlier how the distribution of a sample of observations can be shown as the percentage of the sample with values in each of several small ranges. This was shown in the relative frequency histogram in Figure 3.7. We can take this idea a stage further by considering for each group the proportion of subjects in that group *or a lower one*. Thus we calculate the **cumulative frequency** at each level – the proportion of observations less than or equal to each value. The calculations are shown in Table 3.4. The cumulative relative frequencies can be plotted in a histogram, as in Figure 3.10(a). However, for cumulative frequencies there is no need to group the data like this because we can plot the cumulative frequencies directly, as in Figure 3.10(b). This plot can be used either to see what percentage of

**Table 3.4** Cumulative frequency distribution of 298 IgM values

| IgM g/l | Frequency | Relative Frequency % | Cumulative Frequency | Cumulative Relative Frequency % |
|---|---|---|---|---|
| 0.1 | 3 | 1.0 | 3 | 1.0 |
| 0.2 | 7 | 2.3 | 10 | 3.4 |
| 0.3 | 19 | 6.4 | 29 | 9.7 |
| 0.4 | 27 | 9.1 | 56 | 18.8 |
| 0.5 | 32 | 10.7 | 88 | 29.5 |
| 0.6 | 35 | 11.7 | 123 | 41.3 |
| 0.7 | 38 | 12.8 | 161 | 54.0 |
| 0.8 | 38 | 12.8 | 199 | 66.8 |
| 0.9 | 22 | 7.4 | 221 | 74.2 |
| 1.0 | 16 | 5.4 | 237 | 79.5 |
| 1.1 | 16 | 5.4 | 253 | 84.9 |
| 1.2 | 6 | 2.0 | 259 | 86.9 |
| 1.3 | 7 | 2.3 | 266 | 89.3 |
| 1.4 | 9 | 3.0 | 275 | 92.3 |
| 1.5 | 6 | 2.0 | 281 | 94.3 |
| 1.6 | 2 | 0.7 | 283 | 95.0 |
| 1.7 | 3 | 1.0 | 286 | 96.0 |
| 1.8 | 3 | 1.0 | 289 | 97.0 |
| 2.0 | 3 | 1.0 | 292 | 98.0 |
| 2.1 | 2 | 0.7 | 294 | 98.7 |
| 2.2 | 1 | 0.3 | 295 | 99.0 |
| 2.5 | 1 | 0.3 | 296 | 99.3 |
| 2.7 | 1 | 0.3 | 297 | 99.7 |
| 4.5 | 1 | 0.3 | 298 | 100.0 |
| Total | 298 | 99.9 | | |

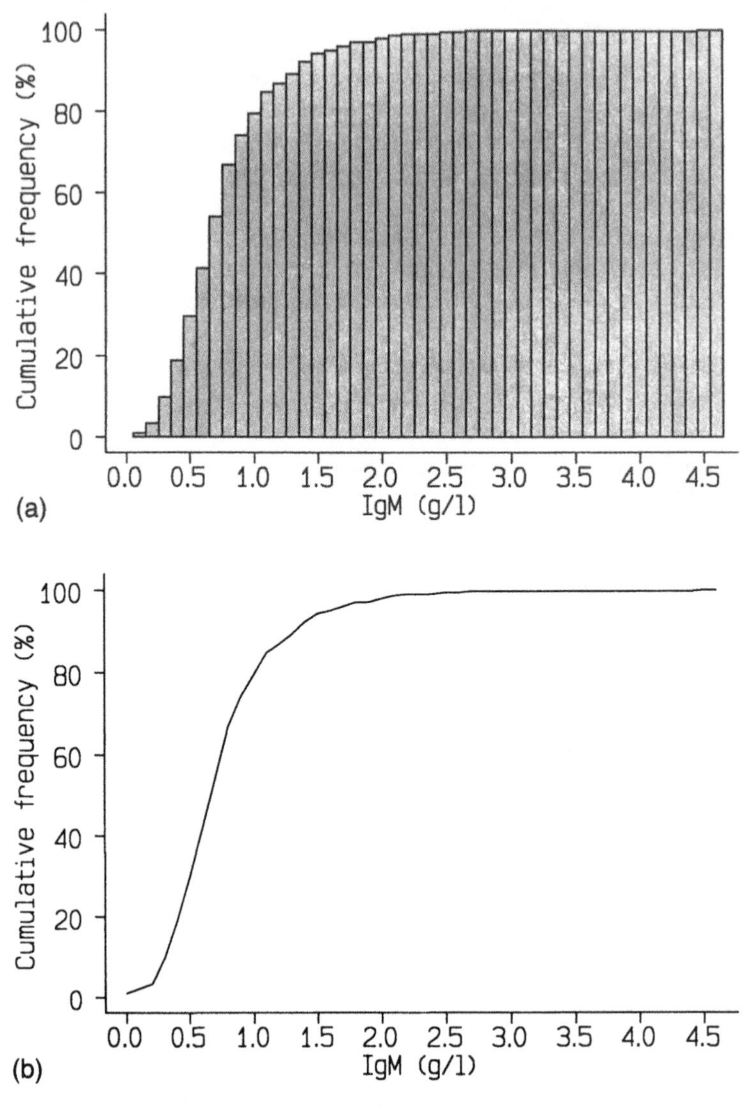


**Figure 3.10** IgM data shown as (a) Cumulative relative frequency histogram, (b) Cumulative distribution.

observations lie above or below any chosen level, or to find the values which a given percentage of children's IgM values lie above or below. For example, we can easily see that the median IgM concentration was 0.7 g/l. This information cannot be obtained from a histogram or cumulative histogram if values have been grouped.

Cumulative frequencies are especially useful for comparing the distribution of values in two or more different groups of individuals. Figure 3.11(a) shows relative frequency histograms for the age at first tooth eruption of 1568 children of smokers and 1576 non-smokers. Figure 3.11(b) shows cumulative histograms of the same data. Figure 3.11(c) shows cumulative frequency polygons of the same data. Because we are considering cumulative frequencies we join the right-hand points of the vertical bars rather than the mid-points as in Figure 3.7(b). This plot shows that the difference between the groups is not as great as was suggested in Figure 3.11(b) – the two groups were side by side in the previous plot, which can lead to a misleading visual impression. We can easily see from Figure 3.11(c) that the median age at first tooth eruption was about one week earlier in the children of smokers.

## 3.4 QUANTIFYING VARIABILITY

Graphical methods are important for examining the variability of data, but it is necessary also to have a numerical way of summarizing the amount of variability. Used in conjunction with the mean, this would provide an informative but brief summary of a set of observations. There are three main approaches to quantifying the variability of a set of data. We can either quote the range of all the values, specific values derived from the cumulative frequency distribution, or we can obtain a numerical measure of the dispersion of the observations around the mean.

### 3.4.1 Range

The simplest way to describe the spread of a set of data is to quote the lowest and highest values. These values are known as the **range**. The range of the IgM data was 0.1 to 4.5 g/l. This is not a satisfactory summary, because it takes account of only the most extreme (and perhaps most peculiar) values at each end of the data, and the way the intermediate values are distributed will not influence the range. Thus for the IgM data we have no idea that 4.5 was considerably more than the second highest value of 2.7 g/l. Mainly for this reason the range is not widely used.

### 3.4.2 Centiles

By specifying two values that encompass *most* rather than all of the data values we get round much of the difficulty. For example, we could calculate the values between which 90% of the observations lie. The value below which a given percentage of the values occur is called a **centile** or **percentile**, and corresponds to a value with a specified cumulative relative frequency.

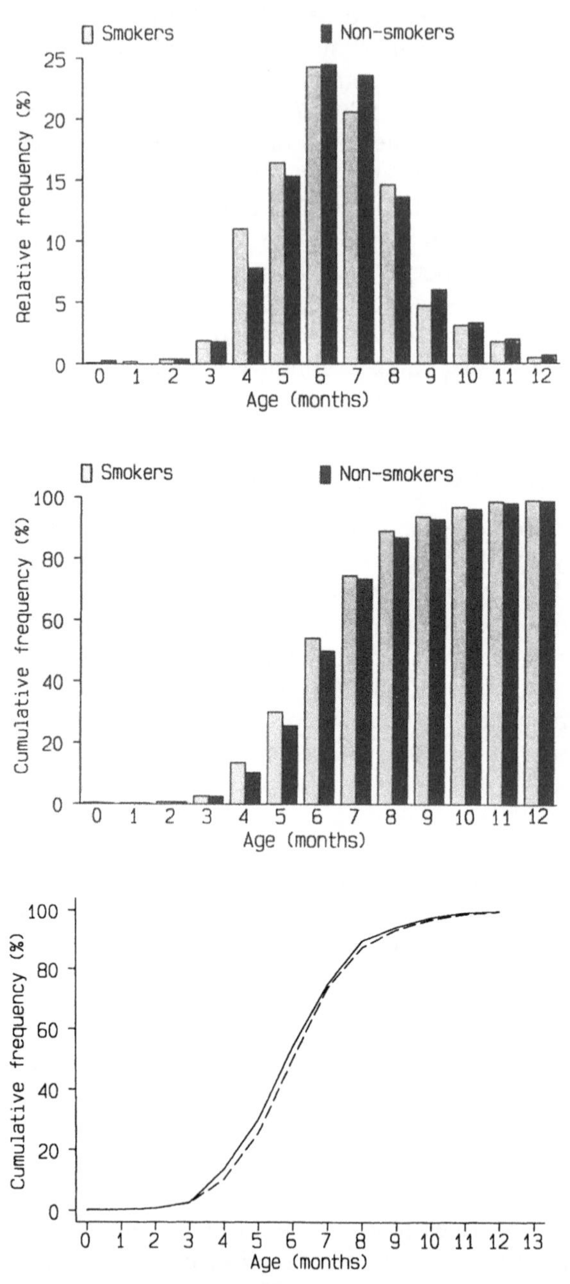


**Figure 3.11** Age at first tooth eruption of children born to smokers (——) and non-smokers (- - - - - -) (Rantakallio and Mäkinen, 1984): (a) Relative frequency histogram; (b) Cumulative relative frequency histogram; (c) Cumulative relative frequency polygon.

We require the 5th and 95th centiles of the distribution of IgM values. From the last column of Table 3.4 we can see that the cumulative relative frequency passes 5% somewhere in the group of IgM values of 0.3 g/l, and 95% is reached at the value of 1.6 g/l.

A more correct general approach is to calculate the ranks of the required observations, which we do by taking the necessary percentages of the sample size plus one. Here we need the values with ranks $0.05 \times 299 = 14.95$ and $0.95 \times 299 = 284.05$. This calculation usually leads to non-integer values, so we may need to interpolate. For example we want the value of IgM 0.95 of the way between the 14th and 15th observations in rank order. As these are, from Table 3.4, both equal to 0.3 g/l the 5th centile is 0.3 g/l, and likewise the 95th centile is 1.7 g/l. However, if we want the 10th centile, we would need the IgM value corresponding to a rank of $0.10 \times 299 = 29.9$. The observations with ranks 29 and 30 are 0.3 and 0.4 g/l and we take the value nine-tenths of the way between these values, by calculating $0.3 + 0.9(0.4 - 0.3) = 0.39$ g/l. The values 0.3 and 1.7 are thus the 5th and 95th centiles of the observed distribution of IgM in this sample of children and these two values thus specify what we can call a 90% **central range**—the range within which the central 90% of values lie (i.e. excluding 5% at each end of the distribution).

Other centiles can be quoted rather than the 5th and 95th. The most common alternative is to quote a 95% central range ($2\frac{1}{2}$th and $97\frac{1}{2}$th centiles), but an 80% central range (10th and 90th centiles) is sometimes used. The 50th centile is another name for the median, as half of the observations are less than (and greater than) this value. The 25th and 75th centiles are known as **quartiles**; these values together with the median divide the data into four equally populated subgroups. The numerical difference between the 25th and 75th centiles is the **inter-quartile range**, and is occasionally used to describe variability.

A simple but useful semi-graphical way of summarizing data using centiles is the **box-and-whisker plot**. Figure 3.12 shows a box-and-whisker plot for the IgM data. The box indicates the lower and upper quartiles and the central line is the median. The points at the ends of the 'whiskers' are the $2\frac{1}{2}$% and $97\frac{1}{2}$% values, although the whiskers sometimes indicate the extreme values. For a single set of data a histogram is more informative, but several sets of data can be summarized economically using the box-and-whisker plot. Sometimes any values outside the range of the whiskers are plotted individually.

### 3.4.3 Standard deviation

The alternative approach to quantifying variability is based on the idea of averaging the distance each value is from the mean. For an individual with

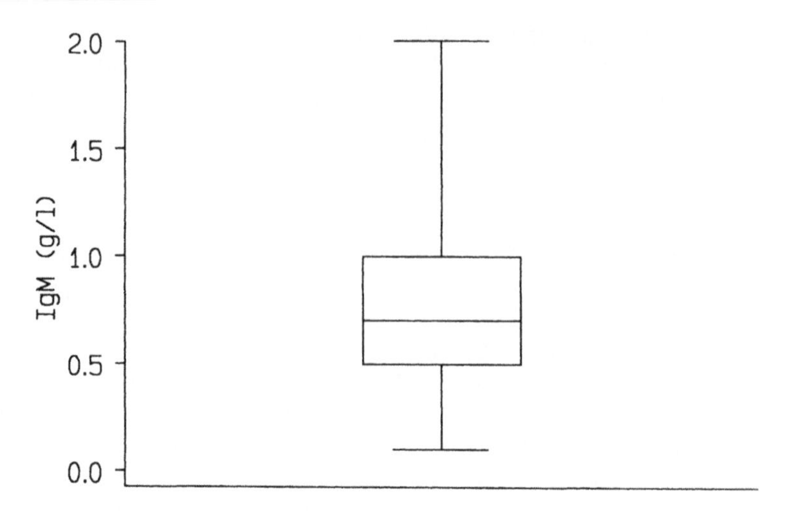


**Figure 3.12** Box-and-whisker plot of the IgM data, showing the $2\frac{1}{2}$, 25, 50, 75 and $97\frac{1}{2}$% cumulative relative frequencies (centiles).

an observed value $x_i$ the distance from the mean $\bar{x}$ is $x_i - \bar{x}$, and if we have $n$ observations we have a set of $n$ such distances, one for each individual. For observations below the mean the difference will be negative. We can calculate the average distance between the observations and their mean, but the sum of these distances, $\Sigma(x_i - \bar{x})$, is always zero because of the way the mean is calculated from the individual observations. However, if we square the distances before we sum them we get a quantity that must be positive. The average of these squared differences thus gives a measure of individual deviations from the mean. This quantity is called the **variance**, and is defined as

$$\frac{\sum_{i=1}^{n}(x_i - \bar{x})^2}{n - 1}.$$

Note that we divide by $n - 1$ rather than the more obvious $n$. Dividing by $n$ gives the variance of the observations around the sample mean, but we virtually always consider our data as a sample from some larger population, and wish to use the sample data to estimate the variability in the population. Dividing by $n - 1$ gives us a better estimate of the population variance, although clearly for large samples the difference is negligible.

The variance will turn up in later chapters, notably when discussing the technique known as **analysis of variance**. For our present purpose, the variance is not a suitable measure for describing variability because it is not in the same units as the raw data. We do not, for example, wish to express the variability of a set of blood pressure measurements in *square* mm Hg. The obvious solution to this problem is to take as our measure the square root of the variance. We call this quantity the **standard deviation**. The standard deviation is usually abbreviated to sd or SD or $s$ or $\sigma$ (the Greek letter sigma), and is defined as

$$\sqrt{\frac{\sum_{i=1}^{n}(x_i - \bar{x})^2}{n - 1}}.$$

Standard deviation is not a good name for this statistic as there is nothing 'standard' about it. It may more reasonably be thought of as approximately the average deviation (or distance) of the observations from the mean.

Many calculators can calculate the standard deviation, by means of a key marked $s$ or $\sigma$. (The use of the Greek $\sigma$ here rather than $s$ is not strictly correct, as will be explained in the next chapter. If there are keys marked $\sigma_n$ and $\sigma_{n-1}$ the latter should be used.)

However, should we wish to do the calculation ourselves there is a much easier formula to use, which is mathematically equivalent:

$$s = \sqrt{\frac{\Sigma x^2 - (\Sigma x)^2/n}{n - 1}}.$$

(Note the simplification of the $\Sigma$ notation, as described in Appendix A.) Using this formula we can calculate the standard deviation from the sum of the observations, $\Sigma x$, and the sum of the squares of the observations, $\Sigma x^2$. We do not need to calculate the individual distances from the mean.

For example, for the PImax data shown in Table 3.1 the sum of the data and the sum of the squares of the data are

$$\sum x = 2315 \qquad \text{and} \qquad \sum x^2 = 229275$$

so the mean PImax is 2315/25 = 92.60 cm $H_2O$ and the standard deviation is

$$s = \sqrt{\frac{229275 - 2315^2/25}{24}}.$$
$$= 24.92 \text{ cm } H_2O.$$

Note that I shall keep an extra decimal place at present for the mean and standard deviation because I shall be doing some further calculations. One decimal place would be sufficient when reporting these results.

The standard deviation has an important role in data analysis, but here we are concerned with its value as a descriptive statistic. In fact, although the standard deviation is widely used for this purpose it is useful only indirectly for describing the variability of a set of data. We can say, for example, that in many circumstances **the large majority (about 95%) of a set of observations will be within two standard deviations of the mean**. The appropriateness of this statement depends on the *shape* of the distribution of the data. If the distribution is reasonably symmetric then the above statement will usually be true.

For the PImax data in Figure 3.8 the mean was 92.60 and the standard deviation was 24.92 cm $H_2O$. The values that are two standard deviations either side of the mean are $92.60 - 2(24.92) = 42.76$ cm $H_2O$ and $92.60 + 2(24.92) = 142.44$ cm $H_2O$. (We often use the expression 'mean ±2SD' to mean both of these values, i.e. the mean 'plus or minus' twice the standard deviation.) All but two of the 25 observations were within this range; we would expect to find on average one observation outside the range mean ±2SD (i.e. about 5% of 25).

### 3.4.4 Skewed distributions

For data which do not have a symmetric distribution we need to be careful when using the standard deviation in the way just described. For example, the IgM data in Figure 3.3 clearly have an asymmetric distribution—there is a long right-hand 'tail'. This is called a **skewed** distribution. The mean and standard deviation of the IgM data are 0.80 and 0.47 g/l respectively. Calculating the mean ±2SD gives the values −0.14 and 1.74. The lower value is negative, which is not a possible value of IgM. The upper value of 1.74 is exceeded by 12 of the observations, 4% of the total. The two values clearly do not describe the range of the bulk of the data very well. Although they still include about 95% of the observations, the exclusions are all in one tail.

For measurements that cannot be negative, which is usually the case, we can infer that the data have a skewed distribution if the standard deviation is more than half the mean. There is no guarantee that the converse is true, however, but a histogram will quickly reveal whether the data are skewed or not. Skewness like that of the IgM data is called **positive** skewness and is common. The opposite phenomenon, with an extended left hand tail, is called **negative** skewness and is rare.

In general, when we have data with a skewed distribution we use other ways of describing the data. There are two main possibilities. The first is to **transform** the data mathematically so that the transformed data have a more nearly symmetric distribution. The most frequent device is to take logarithms (logs) of the data. The rationale for this approach will be discussed in Chapter 7. We can see that it works well here, however, from Figure 3.13 which shows a histogram of $\log_{10}$ IgM values. The mean and SD of the log data are −0.158 and 0.238 respectively, so that the values mean ±2SD are −0.63 and +0.32. These values are indicated in Figure 3.13. They cut off 10 values in the lower tail of the distribution and 6 in the upper tail, and thus give a range of values encompassing 282/298 or 94.6% of the observations. The cut-off values can be 'back-transformed' to the original scale giving 0.23 and 2.08, and reference to Table 3.2 shows the 16 values outside these limits. If we back-transform (or 'antilog') the mean of the log data we get a quantity known as the **geometric mean**. The geometric mean of the IgM data is thus $10^{-0.158} = 0.695$ g/l. Where log transformation successfully removes skewness the geometric mean will be similar to the median, and will be less than the mean of the raw data. The standard deviation of the log data cannot be meaningfully back-transformed.

Note that log data can be negative, and that it does not matter whether logs to base e or base 10 are used. In this example, logs to base 10 were used, with the function $10^x$ used for the back-transformation. Log transformation is only useful for removing positive skewness.

The alternative approach to describing the distribution of skewed data is to calculate the centiles corresponding to a chosen central range. For example, to get the values that enclose 95% of the observations we need to calculate the $2\frac{1}{2}$th and $97\frac{1}{2}$th centiles. Using the method described in the

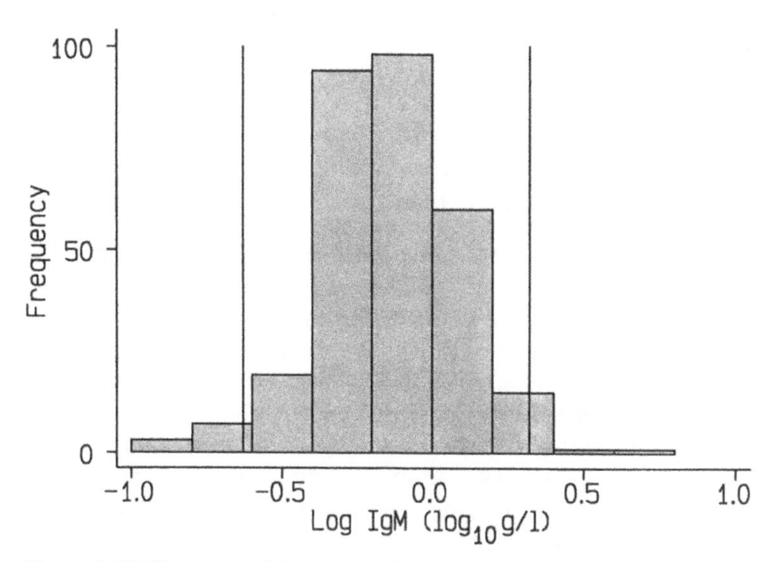


**Figure 3.13** Frequency histogram of $\log_{10}$IgM showing the values of mean ± 2SD.

previous section, these values are obtained by interpolation as 0.2 and 2.0 g/l. These values of 0.2 and 2.0 g/l are called **empirical** centiles as opposed to the earlier values of 0.23 and 2.08 (obtained from the mean ±2SD of the log data), which are estimated centiles. The two methods agree well for these data. Likewise the median IgM value is 0.7 g/l, which is very close to the geometric mean.

### 3.4.5 Comment

The standard deviation is one of the key quantities in statistical analysis. Its value for describing variability is conditional on the distribution of the data. Although it is always valid to calculate the standard deviation we can infer that about 95% of the observations were in the interval mean ±2SD only if we know (or assume) that the distribution of the data was reasonably symmetric. In fact, as happens with the IgM data, the range mean ±2SD may include about 95% of the observations even when the distribution is skewed. However, while we may reasonably use just the mean and SD to summarize such data, the skewness will be hidden. For skewed data, it is preferable to use the median and a 90% or 95% central range to summarize a set of observations. However, it is not practical to quote centiles for small samples, so the range can be given. Otherwise, the standard deviation can be used. It has the advantage of using each observation directly and it is easier to calculate (by computer) for large amounts of data.

The question of the shape of the distribution of one's data is of fundamental importance when choosing a method of analysis, as will be seen in later chapters.

## 3.5 TWO VARIABLES

### 3.5.1 Describing data in two or more groups

In many studies comparisons are made between different groups. For example, two groups of patients may be given different treatments and the outcomes observed. It is desirable in such studies to demonstrate that the characteristics of the two groups of subjects were comparable at the start of the study. As an example, Table 3.5 shows the characteristics of the groups of subjects in a clinical trial comparing short-wave diathermy treatment, osteopathic treatment, and an ineffective placebo treatment in patients with non-specific low back pain (Gibson *et al.*, 1985). The characteristics of the three groups at the start of the study (often called 'baseline' values) are shown as numbers and percentages for categorical variables, and as means and standard deviations for the two continuous variables. This information is usually sufficient to judge the comparability of the groups. I shall consider how we assess whether they *are* comparable in Chapter 15. For the moment we can see that the mean duration of pain had a skewed distribution as the mean is a lot less than twice the standard deviation in all three groups.

**Table 3.5** Details of patients in each treatment group in a study of low back pain (Gibson *et al.*, 1985)

| | Treatment group | | |
|---|---|---|---|
| | Short-wave diathermy | Osteopathy | Placebo |
| Number of patients | 34 | 41 | 34 |
| Sex | 16F/18M | 21F/20M | 11F/23M |
| Mean age (SD) | 35 (16) | 34 (14) | 40 (16) |
| Mean duration of pain in weeks (SD) | 18 (11) | 16 (14) | 17 (11) |
| Median pain score at presentation (range)* | 45 (5–82) | 35 (4–90) | 48 (10–96) |
| Radiological abnormalities of the spine | 12 (34%) | 12 (29%) | 11 (32%) |

*Visual analogue scale

Sometimes we wish to show graphically the distribution of a continuous variable in two or more groups. This can be done by means of a separate histogram for each group, these being aligned vertically, but there is a rather clearer format that shows all the observations. Figure 3.14 shows the distribution of uric acid in a group of women before, during and after pregnancy (Lind *et al.*, 1984). All the data are shown in the graph, and the authors have also given the mean, standard deviation and number of observations at each stage. This informative figure thus effectively incorporates a table while using little extra space. Bar diagrams are often used to show means and standard deviations in each group. This is not a good format – this information is better in a table, or else a more informative display, such as that in Figure 3.14 or a box-and-whisker diagram, should be used.

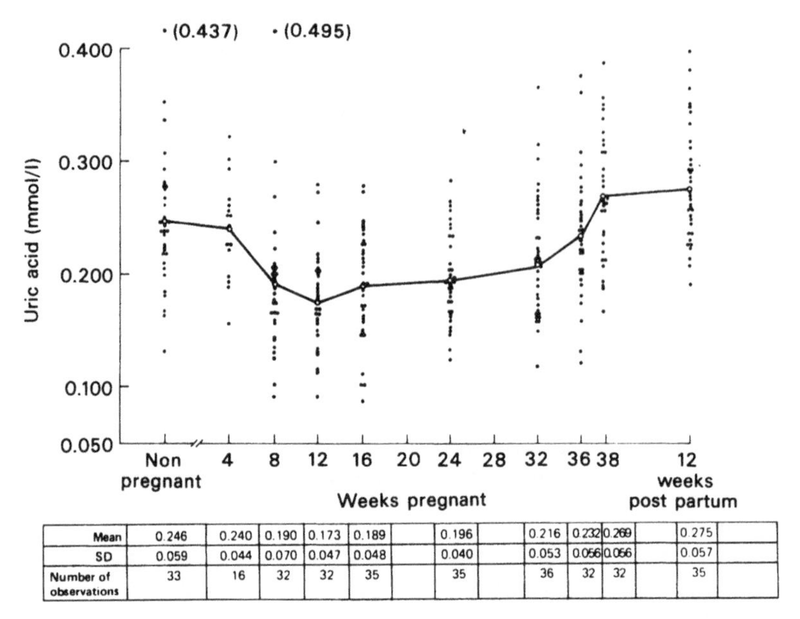


| | Non pregnant | 4 | 8 | 12 | 16 | 20 | 24 | 28 | 32 | 36 | 38 | | 12 weeks post partum | |
|---|---|---|---|---|---|---|---|---|---|---|---|---|---|---|
| Mean | 0.246 | 0.240 | 0.190 | 0.173 | 0.189 | | 0.196 | | 0.216 | 0.232 | 0.269 | | 0.275 | |
| SD | 0.059 | 0.044 | 0.070 | 0.047 | 0.048 | | 0.040 | | 0.053 | 0.056 | 0.056 | | 0.057 | |
| Number of observations | 33 | 16 | 32 | 32 | 35 | | 35 | | 36 | 32 | 32 | | 35 | |

**Figure 3.14** Distribution of serum uric acid in a group of healthy women before, during and after pregnancy (reproduced from Lind *et al.*, 1984, with permission).

### 3.5.2 Relation between two continuous variables

The relation between two continuous variables may be shown graphically in a **scatter diagram**. This is a simple graph in which the values of one variable are plotted against those of the other. For example, Figure 3.15 shows a scatter diagram of the PImax data of Table 3.1 related to age. Scatter diagrams are very simple to produce using statistical computer programs. When there are two (or more) individuals with identical values of both variables this should be shown, preferably by moving one point slightly. Some software packages print the actual number of coincident points up to 9, so that '9' means '9 or more'. It is easy to indicate subgroupings by using different plotting symbols. For example, in Figure 3.15 males and females could have been indicated by closed and open circles. The scatter diagram is a very useful descriptive tool, and is often valuable as a prelude to formal statistical analysis. The graph in Figure 3.14 is really a scatter diagram relating a continuous and a categorical variable.

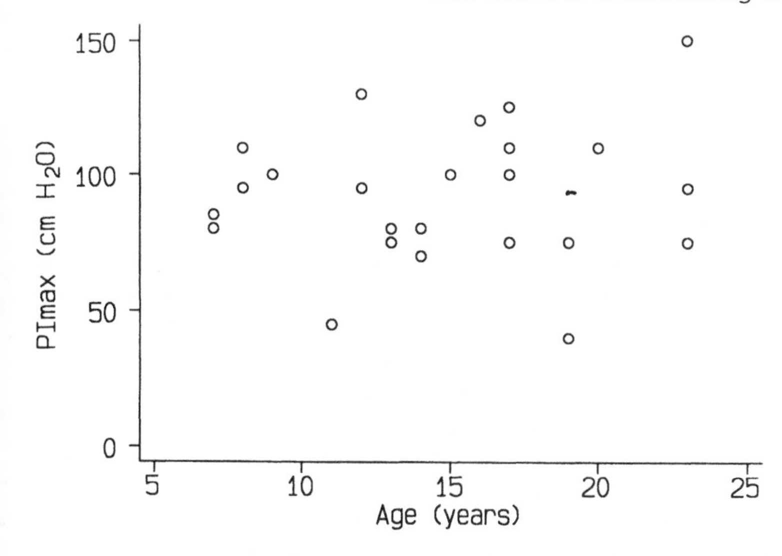


**Figure 3.15** Scatter diagram of PImax by age.

## 3.6 THE EFFECT OF TRANSFORMING THE DATA

If we change our data in some way we will inevitably change the mean and standard deviation too. In some situations we alter, or transform, a complete set of data, in which case the effect on the mean and standard deviation may be predicted.

The simplest case to consider is where we alter the units of measurement. If we change the IgM data from values recorded as g/l to mg/l each observation will be 1000 times as large. It is easy to see that the mean will also be 1000 times bigger, and inspection of the formula for the standard deviation shows that it too will be 1000 times bigger. In contrast, if we add or subtract a constant value from all the observations, the mean of the new data is obtained by the same subtraction or addition but the standard deviation is unaffected. Thus to the mean of a set of temperatures recorded as degrees Celsius we must add 273.15 to give the mean of the equivalent thermodynamic temperature on the Kelvin scale.

Any transformation based on multiplication, division, subtraction or addition is called a **linear** transformation, because if we plot the new values against the original values we get a straight line. The mean and standard deviation of the transformed values are obtained in a simple manner. For other, non-linear transformations, however, we cannot obtain the mean and standard deviation of the transformed data in this way. Examples of non-linear transformation are taking logarithms (illustrated in section 3.4.4) or square roots. Thus the mean of the log data is not the same as the log of the mean of the raw data. The reasons for transforming data are considered in Chapter 7.

## 3.7 DATA PRESENTATION

### 3.7.1 Numerical presentation

Data summary should not be by the mean (or median) alone, but some indication of variability should also be provided. It is common to put the SD in brackets after the mean. When these values are quoted in text the format mean ±SD, as in 'their mean diastolic blood pressure was 102.3 ± 11.9 mm Hg', should be avoided. (Indeed several medical journals no longer allow this notation.) It is much better to write 102.3 mm Hg (SD 11.9) because this format makes it clear what the second number is and also avoids the implication that the range of values from mean −SD to mean +SD is of specific importance. As we have seen, it is the range mean ±2SD which can often be used to describe the spread of the large majority (about 95%) of a set of observations.

It is not possible to give absolute rules for numerical presentation, but the following guidelines will generally be reasonable. It is usually appropriate to quote the mean to one extra decimal place compared with the raw data. The mean should not be presented to ridiculous (and spurious) 'accuracy'. For example, it is clearly absurd to quote the mean length of gestation of a group of babies to the nearest 10 minutes. This is done when quoting weeks of gestation to 3 decimal places. The standard deviation should usually be given to the same accuracy as the mean, or with one extra decimal place.

### 3.7.2 Tables

Whether or not to put descriptive data in tables will depend on the number of variables and groups of subjects. Table 3.5 shows a recommended way of presenting descriptive data, both continuous and categorical. In general it is preferable to put data of a like kind in *columns* rather than *rows* as the eye can scan columns more easily, but this is not always possible. For example, in Table 3.5 the means of the same variables in the three treatment groups are shown in rows, as it is usually more natural that way. However, means and SDs are clearly distinguished side by side, with the latter in brackets for clarity.

Tables can also be used to show raw data, although this is only reasonable when there are not too many observations. Where possible, it is helpful to order the data by one of the variables – after all, there is usually nothing special about the order in which the patients were seen. Many of the tables in this book, such as Table 3.1, have been ordered in this way.

### 3.7.3 Graphs

It is difficult to offer much general advice about when it is appropriate to use a graph rather than a table. Graphs offer the opportunity to show much more data than could be shown in a table, and are thus probably most suited to data that cannot easily be displayed in a table. There is no point in using a graph to show, for example, the means and standard deviations of one variable in two or three groups. Some displays, such as histograms, are in essence graphical – Figure 3.3 is a much clearer display than Table 3.2. It is possible to combine the best features of a table and a figure, and an example was given in Figure 3.14. This form of display should be used more often.

Scatter diagrams are particularly useful for showing the relation between two variables. It is important that all the data points should be shown, which can pose difficulties when there are coincident points (see section 6.7). Different symbols can be used to indicate subgroups of the data.

Graphs are a very powerful way of getting a message across, but the same data can be portrayed in many ways, with a variety of visual effects. For example, Figure 3.16 shows three alternative displays of the data in Table 3.6 showing average amounts of bread consumed per person per week in London from 1960 to 1980. Features visible in one or more figures include a gradual reduction in total bread consumption, a more than proportionate fall in consumption of white bread, and a rise in consumption of brown and wholemeal bread in the last five year period. These features are probably more easily seen in Table 3.6.

**Table 3.6** Amounts of bread consumed in London from 1960 to 1980 (g per person per week) (Sivell and Wenlock, 1983)

| Type of bread | Year<br>1960 | 1965 | 1970 | 1975 | 1980 |
|---|---|---|---|---|---|
| White | 1040 | 975 | 915 | 785 | 620 |
| Brown | 70 | 80 | 70 | 75 | 115 |
| Wholemeal | 25 | 20 | 15 | 20 | 45 |
| Other | 155 | 80 | 85 | 75 | 105 |
| Total | 1290 | 1155 | 1080 | 955 | 880 |

An excellent book on graphical methods in general is that by Tufte (1983), and graphs for statistics are discussed by Moses (1987). Many innovative ideas for descriptive methods are described by Tukey (1977).

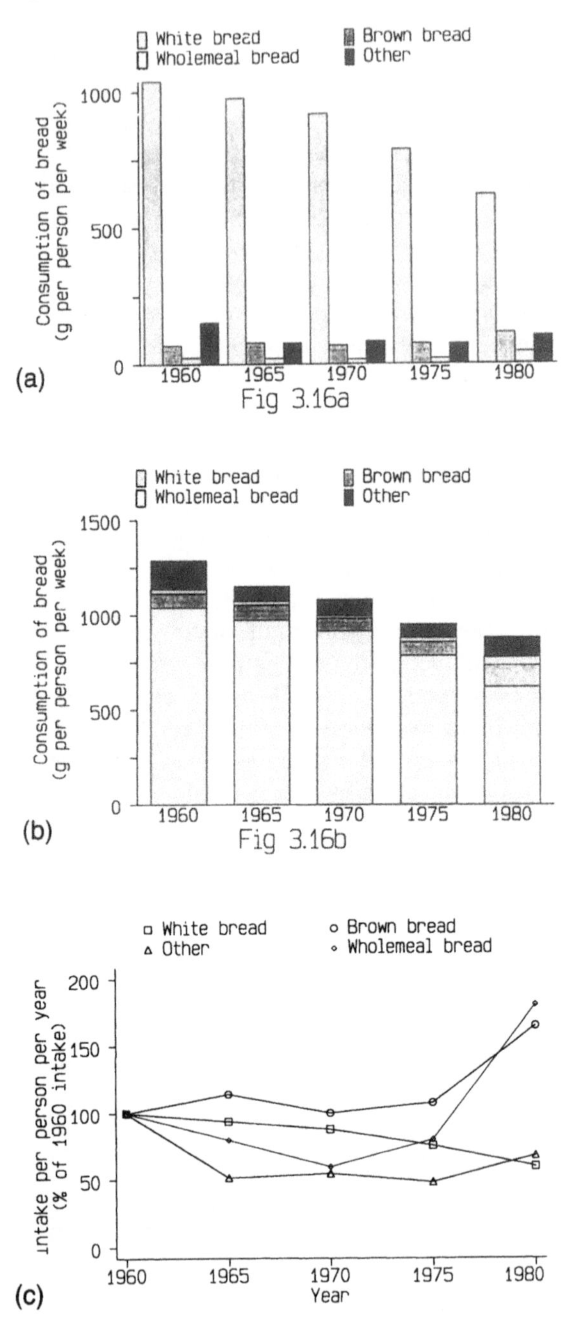


**Figure 3.16** Average amount of bread consumed per person per week in London from 1960 to 1980; three alternative graphs of the data in Table 3.6: (a) adjacent bars, (b) stacked bars, (c) graph of relative changes since 1960.

## EXERCISES

3.1 The table overleaf shows some data for 65 patients with rheumatoid arthritis treated with sodium aurothiomalate (SA) (Ayesh *et al.*, 1987). The total dose of SA is shown, together with values of the sulphoxidation index (SI), which measures the capacity to convert organic divalent alkyl sulphide to its corresponding sulphoxide form. The patients have been separated into 28 without and 37 with major adverse reactions to the drug.

(a) Some values of SI are given as '>80.0'. What is the name given to observations like this?
(b) What is the difficulty about drawing histograms of SI in each group? What shape are the distributions?
(c) Give two reasons why it is preferable to calculate the median rather than the mean to describe the average SI value.
(d) Obtain the median SI for each group of patients. (This should take less than ten seconds.)
(e) Obtain the median total dose of SA for the group with adverse reactions.
(f) Produce stem-and-leaf diagrams to compare the age distributions in the two groups.
(g) Do the data support the idea that patients experiencing adverse reactions were on average older than those without adverse reactions?

| | Without adverse reactions | | | | With adverse reactions | | |
|---|---|---|---|---|---|---|---|
| | Age | Total dose of SA (mg) | SI | | Age | Total dose of SA (mg) | SI |
| 1 | 44 | 1560 | 1.0 | 1 | 53 | 360 | 2.0 |
| 2 | 65 | 1310 | 1.2 | 2 | 74 | 2010 | 2.0 |
| 3 | 58 | 850 | 1.2 | 3 | 29 | 1390 | 2.0 |
| 4 | 57 | 1250 | 1.7 | 4 | 53 | 660 | 3.0 |
| 5 | 51 | 950 | 1.8 | 5 | 67 | 1135 | 3.5 |
| 6 | 64 | 850 | 1.8 | 6 | 67 | 510 | 5.3 |
| 7 | 33 | 1200 | 1.9 | 7 | 54 | 410 | 5.7 |
| 8 | 61 | 1390 | 2.0 | 8 | 51 | 910 | 6.5 |
| 9 | 49 | 1450 | 2.3 | 9 | 57 | 360 | 13.0 |
| 10 | 67 | 3300 | 2.8 | 10 | 62 | 1260 | 13.0 |
| 11 | 39 | 2760 | 2.8 | 11 | 51 | 560 | 13.9 |
| 12 | 42 | 860 | 3.4 | 12 | 68 | 1135 | 14.7 |
| 13 | 35 | 1810 | 3.4 | 13 | 50 | 1410 | 15.4 |
| 14 | 31 | 1310 | 3.8 | 14 | 38 | 1110 | 15.7 |
| 15 | 37 | 1250 | 3.8 | 15 | 61 | 960 | 16.6 |
| 16 | 43 | 1210 | 4.2 | 16 | 59 | 1310 | 16.6 |
| 17 | 39 | 1460 | 4.9 | 17 | 68 | 910 | 16.6 |
| 18 | 53 | 2310 | 5.4 | 18 | 44 | 1235 | 22.0 |
| 19 | 44 | 1360 | 5.9 | 19 | 57 | 2950 | 22.3 |
| 20 | 41 | 1910 | 6.2 | 20 | 49 | 360 | 33.2 |
| 21 | 72 | 910 | 12.0 | 21 | 49 | 1935 | 47.0 |
| 22 | 61 | 1410 | 18.8 | 22 | 63 | 1660 | 61.0 |
| 23 | 48 | 2460 | 47.0 | 23 | 29 | 435 | 65.0 |
| 24 | 59 | 1350 | 70.0 | 24 | 53 | 310 | 65.0 |
| 25 | 72 | 810 | >80.0 | 25 | 53 | 310 | >80.0 |
| 26 | 59 | 1460 | >80.0 | 26 | 49 | 410 | >80.0 |
| 27 | 71 | 760 | >80.0 | 27 | 42 | 690 | >80.0 |
| 28 | 53 | 910 | >80.0 | 28 | 44 | 910 | >80.0 |
| | | | | 29 | 59 | 1260 | >80.0 |
| | | | | 30 | 51 | 1260 | >80.0 |
| | | | | 31 | 46 | 1310 | >80.0 |
| | | | | 32 | 46 | 1350 | >80.0 |
| | | | | 33 | 41 | 1410 | >80.0 |
| | | | | 34 | 39 | 1460 | >80.0 |
| | | | | 35 | 62 | 1535 | >80.0 |
| | | | | 36 | 49 | 1560 | >80.0 |
| | | | | 37 | 53 | 2050 | >80.0 |

3.2 (a) Does Figure 3.1 indicate that professional pilots are more likely to have an aviation accident than other groups?

The following table shows the data that were plotted in Figure 3.1, together with the aviation accident rates per 100 000 hours of recent flight time (Booze, 1977).

| | Number of accidents | Rate per 1000* | Rate per 100 000 hr |
|---|---|---|---|
| Professional pilots | 1302 | 15.9 | 0.2 |
| Lawyers | 57 | 11.0 | 1.5 |
| Farmers | 166 | 10.1 | 1.3 |
| Sales representatives | 137 | 9.0 | 1.2 |
| Physicians | 76 | 8.7 | 1.8 |
| Mechanics and repairmen | 44 | 6.9 | 1.5 |
| Policemen and detectives | 48 | 6.6 | 1.8 |
| Managers and administrators | 643 | 6.0 | 0.7 |
| Engineers | 125 | 4.7 | 1.1 |
| Teachers | 43 | 4.2 | 1.1 |
| Housewives | 29 | 3.7 | 3.2 |
| Academic students | 188 | 3.2 | 3.7 |
| Armed Forces Members | 111 | 1.6 | 0.7 |

*in the specified occupation

(b) The rates per 100 000 hours can also be made into a bar diagram. From such a diagram, or from the figures shown in the table, which two groups of pilots had most accidents? Why do the two sets of figures give different answers? (A scatter diagram is useful to see the relation between the two.)

3.3 Calculate the centiles used to construct the box-and-whisker plot in Figure 3.12 using the method of calculation given in section 3.4.2.

# 4
# Theoretical distributions

## 4.1 INTRODUCTION

The importance of variability in attributes or responses was emphasized in the previous chapter. Without such variability events would be entirely predictable, and there would be no need for statistical methods. Because there is variability, we need statistical analysis to unravel what is going on. For example, while it is now universally accepted that cigarette smoking is hazardous to health, realization that this was so did not come until much careful research was carried out beginning in the 1940s and 1950s (Doll and Hill, 1950). Although the risk of heart disease, lung cancer and other diseases is considerably increased by smoking, the effect was masked because the response to smoking is highly variable. Some heavy smokers live to 80 or 90, whereas many non-smokers die before they are 60. Clearly the ability to detect effects, whether in observational or experimental studies, depends upon both the magnitude of the effect *on average*, and the variability of the effect. We will see that the balance between these ideas is behind a large number of the main statistical methods.

Another essential concept in the application of statistical methods is that of **probability**. We frequently encounter probability in some form in everyday life. It may be reasonably explicit, such as the probability of winning a lottery, or implicit, such as the probability of crossing the road without getting run over. Often we need to judge probability in relation to a decision that has to be taken, for example, whether I take an umbrella when I go out will depend on my perception of the probability of rain. Most aspects of life can be shown to involve some probabilities, and medicine is no exception. What is the probability of a heart transplant patient living for two years? What is the probability that a patient will respond to a particular treatment? What is the probability that a patient with a pain in his stomach has an ulcer? Given appropriate data, statistical methods help to answer many questions like these. It must be remembered, though, that statistical analysis rarely leads to a definite answer, so that we should indicate (or at least be aware of) a degree of uncertainty in our answers.

## 4.2 PROBABILITY

First, we need to consider the mathematical nature of probability. For the purposes of the statistical methods described in this book I shall define the probability of some specific outcome as the proportion of times that that outcome would occur if we repeated the experiment or observation a large number of times. For example, we can estimate the probability that a baby is a boy by observing what proportion of a large number of babies are boys.

By definition a probability lies between 0 and 1; something that cannot happen has a probability of 0, while something that is certain to happen has a probability of 1. A probability is thus somewhat similar to a proportion or a percentage: an outcome with a probability of 0.2 means that there is a one in five, or a 20% chance of it happening. Probabilities are not usually expressed as a percentage. In practice we have to estimate most probabilities, as there is no way of knowing the true value.

There are two simple rules regarding probabilities that we need to consider at this stage:

1. For a given event, for any two outcomes that might happen the probability of *either* occurring is the *sum* of the individual probabilities.

For example, if the probability of an individual being blood group A is 0.43 and of being group B is 0.08, then the probability of being either A *or* B is 0.51. It follows that the probabilities of all possible outcomes must add up to 1, since one of these possibilities *must* occur. For example, the probabilities of being in the different blood groups are approximately

O: 0.46; A: 0.43; B: 0.08; AB: 0.03.

We assume here that all outcomes are mutually exclusive.

2. If we consider two or more different events which are **independent** of each other, then to get the probability of a combination of specific outcomes for each of the events we must *multiply* the individual probabilities of those outcomes.

The idea of **independence** is an essential statistical concept. By independent we mean that if we know the outcome of one event this tells us nothing about the other event. More formally, the probability of each possible outcome for the second event is the same regardless of the outcome for the first event, and so on. For example, if there are three people in a GP's waiting room, the probability that they are all blood group O is $0.46 \times 0.46 \times 0.46 = 0.097$, that is, there is less than one chance in ten. In this context independence requires the three people to be unrelated.

As we would expect, if two events are *not* independent, the multiplicative property does not apply. For example, if the probability of a man being more than six feet tall is 0.2, the probability that both he and his son are over six feet is not $0.2 \times 0.2 = 0.04$ because the heights of children tend to be related to the heights of their parents. This idea is used in reverse in cases of uncertainty to investigate whether two events *are* independent. For example, in a case-control study patients with a disease (cases) are compared with people without the disease (controls) with respect to some possibly hazardous exposure earlier in their life. Women with cervical cancer may be compared with controls with respect to past use of oral contraceptives. If more cases had the exposure than controls then the probability of having been exposed is different for cases and controls and one suspects the exposure as a cause of the disease. Another way of looking at this is to say that having the disease and having had the exposure are not independent events.

## 4.3 SAMPLES AND POPULATIONS

Nearly all statistical analysis is based on the principle that one acquires data on a **sample** of individuals and uses the information to make inferences about *all* such individuals. This idea is probably most familiar in the context of opinion polls. The set of all subjects (or whatever is being investigated) is called the **population** of interest. In the previous chapter data were presented for 25 patients with cystic fibrosis and for 298 normal children aged 6 months to 6 years. Analysing the data from these samples enables us to make inferences about the population. For these studies the populations of interest were, respectively, all patients with cystic fibrosis and all children aged 6 months to 6 years. The way the sample is selected is clearly very important, and is discussed in the next chapter.

We take samples to study because it is rarely, if ever, possible to study the whole population. We might be able to study all patients diagnosed as having cystic fibrosis in one country on a particular date, but they are still only a sample of all people with cystic fibrosis, restricted by time and geography, and undiagnosed cases are excluded. Fortunately we do not need to study the whole population, as a carefully chosen sample can yield reliable answers. We cannot usually count or identify all the members of the population, but the sample allows us to draw inferences about the population, both collectively and individually. For example, a study of the anti-hypertensive effect of a new drug would allows us to estimate (within limits) the possible benefit of the drug to future hypertensive patients not in the study.

The relation between sample and population is subject to uncertainty, and we use ideas of probability to indicate this uncertainty. The idea of a theoretical **probability distribution** is important in this context.

## 4.4 PROBABILITY DISTRIBUTIONS

In the previous chapter I discussed the idea of a distribution of observed data – an empirical distribution. Many statistical methods use the related idea of a **probability distribution** which is specified mathematically. A probability distribution is used to calculate the theoretical probability of different values occurring, and is thus a theoretical equivalent of an empirical relative frequency distribution.

For example, if we know the mean and standard deviation of the height of adult men we can calculate the probability of being more than six feet tall if we assume that the distribution of height in the population is the same as a particular probability distribution. If we know from observation that the proportion of babies that are boys is 0.52, we can use this fact together with some mathematics to find the probability that a woman with four children has four daughters. The value 0.52 is a **parameter** of the probability distribution, as are the mean and standard deviation in the first example. All probability distributions are described by one or more parameters.

Many statistical methods are based on the assumption that the observed data are a sample from a population with a distribution that has a known theoretical form. If this assumption is reasonable (we cannot establish if it is *true*) then the statistical methods of analysis are simple to use and wide-ranging. If the distributional assumption is *not* reasonable and we proceed as if it were, then we may end up with misleading (and invalid) answers. When analysing data we have a choice between methods that make distributional assumptions, called **parametric** methods, and those which make no assumptions about distributions, called **distribution-free** or **non-parametric** methods.

The importance of probability distributions in statistical analysis reflects the dominance of parametric methods. First I shall consider probability distributions for continuous variables, for which one distribution in particular, the **Normal** distribution, is of fundamental importance. Later I shall look at probability distributions for discrete data.

## 4.5 THE NORMAL DISTRIBUTION

The **Normal distribution** is by far the most important probability distribution in statistics. It appears in some form in most of the following chapters, for reasons which are considered more fully in Chapter 8, so an understanding of its nature and role is essential. However, to emphasize that there is no implication that this distribution is more 'normal' than many others, I use a capital N for Normal. (It is also sometimes known as the **Gaussian** distribution, after the mathematician Gauss.)

In the previous chapter I showed how a histogram can be used to depict the distribution of a set of observations of a continuous variable. If there had been thousands of observations, and IgM had been recorded more precisely, the IgM values could be divided into many tiny intervals, and a histogram of the data would appear more like a smooth curve. So it is not difficult to imagine that the histogram or frequency polygon of some observed data is an approximation to some 'underlying' smooth frequency distribution. For example, Figure 4.1 shows a histogram of serum albumin values in 216 patients with primary biliary cirrhosis, and Figure 4.2 shows a

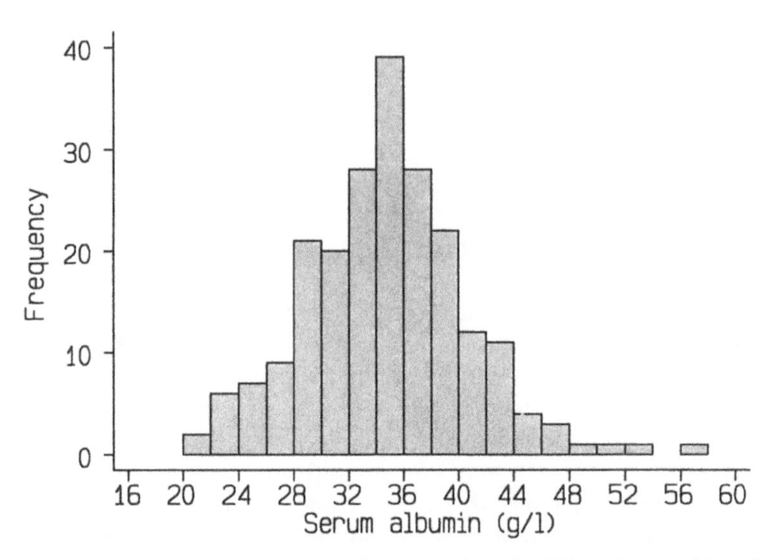


**Figure 4.1** Histogram of serum albumin values in 216 patients with primary biliary cirrhosis (from the study by Christensen *et al.*, 1985)

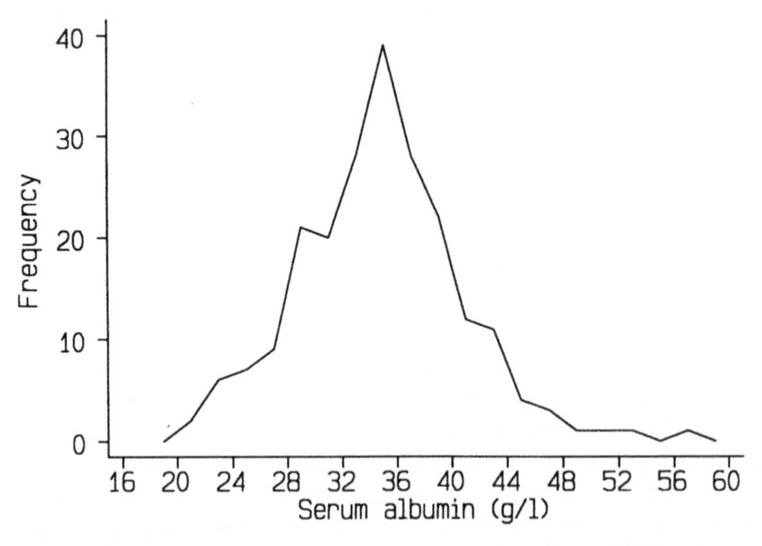


**Figure 4.2** Frequency polygon of serum albumin values in 216 patients with primary biliary cirrhosis.

frequency polygon of the same data, in which the effect is rather clearer.

Frequency distributions for continuous measurements, such as in Figure 4.2, tend to have a single peak: they are called **unimodal**. They may be fairly symmetric, as here, or asymmetric, as with the IgM data discussed in Chapter 3. The Normal distribution is a probability distribution which is unimodal and symmetric; its shape is shown in Figure 4.3. Frequency distributions with two peaks are occasionally seen. These are called **bimodal**, and are usually the result of mixing subgroups with different means.

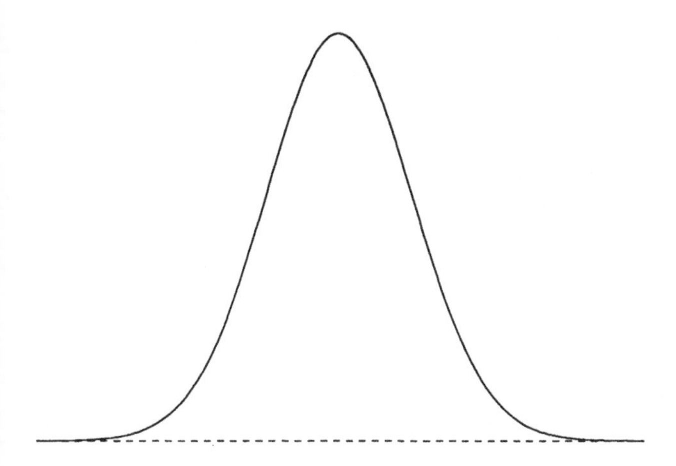

**Figure 4.3** The Normal distribution.

Before considering how we make use of the Normal distribution there are some general points to note about continuous probability distributions. First, they usually have no upper limit and some have no lower limit either. In theory the Normal distribution extends from minus infinity ($-\infty$) to plus infinity ($+\infty$). Second, the height of the frequency curve, which is called the **probability density**, cannot be taken as the probability of a particular value. This is because for a continuous variable there are infinitely many possible values so that the probability of any specific value is zero. The height of a curve is not of any practical use; its value is determined by the fact that the total area under the curve is always taken to be 1. As with histograms of observed data, we use a probability distribution by considering the *area* corresponding to a particular restricted range of values. Because the total area is 1 this area corresponds to the *probability* of those values. To take a simple example, the area to the left of the mean of the Normal distribution is 0.5 (because of the symmetry) and this is the probability of being below the mean.

### 4.5.1 Using the Normal distribution

The mathematical equation of the Normal distribution is unpleasantly complicated, but we do not need to deal with it in order to use the Normal distribution, because the necessary information is readily available in tables. However, it is important to know that the Normal distribution is completely described by two parameters, the mean and the standard deviation. These are usually called $\mu$ (mu) and $\sigma$ (sigma) respectively. Figure 4.4(a) shows the Normal distribution in relation to these parameters. Whatever values the mean and standard deviation have, the Normal distribution is related to the mean and standard deviation in the manner shown in Figure 4.4(a). This feature is illustrated by Figures 4.4(b) and 4.4(c), which show Normal distributions with firstly mean 10 and standard deviation 2 and secondly mean 125 and standard deviation 8. Figure 4.5 shows the histogram of serum albumin shown in Figure 4.1 and the Normal distribution with the same mean and standard deviation. The two are clearly very similar.

As Figure 4.4(a) shows, any position along the horizontal axis can be expressed as a distance of a number of standard deviations (negative or positive) from the mean. This distance is known as a **standard Normal deviate** or **Normal score**. It is equivalent to looking at a Normal distribution with a mean of 0 and a standard deviation of 1, a special Normal distribution known as the **standard Normal distribution**. Any Normal distribution can be converted (or transformed) into a standard Normal distribution by subtracting the mean and dividing by the standard deviation.

One way that we use the Normal distribution is as follows. When a set of observations has a distribution that is similar to a Normal distribution we assume that in the population the distribution of the variable actually **is** Normal, and carry out calculations on this basis. For example, we can calculate the probability that a patient with primary biliary cirrhosis has a serum albumin level greater than 42.0 g/l if we are willing to assume that, among the population of all patients with primary biliary cirrhosis, serum albumin has a Normal distribution.

Table B1 in Appendix B shows the lower tail areas of the standard Normal distribution. The lower tail means the area under the curve from $-\infty$ up to the value of interest. This area is equivalent to the probability of a value lower than the specified value. This idea can also be expressed as the cumulative relative frequency distribution, which is shown in Figure 4.6. Table B1 is simply a more accurate version of the curve in Figure 4.6.

The area below $-1$ is 0.16 and the area below $+1$ is 0.84, so that the

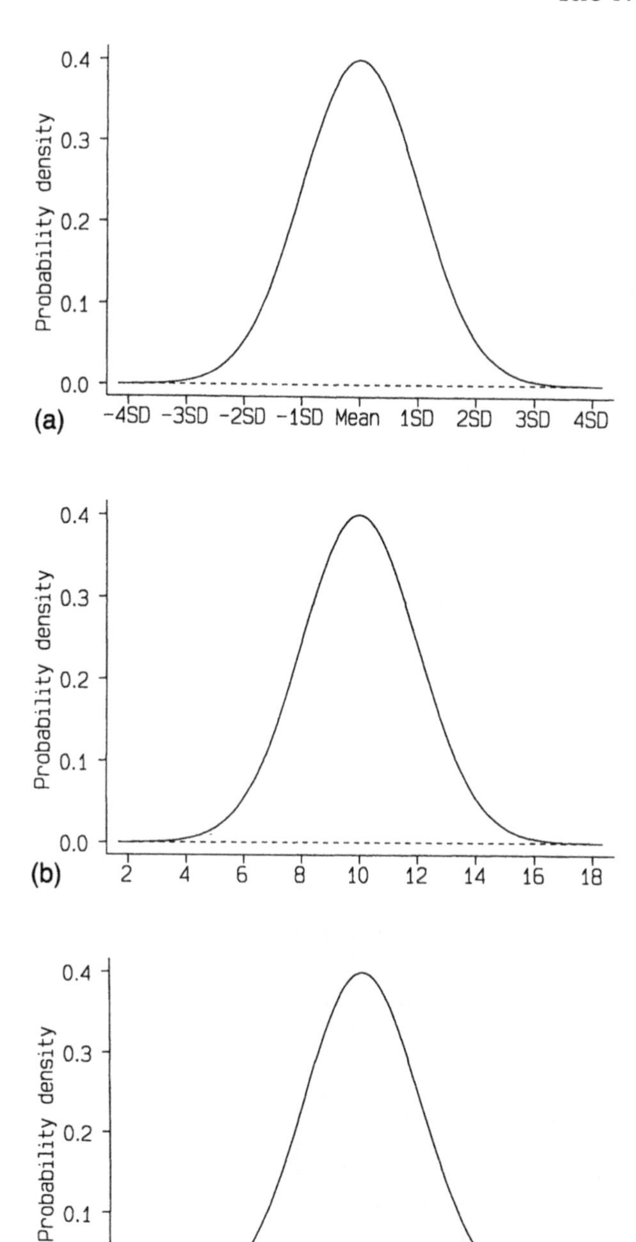


**Figure 4.4** The Normal distribution in relation to its mean and standard deviation. (a) General case; (b) mean = 10, SD = 2; (c) mean = 125, SD = 8.

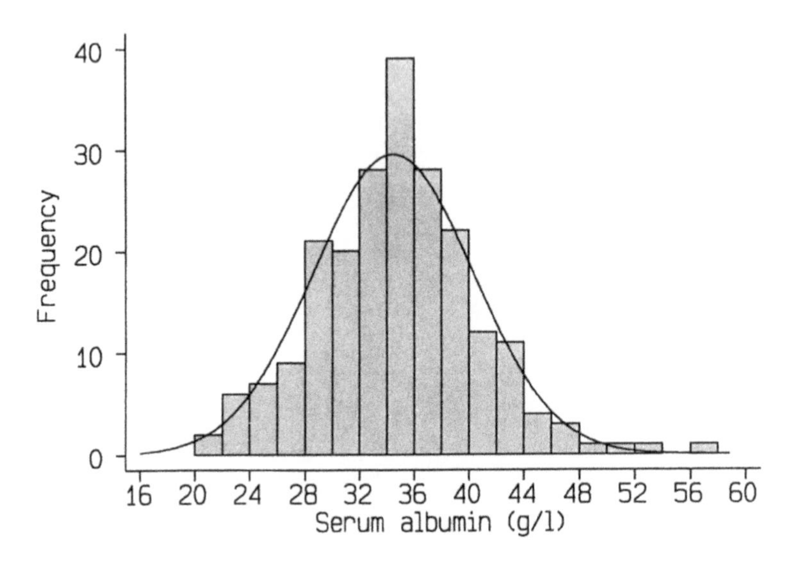


**Figure 4.5** Histogram of 216 serum albumin values and the Normal distribution with the same mean and standard deviation.

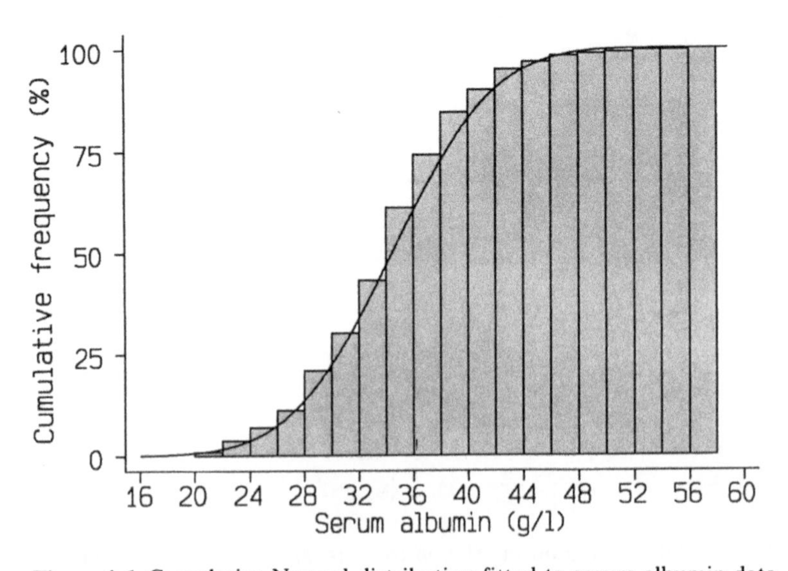


**Figure 4.6** Cumulative Normal distribution fitted to serum albumin data.

area corresponding to the range $-1$ to $+1$ is $0.84 - 0.16 = 0.68$. In other words, for data with an exactly Normal distribution there is a probability of 0.68 of being within one standard deviation of the mean. Repeating these calculations for other numbers of standard deviations we get

| Range | Probability of being within range | Probability of being outside range |
|---|---|---|
| mean ±1SD | 0.683 | 0.317 |
| mean ±2SD | 0.954 | 0.046 |
| mean ±3SD | 0.9973 | 0.0027 |

These values can also be obtained from Table B2. In each case the probability of not being within the stated range is 1 minus the probability of being within the range. We can see that there is a minimal chance – 0.0027 or 0.27%, or about 1 in 400 – that a value from a Normal distribution will be more than three standard deviations above or below the mean, agreeing with the visual impression gained from Figure 4.4. Of course, in very large samples we would expect several values to be this extreme.

The probability of being within two standard deviations of the mean is just over 0.95. In other words, about 95% of observations from a Normal distribution will be within the range mean −2SD to mean +2SD, which agrees with the more general statement in the previous chapter. As we will see later, exactly 95% of the area under the Normal distribution curve actually falls in the slightly narrower range of mean ±1.96SD.

### 4.5.2 An example

Returning to the serum albumin data, we can calculate the probability of a value being above 42.0 on the assumption that the true distribution is Normal. The mean serum albumin level was 34.46 g/l and the standard deviation was 5.84 g/l. We first calculate how many standard deviations from the mean the value of 42 g/l is, which is given by

$$\frac{42 - 34.46}{5.84} = 1.29.$$

From Table B1 we find that the probability of being greater than 1.29 is 0.0985, so the probability of a value above 42 g/l is 10%.

From Table B3 we can find the values which enclose a given percentage of the distribution – the central range. For example, 90% of the distribution lies within the range mean ±1.645SD, 95% within mean ±1.96SD, and

99% within mean ±2.576SD. For the serum albumin data we get the following ranges:

| Central range | Serum albumin (g/l) |
|---|---|
| 90% | 24.85 to 44.07 |
| 95% | 23.01 to 45.91 |
| 99% | 19.39 to 49.53 |

We can thus use the Normal distribution to estimate the centiles of the distribution of the variable in the population. We could have calculated the observed centiles of the sample data and used these values as estimates of the population centiles, but when the data are near to Normal the use of the Normal distribution is more reliable, especially in the tails of the distribution. It is also easier, requiring just two values and a table of the Normal distribution rather than the complete set of raw data values. Figure 4.5 showed that the distribution of the 216 serum albumin values was very similar to the Normal distribution with the same mean and standard deviation. We can use the procedure just described to calculate from the Normal distribution the number of values expected in each interval of the histogram. For example, the number expected in the interval 26.0 to 28.0 g/l is the probability of being in that interval multiplied by 216. The standard Normal deviates for 26.0 and 28.0 are

$$\frac{26.0 - 34.46}{5.84} = -1.45$$

$$\frac{28.0 - 34.46}{5.84} = -1.11$$

From Table B1 we get lower tail areas of 0.0735 and 0.1335, giving a probability of $0.1335 - 0.0735 = 0.0600$ of being between 26.0 and 28.0. The expected number of observations in this interval is thus $216 \times 0.0600 = 13.0$. Table 4.1 shows the results of similar (but more precise) calculations for the whole range of values, giving observed frequencies and the frequencies expected if the population distribution of serum albumin was a Normal distribution with the same mean (34.46 g/l) and standard deviation (5.84 g/l). Note that expected numbers are usually quoted as fractions even though the observed frequencies must be whole numbers.

I observed in section 4.4 that the widely-used parametric methods of statistical analysis incorporate important assumptions about the distribution of data. In most cases the distribution involved is the Normal distribution, which is one of the reasons why it is the most important distribution in

**Table 4.1** Distribution of serum albumin in 216 patients with primary biliary cirrhosis together with expected frequencies based on a Normal distribution with the same mean and standard deviation

| Serum albumin (g/l) | Observed frequency | Expected frequency |
|---|---|---|
| < 20 | 0 | 1.4 |
| 20– | 2 | 2.1 |
| 22– | 6 | 4.4 |
| 24– | 7 | 8.0 |
| 26– | 9 | 13.1 |
| 28– | 21 | 19.1 |
| 30– | 20 | 24.7 |
| 32– | 28 | 28.5 |
| 34– | 39 | 29.2 |
| 36– | 28 | 26.7 |
| 38– | 22 | 21.8 |
| 40– | 12 | 15.8 |
| 42– | 11 | 10.2 |
| 44– | 4 | 5.9 |
| 46– | 3 | 3.0 |
| 48– | 1 | 1.4 |
| 50– | 1 | 0.6 |
| 52– | 1 | 0.2 |
| 54– | 0 | 0.1 |
| 56– | 1 | 0.0 |
| Total | 216 | 216.2 |

statistics. Although many measurements do have a reasonably Normal distribution, such as human height, many do not, such as human weight or serum cholesterol. There are various ways in which data may deviate from Normality, notably by being asymmetric or skewed. The IgM data shown in Figure 3.3 illustrated positive skewness. It should not be assumed that a set of observations is approximately Normal – this must be established. One common type of skewed distribution closely related to the Normal distribution is the Lognormal distribution, which is discussed in the next section.

### 4.5.3 Sampling variation

Figure 4.5 showed a visual comparison of a set of observations of serum albumin and the Normal distribution having the same mean and standard deviation. The question of whether data are close enough to a Normal distribution is important, and will be considered at various points in the following chapters.

Although formal methods can be used (described in Chapter 7), whether a set of observations are reasonably Normal is often a matter of judgement, usually by visual inspection of a histogram. It is instructive to look at distributions obtained by taking random samples from a Normal distribution to give a reference against which to judge a set of observed data. Figure 4.7 shows frequency histograms of 16 samples of 50 observations sampled at random from the standard Normal distribution. Each sample is equivalent to considering 50 individuals sampled from a population *known* to have a Normal distribution for the variable of interest. There is considerable irregularity in the distributions of these samples, with the key properties of unimodality and symmetry generally absent. This figure should be borne in mind when considering whether observed data might have come from a Normal distribution, especially when the sample size is small.

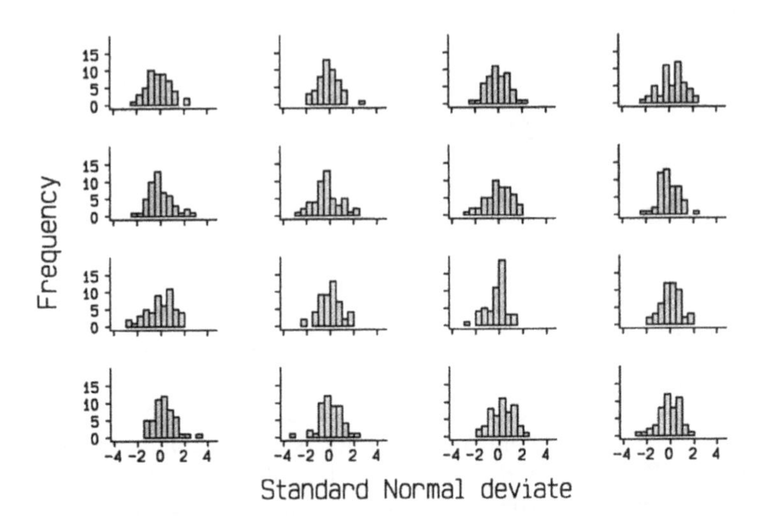


**Figure 4.7** Distributions of 16 samples of size 50 from the Normal distribution.

## 4.6 THE LOGNORMAL DISTRIBUTION

In section 3.4 we saw that in some circumstances a set of data with a positively skewed distribution can be transformed into a symmetric distribution by taking logarithms. Taking logs of data with a skewed distribution will often give a distribution that is near to Normal. Figure 4.8 shows a histogram of serum bilirubin levels in the same 216 patients with primary

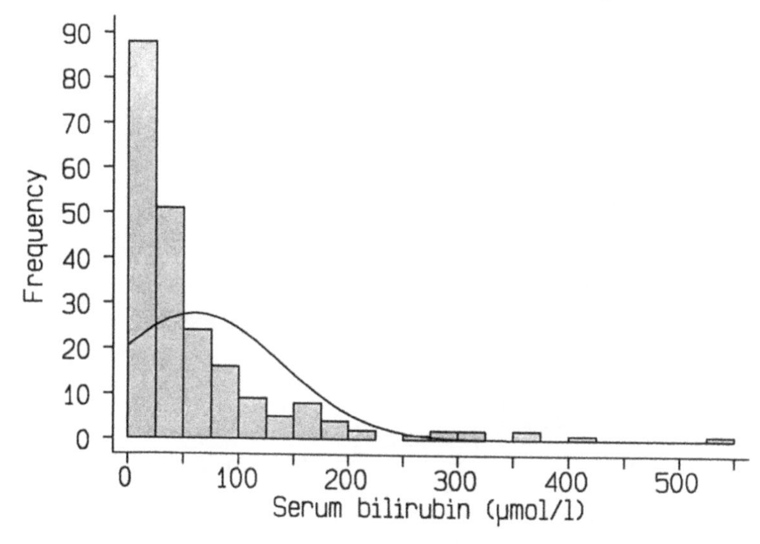


**Figure 4.8** Histogram of serum bilirubin values in 216 patients with primary biliary cirrhosis with fitted Normal distribution (from the study by Christensen *et al.*, 1985).

biliary cirrhosis (PBC). The mean and standard deviation are 60.7 and 77.9 μmol/l respectively. The superimposed best-fitting Normal distribution (with the same mean and standard deviation) is a terrible fit to the data because of the extreme skewness. If we take logs (to base e) of the data we get a much more symmetric distribution with a mean of 3.55 and a standard deviation of 1.03 log μmol/l. Figure 4.9 shows a histogram of $\log_e$ serum bilirubin with the fitted Normal distribution, which is a much better fit. Figure 4.10 shows the raw data with the 'back-transformation' of the fitted Normal distribution function. The fitted curve is an example of the **Lognormal distribution** function. Data with a Lognormal distribution can be transformed to Normality by taking logarithms.

With skewed data like the serum bilirubin measurements log transformation will often produce approximate Normality. We can then perform our calculations on the log data and transform the answers back to the original scale. For example, we may wish to use our data to estimate the values enclosing 95% of serum bilirubin levels for all patients with PBC. Assuming a Lognormal distribution, we can make our calculations from the Normal distribution with mean 3.547 and standard deviation 1.030 (these being more accurate values than those shown above). In log units, 95% of the distribution will be expected to be between mean $-1.96$SD and mean $+1.96$SD. These values are

$$3.547 - (1.96 \times 1.030) = 1.528 \qquad \text{and} \qquad 3.547 + (1.96 \times 1.030) = 5.566.$$

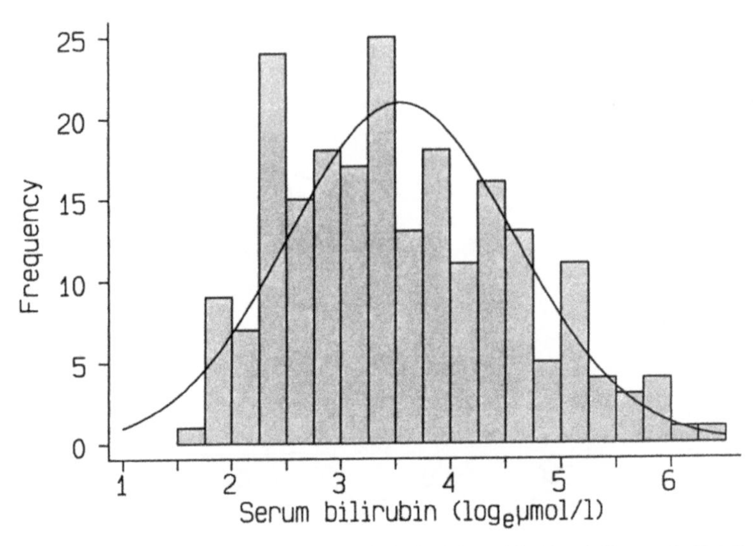


**Figure 4.9** Histogram of log serum bilirubin with fitted Normal distribution (logarithms to base e).

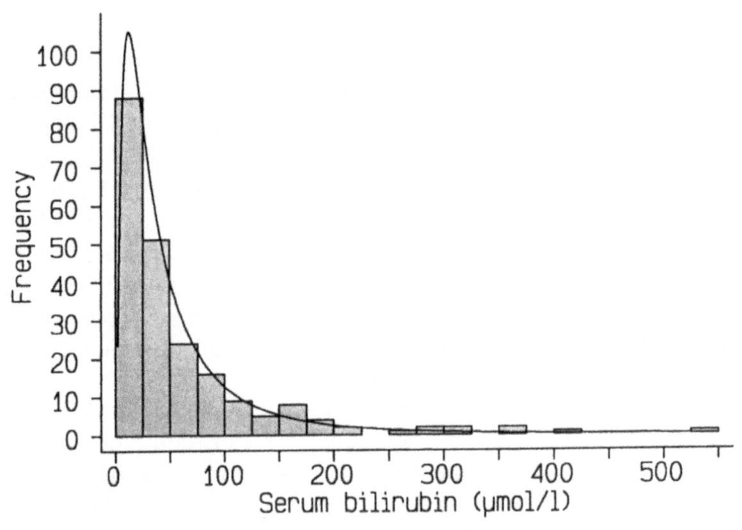


**Figure 4.10** Histogram of serum bilirubin with fitted Lognormal distribution.

The antilogs of these values (using the function $e^x$) are $e^{1.528} = 4.61$ and $e^{5.566} = 261.4$ $\mu$mol/l. The antilog of the mean of the log data is $e^{3.547} = 34.7$ $\mu$mol/l, which is the geometric mean of the data. All of these values are depicted in a box-and-whisker diagram in Figure 4.11.

It should not be *assumed* that data with a skewed distribution can be transformed to approximate Normality. This must be established, perhaps visually as in Figure 4.9 or formally using the methods described in section 7.5.

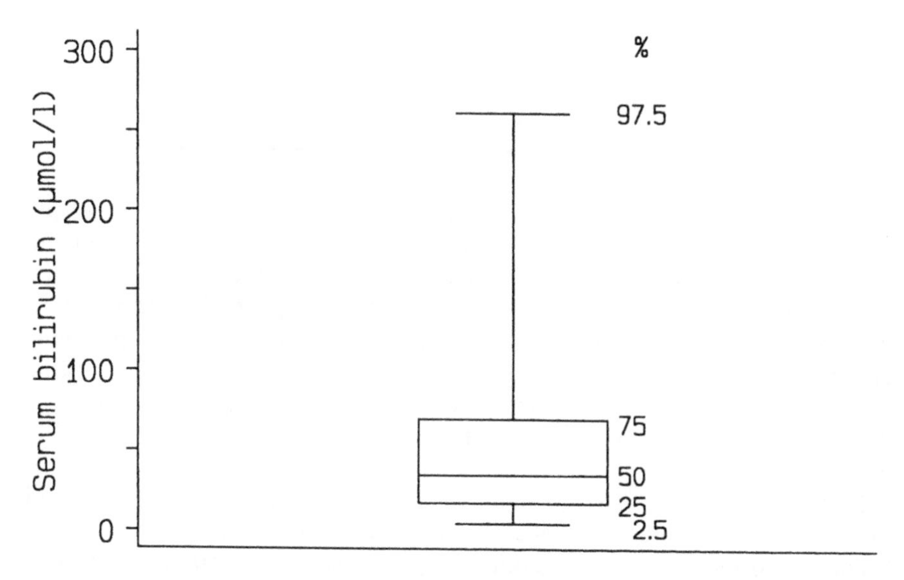


**Figure 4.11** Box-and-whisker diagram of serum bilirubin showing 95% central range derived from fitting a Normal distribution to log data.

## 4.7 THE BINOMIAL DISTRIBUTION

The simplest probability distribution for discrete data is when there are only two possibilities. The probability of being in blood group B is about 0.08 so the probability of being group O, A or AB is 0.92. For a group of unrelated people, we can work out the probability of different numbers of people being in blood group B. The probability of two people both being in blood group B is thus $0.08 \times 0.08 = 0.0064$, and the probability of neither being in blood group B is $0.92 \times 0.92 = 0.8464$. We multiply the probabilities because the blood groups of two unrelated people are independent. The probability of only one of the two being in blood group B is more complicated, because there are two ways in which this could happen. Thus the probability of exactly one of two people being in blood group B $= 2 \times 0.08 \times 0.92 = 2 \times 0.0736 = 0.1472$.

We can summarize the possibilities as follows:

| | | Number in blood group B | Probability |
|---|---|---|---|
| B | B | 2 | 0.0064 |
| not B | B | 1 | 0.0736 |
| B | not B | 1 | 0.0736 |
| not B | not B | 0 | 0.8464 |
| Total | | | 1.0000 |

Figure 4.12 shows the probability distribution of the number of people out of two in blood group B. This distribution is a simple example of the **Binomial distribution**. To get the three probabilities shown we had to make three simple calculations. However, if we extend this simple calculation to consider the number of people out of four it is not so easy. Each person is either group B or not group B so there are $2 \times 2 \times 2 \times 2$ possible orderings, which is 16. The number of possible orderings for $n$ people is $2^n$, so if we have seven people for example, there are 128 possible orderings.

Fortunately, we can bypass most of the calculations by using a general formula. As it is rather complicated, the details are given in section 4.9. Using the formula one can calculate the probability of different numbers of outcomes of a particular type in a series of events from the probability of one such outcome. For example, Figure 4.13 shows the probability

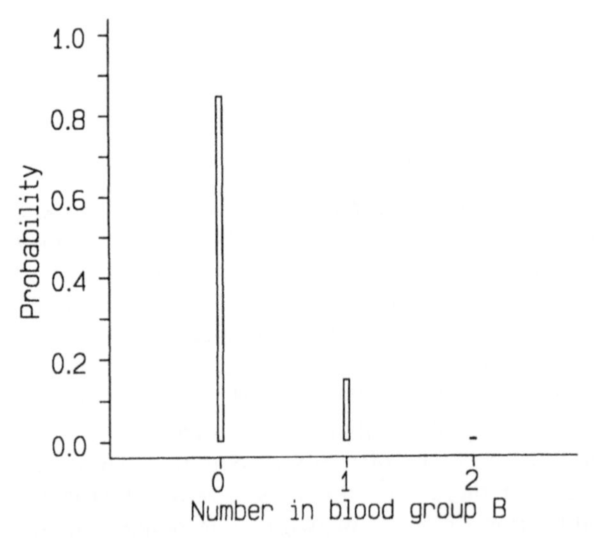


**Figure 4.12** Binomial distribution of number of people out of two in blood group B.

distribution for the number of individuals out of 10 being of blood group B. (The calculations are shown in section 4.9.) The distribution is asymmetric, but as the sample size increases the Binomial distribution becomes

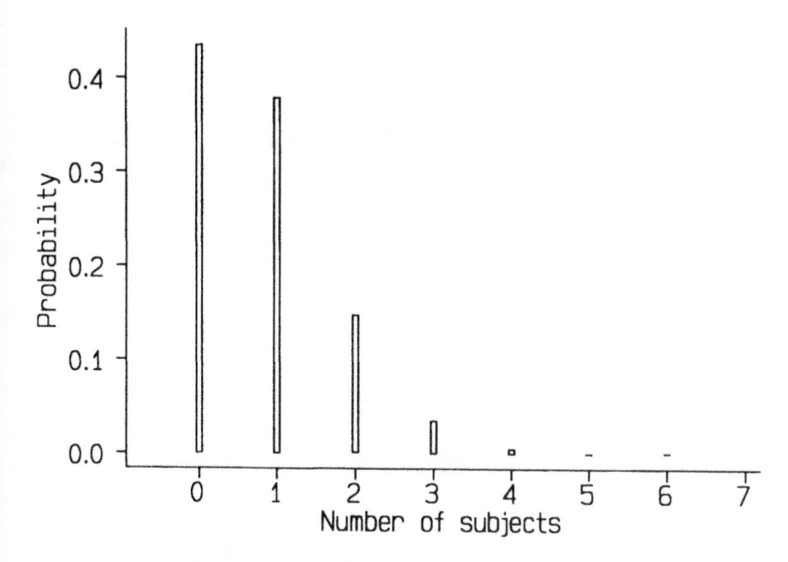


**Figure 4.13** Binomial distribution showing the number of subjects out of ten in blood group B based on the probability of being in blood group B of 0.08.

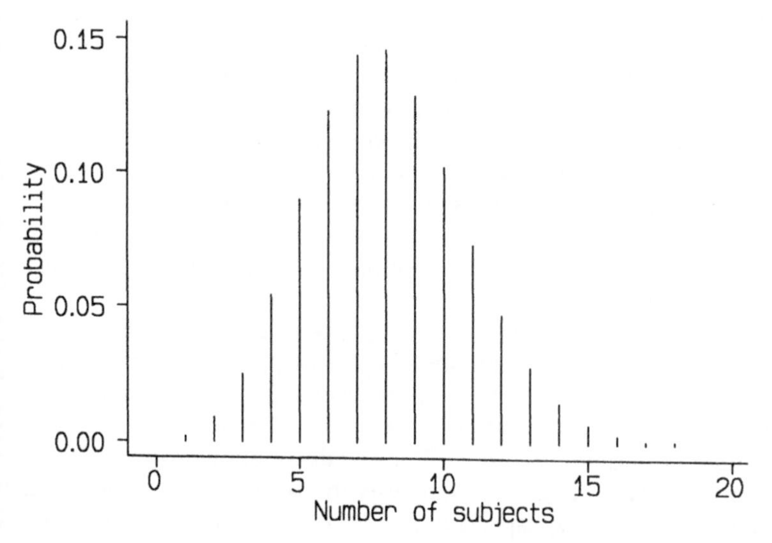


**Figure 4.14** Binomial distribution showing the number of subjects out of 100 in blood group B based on the probability of being in blood group B of 0.08.

more symmetric and gradually begins to look like a Normal distribution. Figure 4.14 shows that the Binomial distribution for the number of people in blood group B in a sample of 100 is almost symmetric.

The Binomial distribution is sometimes used to compare an observed set of data with the expected distribution. Its main use, however, is in the analysis of data where there are only two possibilities, such as whether or not someone suffers from asthma. Here we are interested in the *proportion* of subjects with asthma. Data of this type occur frequently in medical research, and we often wish to compare the proportion of events of a certain type occurring in different groups of subjects. The sample sizes in the groups are often large enough for the Binomial distribution to be very like a Normal distribution with the same mean and standard deviation, which simplifies analysis (see Chapter 10).

## 4.8 THE POISSON DISTRIBUTION

A different type of discrete data arises when we count the number of occurrences of an event, perhaps for different subjects or for units of time. Examples of data like this are the daily number of new cases of breast cancer notified to a cancer registry, and the number of abnormal cells in a fixed area of histological slides from a series of liver biopsies.

The theoretical situation giving rise to data of this type is easiest to describe in relation to events occurring over time (or space) at a fixed rate on average, but where each event occurs independently and at random. Such data will have a **Poisson distribution**. For example, the daily number of new registrations of cancer may be 2.2 on average, but on any day there may be no new cases or there may be several. If we assume that the conditions for a Poisson distribution hold, we can calculate the probability of any number of new cases on a single day. These probabilities are shown in Figure 4.15 (and the calculations are shown in section 4.9).

The Poisson distribution is very asymmetric when its mean is small, as here, but with a large mean, such as 50, it becomes nearly symmetric. In fact, like the Binomial distribution, it becomes more like a Normal distribution. Note that the Poisson distribution has no theoretical maximum value, but the probabilities tail off towards zero very quickly.

Table 4.2 shows some data that might be expected to follow a Poisson distribution. The table gives the number of crimes per day in three small areas of India from 1978 to 1982, on days where there was either a full moon or a new moon. Also shown are the expected number of days with different numbers of crimes, based on Poisson distributions with the same means as the observed data. The similarity between the observed and expected frequencies is clear, especially for the new moon days, demonstrating that these data are close to a Poisson distribution.

The Poisson distribution is completely described by a single parameter,

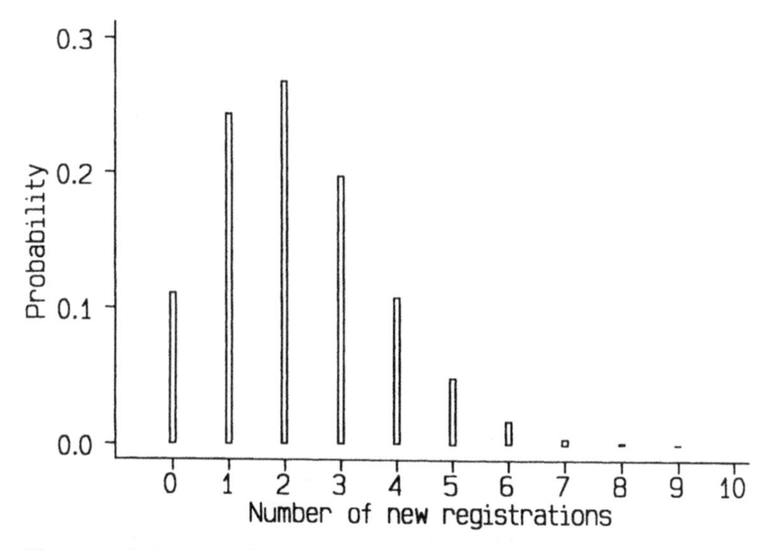


**Figure 4.15** Poisson distribution with mean 2.2.

**Table 4.2** Number of crimes per day in three areas of India during 1978 to 1982 (Thakur and Sharma, 1984) showing observed frequencies (Obs) and expected frequencies using the Poisson distribution (Exp)

| Number of crimes | Full moon days | | New moon days | |
|---|---|---|---|---|
| | Obs | Exp | Obs | Exp |
| 0 | 40 | 45.2 | 114 | 112.8 |
| 1 | 64 | 63.1 | 56 | 56.4 |
| 2 | 56 | 44.3 | 11 | 14.1 |
| 3 | 19 | 20.7 | 4 | 2.4 |
| 4 | 1 | 7.1 | 1 | 0.3 |
| 5 | 2 | 2.0 | 0 | 0.0 |
| 6 | 0 | 0.5 | 0 | 0.0 |
| 7 | 0 | 0.1 | 0 | 0.0 |
| 8 | 0 | 0.0 | 0 | 0.0 |
| 9 | 1 | 0.0 | 0 | 0.0 |
| Total | 183 | 183.0 | 186 | 186.0 |
| Mean | | 1.40 | | 0.50 |
| SD | | 1.16 | | 0.75 |

the mean, as is shown in section 4.9, because the variance of the Poisson distribution turns out to be the same as the mean. It follows that data from different sources will have very similar distributions if they can both be

**Table 4.3** Comparison of distributions of crimes on new moon days (Thakur and Sharma, 1984) and number of deaths per day in a Montreal hospital in 1971 (Zweig and Csank, 1978)

| | Crimes on new moon days in India | | Deaths per day in a hospital in Montreal | | Expected distribution Poisson (0.51) |
|---|---|---|---|---|---|
| $n$ | % | Frequency | % | Frequency | % |
| 0 | 61.3 | 114 | 60.3 | 220 | 60.0 |
| 1 | 30.1 | 56 | 31.0 | 113 | 30.6 |
| 2 | 5.9 | 11 | 6.3 | 23 | 7.8 |
| 3 | 2.2 | 4 | 2.2 | 8 | 1.3 |
| 4+ | 0.5 | 1 | 0.3 | 1 | 0.2 |
| Total | 100.0 | 186 | 100.0 | 365 | 99.9% |
| Mean | | 0.505 | | 0.512 | |
| SD | | 0.752 | | 0.736 | |

considered to be close to Poisson and have the same mean. Table 4.3 shows that the relative frequency distribution of the number of crimes on new moon days in India is virtually identical to the distribution of the number of deaths per day in a hospital in Montreal. Both observed sets of data are very close to a Poisson distribution with a mean of 0.51.

The Poisson distribution is appropriate for studying rare events. We can consider the problem as being the same as that of the Binomial distribution where the probability of the outcome of interest is very small but there are a large number of events. The Poisson distribution is not used greatly in medical research although, like the Binomial distribution, it is used implicitly in some other types of statistical analysis.

## 4.9 MATHEMATICAL CALCULATIONS

*(This section gives the mathematical calculations relating to the sections on the Binomial and Poisson distributions. It can be omitted without loss of continuity.)*

### 4.9.1 Binomial distribution

To take an example, suppose we wish to calculate the probability of different numbers of individuals out of ten being blood group B, for which $p = 0.08$. The probability of, say, a particular 4 of the 10 people being blood group B is $p^4(1-p)^6$, so that the probability of *any* 4 being blood group B is this probability multiplied by the number of ways of choosing 4 people from 10.

In general, suppose we have $n$ 'events' and wish to calculate the probability of 0, 1, 2, up to $n$ of them being a specific type, where $p$ is the overall probability of this type of outcome. Then the Binomial probability of $r$ such events is given by

$$\binom{n}{r} p^r (1 - p)^{n-r}$$

where $\binom{n}{r}$ is the number of ways of choosing $r$ items from $n$, and is a number we have to calculate.

We can evaluate $\binom{n}{r}$ simply by using the following relations:

(i) $\binom{n}{0} = 1;$

(ii) $\binom{n}{r} = \binom{n}{r-1} \times (n - r + 1)/r;$

and

(iii) $\binom{n}{n-r} = \binom{n}{r}.$

So we have

$$\begin{aligned}
\binom{10}{0} &= 1 &&= \binom{10}{10} \\
\binom{10}{1} &= \binom{10}{0} \times 10/1 = 10 &&= \binom{10}{9} \\
\binom{10}{2} &= \binom{10}{1} \times 9/2 = 45 &&= \binom{10}{8} \\
\binom{10}{3} &= \binom{10}{2} \times 8/3 = 120 &&= \binom{10}{7} \\
\binom{10}{4} &= \binom{10}{3} \times 7/4 = 210 &&= \binom{10}{6} \\
\binom{10}{5} &= \binom{10}{4} \times 6/5 = 252
\end{aligned}$$

The probability that 4 of the 10 people are blood group B is thus

$$210(0.08)^4(0.92)^6 = 0.00522$$

or 0.5%. Figure 4.13 shows the complete distribution.

The general formula for the coefficients $\binom{n}{r}$ is

$$\binom{n}{r} = \frac{n!}{r!(n-r)!}$$

where $n!$ (pronounced n **factorial**) is equal to $1 \times 2 \times 3 \times \ldots \times n$ (see Appendix A). Note that $0! = 1$ (see Appendix A). The coefficients $\binom{n}{r}$ can be obtained from tables of $\log\binom{n}{r}$ (Lentner, 1982, pp. 74–81), or calculated in the way described above.

If the true proportion of events of interest is $p$, then in a sample of size $n$ the mean of the Binomial distribution is $np$ and the standard deviation is $\sqrt{np(1-p)}$.

### 4.9.2 Poisson distribution

The general Poisson formula for the probability of $k$ events is $e^{-\mu} \mu^k/k!$ where $\mu$ (the greek letter mu) is the mean and e is a mathematical constant approximately equal to 2.718 (see Appendix A). The standard deviation is $\sqrt{\mu}$.

If the conditions for a Poisson distribution hold, the probability of getting no new cases on a day is

$$P(0) = e^{-\mu}.$$

The Poisson distribution that will fit the data best has the same mean as that of the observations: 2.2. So here $P(0)$ is $e^{-2.2} = 0.111$. Rather than use the complicated formula above we can calculate $P(1)$, $P(2)$, etc. from the relation $P(i) = mP(i-1)/i$, where $m$ is the sample mean. So we have

$$P(1) = 2.2 \times 0.111/1 = 0.244$$

$$P(2) = 2.2 \times 0.244/2 = 0.268$$

$$P(3) = 2.2 \times 0.268/3 = 0.197$$

$$P(4) = 2.2 \times 0.197/4 = 0.108$$

$$P(5) = 2.2 \times 0.108/5 = 0.048$$

$$P(6) = 2.2 \times 0.048/6 = 0.017$$

$$P(7) = 2.2 \times 0.017/7 = 0.005$$

$$P(8) = 2.2 \times 0.005/8 = 0.002$$

and so on. The distribution is shown in Figure 4.15.

Note that this is a good example of the need to keep full numerical precision through a series of calculations, because any error caused by rounding would affect all subsequent calculations. The figures shown above have, however, been rounded to clarify the presentation.

## 4.10 THE UNIFORM DISTRIBUTION

A different problem is that of determining whether there is a seasonal variation in the onset of a disease. If there is no seasonal variation we would expect little variation in the number of new cases each month. For example, if a diabetes clinic in a district general hospital registers 126 new cases in a year, and if there were no seasonality for the onset of diabetes, then we would expect to have one-twelfth of 126 or 10.5 new cases in every month. (We could make a slight correction for the variation in the number of days in a month.) In practice natural variability will lead to some variation in the monthly accrual of new cases, but this will be unsystematic if there is no seasonality, whereas there will be some systematic trend if there is seasonality. The theoretical **Uniform distribution**, which has the same relative frequency for each month, is used for examining such data. Statistical analysis of periodic variation is discussed in section 14.7.

## 4.11 CONCLUDING REMARKS

Theoretical distributions feature in some way in a large proportion of statistical analysis. The Normal distribution is by far the most important of those discussed. Apart from the assumptions of many analyses that the data follow a Normal distribution, there is also a central role for the Normal distribution in many methods of statistical inference, as described in Chapter 8.

There are many other probability distributions not discussed in this chapter. Most of these are of specialized use and will not appear in this book, but three are important in statistical analyses described in later chapters: the $t$ distribution, the $F$ distribution and the Chi squared distribution.

## EXERCISES

4.1 Assuming that the height of adult males has a Normal distribution, what proportion of males will be more than two standard deviations above the mean height?

4.2 The probability of being blood group B is 0.08. What is the probability that if one pint of blood is taken from each of 100 unrelated blood donors fewer than three pints of group B blood will be obtained?

4.3 The probability of a baby being a boy is 0.52. For six women delivering consecutively in the same labour ward on one day, which of the following exact sequences of boys and girls is most likely and which least likely?

GBGBGB    BBBGGG    GBBBBB

4.4 The Binomial distribution with $p = 0.15$ and $n = 10$ is as follows:

| $r$ | Probability | $r$ | Probability |
|---|---|---|---|
| 0 | 0.1969 | 6 | 0.0012 |
| 1 | 0.3474 | 7 | 0.0001 |
| 2 | 0.2759 | 8 | 0.0000 |
| 3 | 0.1298 | 9 | 0.0000 |
| 4 | 0.0401 | 10 | 0.0000 |
| 5 | 0.0085 | | |

(a) If 15% of all pregnancies result in miscarriages, what is the probability that more than half of a group of ten pregnant women will have a miscarriage?

(b) Among groups of users of video display terminals there are 20 000 large enough for ten women to become pregnant in one year. If we call six or more miscarriages out of 10 a 'cluster', how many clusters would we expect in one year, assuming that there is no increased risk of miscarriage associated with using a terminal? (Based on Blackwell and Chang, 1988)

4.5 If an infection is present in a school it would be expected to spread to 10% of the children

(a) How many children should be tested to have a probability of 0.95 (95%) of detecting the infection if it is there? (Hint: consider the probability of all the children in the sample being negative to the test if the infection is present in the school.)

(b) What is the effect of the number of children in the school on this calculation?

4.6 Over a 25 year period the mean height of adult males increased from 175.8 cm to 179.1 cm, but the standard deviation stayed at 5.84 cm. The minimum height requirement for men to join the police force is 172 cm. What proportion of men would be too short to become policemen at the beginning and end of the 25 year period, assuming that the height of adult males has a Normal distribution?

4.7 A researcher plans to measure blood pressure in a number of subjects. He proposes to take three measurements, but intends to discard the third measurement as unreliable if it does not fall between the first two measurements. Assuming that the subjects' blood pressure stays constant during the measuring, what is the probability that for a given subject the third value will not lie between the other two? (Hint: the answer does not depend upon the variability of blood pressure measurements.) Comment on the researcher's proposal.

4.8 In Britain the commonest autosomal recessive disorder is cystic fibrosis, with about one in 2000 live births being affected. If both parents are heterozygous for the abnormal gene there is a 1 in 4 chance of their child having cystic fibrosis.

(a) What is the probability that a couple who are both heterozygous will have two unaffected children?
(b) If they have four unaffected children, what is the probability that their fifth child would be unaffected?
(c) About one in 22 people is heterozygous for cystic fibrosis. In a hospital where there are 3500 births a year, what is the expected number of babies per year affected by cystic fibrosis (assuming that there is no genetic counselling)?

# 5

# Designing research

> Probably no aspect of clinical research is as neglected as study design. Eager young investigators attend classes on medical statistics, find dozens of ways to compute 'P' values, but rarely learn how to organize a clinical research project properly. Yet careful study design is the foundation of quality clinical research.
>
> Noller and Melton (1985)

> There are only a handful of ways to do a study properly but a thousand ways to do it wrong.
>
> Sackett (1986)

## 5.1 INTRODUCTION

All medical research is carried out in relation to one or more objectives, which should focus the plan or **design** of the research. In some cases there is a clear best way to proceed, but more often there is a choice of reasonable ways of designing a study. The statistical aspects of design relate mainly to the structure of the study and all aspects of the collection of data, including the choice of measurements to make and their frequency. Although many of the general issues covered in this chapter apply to clinical trials, these have many special features and are discussed in detail in Chapter 15.

Research can be crudely divided into **observational** and **experimental** studies. In observational studies we collect information about one or more groups of subjects, but do nothing to affect them. Observational studies can be **prospective**, where subjects are recruited and data are collected about subsequent events, or **retrospective**, where information is collected about past events. Observational studies include censuses, surveys, case-control studies and cohort studies; they are considered in sections 5.9 to 5.12.

Experimental studies are those in which the researcher affects (controls) what happens to all or some of the individuals. Similar problems arise in studies of humans, animals and laboratory samples, although the emphasis in this chapter is on clinical studies. Sections 5.4 to 5.8 consider the design of experimental studies.

Most studies aim to answer fairly simple questions but it does not necessarily follow that they require fairly simple designs. The key point is to tailor the research design to the study objective(s). Without adequate planning the researcher cannot expect to be able to make meaningful conclusions. Some important general principles of design are discussed later in this chapter.

In most research we wish to extrapolate the results from a study to the population in general. There are two aspects that require particular attention in this respect. First, the sample(s) studied should be representative of the population(s) of interest; this applies especially to observational studies. Secondly, groups being compared should be as alike as possible apart from the features of direct interest; this applies particularly in experimental studies, such as clinical trials, but is also relevant in many observational studies, such as case-control studies. I return to these issues below.

Research design is arguably the most important aspect of the statistical contribution to medicine. It is for this reason that for over 50 years statisticians have been urging medical researchers to consult them at the planning stage of their study, rather than at the analysis stage. The data from a good study can be analysed in many ways, but no amount of clever analysis can compensate for problems with the design of a study.

## 5.2 CATEGORIES OF RESEARCH DESIGN

Research designs can be classified in several ways, some of which are:

1. observational or experimental;
2. prospective or retrospective;
3. longitudinal or cross-sectional.

These terms are explained below. The first classification relates to the purpose of the study, while the others describe the way in which the data are collected. Not all combinations of these classifications are possible, but most are.

### 5.2.1 Observational or experimental

In an **observational** study the researcher collects information on the attributes or measurements of interest, but does not influence events. An example would be a study to discover the prevalence of hearing difficulties in small children. Observational studies include surveys and most epidemiological studies. By contrast, in an **experimental** study the researcher deliberately influences events and investigates the effects of the intervention. Experimental studies include clinical trials and many animal and laboratory studies. In general stronger inferences can be made from experimental studies than from observational studies. Experimental studies are usually carried out to make comparisons between groups; observational studies may also be comparative, but they are often essentially descriptive.

### 5.2.2 Prospective or retrospective

There is a clear distinction between **prospective** studies, in which data are collected forwards in time from the start of the study, and **retrospective** studies, in which data refer to past events and may be acquired from existing sources, such as hospital notes, or by interview. Experiments are prospective, but observational studies may be prospective or retrospective. Of course, retrospective data can be obtained to compare different treatments, for example different types of mastectomy, but such a study would not be an experiment as it was not a pre-specified study performed under standardized conditions. Retrospective studies include case-control studies (see section 5.10).

### 5.2.3 Longitudinal or cross-sectional

**Longitudinal** studies are those which investigate changes over time, possibly in relation to an intervention. Observations are taken on more than one occasion, although they may not all be used in the analysis. Clinical trials are longitudinal because we are interested in the effect of treatment commencing at one time point on outcome at a later time. **Cross-sectional** studies are those in which individuals are observed only once. Most surveys are cross-sectional, as are studies to construct reference ranges. Observational studies may be longitudinal or cross-sectional, but experiments are usually longitudinal.

There is also the 'pseudo-longitudinal' study in which each subject is seen at only one time, but the data are used to describe changes over time. Examples are studies to derive cross-sectional growth charts for children and studies of hormone levels during the menstrual cycle (see section 5.13).

### 5.2.4 Summary of inter-relationships

Figure 5.1 summarizes the most likely possible combinations of design features. There is a clear distinction between experimental studies which are nearly all prospective and longitudinal, and observational studies which can be either retrospective or prospective and also either cross-sectional or

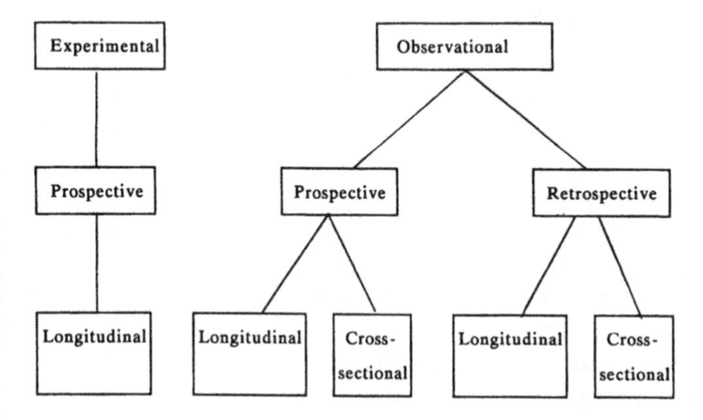


**Figure 5.1** Types of research design.

longitudinal. For this reason experiments and observational studies are considered separately later in this chapter.

It is possible to construct more complex categorizations of research designs (Bailar *et al.*, 1984), but Figure 5.1 describes the main features of most research studies.

So far discussion of design has related to broad issues. The following sections look at design in more detail with particular emphasis on two important aspects of statistical inference from the sample to the population – the representativeness of the sample and the interpretation of any associations found.

### 5.2.5 Control

Whatever the experiment, it is essential to have a comparison, or **control**, group to which the experimental procedure is not applied. It is not usually scientifically or ethically acceptable to say 'Let's try this new treatment on some patients and see what happens'. It is far better to have a control group who are treated normally (or in some way differently), against which comparisons can be made. If we wish to evaluate the benefits of mothers counting fetal movements in pregnancy we should have a concurrent control group of mothers who do not count movements. This is a key component of the evaluation of new therapies or procedures in medicine.

Controls are also advisable in observational studies. If we ask users of visual display terminals (VDTs) if they get eye strain or backache, we should also ask the same questions of a group of comparable employees who do not use VDTs.

In each case the presence of the control group strengthens the inferences that may be made from the results of the study. However, as I shall discuss below, the choice of suitable controls in observational studies is not easy.

## 5.3 SOURCES OF VARIATION

Chapters 3 and 4 both began with comments about the importance of variability to the statistical approach. Variability in behaviour or response to some stimulus, be it tobacco or an antibiotic drug, is the norm. As noted in Chapter 3, some sources of variability may be known, or suspected, but much remains unexplained. For example, we know several variables that affect birth weight, such as length of gestation, fetal sex, parity, maternal smoking, height above sea level, and so on, but statistical models incorporating such information explain only about a quarter of the variability in birth weight. While there are undoubtedly other factors not yet identified that contribute to the variability, it is most unlikely that any important factors remain unidentified. The bulk of the observed variability must therefore be considered unexplainable, which we call random variation. There is considerable random variation in most clinical measurements. For some, such as body temperature, there is relatively little variation, but for others, such as birth weight, blood pressure, or many serum constituents, there is enormous variation. When we are designing a study to compare groups with respect to levels of some clinical measurement, this natural variability must be borne in mind. We can think of this random variability as 'background noise', against which we are trying to detect some effect, or 'signal', of interest. There is a good analogy here with the concept of the 'signal to noise' ratio used in other fields. If the outcome measurement is highly variable we will need a larger study to be able to detect a systematic effect of interest. Another possible design to consider is that in which we remove between subject variation by studying within subject changes from a baseline level.

Further, individuals will exhibit similar variation in other characteristics not directly being studied but which might affect the variables of interest. Many of the principles of experimental design are aimed at trying to control variation that we are not interested in, so that we can focus our attention on the variability that we are interested in. Two consequences of this general variability relevant to the design of studies are:

1. Care is needed to make samples representative of the population.
2. In comparative studies care is needed in making groups similar with respect to known sources of variation.

In addition, we need to bear in mind that when the measurement of interest is highly variable, large samples are needed to get reliable results.

These issues are discussed below, firstly for experimental studies and then for observational studies. However, methods for calculating the appropriate sample size for comparative studies are given in Chapter 15, as they are most often used when designing clinical trials.

Before examining different types of experimental design in detail it should help to consider a real study that illustrates many of the issues.

## 5.4 AN EXPERIMENT: IS THE BLOOD PRESSURE THE SAME IN BOTH ARMS?

Blood pressure is a particularly variable measurement. Not only does it vary considerably between individuals, for which we have partial explanation, but it varies greatly over time for each individual. There is marked variation over 24 hours (circadian variation) as well as day-to-day variation. In addition, blood pressure is difficult to measure. In recent years new technology has been developed to allow continuous recording of blood pressure via an indwelling catheter in the arm linked to a small tape recorder. Ambulatory blood pressure monitoring is more informative, as it gives data for 24 hours, and also potentially more accurate as it measures blood pressure directly and without observer error. Many people regard this intra-arterial technique as the 'gold standard' against which to judge new methods, in particular indirect (i.e. non-invasive) ambulatory recorders. Because of the variability referred to it is important to take simultaneous measurements using the two devices, and thus to use both arms. The question then arises as to whether there might be any systematic difference in blood pressure between the left and right arms.

A study to answer this question was described by Gould *et al.* (1985). The design was as follows. The equipment used to measure the blood pressure was a 'random zero' sphygmomanometer, a machine designed to remove observer bias. (To the reading observed must be added another 'random' quantity not known until afterwards.) A cuff was attached to each arm, and both were connected to the same sphygmomanometer. An electric air pump was used to equalize the pressure to the two cuffs. Clearly it was necessary to have two observers – one to each arm. Despite the use of a special sphygmomanometer it was important that the observers did not measure only one arm in case there was a systematic difference between the observers. Thus each observer had to take half of the observations on the left arm and half on the right, and it was felt sensible (although it was not essential) for each observer to measure both arms of each patient. A similar argument applied to the two cuffs, which might have been slightly different. Thus each cuff had to be applied equally to each arm and again this was carried out for each patient. In view of the known variability of blood pressure it was decided that each observer would take two measurements using each cuff on each arm of each patient, giving 16 measurements per patient. Finally, there might have been a tendency for a patient's blood pressure to change systematically during the series of measurements. Thus the order in which the cuffs were applied to the arms and the order in which the observers measured the two arms was varied using **randomization**. A detailed explanation of randomization is given in section 5.7. There was no communication of results between observers.

The study was carried out on 91 subjects with essential hypertension.

The above design was used to try to get as pure a comparison as possible of the blood pressure in the left and right arms. In addition the circumference of each arm was recorded, and a record was kept of the order in which the measurements were taken for each subject. This study illustrates many features of the design of an experiment, some of which will be discussed in more detail in section 5.5:

*Number of observers* It was necessary to have two observers per subject, but it is often a good idea to have more than one observer even when it is not necessary, as it allows the differences between observers to be quantified (see section 14.2).

*Replicated measurements* It is desirable to take more than one reading in each combination of experimental conditions as it gives greater precision for estimating the effects of interest. The replicates need to be independent readings, however. They were independent in the arm comparison study because the type of machine used meant that the observers did not know what their previous measurement was.

*Balanced design* It is not essential that the same number of observations is taken for each combination of experimental factors, but if everything is balanced, as in the above study, the analysis is very much simpler.

*Randomization* The order in which the observers and cuffs were allocated to the two arms for each patient was determined at random. Randomization is one of the key elements of experimental design.

*Covariates* Sometimes there are non-experimental features (**covariates**) that need to be recorded as they might have affected the results. While they may vary from observation to observation, such as ambient temperature, they may vary only from subject to subject, such as age. In this study arm circumference was considered to be a possible covariate as it affects the fit of the cuff. Arm circumference is intermediate between the two examples given, varying within subject (i.e. between arms) but not from observation to observation. Another potential covariate was the order of observations. The design was randomized and balanced because it was anticipated that recorded blood pressure would fall over repeated measurements. However, it is possible to take account of the order of measurements in the analysis to improve precision.

*Sample size* A large sample was taken to provide a precise estimate of the difference between the arms.

## 5.5 THE DESIGN OF EXPERIMENTS

An experiment should be designed to answer the question of interest as simply and clearly as possible. It is important to consider the way the data will be analysed when designing an experiment as this can save complications later. This chapter considers experiments in general. Chapter 15 considers clinical trials in depth, as there are many special issues involved.

In this section I discuss some of the more important aspects to consider when designing an experiment.

### 5.5.1 Bias

Any study, whether experimental or observational, will be set up to answer one or more specific questions. The reliability of the results, and thus the interpretation of the findings, is crucial. An experiment provides the best opportunity to get at the truth, but there are several precautions that should be taken to ensure that the results are not biased. For example, in a comparative experiment, such as the arm comparison study, it is important that the groups of observations being compared are comparable in all aspects other than that being manipulated by the experimenter. Several of the design features of the arm comparison study were included for this reason.

Bias can occur through structural deficiencies in a study. For example, if one observer had taken all measurements on the left arm and the other all those on the right arm, the between arm differences would have been inseparable from any between observer differences, an effect called **confounding**. In fact, that study was carried out expressly to see if there would be confounding when different machines were compared one to an arm. Making sure that the different observer-arm-cuff combinations were used equally in the 1st, 2nd, 3rd and 4th orders is another example of avoiding bias.

### 5.5.2 Randomization

An important possible source of bias is the way in which subjects vary in features that are not part of the design. For example, if we had measured blood pressure in the left arm only in one group of patients and in the right arm only in another group, then the average difference observed between left and right arms could be affected by differences between the groups with respect to any variable related to blood pressure, such as age. Clearly it is better to use both arms in the same patients, but in most studies the procedures or treatments cannot be given to the same individuals. The usual approach here is to allocate treatments to patients **at random**. As described in section 5.7, the word random has a specific statistical meaning. Random allocation is one of the fundamental principles of experimental design. Another device is to find pairs of subjects with closely similar characteristics and allocate treatments to the matched pair at random. Matching is discussed in section 5.8.

In the arm comparison study the order in which the observers measured the left and right arms and the order of use of the two cuffs were randomized. There was no specific reason to expect a bias from, for example, observer 1 always starting on the left arm, but random ordering was used as a safeguard against possible subtle unknown effects.

### 5.5.3 Blinding

Bias can also occur through subconscious effects. For example, observers' judgements may be affected by knowing the treatment that a subject is getting, or by knowledge of a previous measurement for that subject. The latter problem was avoided in the arm comparison study by the choice of blood pressure measuring machine. The former problem is especially relevant in clinical trials, where it is desirable to keep both patients and assessors in ignorance of the treatment given, a procedure known as **blinding** (see Chapter 15).

### 5.5.4 Replication

For measurements that are highly variable or difficult to measure accurately it may be useful to take more than one measurement on each individual. These **replicates** can be treated in the analysis as separate observations, which may make the analysis more complicated but gives greater potential to detect effects of interest. This analysis is only valid if the replicates are independent, which is often not the case if the observer knows what measurement they obtained the first time.

More often the average of the replicates is used in the analysis. This latter approach may mirror clinical practice – some 'noisy' variables such as blood pressure, peak expiratory flow rate, and ultrasound measurements are usually repeated.

### 5.5.5 Sample selection

It is always desirable for the sample in a study to be representative of the population of interest, but this is not as important in experiments as in observational studies. For example, it is unlikely that the choice of the sample for the arm difference study would have affected the results. It is much more important to ensure that the sub-groups being compared are as similar as possible.

Although in principle representative samples are best obtained by random selection from the population, this ideal is virtually never met in practice. However, the sample should be chosen to be as similar as possible to the relevant population, so it is essential to be able to describe just how the sample was chosen.

These considerations are probably irrelevant for most animal experiments.

### 5.5.6 Sample size

Another way of combating variability is to increase the sample size. Larger samples enable us to evaluate effects of interest more precisely. The determination of an appropriate sample size is most common in clinical trials and section 15.3 describes formal methods for choosing an appropriate sample size in comparative studies. Similar principles apply to all studies, but the methods can be complicated so expert assistance is required.

## 5.6 THE STRUCTURE OF AN EXPERIMENT

In a designed experiment such as the arm comparison study there may be several conditions (called **factors**) being controlled by the investigator. It may be helpful to draw a diagram to show the structure of the design. As well as clarifying the design the diagram will show how the data should be analysed.

A simple example is an experiment to compare three separate groups of subjects given different analgesics to combat migraine. Figure 5.2 shows the simple structure of this design. Each x denotes an observation. In this design there is no need for the three groups to be of equal size but in more complicated designs equal sizes are highly desirable. If the study design

| | Analgesic | |
|---|---|---|
| A | B | C |
| x | x | x |
| x | x | x |
| x | x | x |
| x | x | x |
| x | x | x |
| x | x | x |
| | x | x |
| | x | x |
| | x | |
| | x | |

**Figure 5.2** Structure of a study to compare three groups of subjects receiving analgesics A, B or C. Each x indicates one subject.

were changed so that each subject received all three analgesics in random order, the design would be as shown in Figure 5.3. Here observations on the same subject are connected.

A study may combine both these features, so that subjects are examined more than once but different groups of subjects are treated differently. For example, we may wish to compare subjects' weights before and after different diets; Figure 5.4 shows the appropriate design. Figures 5.2 to 5.4 illustrate the important distinction between **within subject** and **between subject** comparisons.

The study comparing blood pressure in the left and right arms was more complicated. There were three factors – arms, observers and cuffs – and two measurements (replicates) were taken for each combination. The design of this study, which is shown in Figure 5.5, is known as a **factorial design** as all combinations of factors are used.

It is not possible to say what the best design is in any given circumstance. The choice of factors to control, which factors are between subject and which within, and how many observations to take for each subject is difficult, and it will often take much thought to arrive at a satisfactory design. Expert statistical help is particularly valuable at this stage. Any weaknesses in the design cannot be rectified later.

```
        Analgesic
  A         B         C
---------------------------
  x---------x---------x
  x---------x---------x
  x---------x---------x
  x---------x---------x
  x---------x---------x
  x---------x---------x
  x---------x---------x
  x---------x---------x
  x---------x---------x
  x---------x---------x
  x---------x---------x
  x---------x---------x
  x---------x---------x
---------------------------
```

**Figure 5.3** Structure of a study to compare three treatments in one group of subjects. Lines join observations on the same subject, which are made in random order.

| Diet 1 | | Diet 2 | | Diet 3 | |
|---|---|---|---|---|---|
| Before | After | Before | After | Before | After |
| x-----x | | x-----x | | x-----x | |
| x-----x | | x-----x | | x-----x | |
| x-----x | | x-----x | | x-----x | |
| x-----x | | x-----x | | x-----x | |
| x-----x | | x-----x | | x-----x | |
| x-----x | | x-----x | | x-----x | |
| x-----x | | x-----x | | x-----x | |
| x-----x | | x-----x | | x-----x | |
| x-----x | | x-----x | | x-----x | |

**Figure 5.4** Structure of a study to compare two groups measured before and after treatment.

| Left arm | | | | Right arm | | | |
|---|---|---|---|---|---|---|---|
| Observer 1 | | Observer 2 | | Observer 1 | | Observer 2 | |
| Cuff 1 | Cuff 2 | Cuff 1 | Cuff 2 | Cuff 1 | Cuff 2 | Cuff 1 | Cuff 2 |

x-x----x-x-----x-x----x-x-----x-x----x-x-----x-x----x-x
x-x----x-x-----x-x----x-x-----x-x----x-x-----x-x----x-x
x-x----x-x-----x-x----x-x-----x-x----x-x-----x-x----x-x
x-x----x-x-----x-x----x-x-----x-x----x-x-----x-x----x-x
etc (91 rows)

**Figure 5.5** Structure of the study to compare blood pressure in the left and right arms – a three way factorial design.

## 5.7 RANDOM ALLOCATION

There have been several mentions of random allocation earlier in this chapter. The rationale for and methods of randomization in experimental studies are discussed in this section.

There are two main reasons for using randomization. The first reason is to prevent bias. As noted earlier, we want to compare treatments between groups which do not differ in any systematic way. If subjects receive treatments chosen by the investigator (or indeed the subject) there is the likelihood of bias arising – usually subconscious but occasionally intentional. We can avoid this possibility by allocating treatments to subjects at random. There is further discussion of this issue with regard to clinical trials in section 15.2.2.

Bias can also arise through unknown effects. For example, when two or more treatments (or experimental conditions) are used for each subject it is advisable to randomize the order in which they are applied to each subject in case there is any unknown bias associated with time or the order of measurements. This argument was behind the randomization of the order of measurements in the arm comparison study.

The other reason for randomizing is that statistical theory is based on the idea of random sampling. In a study with random allocation the differences between treatment groups behave like the differences between random samples. As noted in Chapter 4, we know how random samples are expected to behave, and so can compare the observations with expectation, for example assuming that the treatments are equally effective.

### 5.7.1 Simple randomization

It is not always appreciated that **random** does not mean the same as **haphazard**. By random allocation we mean that each patient has a known chance, usually an equal chance, of being given each treatment, but the treatment to be given cannot be predicted. Thus alternately allocating two treatments to a series of patients is not random allocation. The simplest method of random allocation is tossing a coin – heads is treatment A, tails is treatment B. An equivalent method is to use a table of random numbers, such as that in Table B13. In these tables each number occurs equally often, and the ordering is random, and so completely unpredictable. Another option is to use a **random number generator** on a computer.

The first step is to decide the correspondence between the random numbers and the different experimental groups. For example, if we wish to allocate equally two treatments to subjects using Table B13 we could take odd numbers to indicate one treatment and even numbers to indicate the other. We must then choose a place to start, and this can be done using a pin or some equally arbitrary method. In addition we can choose the direction in which to read the table.

Suppose that the first two digit numbers in the table from our starting place are

12 19 20 52 81 30 74 93 02 67 41 50, etc.

If we take odd numbers for treatment A and even numbers for treatment B, then these numbers indicate the sequence

BABBABBABAAB

for the first 12 subjects. Alternatively we could take each digit on its own, to give

ABAABBABBAABABAABBBABAAB

for the first 24 subjects. A third approach would be to take numbers 00 to 49 for A and 50 to 99 for B, and there are countless other possible strategies. It makes no difference which is used.

We can easily generalize the last approach to situations with more than two treatments or experimental conditions. For example, we could use the following scheme for three groups:

01 to 33: treatment A

34 to 66: treatment B

67 to 99: treatment C

00 : ignored

and similarly for other designs. Notice that at any point in the sequence the numbers of patients allocated to each treatment will probably differ. We sometimes wish to keep the numbers in each group very close at all times, which we can achieve by **block randomization**. Further, with simple randomization the distribution of the characteristics of the subjects in each group is left completely to chance. We often know or suspect that some subjects will behave differently, for example they may have different prognoses, and so it is desirable to keep the numbers within these classes similar in the different treatment groups. We can achieve this by **stratified randomization** or **minimization**. These techniques are all described below.

Clearly it is very easy to adapt the above method to give a **weighted randomization**, leading to unequal numbers in the different groups. For example, we could allocate treatments A and B in proportions 2 to 1 by using 01 to 66 for A and 67 to 99 for B.

### 5.7.2 Block (or restricted) randomization

Block (or restricted) randomization is used to keep the numbers of subjects in the different groups closely balanced at all times. For example, if we consider subjects in blocks of four at a time, there are six ways in which we can allocate treatments so that two subjects get A and two get B:

| | |
|---|---|
| 1 AABB | 4 BBAA |
| 2 ABAB | 5 BABA |
| 3 ABBA | 6 BAAB |

If we use combinations of only these six ways of allocating treatments then the numbers in the two groups at any time can never differ by more than two, and they will usually be the same or one apart. We choose blocks at random to create the allocation sequence. Using the previous random sequence beginning

121920528130749302674150

we can omit those numbers outside the range 1 to 6 to get

12122134326415

from which we can construct the block allocation sequence

AABB ABAB AABB ABAB ABAB AABB ABBA BBAA ABBA

and so on. Notice the apparently non-random beginning of the sequence – 121221 – in which only two of the six numbers appear. Lists of random numbers always throw up peculiar sequences like this one – they would not be random if they did not. Inspection of Table B13 shows many such sequences.

Randomized blocks can be of any size, but using a multiple of the number of treatments is more logical. Large blocks are best avoided as they control balance less well. In clinical trials it is highly desirable for the randomization sequence to be kept hidden from those actually giving the treatments. This is often achieved by creating a pile of opaque numbered sealed envelopes each containing the allocation for one patient. Even so, with the knowledge that restricted randomization is being used, it is possible to deduce in advance the treatment to be given to every fourth patient. For this reason it is better for the users of the random numbers not to know how the sequence was constructed, and it may also be desirable to vary the block length, again at random, perhaps using a mixture of blocks of size 2, 4, or 6. A similar approach is used when there are more than two treatments. For example, blocks of size 3, 6, or 9 can be used for three treatments. Obviously these considerations do not apply to experiments on animals or laboratory experiments on human samples.

There is further discussion in section 15.2 of the problems associated with treatment allocation in clinical trials.

### 5.7.3 Stratified randomization

While simple randomization removes bias from the allocation procedure, it does not guarantee, for example, that the subjects in each group have similar age distributions. Indeed in small studies it is highly likely that some chance imbalance will occur, which might complicate the interpretation of results. Even in studies with over 100 subjects there may be some substantial variations by chance, especially for characteristics that are quite rare. In many clinical studies it is known beforehand that subgroups of patients are expected to respond differently to treatment. Here it is advisable to ensure that the subjects receiving each treatment have similar characteristics.

We can use **stratified randomization** to achieve approximate balance of important characteristics without sacrificing the advantages of randomization. The method is to produce a separate block randomization list for each subgroup (stratum). For example, in a study to compare two alternative treatments for breast cancer it would be important to stratify by menopausal status. Two separate lists of random numbers should be obtained, from which two separate piles of sealed envelopes can be prepared, for premenopausal and postmenopausal women. It is essential that stratified treatment allocation is based on block randomization within each stratum rather than simple randomization; otherwise there will be no control of balance of treatments within strata, and so the object of stratification will be defeated.

Stratified randomization can be extended to two or more stratifying variables. For example, we might wish to extend the stratification in the breast cancer trial to tumour size and number of positive nodes. We have to produce a separate randomization list for each combination of categories. If we had two tumour size groups (say $\leq 4$ and $> 4$ cm) and three groups for node involvement (0, 1–4, $> 4$) as well as menopausal status, then we have $2 \times 3 \times 2 = 12$ strata, which may exceed the limit of what is practical. There is the further problem with multiple strata that some of the combinations of categories may be rare, so that the treatment balance expected from the use of block randomization does not occur.

Some thought should be given to which variables are used for stratification, restricting the choice to variables known to be prognostically important. Many trials stratify using age and sex. While age is frequently known to be prognostic, sex is often not prognostic and need not be used for stratification.

In a multicentre study the patients within each centre will need to be randomized separately unless there is a central coordinated randomizing service. Thus 'centre' is a stratifying variable, and there may be other stratifying variables as well.

In small studies it is not practical to stratify on more than one or perhaps two variables, as the number of strata can quickly approach the number of subjects. When it is really important to achieve close similarity between treatment groups for several variables **minimization** can be used (see section 5.8).

### 5.7.4 Other uses of randomization

In some studies it is either impossible or impractical to allocate treatments to individual subjects. Suppose that we wish to evaluate the effectiveness of a health education campaign on television or in the newspapers to increase awareness of the dangers of drugs, or indeed to change behaviour. We cannot target *individuals* at random, but rather we can randomly assign whole *areas* to receive different media coverage. With a large number of small areas this **cluster randomization** should give reliable results, but with a small number of very large areas, as would be likely in the example given, there are problems in ensuring the comparability of the areas. Here it is valuable to obtain baseline data before the study starts so that changes within areas over the time of the study can be compared. Other clusters sometimes used in experimental research are schools, hospitals and families.

As with treatment comparisons on individuals, randomized studies on areas will give more reliable results than non-randomized studies, but randomization is often impossible. Much of the controversy over the possible association between the fluoridation of drinking water and cancer in the United States was due to the different characteristics of areas which did or did not have fluoride.

Randomization can also be used in other ways in experiments. In the arm comparison study the order in which the two observers and two cuffs were used on each arm was randomized in case there was some systematic order effect. It is a good idea to use balanced randomization in situations where there is the possibility of some systematic unwanted effect (that is, a bias). No harm will be done if it turns out that there was no such effect.

It is also advisable to use randomization in animal experiments (Gart *et al.*, 1986). For example, if mice are to be given one of two or more different treatments it is best to select them one at a time and use a random sequence to determine the treatment. There are likely to be size differences between those animals pulled out first from the cage and those left to the end (Festing, 1981). There may also be systematic differences between animals in different cages, so that each cage should contain some animals given each treatment.

Likewise randomization has a role in laboratory experiments, such as when analysing samples that have been treated differently (e.g. by irradiation). If the samples are analysed in a continuous process, such as when using a Coulter counter to measure haemoglobin and white cell counts in samples of whole blood, then the order of analysis should preferably be randomized in relation to the differently treated samples.

In some experiments samples are analysed in batches and there are physical constraints on the number that can be dealt with in one go. It is advisable to have equal numbers of each type of sample in each batch. Further, if there is the possibility of systematic differences between the different locations, then the positions of the samples should also be randomized. For example, different types of sample can be randomly allocated to the numbered wells in a $6 \times 6$ plate.

## 5.8 MINIMIZATION

The only form of allocation that is an acceptable alternative to randomization is **minimization**, which is a clever method of ensuring excellent balance between the groups for several prognostic factors, even in small samples. It is based on the idea that the next patient to enter the trial is given, with probability greater than 0.5, whichever treatment would minimize the overall imbalance between the groups at that stage of the trial. Often the probability is taken as 1, but a value greater than, say 0.75, should achieve much the same result with the advantages of a random component. Details of the method are given in section 15.2.3, as the technique is mainly used in clinical trials.

## 5.9 OBSERVATIONAL STUDIES

As shown in Figure 5.1, observational studies can take different forms. Many studies are carried out to investigate possible associations between various factors and the development of a particular disease or condition. Examples are studies of the relation between passive smoking and lung cancer, the use of visual display terminals and miscarriage, and alcohol consumption and suicide. There is no logical difference between comparing the outcome of two groups of patients given alternative treatments and comparing the outcome of groups receiving different exposures. In general, however, areas of **epidemiological** research such as those listed above are not amenable to being investigated by randomized trials. We cannot randomize individuals to smoke or not to smoke nor to work in particular jobs, and other factors such as age and race are not controllable by the individual. We must use **observational studies**, therefore, to study factors or exposures which cannot be controlled by the investigators. Nevertheless, as stated by Gray-Donald and Kramer (1988), 'the goal of an observational study should be to arrive at the same conclusions that *would* have been obtained by an experimental trial'.

There are two main types of observational study that are used to investigate causal factors – the **case-control** study and the **cohort** study. Figure 5.6 indicates the basic structure of these designs. In a retrospective case-control study a number of subjects with the disease in question (the cases) are identified along with some unaffected subjects (controls). The past history of these groups in relation to the exposure(s) of interest is then compared. In contrast, in a prospective cohort study a group of subjects is identified and followed prospectively, perhaps for many years, and their subsequent medical history recorded. The cohort may be subdivided at the outset into groups with different characteristics, or the study may be used to investigate which subjects go on to develop a particular disease. (There is also the **historical cohort** study, in which a past cohort is identified, and

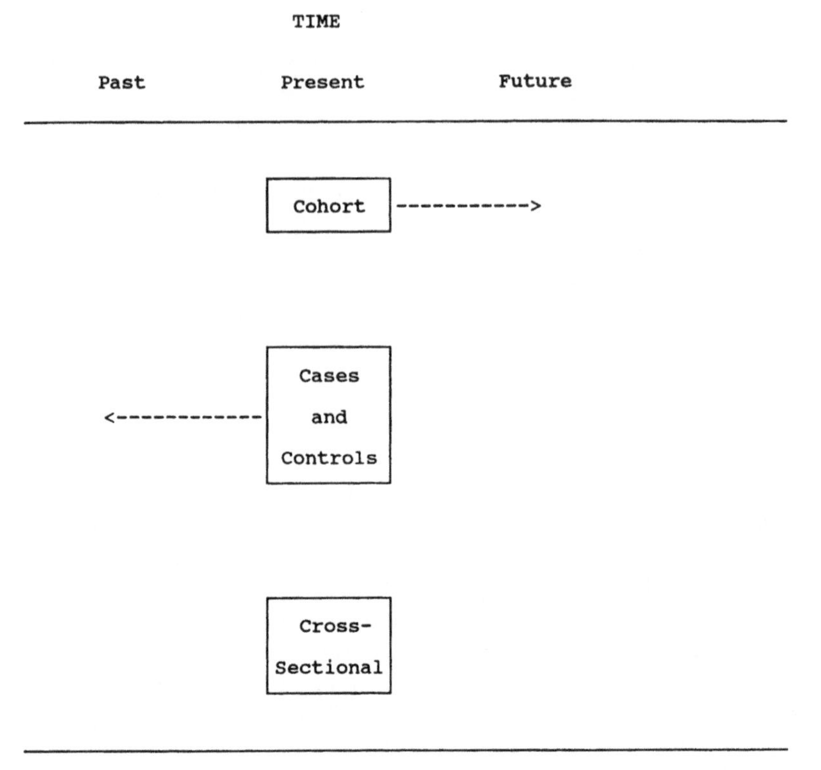


*Cohort Study*:

disease experience is collected prospectively

*Case-Control Study*:

past experience of cases and controls is recalled

*Cross-Sectional Study*:

past experience and current disease status are collected at the same time

**Figure 5.6** Basic structure of the case-control study, the cohort study and the cross-sectional study.

their experience up to the present is obtained. Few studies like this are carried out as the necessary data are rarely available.) Also shown in Figure 5.6 is the **cross-sectional** study, in which subjects are investigated on one occasion only. The advantages and disadvantages of the retrospective case-control study, the prospective cohort study and the cross-sectional study are described in the next three sections.

## 5.10 THE CASE-CONTROL STUDY

As shown in Figure 5.6, in the **case-control** study we identify a group of subjects (cases) with the disease or condition of interest, say lung cancer, and an unaffected group (controls), and compare their past exposure to one or more factors of interest, such as consumption of carrots. If the cases report greater exposure than the controls we may infer that exposure is causally related to the disease of interest, for example that consumption of carrots affects the risk of developing lung cancer.

The prime advantages of the case-control approach are practical: it is relatively simple, and thus quick and cheap. The case-control design is also valuable when the condition of interest is very rare. The disadvantages of this design are important, however, and relate to possible biases in the comparison of cases and controls. Sackett (1979) identified as many as 35 different biases that can occur with case-control studies; some of the main ones are described below.

### 5.10.1 Selection of controls

The main difficulty with the case-control study is the selection of an appropriate control group. If we follow the analogy with the randomized clinical trial, we want the controls to be as similar as possible to the cases, except that they do not have the disease being investigated. Obtaining such a group, however, is not straightforward. Subjects who do not have the outcome of interest may well differ in other ways from the cases, and in particular may be atypical with regard to the exposure of interest. For example, when the cases are hospital patients with a particular condition it is common to take as controls patients in the same hospital(s) with different conditions. Patients in hospital may be expected to have other conditions that are also affected by the exposure of interest. For example, in a study of lung cancer and smoking, use of hospital controls may well lead to an underestimate of the relation because many other medical conditions are related to smoking. This bias would not appear so likely in a study of lung cancer and consumption of carrots (Pisani *et al.*, 1986), but diet may be affected by or may lead to other medical conditions.

In particular, problems can arise from different hospital admission rates among four groups: exposed and unexposed cases and exposed and unexposed controls. This bias was postulated on theoretical grounds by Berkson in 1946, but was not demonstrated empirically until 1978 (Roberts *et al.*, 1978).

The alternative approach is to select community controls, choosing subjects from the non-hospitalized population. It is, however, not straightforward to select a representative control group from the general population, especially if, for example, a certain age and sex distribution is required.

There is also likely to be less willingness among healthy people to participate in a study than among hospital patients, which would introduce a further bias. Some studies use both hospital controls and community controls, which is a desirable approach when there is doubt about the validity of hospital controls.

One way to make the cases and controls more comparable is to **match** for some variables that might confuse the comparison. Matching means that each case is *individually* paired with a control subject. For example, for each case we might seek a control subject of the same age, sex and occupation. Matching is only useful, however, for variables that are strongly related to both the exposure and the outcome of interest. Further, it is important to appreciate that any variable used for matching cannot be investigated as a possible risk factor for the outcome. Thus if we individually match post myocardial infarct (MI) patients (cases) with non-MI controls with respect to whether or not they are vegetarian, we cannot find an association between MI and meat-eating if there is one.

For rare events, the strength of the study can be increased by having more controls than cases. Where matching is used each case can have several matched controls. For example Cuckle *et al*. (1986) compared the level of alpha-fetoprotein in stored serum from the umbilical cords of Down's syndrome babies and controls. For each Down's baby they took three controls matched for the baby's gestational age at delivery and duration of storage of the serum samples.

### 5.10.2 Selection of cases

The selection of controls is a major problem, but the selection of cases should also be considered carefully. While it may be reasonable to group together all diabetics, many diseases such as most cancers are heterogeneous in cause, nature and degree. The choice of cases with respect to type of disease and other factors such as age determines the degree of generalizability of results.

### 5.10.3 Recall bias

Another important source of bias is that due to differential recall by cases and controls. In many case-control studies retrospective information is obtained by interviewing the subjects. People with a particular disease or condition may have thought a lot about a possible link with their past behaviour, especially with respect to widely publicized risk factors. For example, women having a miscarriage may be more likely to report exposure to possible hazards, such as use of a video display terminal, than women whose pregnancies went to term. Such a study may thus reflect perception of risk rather than a true risk.

Although it may not always be present (Mackenzie and Lippman, 1989), there is enormous scope for recall bias in case-control studies. In general the bias is due to under-reporting of exposure in the control group. Usually there are no records against which to check reports, but efforts should be made to evaluate and minimize the effect of recall bias.

### 5.10.4 Inaccuracy of retrospective data

In addition to biased recall of events, there is the possibility of a general inaccuracy in recalled information. Studies requiring recall of detailed dietary or smoking habits are prone to this problem, as are those requiring a precise breakdown of subjects' working history to evaluate total exposure to a hazard.

While there may be no general tendency to over- or under-estimate exposure in the recalled information from a large number of subjects, the 'noise' introduced by errors in recall do have the effect of leading to an underestimate of the association between the exposure and the outcome of interest (Breslow and Day, 1987, p. 41). There is not usually much that can be done to improve the accuracy of long-term recall data.

A related problem is that data obtained from hospital notes will suffer from incompleteness due to missing information and missing notes.

### 5.10.5 Ascertainment bias

Another form of bias can arise through a relation between the exposure and the probability of detecting the event of interest. For example, women taking the oral contraceptive pill will have more frequent cervical smears than women not on the pill, and as a consequence are more likely to have cervical cancer detected if it is present (and it is likely to be detected at an earlier stage). Thus in a case-control study comparing women with cervical cancer and a control group, an excess of pill taking among the cases may be (at least partly) due to the **ascertainment bias** (or **detection bias**) related to more frequent screening.

### 5.10.6 Comment

The problems discussed are only the most obvious difficulties associated with case-control studies. More detailed discussion can be found in epidemiology textbooks, such as Breslow and Day (1980) and Schlesselman (1982). Case-control studies can be very valuable, but much care is needed in their planning, analysis and interpretation. The considerable scope for bias is a strong reason for seeking expert epidemiological and statistical collaboration at the planning stage. It has been suggested that many contradictory results from case-control studies of the same topic are due to the lack of adherence to rigorous scientific principles in their design (Mayes *et al.*, 1988).

However carefully sources of bias have been excluded the observation in a case-control study of an association between an outcome and a risk factor must be interpreted with much care. Specifically, it is wrong to take such a finding as necessarily indicating a causal link. Observational studies cannot do more than suggest possible causal links – other research is needed to investigate these ideas more deeply. For example, Mattila *et al.* (1989) found an association between poor dental health and acute myocardial infarction. While the authors advanced a possible explanation for a causal link, the observed association might be because people with poor dental health tend to look after themselves poorly in general, for example with respect to their diet. Clearly it helps to collect information on possible confounding variables, which can be incorporated into the analysis.

## 5.11 THE COHORT STUDY

The prospective **cohort** study (or **follow-up** or **longitudinal** study) is the method of choice for an observational study, but there are certain difficulties with this design too. The essence of the cohort study is to identify a group of subjects of interest and then follow them up to see what happens. Because of the need to observe unaffected individuals until a fair proportion develop the outcome of interest, cohort studies can take a long time and may thus be very expensive. They are usually unsuitable for studying rare outcomes as it would be necessary to follow a huge number of subjects to get an adequate number of events.

There is usually one particular event of interest, such as death or recurrence of disease, but there may be several. There may be subgroups of subjects identified at the outset whose experience is to be compared, such as smokers and non-smokers or patients with different stages of breast cancer. Alternatively the purpose of the study may be to use the information gained to try to identify those subjects most at risk of developing the outcome of interest. For example, we could follow patients with cirrhosis of the liver, identify those developing carcinoma of the liver over, say, ten years, and compare their characteristics with those who do not get a carcinoma. Because the study is prospective the nature and quality of the data recording can be carefully controlled.

Breslow and Day (1987, pp. 15–20) summarize the advantages of cohort studies over case-control studies. There are some problems with cohort studies, however. Selection of the subjects to study is a common problem with all research, and is discussed below along with three problems specific to follow-up studies.

### 5.11.1 Selection of subjects

The selection of subjects to study is important in all research. In follow-up studies the probability of the event of interest occurring may be strongly related to how the sample was obtained. The issues are clearly seen in a review by Ellenberg and Nelson (1980) of published studies of the frequency of an adverse prognosis in children having a febrile seizure. They observed that such seizures occur in 2% to 4% of all young children, and as there may be harmful consequences of long-term anti-convulsant therapy it was important to quantify the risk of further seizures.

They reviewed 23 studies in which the risk of subsequent nonfebrile seizures had been ascertained. In 17 studies the children had been identified in special clinics or hospital emergency rooms. The other six had taken population samples, in which the investigators attempted to identify and follow up all children in a defined population who experienced a febrile seizure in a certain time period. It is likely that the prevalence of febrile seizures varies from one area to another, and we would expect some effect of different protocols in the different studies. Nevertheless we would expect different population-based studies to give similar results. In contrast, the clinic-based studies will inevitably be biased towards higher risk children because they will only see the more serious cases. The extent of the bias will be variable according to local referring patterns and alternative facilities. We would thus expect the clinic-based studies to show higher and more variable recurrence rates than the population based studies, and this is exactly what Ellenberg and Nelson found. The seven population-based studies obtained recurrence rates of from 1.5 to 4.6% (median 3.0%), whereas the 17 clinic-based studies found rates between 2.6% and 76.9% (median 16.9%). These large estimated recurrence rates had led to many children being treated prophylactically; the much smaller rates obtained in the population-based studies argued against such treatment.

Similar differences in outcome in relation to sample selection would be likely in follow-up studies of other medical conditions. In some cases, however, studying attenders at special clinics may give an optimistic picture. Examples are cystic fibrosis in newborn babies and myocardial infarction, for both of which some cases will not live long enough to be able to attend a clinic. Population samples are difficult and expensive to carry out, but studies of highly selected subjects may well give misleading results, especially regarding the natural history of disease.

### 5.11.2 Loss to follow-up

The main difficulty specifically encountered in cohort studies is that some subjects will not be followed up for the full length of the study. They may move to another area or lose interest, or they may even die. The longer the study, the more subjects will be lost. Losses to follow-up reduce the numbers supplying information, and thus weaken the analysis slightly. The main worry, however, is that subjects are lost to follow-up for some reason that is related to the outcomes being studied or to pre-defined risk categories. There is a considerable risk of this type of bias, and so strenuous efforts are needed to try to contact as many people as possible. Some losses are inevitable, and it is useful to compare the characteristics of these subjects on entry to the study with those with whom contact is maintained.

Even with a short follow-up period there will be losses for various reasons, some of which might be related to the aim of the research. Martin and Bracken (1987) identified 6219 pregnant women in New Haven for possible inclusion in a study to investigate the relation between maternal caffeine consumption and birth weight. Of these, 5331 women agreed to be contacted, and 4926 were eligible for the study. The number yielding data for the main analysis was reduced to 3858, with the following reasons for exclusion:

**4926** eligible and willing to be in study
473 refused to be interviewed
263 could not be reached
4 unreliable interviews
**4186** valid interviews obtained
76 pregnancy outcome not ascertained
56 delivered at a different hospital
116 not a live birth
46 not singleton deliveries
33 birth weight not recorded
**3858** caffeine consumption and birth weight obtained.

This study illustrates the wide range of reasons for incomplete follow-up. It may not seem likely that any of these reasons for loss to follow-up would have been related to either caffeine consumption or birth weight to an important degree, but the possibility of bias should always be considered.

In studies carried out over many years large numbers of subjects may be lost, especially in highly mobile populations, severely weakening the reliability of the results. Non-response to postal questionnaires is particularly common. If the outcome of interest is death, however, national registers can provide information about subjects who have not maintained contact. Similarly, in some countries disease registers allow virtually complete follow-up. For example, in a study of all Swedish conscripts in

1969–70, registers were used to identify both admissions for psychiatric care and deaths (Andréasson *et al.*, 1987).

### 5.11.3 Other problems

Long-term studies may suffer from problems associated with change in habits. For example, people may change jobs (and hence exposure to risk) or become unemployed, or may change the consumption of cigarettes, alcohol or specific items of food. It is, though, a strength of the cohort study that repeated assessments of risk status can be made.

Perhaps a more serious problem is that different groups may not be investigated equally closely. In particular a high risk group may be studied more carefully, resulting in advantageous earlier detection of medical problems. Conversely, intensive investigation of the high risk group may lead to the greater discovery of conditions that are actually equally common in the low risk group. **Surveillance bias** is eliminated when all subjects are investigated identically, preferably with the assessors being unaware of each person's risk status.

## 5.12 THE CROSS-SECTIONAL STUDY

In a cohort study subjects with different characteristics are identified and followed to see what happens. By contrast, in a **cross-sectional** study all the information is collected at the same time because subjects are only contacted once. Many cross-sectional studies are descriptive, and these are often called **surveys**. For example, we might ask undergraduates about their alcohol consumption, carry out a survey of the use of alternative medicine in a particular area, or investigate the ability of a particular blood test to give a correct 'diagnosis' in inpatients with certain symptoms.

Some cross-sectional studies are, however, carried out to investigate associations between a disease and possible risk factors, so that this design is an alternative to the case-control and cohort approaches. The cross-sectional study does not suffer from many of the difficulties that affect these other designs, such as recall bias and loss to follow-up. It is relatively cheap and easy to carry out. Needless to say, there are different special problems associated with cross-sectional studies.

### 5.12.1 Sample selection

Cross-sectional studies share the problems of sample selection with cohort studies. Although research is carried out on a limited number of individuals, the interpretation of results is usually extended widely. A survey of GP referral practices or health education in one county will probably be taken as an indication of what happens nationally. However, the nature of hospital inpatients, clinic attenders, general practice attenders and those not attending anywhere may vary enormously. Apart from affecting the observed prevalence of a disorder, the choice of sample may have a strong effect on the observed relation with other factors. Clearly, the validity of the extrapolation depends crucially on the representativeness of the sample. It is an inherent weakness of most observational studies that the sample is not representative of the population. In some cases, however, we can select a random sample for a survey, which is the ideal method.

### 5.12.2 Response rates

Many cross-sectional studies obtain all or most of their information from postal questionnaires. Non-response can be a big problem, with perhaps only 50% to 80% of questionnaires being returned. Many studies have found that there are marked differences (demographic and health-related) between those who do or do not respond to a questionnaire, with the non-responders usually being less healthy. This is sometimes known as **volunteer bias**. If some information is available for non-responders – perhaps basic demographic details – it is valuable to assess whether there are any apparent differences between responders and non-responders. Similar age and sex distributions will not, however, necessarily indicate a lack of bias.

For example, in a health status survey of elderly people the response rate was age related, being highest in those aged 85 and over (84%) and lowest in those aged 65 to 74 (74%) (Rockwood *et al.*, 1989). However, non-responders were found to spend more time in hospital than responders, and this difference was most marked in the oldest group.

In any study strenuous efforts should be made to get as high a response rate as possible. For example, in studies collecting data by postal questionnaire it is common to have second and third mailings for those who do not respond to the first letter.

### 5.12.3 Cause or effect?

The particular difficulty associated with cross-sectional studies looking at associations with disease concerns the sequence in time of the disorder of interest and the possible risk factor. For example, if we were to carry out a study of the relation between employment status and health we would probably find that the unemployed have worse health than those in employment. We might conclude that being unemployed leads to poorer health, but an equally valid possibility is that poor health leads to being unemployed, or both statements might be true. Because we have collected both sets of information at the same time we cannot draw a clear inference of causality. Similar situations arise in many circumstances where either the disorder develops slowly or the exposure is long-term (or both). Some case-control studies suffer from the same weakness. A prospective study is the best way to investigate such questions.

## 5.13 STUDIES OF CHANGE OVER TIME

The last type of study design considered in this chapter is that in which two or more independent sets of cross-sectional data are used to make inferences about changes over time. Two situations where this design is used will illustrate many of the difficulties.

The first example is in the study of growth patterns when it is not possible to take many measurements from each individual. For example, ultrasound measurements of the fetus are now routine in many hospitals, and it is important to know the usual variability of the various measurements of fetal size such as head circumference. Many such studies have been performed. Apart from the usual problem of sample selection these studies often include variable numbers of measurements from different fetuses. Most pregnant women have just a single ultrasound scan at about 15–20 weeks of gestation. Repeat scans are usually performed only if there is some reason for clinical concern, such as apparently poor growth. Inclusion of such data will therefore bias the sample towards these fetuses, which will particularly affect data in the second half of pregnancy. A further problem is that data collected in this way are usually plotted and the line joining the means at each week of gestation is taken as the average 'growth curve'. The means do not, however, indicate average growth but average size; by definition we need measurements of each fetus on two or more occasions in order to study growth. We cannot make valid inferences about growth from single measurements of size; we cannot create a longitudinal study from cross-sectional data.

The same applies when we consider populations rather than individuals, and further problems arise when we are concerned with a possible causal relation. For example, the change in the death rate from motoring accidents has been compared in several countries for the periods before and after the introduction of seat-belt legislation. The inference of such studies is that any reduction in the death rate is due to the introduction of seat-belts, but there may have been other differences between the two time periods, such as a reduction in drinking and driving. The problem is seen more clearly when data for many time periods are examined. Data from 1950 to 1984 show a steady rise in the average daily prison population and a fall in the number of patients in psychiatric beds. This was interpreted as a causal link, with discharged long-stay psychiatric patients ending up in prison (Weller and Weller, 1986). However, any two quantities changing over time will show a statistical association, such as the price of beer and the salaries of priests (Gibbons and Davis, 1984) or the proportion of unmarried mothers and the rate of Caesarean section. Association is not necessarily causation; very careful statistical analysis of such data is required.

## 5.14 CHOOSING A STUDY DESIGN

The choice between an experiment and an observational study is usually straightforward. If it is possible, both ethically and logistically, to carry out an experiment, then this is the preferred approach. In particular, the evaluation of alternative treatments is best addressed by a randomized controlled trial (see Chapter 15). Most studies are not experiments. A review of papers published in the *New England Journal of Medicine* in 1978–79 found that only 90 of 332 original articles were controlled experiments (Bailar *et al.*, 1984), and the proportion is probably unusually high in that journal. The majority of the remainder were observational studies, and most of those were cross-sectional studies. The previous sections have discussed the advantages and (especially) the disadvantages of case-control, cohort and cross-sectional studies. All have their weak points, although the prospective cohort study is usually the best bet if feasible.

The large number of possible biases in observational studies can lead to considerable variation in the findings from similar studies of the same phenomenon. This is seen in the regular series of scares about an increased risk of cancer associated with high consumption of coffee, beer, tea, sweeteners, and so on. Feinstein (1988) argued that much of the confusion can be attributed to the failure to develop adequate scientific standards for observational epidemiological studies. Lichtenstein *et al.* (1987) gave guidelines for reading reports of case-control studies.

The choice of the most appropriate design is not easy, as there are many considerations to weigh up. The involvement of a statistician at the planning stage is strongly recommended. As well as advising on the choice of design, they can give valuable assistance regarding the selection of suitable samples of individuals for study, a problem that must be confronted with any study design but is especially important in observational studies. The statistician can (and should) also advise on the appropriate sample size. Chapter 15 describes sample size calculations for clinical trials; similar methods are available for observational studies.

A recurring theme in this and later chapters is the considerable gulf between an observed association and inference of a causal mechanism. Only in randomized trials and other experiments can we reasonably ascribe an observed effect to be causal, because of the controlled nature of the investigation. (But Chapter 15 describes some of the possible problems that can arise in clinical trials.) When planning an observational study it is important to bear in mind the information that will be obtained, and how easily the results will be able to be interpreted. In observational studies the interpretation of observed associations needs great care. For example, the study of Swedish conscripts found a strong association between cannabis consumption and subsequent schizophrenia (Andréasson *et al.,* 1987). The authors of the report were very careful, however, to consider whether the relation was causal or not. In particular they considered, but cautiously rejected, the possibility that cannabis consumption might be caused by emerging schizophrenia. The study of longevity and left-handedness referred to in section 1.1 is a contrasting example (Halpern and Coren, 1988). Although the authors acknowledged that the observed small reduction in longevity of left-handers is not necessarily causal, they did not consider the possibility of bias as an explanation. Their finding could well be explained by having analysed age at death, ignoring those still alive, for baseball players born over a long period during which the prevalence of left-handedness would have risen through changes in social attitudes. Those left-handers who died would thus be expected to have died younger than right-handers who had died. (The correct way to analyse this type of data is described in Chapter 13.)

This chapter has introduced various issues in the design of research, but is by no means comprehensive. Lengthier discussion can be found in Gehlbach (1982) for a general discussion of design issues, Pocock (1983) for clinical trials, Breslow and Day (1980) or Schlesselman (1982) for case-control studies, and Breslow and Day (1987) for cohort studies.

## EXERCISES

5.1 In 1978–79 a random sample of 1007 residents (608 men and 399 women) of the Lothian region (around Edinburgh) had been asked precisely what alcohol they had drunk in the previous seven days. In March 1981 the combination of an increase in taxation and brewers' prices meant that, for the first time in over 30 years, the price of alcoholic beverages increased faster than the retail price index. So in the autumn of 1981 the 676 respondents (484 men and 192 women) who had had at least one alcoholic drink in the seven days on which the original survey had been based – the so-called 'regular drinkers' – were reinterviewed.

The first survey was carried out between July 1978 and February 1979 and the second between September 1981 and March 1982. Over the three years, the cost of alcoholic beverages had risen by 61% while the retail price index had risen by 52%. Average earnings (and disposable income) had risen more than the retail price index, suggesting that those in regular employment were marginally better off than in 1981. Unemployment in the Edinburgh area, however, had risen steeply between 1978 and 1982 for both men and women.

The results of the second survey were reported as follows:

'Of the original 676 regular drinkers, 463 (69%) were successfully interviewed. Of the 213 who were not, 85 could not be traced, 48 were known to have left the region, 39 refused, and 23 were either dead or too ill to be interviewed. A disproportionate number of lost respondents were under the age of 30, unmarried, and not in regular employment. Nevertheless, the sex ratio and both male and female alcohol consumption at the time of the first survey of the 463 who were reinterviewed were representative of the original sample.' (Kendell *et al.*, 1983)

(a) The authors were interested in reduction in alcohol intake, and so did not interview those subjects not reporting drinking in the first survey. Is this reasonable?
(b) What was the response rate to the second survey? How might non-respondents differ from respondents? What is the likely effect on the interpretation of the results of the survey?
(c) Does it matter that the two surveys were not carried out at exactly the same time of year?
(d) If the data showed a reduction in alcohol consumption among the 463 reinterviewed subjects, could the authors reasonably conclude that it was due to the rise in excise duty on alcohol?

The Discussion of the paper begins:

'The central finding of this before and after survey is that a representative population of 463 regular drinkers in the Lothian region reduced their alcohol consumption by 18% between 1978–9 and 1981–2 and simultaneously experienced a 16% reduction in adverse effects. The main cause of this fall in consumption was probably the rising cost of alcoholic beverage relative to the cost of living and average incomes during that three year period.'

(e) Were the 463 'regular drinkers' really a 'representative population'?
(f) Comment on the authors' interpretation of the results. Would your opinion be different if they had interviewed all 1007 subjects in the second survey?

In the final paragraph the authors wrote:

'The findings of this study indicate, therefore, that an increase in excise duty on alcoholic beverages can be an effective means of reducing the ill effects of excessive alcohol consumption.'

(g) Do these conclusions have any validity?

5.2 A researcher wished to see if women who have taken the oral contraceptive pill have an earlier or later menopause than other women. He decided to study a group of women born in 1930 as these would be young enough for some to have taken the pill but old enough for some to have reached the menopause. He obtained the names of all 132 women in one general practice who were born in 1930, using the practice's age–sex register. Women claiming to have had the menopause were checked by measuring their follicle stimulating hormone (FSH) levels.

Of the 132 women, 101 were excluded from the study for the following reasons:

22 not available (21 not contactable, 1 refusal)
60 premenopausal
14 hysterectomy
1 radium-induced menopause
2 unmarried
2 FSH $< 30$ IU/l

(a) What was the design of this study?
(b) Is the sample of 31 women representative of the population of interest?

The researcher found that 12 of the 31 women had taken the oral contraceptive pill at some time, while 19 had not. He obtained the following results relating to age at menopause in the two groups, and concluded that taking the pill does not delay the menopause:

| | | Age at menopause (years) | |
|---|---|---|---|
| | *n* | Mean | SD |
| Pill users | 12 | 47.2 | 2.1 |
| Non pill users | 19 | 47.5 | 2.1 |

(c) What was the fundamental error in the design of this study?
(d) What design is needed to answer the question originally posed?

(This exercise is based on a frank account of a flawed research project by Davis, 1985.)

5.3 Halpern and Coren (1988) wished to see if there was a difference in longevity between left-handed and right-handed people. One of the few sources of handedness of individuals is a baseball encyclopaedia. From an encyclopaedia they recorded the dates of birth and death of 1472 right-handed and 236 left-handed players.

(a) Was this a representative sample of the population?
(b) The authors did not state the time span of the data, but as they note deaths up to age 99 it is likely to cover the whole of the twentieth century. How might the long time span bias the comparison of left- and right-handers?
(c) They compared the mean age at death in the two groups. Why is this a misleading comparison?
(d) What would be a better design to answer this question, assuming that handedness data were more widely available?

# 6
# Using a computer

> The good news is that statistical analysis is becoming easier and cheaper. The bad news is that statistical analysis is becoming easier and cheaper.
>
> Hofacker (1983)

## 6.1 INTRODUCTION

Recent technological advances have provided many medical researchers with access to a computer. This change has largely been beneficial, but Hofacker's words above should be borne in mind. Computers remove most of the tedious aspects of statistical analysis, and should give us correct answers, but they do not guarantee that we will obtain correct and valid results. In this chapter I shall consider the advantages and disadvantages of using computers for statistical analysis, and suggest ways to approach the analysis of data. I shall also consider the design of forms for collecting data to be analysed by computer.

## 6.2 ADVANTAGES OF USING A COMPUTER

There are many advantages in using a computer to carry out statistical analyses. Most obviously it enables us to do things we couldn't otherwise do, but there are many other benefits:

### *(a) Accuracy and speed*

Good computer programs (known as **software**) will give the correct answers quickly. Analysis by hand is prone to arithmetical errors, and is painfully slow for all but the simplest tasks.

### *(b) Versatility*

A computer gives access to a wide range of statistical techniques, many more than are described in this book. Even complex analyses can be performed quickly.

*(c) Graphics*
Computer programs enable plots of observations or statistical results to be obtained easily. Full advantage should be taken of this facility. Histograms and scatter diagrams can be used to inspect the raw data (see Chapter 7), and plots can also be used to study the results from an analysis. Section 6.8 discusses some practical issues relating to computer plots.

*(d) Flexibility*
A major advantage is the ability to make small changes and repeat the analysis. For example, it is simple to rerun an analysis after transforming the data, perhaps by taking logs (see Chapter 7), to perform the same analysis on a subset of the data, or to add some new observations.

*(e) New variables*
It is simple to generate new variables. We may calculate a subject's age from their date of birth and the date of the study, or the change in a measurement by taking the difference between pre- and post-treatment values, or count the number of symptoms a patient has. Such calculations should always be done on the computer, which is faster and more accurate than doing the calculations by hand. Of course, if the instruction to create a new variable is incorrect or is typed wrongly all of the observations will be wrong.

*(f) Volume of data*
Vast amounts of data can be handled. Indeed for some programs there is no limit to the number of subjects (cases) that can be analysed.

*(g) Easy transfer of data*
Once data have been entered into a computer file they can easily be transferred between researchers either electronically (by telephone line) or by sending a 'floppy disk' by post. It should never be necessary to enter the same data into a computer twice, but unfortunately computers use a variety of disk formats and sizes.

## 6.3 DISADVANTAGES OF USING A COMPUTER

To counterbalance the major benefits there are several potential problems that users of statistical software should be aware of.

*(a) Errors in software*
Not all statistical programs are well-written. Some may give incorrect answers in certain circumstances, either through poor programming or inadequate understanding of the statistical theory. It is advisable to use programs that are reputable and have been around long enough for errors

to be found, the best known of which are BMDP, Minitab, SAS and SPSS. Since the advent of microcomputers (PCs) there has been a huge increase in the number of statistical programs on the market, some of which are poor and some incorrect (Bland and Altman, 1988; Dallal, 1988). Sections 6.4 and 6.5 give advice about choosing and evaluating statistical software.

*(b) Versatility*

Versatility was given as one of the advantages of using a computer, but it can lead to difficulties too. Because of the wide variety of analyses available, it is easy to use an inappropriate method. It is essential to be aware of the limits of your statistical knowledge, and to use only methods that you understand. If your problem seems to require methods you are not familiar with you should seek expert advice.

*(c) The black box approach*

Using a computer may distance you from your data. It is possible to perform statistical analyses automatically: the data go in at one end and the results come out at the other, untouched by human thought. Because much statistical analysis is concerned with average effects you may get no feel for the way individuals respond.

*(d) Garbage in garbage out*

'Garbage in garbage out' refers to the fact that sensible answers follow only from sensible questions. If the data input or the specification of the analysis was wrong then the results will be wrong. For example, a common problem is what to do about missing observations. When data are entered into the computer such values are sometimes left blank, in which case the value will automatically be taken as zero, or they are given a numerical 'missing value code', such as 99. It is common to use values like 9, 99, 999, etc. as missing values, or perhaps a negative number – any value will do as long as it clearly could not be a genuine observation.

Table 3.1 showed the PImax values of 25 patients with cystic fibrosis; the mean and standard deviation were 92.6 and 24.92 cm $H_2O$ respectively. Suppose that there had been five other patients in the study whose PImax was unknown. If their values were left blank (zero) or coded 999 and all 30 values analysed by a computer program then the results would have been as follows:

| Value for missing data | Result for 30 subjects Mean | SD |
|---|---|---|
| 0 | 77.2 | 41.79 |
| 999 | 243.7 | 344.32 |

both of which are major distortions of the truth. The computer will accept the values 0 or 999 as genuine observations, and so will give false answers. Missing data must be identified as such to the program (see section 6.6).

A similar problem may arise when information is not appropriate for some individuals rather than actually missing. For example, the number of pregnancies is only appropriate for women, and may be recorded as 9 or 99 for all males in a study. These examples show the importance of checking the data before analysis, as discussed in section 6.6 and in the next chapter.

## 6.4 TYPES OF STATISTICAL PROGRAM

Commercially available statistical software is generally capable of performing many types of statistical analysis. Statistical programs, often called packages, vary in their capability and the way in which they work. Some of the more important aspects to consider are:

1. statistical methods available
2. accuracy
3. maximum amount of data that can be analysed
4. facilities for data manipulation (including editing)
5. ability to accept missing data
6. ease of use (is it 'user-friendly'?)
7. maturity (is it tried and tested?)
8. speed
9. documentation
10. error handling
11. graphics capability
12. quality of output
13. cost.

The most important considerations are the first two in the above list, because you obviously need a package that will perform the analyses desired and achieve correct results. However, assessing accuracy is not easy. Other key issues are the ability to create plots simply, and helpful error messages when you make a mistake, as you often will. In addition, there are different ways of telling the program what you want done. In some packages one enters commands such as

plot height age

but in others one chooses from a **menu** of options. This is known as an **interactive** system. For programs that use commands it is usually possible to create a file of commands which can then be executed as a block. This has the advantage that possibly complicated instructions only have to be typed once, and that it is easy to edit the file to produce slightly different analyses.

As well as statistical packages, which cover a wide range of analyses, there are also some specialized programs for particular purposes, such as calculating sample sizes or confidence intervals. These are subject to some of the above requirements too, but should be judged mainly on their specific ability to do things that cannot be done in the usual packages.

It is worth seeking advice from a colleague or from a statistician before choosing a package to use, or buy. I strongly recommend that you use the same package for all your analyses, as it takes a considerable effort to become fully acquainted with even one package. So it is important to choose your software carefully. Few, if any, packages will perform all the analyses in this book, so that it is necessary to know all the types of analysis you might wish to do, which is not at all easy. There are many microcomputer statistics programs on the market (or even free) that can give incorrect results (Dallal, 1988), so if you have doubts about a particular statistical program it is advisable to compare its output with that from another.

The next section discusses some aspects of evaluating statistical software. If you know that you have reliable software then you can go on to section 6.6, which describes a general strategy for analysis.

## 6.5 EVALUATING A STATISTICAL PACKAGE

*(This section can be omitted without loss of continuity.)*

The main concerns when evaluating a statistical computer program are:

1. Does it perform all the desired functions?
2. Is it easy to use?
3. Does it give the correct answers?

Advice from colleagues or from a statistician can be of great assistance in answering the first two questions, because it takes some familiarity with a package before one can really judge its value and ease of use. The list of features given in section 6.4 can aid evaluation. The purpose of this section is to give limited assistance in relation to (3.) above.

A computer program may give the wrong answers either because it uses an incorrect formula or because it is not well written. The former is unlikely but possible. More often problems occur because of the way in which the program was written. The procedure by which a computer program performs a given calculation is known as an **algorithm**. Some algorithms are inferior in that they lose accuracy in some circumstances. To take a simple example, it can be shown that the standard deviation of three numbers $x$, $x + c$ and $x + 2c$ is $c$, whatever values we give $x$ and $c$. I calculated the standard deviations of sets of three numbers where $x$ increases but $c$ is held at 0.1 using two pocket calculators. For each of the four sets of numbers

(a) 7.0 7.1 7.2
(b) 77.0 77.1 77.2
(c) 777.0 777.1 777.2
(d) 7777.0 7777.1 7777.2

both gave the correct answer of 0.1, but for the set

(e) 77777.0 77777.1 77777.2

one calculator gave the standard deviation as 0.0 while the other gave an error – it would not calculate the standard deviation. The reason for this problem is that in extreme circumstances the calculator loses accuracy because it cannot store the large numbers obtained when the data are squared. There are algorithms that avoid this problem, and while we may not expect them to be used on a pocket calculator we would certainly expect a computer program to give the correct answers for such data. However, many microcomputer packages use the inferior algorithm (Dallal, 1988). There is also a risk of losing numerical accuracy in some complex analyses; problems with regression analysis are discussed in Chapter 12.

Increasing use is being made of **spreadsheet** software for performing simple statistical analyses. These programs are not well suited to statistics, and may use inferior or incorrect methods. I do not recommend them for serious statistics.

Another aspect to consider for some types of analysis is which form of a test is used when there are different forms available. Subsequent chapters will discuss matters such as one and two-sided tests, the use of continuity corrections, and the adjustment for ties in analyses of ranks (non-parametric methods). It is important to know precisely what method the program uses, and this is not always clear from the manual. Indeed some manuals are positively misleading (Bland and Altman, 1988).

When using a package to perform a particular analysis for the first time it is advisable to begin by analysing some sets of data for which you already know the answers. In this book the raw data are given for the worked examples wherever possible to enable you to do this.

## 6.6 STRATEGY FOR COMPUTER-AIDED ANALYSIS

This section contains a broad strategy for analysing data on a computer. Notice that there are several steps to pass through before moving to the analysis of the data.

*(a) Data collection*

Section 6.7 describes several aspects of preparing a coding sheet for data that are going to be typed into a computer. Data entry will be much quicker and more accurate if there is a well-designed coding form to work from.

*(b) Data entry*

Data should be typed into a **file** on the computer. This may be possible within the statistics package or using a general purpose editing program. The reason for storing the data is that you will often need to carry out further analyses at a later date, and you only want to enter the data once. Also it is easy to list the data and check that the values have been entered correctly. I consider formats for data files in section 6.7. A statistical package that cannot read data from a file should be rejected.

*(c) Data checking*

There is a tendency to believe that once the data are on the computer they must be correct. In fact it is all too easy to make errors when entering (typing) data, however careful one is. It is essential to check that the data have been typed correctly, however tedious this may be. The best way to minimize errors is to have the data entered twice, preferably by two different people. Here it is useful to have a program for comparing files. Any differences between the two files are checked and the correct value obtained. Data checking is discussed in section 7.2.

*(d) Data screening*

Before starting the main statistical analysis it is important to look at the data. It is a simple task to produce a histogram of each variable, and pairs of variables can be inspected by scatter diagrams. These plots will give a first idea of the average value, the variability, the shape of the distribution, and whether there are any outlying or missing values. Data screening is discussed in section 7.5.

*(e) Data analysis*

The appropriate form of statistical analysis will often follow directly from the design. In particular, values of a variable may be compared between groups or within a group, as discussed in Chapter 5. Within group comparisons must make use of techniques intended for that type of data.

The objectives of the study should indicate a few main analyses of interest. Although the pre-specified analyses are the most important ones, inspection of the data may suggest some additional analyses of interest. The results of these 'exploratory' analyses should be interpreted cautiously (see Chapter 8).

Many statistical methods are based on certain assumptions about the data. These may require further analyses to verify them.

I strongly recommend that you keep a 'log' of the computing session if the software has the facility, in which both the input commands and results are shown. This is especially important when the commands are not stored on a file.

*(f) Checking results*

You should check that the results relate to the correct number of observations – it is surprisingly easy to lose or gain a few cases unwittingly. It is important to appreciate that the results obtained from a computer should not be taken as automatically correct. Simple preliminary inspection of the data should give you some idea of what results to expect. If the results obtained differ markedly from expectation, then you should check that there are no errors in the data, and that the proper analysis has been performed. It is easy to make mistakes when trying to analyse data, especially with complex analyses. The computer will give you the correct answer only if you ask the correct question. Clearly it is much easier to check results when there is a log of the analysis, as suggested above.

*(g) Interpretation*

Interpretation of results is discussed in subsequent chapters.

## 6.7 FORMS FOR DATA COLLECTION

When data are to be collected for subsequent analysis using a computer, it is a good idea to use a standard form with assigned boxes for each digit. This applies to studies where data are to be extracted from existing records, such as hospital notes, as well as to prospective studies. It is especially important when information on many variables is collected for each individual.

I shall first consider alternative ways in which computer programs can accept (read) data from a file, and then aspects of form design. Further discussion of form design is given by Pocock (1983, pp. 160–6), De Pauw and Buyse (1984) (with special reference to cancer trials) and Armitage and Berry (1987, pp. 8–14).

### 6.7.1 Formats for input to computer programs

A standard format (called **free format**) that most packages will read is shown in Figure 6.1 which illustrates the first part of the data from a trial comparing two antihypertensive drugs. Here each row of the file contains several variables for one individual and each item of information is separated from the next by one or more spaces. There is no necessity for the columns to line up vertically as in this example, but I recommend this

```
001 17 02 89 25 11 33 1 2 170.2  77.1 141  82 129  79
002 21 02 89 02 02 44 1 1 162.3  80.8 150  85 144  81
003 28 02 89 14 06 40 2 2 151.9  72.2 142  79 142  76
004 05 03 89 01 12 28 1 1 178.8  91.4 181 101 155  87
005 11 03 89 18 05 48 1 1 166.0  81.8 170  90 158  84
006 12 03 89 24 09 37 2 1 171.4  73.3 139  82 134  78
007 17 03 89 07 04 36 2 2 155.8  61.5 184 107 177 102
008 20 03 89 12 02 38 1 2 185.2 100.6 157  93 150  88

                              etc
```

**Figure 6.1** An example of a generally applicable style of data layout for entry into a statistical computer program. Different items are separated by one or more spaces and the figures in each column are aligned. The columns contain, in sequence, patient number, date of entry to study, date of birth, sex, treatment, height, weight, initial blood pressure (systolic and diastolic) and final blood pressure.

practice as it makes it easy to check visually that all information has been entered correctly. I strongly recommend that a code number is used to identify each subject, as in Figure 6.1. This makes it easy to check any suspicious values, to add extra variables at a later date, to check that nobody is in the study twice, and so on.

The alternative to free format is **fixed format**, in which items need not be separated by spaces in the data file. The disadvantage of this format is that it is necessary to tell the program the precise format used, and this can be complicated if you are unused to computer programming. With fixed format you can use blanks to indicate missing data, but this is a bad idea as a blank cannot be distinguished from an omission due to oversight. Also, most programs will interpret blanks as zero, which is potentially disastrous (as shown in section 6.3). Fixed format files occupy slightly less space on the disk, but this is of no real practical consequence. Not all packages can accept data in fixed format, and in any case free format is easier to deal with.

Statistical programs require a value for every variable for each subject, so a good feature of free format is that you will need to enter some quantity even when a value is missing. A blank cannot be used because blanks are used to separate adjacent items. Some programs have the useful facility of letting you indicate missing data in the file by a special symbol, such as ? or *. Otherwise you must give missing data a numerical value which is impossible for that variable, perhaps −1 or 99, and then remember to give the appropriate instruction to the program to indicate the missing value code. The absence of a missing value code facility would make a statistical package unacceptable.

There is a variety of ways in which programs can handle the situation where you have too much data for each individual to fit onto the width of your screen (80 characters). You will need to consult your manual.

### 6.7.2 Form design

Figure 6.2 shows a form that could have been used to collect the data shown in Figure 6.1. Some of its features have been described already, such as the subject's identifying code number. The numbers associated with each group of boxes indicate the number of characters from the start of the line when the data are typed into the computer. The missing numbers mean that there is a blank between each piece of information, indicating that the data will be in free format. Note that the patient's name should not be entered into the computer file.

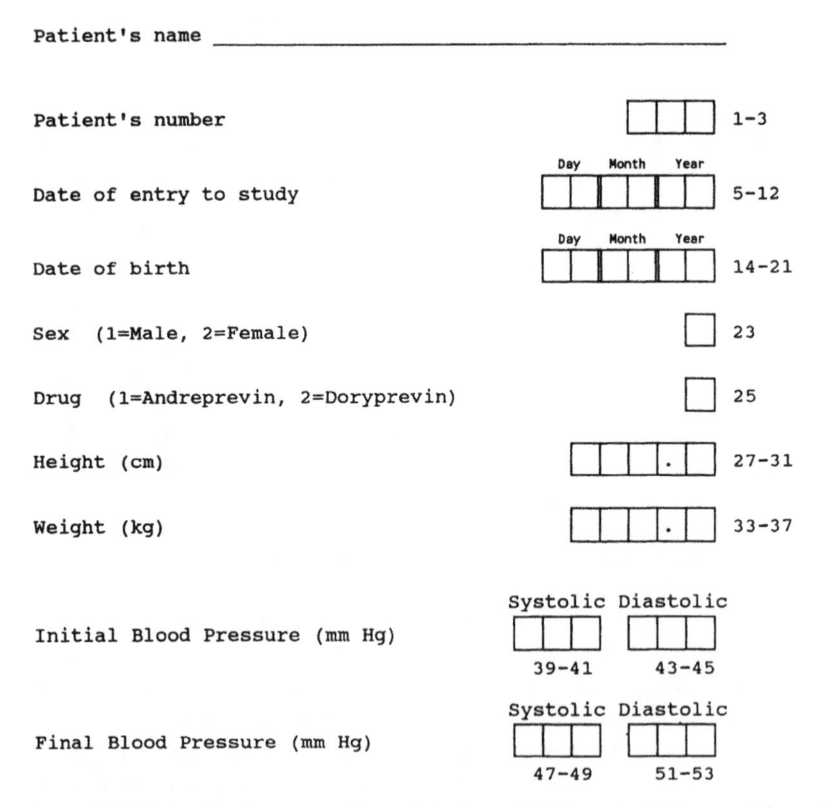

Patient's name ______________________

Patient's number [ ][ ][ ] 1-3

Date of entry to study Day [ ][ ] Month [ ][ ] Year [ ][ ] 5-12

Date of birth Day [ ][ ] Month [ ][ ] Year [ ][ ] 14-21

Sex (1=Male, 2=Female) [ ] 23

Drug (1=Andreprevin, 2=Doryprevin) [ ] 25

Height (cm) [ ][ ][ ].[ ] 27-31

Weight (kg) [ ][ ][ ].[ ] 33-37

Initial Blood Pressure (mm Hg) Systolic [ ][ ][ ] 39-41 Diastolic [ ][ ][ ] 43-45

Final Blood Pressure (mm Hg) Systolic [ ][ ][ ] 47-49 Diastolic [ ][ ][ ] 51-53

**Figure 6.2** Part of a form to collect data for a trial comparing two antihypertensive drugs, corresponding to the data in Figure 6.1.

The way in which forms are designed for recording data needs careful thought. Categorical and continuous variables pose different problems.

*(a) Categorical data*
A number should be assigned to each possible category, as in the following examples:

Diabetes: 1=Yes, 2=No
Blood group: 1=A, 2=B, 3=AB, 4=O

I strongly recommend that all the codes are on the form itself rather than on a separate sheet. Two simple examples are shown in Figure 6.2. If it is necessary to use codes higher than nine, a second box will be needed.

It is advisable to avoid zero as a code when fixed format is used, as some programs do not distinguish 0 from a blank corresponding to a box which has not been filled in. This is not a problem for free format input, as some number must be entered for every variable.

Some variables have several possible non-mutually exclusive answers, such as prior or concomitant therapy. Here it is necessary to have one yes/no box for each possible answer of interest. It is desirable to have consistent codes where possible. For example, all questions with yes or no answers should use the same codes.

It is possible with some programs to use letters instead of numbers for categorical data. Thus sex could be entered as M or F, and drug as, say, A or D. This has some advantages, but means that the data file will not be acceptable to all programs.

*(b) Continuous data*
Measurements should be recorded to the same accuracy as that to which they are measured – there is no advantage in rounding values before recording them. Nor is it usually a good idea to categorize continuous variables when recording data, for example by allocating numeric codes to ranges of values. For statistical analysis it is desirable to have the data recorded as precisely as possible. One box should be allowed for each digit, and the location of the decimal point should be shown if relevant, as for height and weight in Figure 6.2. The decimal point does not have to have its own box; if it were omitted here we would need to divide all heights and weights by 10 before analysis. It is useful to indicate on the form the units used, especially where there are alternatives in common use.

Only one digit should go in each box, so it is essential to allow enough boxes for the largest value that could be recorded. Thus we ought to allow three boxes before the decimal point for adult body weight in kg because some people weigh more than 100 kg. It will not matter if it turns out that the first box is never used.

Whoever fills in the forms should understand the importance of using the right-hand boxes when not all boxes are needed. Thus diastolic blood pressure below 100 must be written in the second and third of the three available boxes.

*(c) Dates*

The usual British ordering of dates is day, month, year, as shown in Figure 6.2, but in the USA it is month, day, year. It is important to indicate on the form which order is required.

In fact the order year, month, day is a good option, apart from its unfamiliarity, as it allows the data to be sorted simply by using the date as a six digit number.

*(d) Missing data*

If your program will accept a symbol for this purpose, such as *, then this can be used, but it will mean that your file may not be readable by any other statistical program. Otherwise a special numeric code should be used. The most common method is to fill each box with nines, so that unknown blood pressure is recorded as 999 and unknown sex as 9.

### 6.7.3 Multiple forms

Clinical data are often obtained from a subject each time they are seen, for example during pregnancy. When patients are not seen equally often there will be varying amounts of information among the subjects being studied. It is implicit in Figure 6.1 that there should be the same amount of information about each subject. Although unequal amounts of data per subject can be stored using a type of software known as a **database**, most statistical computer programs can only deal with data sets where the same information is available for all subjects (called **rectangular** data). Some summarizing of such data sets will be necessary before analysis can begin.

The simple expedient of treating each visit as a separate data set should never be adopted – it is completely invalid to treat multiple records from one patient as if they were from several patients. The amount of data should be considered when the study is being planned, even for retrospective studies based on examining case notes. This type of data can be extremely difficult to organize appropriately for statistical analysis. I recommend expert assistance if it is necessary to collect multiple sets of data from each subject.

### 6.7.4 Analysis of data on a file

A consequence of the formats described above is that on the computer file each row represents an individual, with different variables in columns. In many analyses we wish to compare subgroups of subjects, so it is necessary for the program to accept data where all the values are in a single column, and an indicator of the subgroup is in a different column. For example, for the data shown in Figures 6.1 and 6.2 we would wish to compare final blood pressures for patients receiving the different treatments. Some programs expect sets of data to be compared to be in different columns, in which case they would be unsuitable for statistical analysis of data stored in files in the manner described. This is a further feature to be considered when evaluating statistical software.

## 6.8 PLOTTING

The ability to plot data is a major advantage of using a computer. There are two types of plot that can be produced, whether plotting on the screen or on paper – a **line** plot or a **high-resolution** plot. The first method uses the usual 'alphanumeric' character set and places each point as near as possible to its correct location, while the second uses the graphical capability of the computer to give a much more accurate plot. Figure 6.3 shows a line plot of the data shown in Figure 11.4; line plots can be produced by most statistical packages. Coincident points are usually indicated by showing the number of points (up to 9). It is often difficult to specify the scaling of axes and to indicate different groups. Most statistical packages can plot histograms and scatter diagrams, and some can produce box-and-whisker or stem-and-leaf plots. Line plots are very useful when analysing data, but they are not of top quality. Until recently few statistical packages could produce high-resolution plots, but improved graphical facilities are becoming more common. The figures in this book were

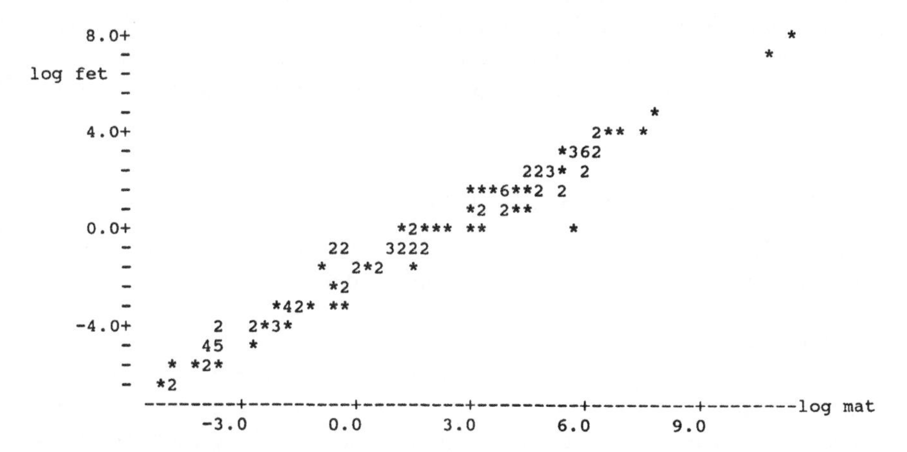


**Figure 6.3** Line plot of data shown in Figure 11.4 relating log maternal weight to log fetal weight in mammals.

produced on a personal computer (using the package STATA) and printed on a high-resolution laser printer.

## 6.9 OTHER USES OF COMPUTERS

The obvious main statistical value of computers is in the analysis of data and, as just indicated, for producing graphs. However, there are some other applications which can be useful, mostly relating to random numbers.

We saw in Chapter 5 the importance of random allocation in research, especially for allocation of treatments in clinical trials. Table B13, which can be used for this purpose, was generated by a computer program using an algorithm that produces a sequence of numbers which have virtually the same properties as random numbers. The disadvantage of using a table is that you must use the same set of numbers each time, although you can start at an arbitrary place in the table. It is better to generate new random numbers each time using a suitable algorithm, and many statistical programs can do this. Algorithms vary in quality, but all are likely to be good enough for treatment allocation.

The numbers in Table B13 are digits in the range 0 to 9, and are thus a random sample from a Uniform distribution, as described in Chapter 4. Sometimes we wish to obtain a random sample from some other distribution, especially the Normal distribution, in order to study variability under known conditions. An example of this use was seen in Figure 4.7 which showed random samples of size 50 from a standard Normal distribution. Several programs can generate random samples from a Normal distribution.

Investigating what happens in a defined situation is a simple example of an approach known as **simulation**. The idea is to study what happens under certain assumptions about the nature of a process, and what the effect is of varying the assumptions. Simulation is used in Chapter 8 to illustrate variability among samples drawn from a population with specified characteristics.

## 6.10 MISUSES OF THE COMPUTER

Some disadvantages of using computers were given earlier in this chapter. There are three further misuses of computers that should be avoided.

### *(a) 'Data-dredging'*

Many studies have clearly defined objectives, but other information is collected because it 'may be interesting'. It is easy to perform a large number of statistical analyses in the hope that something interesting will turn up, especially in studies without clear objectives. As we will see in Chapter 8, there is a good chance of finding some apparent relationship in a sample purely by chance when there is no real relationship in the population. For this reason I stressed in Chapter 5 that the main objectives, and thus the principal analyses, should be clearly identified in advance. Any exploratory analyses should be considered as useful, if at all, only for generating hypotheses for examination in further studies.

*(b) Over-complexity*

It may be tempting to subject your data to a complex statistical analysis because the methodology is available, but this is not good statistical practice. The analysis should be restricted to the minimum necessary to answer the relevant questions. One important reason for keeping analyses simple is that it is much easier to explain to other researchers what you did and what you found.

*(c) Spurious precision*

Computers usually produce results to many significant figures, but they should nearly always be rounded before being reported. I have seen published examples of equations purporting to predict birthweight to the nearest 1/10 000 g and length of gestation to the nearest ten minutes, results which appeared to have come straight from computer output. Some guidance on the appropriate numerical presentation of the results of statistical analysis was given in section 2.8, and there are further comments in subsequent chapters.

## 6.11 CONCLUDING REMARKS

For all but the smallest data sets it is desirable to use a computer for statistical analysis because of all the benefits indicated. However, while computers remove the drudgery and errors associated with hand calculations, there is a danger that the raw data are never examined properly. The next chapter discusses the preliminary inspection of data. Also, it is easy to perform statistical analyses without a true understanding of the methods used. Properly used, computers are enormously beneficial for statistical analysis, but they do not obviate the need for expert advice when appropriate.

# 7

# Preparing to analyse data

No statistical technique will ever yield 'good' results from data of dubious quality.

Buyse (1984)

## 7.1 INTRODUCTION

Before analysing a set of data it is important to check as far as possible that the data seem correct. Errors can be made when measurements are taken, when the data are originally recorded, when they are transcribed from the original source (such as from hospital notes), or when being typed into a computer. We cannot usually know what is correct, so we restrict our attention to making sure that the recorded values are plausible. This process is called **data checking** (or **data cleaning**). We cannot expect to spot all transcription and data entry errors, but we hope to find the major errors. As we will see, it is the large errors that can influence statistical analyses. If the data are being analysed on a computer, then checking should take place *after* the data have been entered into the computer. For very large surveys or clinical trials cleaning the data may be a lengthy process.

It is also important to **screen** the data to identify features that may cause difficulties during the analysis. Three specific aspects are considered in this chapter – missing data, outlying values, and the possible need for data transformation. Aspects of checking and screening are similar and in practice they can be carried out at the same time.

The ideas in this chapter are particularly aimed at studies with many variables or subjects or both, but the general principles apply to any study. It is important to examine the data carefully before proceeding to the substantive analysis.

## 7.2 DATA CHECKING

Errors in recorded data are common. For example the recorded values may be wrong because of confusion over the correct units of measurement, digits may be transposed when data are transcribed, or data may be mistyped when being entered onto a computer. Data checking aims to identify and, if possible, rectify errors in the data. Clearly errors in the original data cannot usually be rectified, but errors introduced at a later stage can be put right if the original record is consulted.

As noted in section 6.6, an important first step is to check that the data have been typed into the computer file correctly. For large files double entry is best, whereby the data are retyped and compared with the first version, preferably using a computer program designed for this purpose. For small data sets the simplest way is for one person to read aloud the data from the computer with another person checking against the original data.

Checking the data is likely to reveal some observations that, while plausible, are distant from the main body of the data. It is also likely to reveal that a number of intended observations are missing. These problems are discussed in sections 7.3 and 7.4.

### 7.2.1 Categorical data

For categorical variables it is simple to check that all recorded data values are plausible because there is a fixed number of pre-specified values. For example, if we have four codes for blood group, as follows

1 = A
2 = B
3 = O
4 = AB

then we expect to find only values 1, 2, 3 or 4 in the data, except for any subjects with missing information. If missing values are coded as 9, as recommended in Chapter 6, then we know that any blood group coded as 0, 5, 6, 7, or 8 is clearly wrong.

Values of 0 obtained from computer analysis may indicate that the blood group was left blank – most computer programs do not distinguish blanks and zeros. In this example it is possible that O might be coded as 0 rather than 3. Erroneous values should be checked as far as is possible (if necessary, back to the original source of the information). If a mistake is found the value should be changed to one of the valid codes, here 1, 2, 3, or 4; if not, the missing value code should be used.

### 7.2.2 Continuous data

For continuous measurements we cannot usually identify precisely which values are plausible and which are not, and it is not important to do so. It should, however, always be possible to specify lower and upper limits on what is *reasonable* for the variable concerned. For example, in a study of pregnancy we might put limits of 14 and 45 on maternal age, or in a study of adult males we may use limits of 70 and 250 mm Hg for systolic blood pressure. We then need to identify values outside the limits, a procedure known as **range checking**. Unlike the categorical data case, however, these values are not necessarily wrong. Suspicious values should be checked and any errors found should be corrected. Values remaining outside the prespecified range must either be left as they are, or recorded as 'missing' if they are felt to be impossible rather than just unlikely. It may, therefore, be advisable to have two sets of limits for each variable, denoting suspicious (or unlikely) values and impossible values. Defining what is impossible may be extremely difficult. What values of maternal age or systolic blood pressure are impossible? And at what point is 'impossible' reached?

A common cause of error is misplacing the decimal point, perhaps because of confusion over the right units of measurement to use or a transcription error. Often an error by a factor of ten will give an impossible value, but if the recorded value is plausible a misplaced decimal point may well go undetected. Plausible but unlikely values should be corrected only if there is evidence of a mistake.

### 7.2.3 Logical checks

Checking the data is more complicated when the values of a variable that are reasonable depend on the value of some other variable. We call these **logical checks**. Firstly, it is common for some information to be sought only in certain cases. For example, in a study of survival after a kidney transplant, information on number of previous pregnancies is relevant only for women, and so for men should be set to missing or to a different code indicating 'not applicable'. (Some computer programs allow for different types of missing information.)

If there were restrictions on who should be in the study (for example, entry criteria in a clinical trial – see Chapter 15), then the data should be checked as far as possible to see that everyone really was eligible. A common example is in studies of anti-hypertensive agents, in which there is a range of blood pressures for which subjects can be entered in the study. Many studies have restrictions on the age of participants.

A different problem occurs when two variables are used to construct another variable. The value of the new variable may be impossible even though the values of the original variable were both reasonable. For example, a common measure of body size (a crude measure of fatness) is the 'body mass index' or 'Quetelet's index', defined as Weight/Height$^2$. If such **derived** variables are especially important they should be checked along with recorded variables before beginning the main analysis.

More generally, there may be subjects who have a combination of values of two variables that is very unlikely even though each is within acceptable limits. If we have two closely related variables, such as systolic and diastolic blood pressure, we do not expect a subject at the 5th centile of the distribution of systolic pressure to be at the 95th centile for diastolic pressure. In a large study it is impracticable to consider all pairs of variables in this way, but those of major importance, such as blood pressure in anti-hypertensive drug trials, should be studied closely, most simply by examining scatter diagrams.

Lastly in this section, there is the case where the same variable is measured several times on each subject. It is valuable to plot each person's sequence of recorded values to ensure that they behave reasonably. Sometimes we will expect each measurement to be larger than the previous one, such as annual height measurements of children, and this is easily verified. Unfortunately it may be difficult to produce such plots using statistical software, as few programs can cope with serial data on each subject.

### 7.2.4 Dates

Recorded dates are important when they are used to calculate the time between two events. For example, we can calculate a subject's age at some event, such as surgery or death, from the date of the event and the subject's date of birth. Other common calculations are the time between an event and the patient's death (their **survival time**) or the time between the first symptom and the diagnosis of the disease. As recommended in Chapter 6, it is preferable to record all the relevant dates, as mental calculation of time intervals is extremely unreliable. However, recording dates also causes problems as they are especially prone to transcription errors.

Dates should be checked as follows:

1. Check that all dates are within a reasonable time span. Dates of birth may relate to the age range for inclusion in a study. Note that studies including elderly people may include dates of birth before 1900. Dates of other events, such as surgery or death, will probably lie within the time span of the study.
2. Check that all dates are valid. The day of month should lie in the range 1 to 31, and so on, but dates such as 30 February are impossible. Some computer programs have routines for checking the validity of dates.

3. Check that dates are correctly sequenced. Often dates of different events should fall in a certain sequence, such as dates of birth, surgery, and death.
4. Check derived ages and time intervals. After checks (1) and (2) the dates should be used to calculate ages and time intervals of interest, such as age at surgery or time between surgery and death. These should then be range checked as described earlier.

## 7.3 OUTLIERS

Checking the data for continuous variables may reveal some outlying values that are incompatible with the rest of the data. Typically there may be one or two outliers for a few variables, although for most variables there will not be any.

As already discussed, suspicious values should be carefully checked. If there is no evidence of a mistake, and the value is plausible, then it should not be altered. An exception to this rule is where the value is correct but investigation reveals that there is something special about that individual, such as a concurrent illness. Here it may be reasonable to exclude the observation. In contrast, it is especially dangerous to remove values simply because they are largest or smallest. Also, there is no justification behind automated procedures such as removing all values more than three standard deviations away from the mean. Statistical techniques can be used to detect suspicious values, but should not be used to determine what happens to them.

Outliers are particularly important because they can have a considerable influence on the results of a statistical analysis. Because by definition they are extreme values, their inclusion or exclusion can have a marked effect on the results of an analysis. To take a simple example, Table 7.1 shows numbers of $T_4$ cells per $mm^3$ in blood samples from 20 patients in remission from Hodgkin's disease. The mean of the values is 823.2 and the standard deviation is 566.4. If we consider that the highest value of 2415 is an outlier and discard it, the mean of the remaining 19 values is 739.4 and the standard deviation is 436.4 – both must fall when the largest value is omitted. The effect of excluding a single observation can, as here, be quite marked, which is why decisions about which data are to be analysed should be made before the full analysis starts.

A histogram of the $T_4$ data shows that the distribution is skewed (Figure 7.1a), whereas that for the logarithm of the cell counts is symmetric (Figure 7.1b). Further, the apparent outlier is seen in the log scale to be very reasonable. Transformations are considered in section 7.6.

Outliers can be influential in regression analysis, a technique described in Chapter 11 for finding the best straight line describing the relation

**Table 7.1** Numbers of $T_4$ cells/mm$^3$ in blood samples from 20 patients in remission from Hodgkin's disease and 20 patients in remission from disseminated malignancies (non-Hodgkin's) (Shapiro *et al.*, 1986)

| | Hodgkin's | non-Hodgkin's |
|---|---|---|
| | 171 | 116 |
| | 257 | 151 |
| | 288 | 192 |
| | 295 | 208 |
| | 396 | 315 |
| | 397 | 375 |
| | 431 | 375 |
| | 435 | 377 |
| | 554 | 410 |
| | 568 | 426 |
| | 795 | 440 |
| | 902 | 503 |
| | 958 | 675 |
| | 1004 | 688 |
| | 1104 | 700 |
| | 1212 | 736 |
| | 1283 | 752 |
| | 1378 | 771 |
| | 1621 | 979 |
| | 2415 | 1252 |
| Mean | 823.2 | 522.1 |
| SD | 566.4 | 293.0 |

between two continuous variables. Figure 7.2 shows the change in plasma protein levels after haemodialysis in 12 patients with chronic renal failure, in which the youngest patient is a possible outlier. Also shown are the fitted regression lines for all the data and with that patient excluded. They illustrate that the regression line gets 'pulled' towards outlying values, regardless of the distribution of the rest of the data, especially in small samples. A single outlying point can have a considerable effect on the visual impression. If we cover the suspicious value it is clear that there is no apparent relation in the rest of the data. In Chapter 11 I suggest that a scatter diagram should always accompany regression analyses.

Outliers can affect many types of statistical analysis, often by inflating the variance of a set of observations and so obscuring the effect of interest. Awareness of any outliers is a highly beneficial spin-off from checking the data.

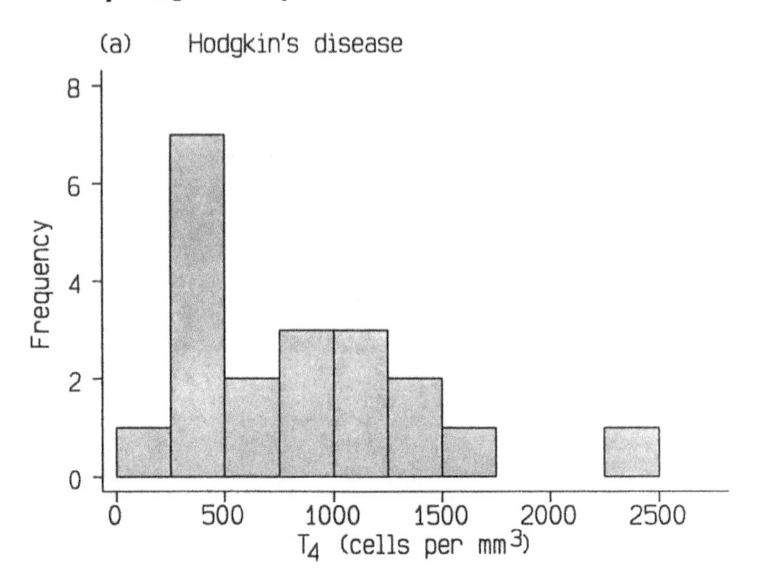
(a) Hodgkin's disease
Frequency
0
2
4
6
8
0
500
1000
1500
2000
2500
$T_4$ (cells per mm$^3$)

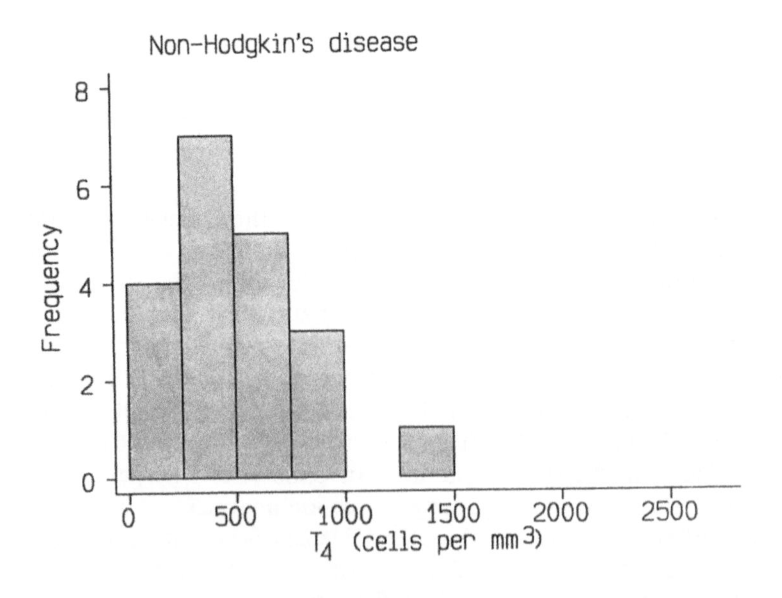
Non-Hodgkin's disease
Frequency
0
2
4
6
8
0
500
1000
1500
2000
2500
$T_4$ (cells per mm$^3$)

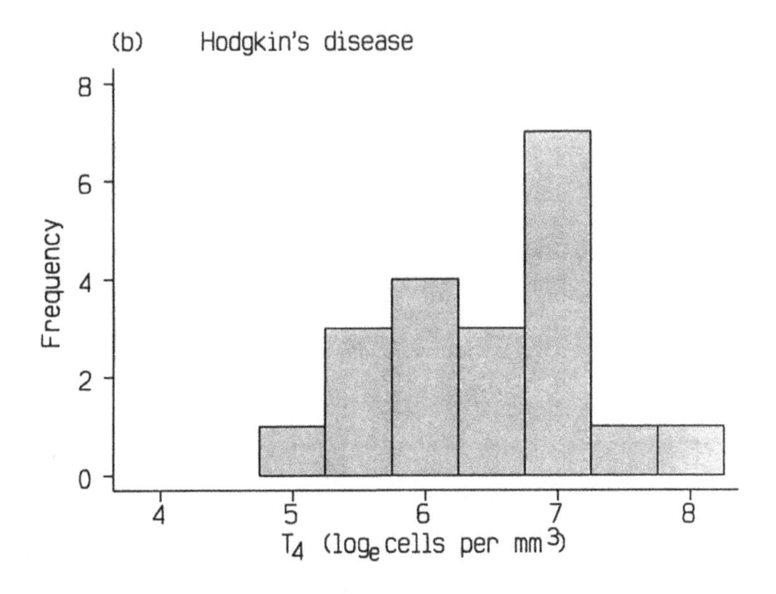


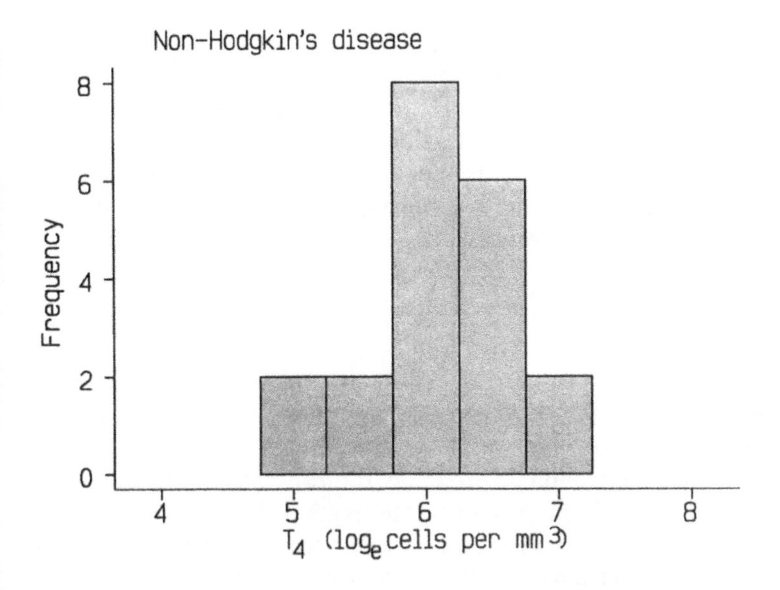


**Figure 7.1** Histograms of $T_4$ cell counts/mm$^3$ in patients with and without Hodgkin's disease shown in Table 7.1 (a) raw data; (b) after $\log_e$ transformation.

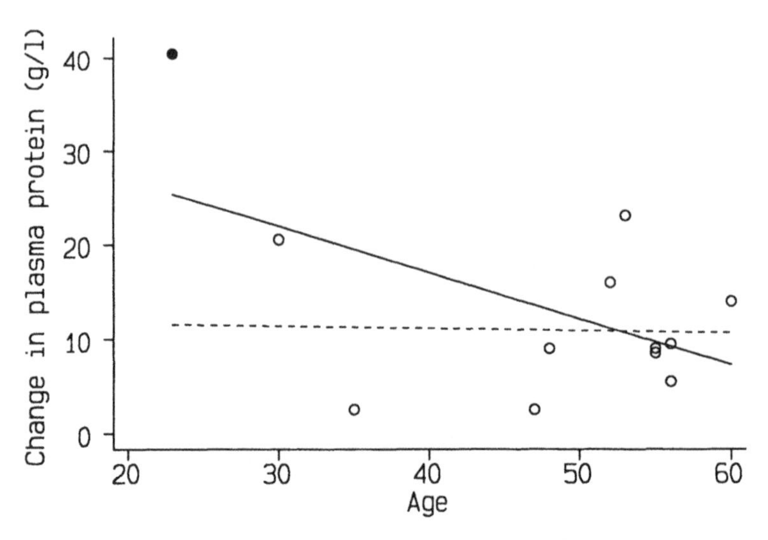


**Figure 7.2** Data showing the relation between change in plasma protein (g/l) after haemodialysis and age in 12 patients with chronic renal failure, showing regression lines for all data (——) and excluding the youngest patient (- - - - - -). Data from Toulon *et al.* (1987).

A useful strategy to adopt when analysing data is to carry out the analysis both including and excluding the suspicious value(s), as in Figure 7.2. If there is little difference in the results obtained then the outlier(s) had minimal effect, but if excluding them does have an effect it may be better to find an alternative method of analysis. Rank methods, introduced in Chapter 8, may be a good approach here. This is an area where expert statistical advice is valuable.

## 7.4 MISSING DATA

Another by-product of checking your data is that any missing observations will be identified. As noted in Chapter 6, the most common device is to use codes such as 9, 99, 999, or 99.9, according to the nature of the variable, although some computer programs (unfortunately few) allow * or some other symbol to indicate a missing observation. If a numeric value is used it is essential to identify the value as a missing value to the statistical software before analysing the data. It is very easy to forget that one or two values are missing, perhaps coded as 999, when carrying out an analysis. The effect on the analysis can be severe, as was illustrated in section 6.3.

The advantage of using * is that there is no danger that subsequent analysis will treat the missing value code as a real observation.

For categorical variables *missing* is just an additional category and so these individuals can be included in any cross-tabulations. However, it is still important that the code (say 9) is identified as missing in a computer program when performing a statistical analysis. For continuous variables it is essential that missing data are identified.

It is important to remember the possibility of missing value codes when creating a new 'derived' variable. For example, if we use height and weight to derive the body mass index (BMI) (described in section 7.2.3), and either or both variables are missing we can get very misleading answers if we have not identified the codes as missing:

| Height (m) | Weight (kg) | BMI (Wt/Ht$^2$) |
|---|---|---|
| 1.62 | 68.2 | 26.0 |
| 1.62 | 999.9 | 381.0 |
| 9.99 | 68.2 | 0.7 |
| 9.99 | 999.9 | 10.0 |

In this case the derived values if either variable is missing are impossible, but this will not always be the case. Missing value codes should be identified before derived variables are constructed. Good computer programs will set the value of a derived variable to missing if any of its components is missing.

Dates are sometimes only partially recorded. If the day is missing it can be set to 15 (halfway through an average month), and a missing month can be set to 6 or 7 (halfway through the year) to minimize the possible error. Substitutions like these are reasonable if the effect is very small compared with the time span being investigated. However, care should be taken that this substitution does not result in a reversal of the sequence of two dates. For example, if date of surgery is given as 08–89, with the day missing, and date of death is 13–08–89, then setting the day of surgery to 15 will make the patient's survival time −2 days.

### 7.4.1 Why are data missing?

It is worth thinking about why the data are missing; in particular we ought to know if there is a reason related to the nature of the study. As with impossible values, it may be possible to check with the original source of the information that missing observations are really missing. Frequently values are missing essentially at random, for reasons not related to the study. For example, some patients may not have been asked a particular question, or a blood sample may have been lost or destroyed. Most large studies will have some missing data for reasons like these. The lack of information may, however, be informative. In a study in which information about a patient is collected on several occasions, lack of information for the later times may be because the patient was withdrawn from the study due to side-effects, or even because they died. Another possibility is that they may have been withdrawn from the study because the variable of interest responded inappropriately. For example, it is common in studies in hypertension to withdraw patients if their blood pressure rises above a pre-selected level, which must compromise an analysis of change in blood pressure. There is further discussion of this type of data in section 14.6.

For information that is coded as 'yes' or 'no', such as the presence of a particular symptom, it may be tempting to consider replacing missing values by 'no', on the grounds that the information would have been recorded if the symptom had been present. This assumption is usually unwarranted, and should not be made lightly. This problem is most likely in retrospective studies, for example when data are obtained from patients' hospital notes.

## 7.5 DATA SCREENING

So far in this chapter I have considered various aspects of checking, as far as possible, that the data are correct. The other important aspect of preliminary data examination is to see how suitable the data are for the type of analysis that is intended, a process sometimes called **data screening**. As already indicated, the presence of one or more outliers can markedly affect, and perhaps invalidate, an analysis. Data screening is concerned largely with the distribution of continuous data, outliers being just one of the aspects considered in this section.

### 7.5.1 The distribution of observations

As subsequent chapters will show, many types of statistical analysis of continuous data are based on the assumption that the data are a sample from a population with a Normal distribution. Alternative methods based on ranks are usually available that do not make that assumption, but they have certain disadvantages. It is important to know the distribution of the data before embarking on an analysis based on the assumption of Normality. Data that are not compatible with a Normal distribution can often be

**transformed** to make them acceptably near to Normal, as described in section 7.6.

For each continuous variable the mean and standard deviation (SD) should be calculated. If possible a histogram should be produced to see the shape of the distribution. If this is not possible then quantiles of the distribution (for example, the 10th, 50th and 90th centiles) can be examined to see if the distribution appears symmetric.

For small samples especially it may be difficult to judge the degree of Normality of a set of data. As Figure 4.7 showed, even samples of size 50 from a Normal distribution may look non-Normal. The graphical technique called a **Normal plot**, described below, gives a much better idea of Normality.

A good way of checking many variables visually is to produce a 'matrix' of scatter plots of all pairs of variables. An example is given in Figure 12.2.

### 7.5.2 The Normal plot

The Normal plot is based on two ideas. First, the cumulative frequency distribution gives a better idea of the shape of the data than does the frequency distribution. It is much less affected by the small fluctuations that were seen in Figure 4.7. The cumulative frequency distribution for data that are Normally distributed has an S shape, as shown in Figure 4.6. It is, however, difficult to judge Normality from the cumulative frequency distribution, which is where the second idea comes in. Because all Normal distributions are precisely the same shape (Figure 4.4) we can stretch the vertical scale to make the cumulative distribution function a straight line if the data are Normal. Departures of the sample data from Normality are thus easily seen as departures from a straight line.

Suppose we have a variable whose values in the population have a Normal distribution with a mean of 34.46 and a standard deviation of 5.84. Figure 7.3 shows (a) the frequency distribution, (b) the cumulative frequency distribution, and (c) the Normal plot. The horizontal axis of the Normal plot shows the numerical value of the observation, and the vertical axis gives the relative frequency in terms of the number of standard deviations from the mean. The values labelled on the vertical axis of the Normal plot correspond to cumulative percentages of 0.1%, 2.3%, 16%, 50%, 84%, 97.7% and 99.9% (see section 4.5.1). The calculation of the plotting coordinates is explained below. Figure 7.3 shows what happens in theory, and Figure 7.4 shows the same process for a sample of size 216 chosen at random from the same population. The top panel shows a histogram of the data, which exhibits some irregularities. The second shows the cumulative frequency distribution and the last the Normal plot. The data are close to a straight line in the Normal plot.

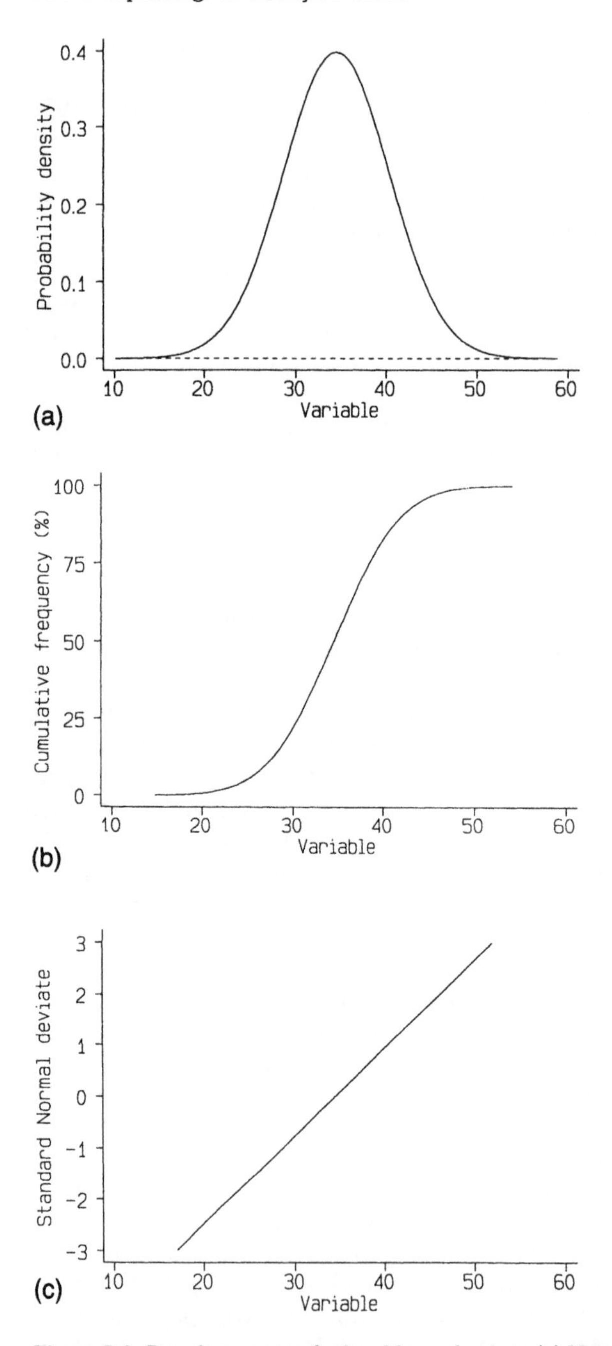


**Figure 7.3** Development of the Normal plot (a) Normal frequency distribution (mean = 34.46, SD = 5.84); (b) Normal cumulative frequency distribution; (c) Normal plot.

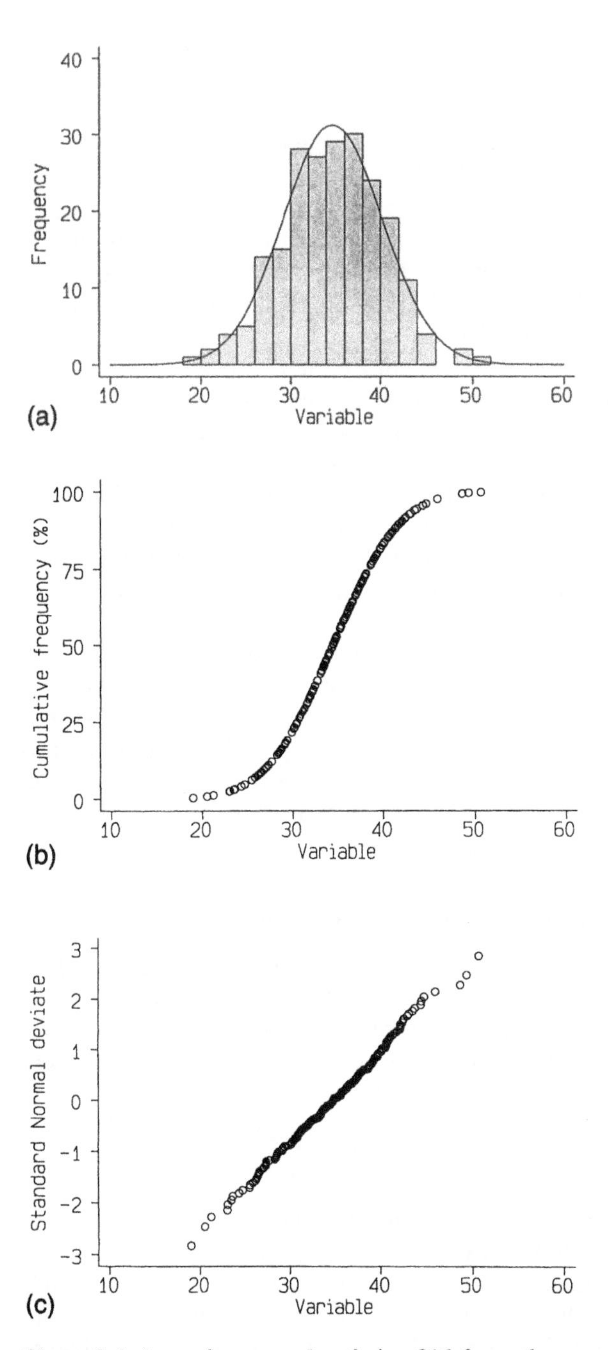


**Figure 7.4** A random sample of size 216 from the population shown in Figure 7.3 (a) frequency histogram (b) cumulative frequency distribution (c) Normal plot. Figure 7.4(a) also shows the corresponding Normal population.

Now that we know what sort of picture to expect when the data really do come from a Normal distribution, we have some basis for judging some real data. Figure 7.5 gives a Normal plot for the serum albumin values from the study of 216 patients with primary biliary cirrhosis previously discussed. These data had a mean of 34.46 g/l and the standard deviation was 5.84 g/l. Figures 7.3, 7.4 and 7.5 are thus directly comparable. When we produce a Normal plot for some data this is the comparison that is implicitly being made. The Normal plot in Figure 7.5(c) is very near to a straight line, indicating that the distribution of serum albumin values in these patients is near to a Normal distribution, in agreement with Figure 4.5. I shall consider below how we can quantify the nearness.

By contrast, the distribution of serum bilirubin values in the same patients was shown in Figure 4.8 to be highly skewed and not near to a Normal distribution. The markedly curved Normal plot of the data in Figure 7.6(a) confirms this finding. However, as described in Chapter 4, after log transformation the data have a nearly Normal distribution, as shown by the Normal plot in Figure 7.6(b). The reasons why we might wish to transform a set of data to get an approximately Normal distribution are discussed in section 7.6.

While the Normal plot is a very useful graphical device for judging the Normality of a set of data, it only allows for a subjective assessment. Because of sampling variation we know that samples from Normal distributions will not be exactly Normal (see Figure 4.7) especially if the sample is small. Where it is important for the data to be close to Normal it is useful to have a method for quantifying the deviations from Normality.

### 7.5.3 Evaluating departures from a Normal distribution

One way of measuring non-Normality is to calculate what are called 'higher moments' of the distribution of data. The first two moments have already been described – they are the mean and variance. However, these values give no information about the *shape* of the distribution. We can measure shape by means of quantities based on

$$\sum \frac{(x_i - \bar{x})^3}{n - 1} \quad \text{and} \quad \sum \frac{(x_i - \bar{x})^4}{n - 1}$$

which are obvious extensions to the formula for the variance. From these we can derive quantities called **skewness**, which is a measure of asymmetry, and **kurtosis**, which is a measure of flatness or peakedness. These values can then be compared with the theoretical values for a Normal distribution. I do not recommend this approach, however, as it is preferable to have a single assessment of Normality rather than two.

Situations in which we may wish to assess the Normality of a set of data

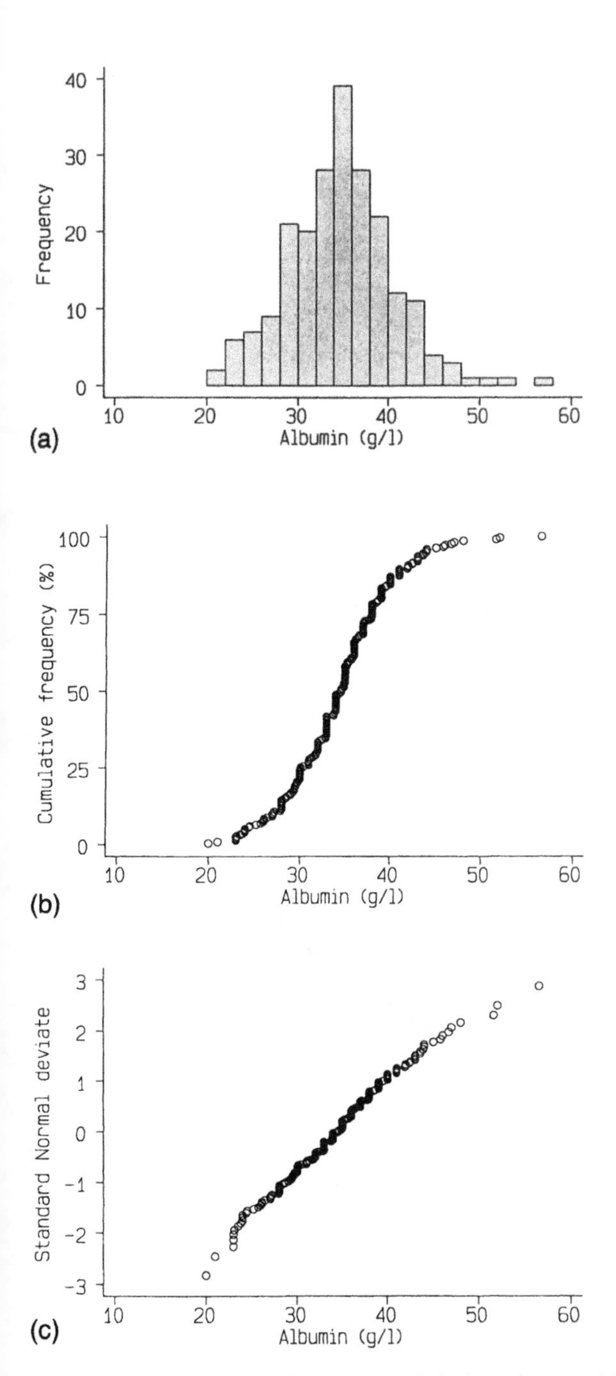


**Figure 7.5** Serum albumin values of 216 patients with primary biliary cirrhosis expressed as (a) frequency histogram; (b) cumulative frequency distribution; (c) Normal plot.

(a)

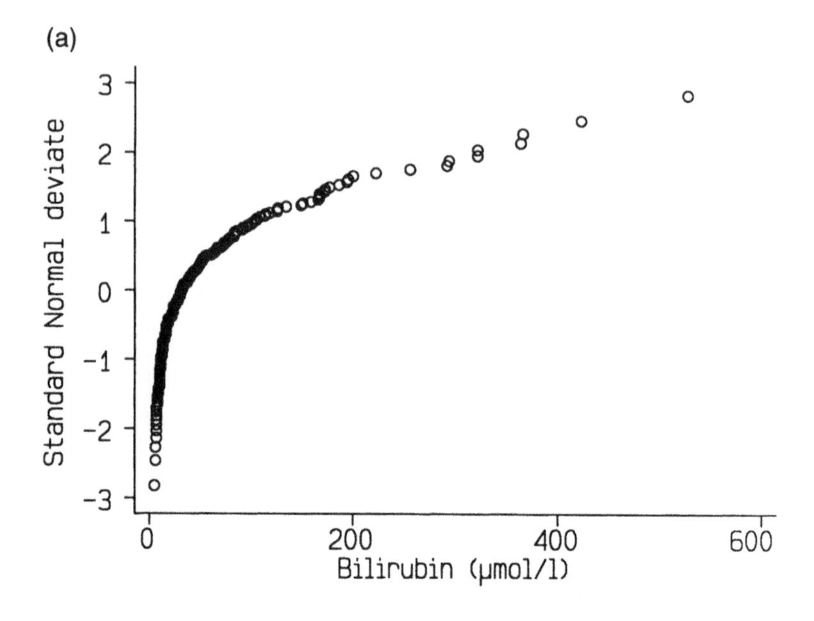


(b)

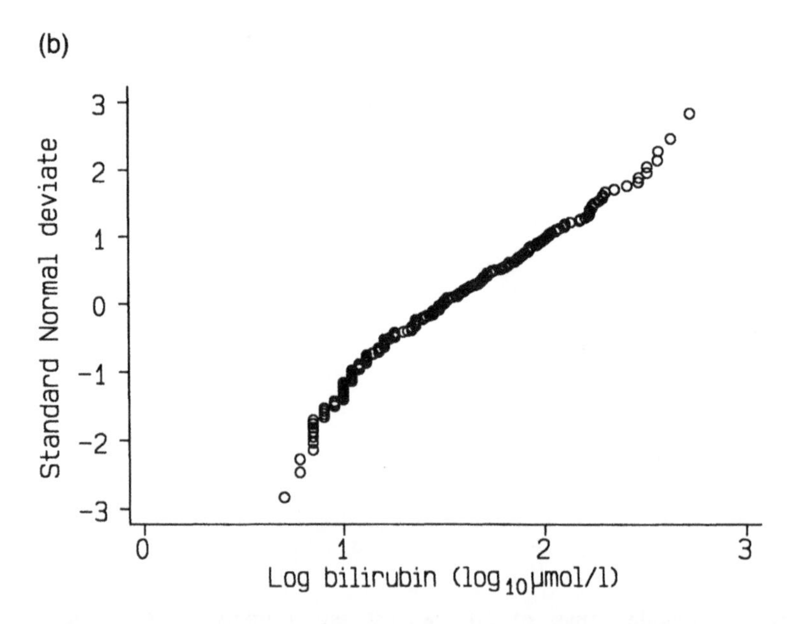


**Figure 7.6** Normal plots of serum bilirubin values in 216 patients with primary biliary cirrhosis (a) raw data; (b) after $\log_{10}$ transformation.

arise in subsequent chapters. For many purposes it is not necessary to do more than check the Normal plot by eye, but if something more is required then a more useful approach is based on measuring the straightness of the Normal plot. We can then calculate the probability that such a value would be obtained in a sample if the population had a Normal distribution, and if this probability is large enough, say greater than 0.05 (1 in 20), we conclude that the data are reasonably near to a Normal distribution. This procedure is an example of a standard statistical approach to inference which is introduced properly and discussed in detail in the next chapter.

The **Shapiro-Wilk *W* test** for Normality is available in several statistical computer programs. However, if it is unavailable the closely related **Shapiro-Francia *W′*** can be calculated fairly easily. It is, however, not described until section 11.6 as it requires a method of analysis introduced in that chapter. For the albumin data shown in Figure 7.5 the Shapiro-Wilk *W* test yields a large probability of 0.76, while the bilirubin data in Figure 7.6 yield a very small probability (Table 7.2). Clearly the serum albumin data are compatible with a Normal distribution, while the raw serum bilirubin values are not. The Normal plot of the log serum bilirubin values (Figure 7.6b) is straight except for a few values at the lower end, but the *W* test shows that the data are not at all compatible with a Normal distribution (Table 7.2). This illustrates the fact that in large samples the test is able to detect small amounts of non-Normality, that in most circumstances would be unimportant. As Figure 4.9 showed, the log bilirubin data are very similar to a Normal distribution. Thus some judgement is required in assessing the Normal plot and the *W* test.

**Table 7.2** Shapiro and Wilk's *W* test applied to 216 values of serum albumin, serum bilirubin and log serum bilirubin (from the study by Christensen *et al.*, 1985)

| Variable | *W* | Probability (P) |
|---|---|---|
| Serum albumin | 0.986 | 0.76 |
| Serum bilirubin | 0.668 | $< 0.0001$ |
| Log serum bilirubin | 0.956 | $< 0.0001$ |

Non-Normality is usually most marked in the tails of the distribution. Outliers will show up in a Normal plot as one or more points lying away from the general linear trend of the rest of the data. Even one outlier can make the data fail the Shapiro-Wilk test. Systematic curvature, as seen in Figure 7.6(a), indicates skewness (to the right), while an S shaped plot will indicate either too many or too few values in both tails of the distribution in comparison with a Normal distribution, as shown in Figures 7.7 and 7.8

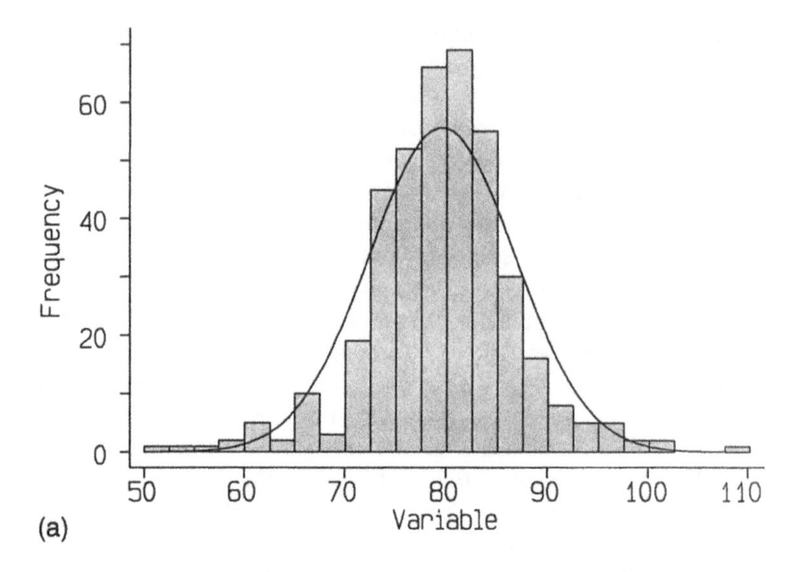


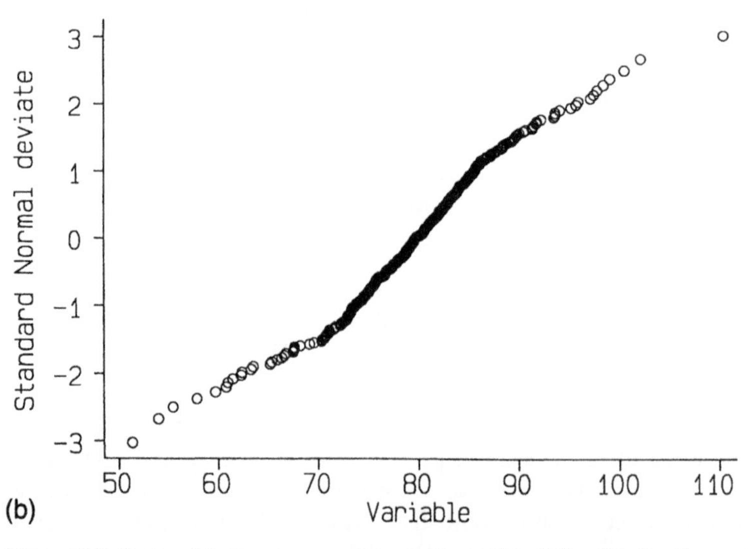


**Figure 7.7** Data with too many values in the tails of the distribution compared with a Normal distribution ($n = 400$, mean = 80, SD = 7.2) (a) histogram; (b) Normal plot.

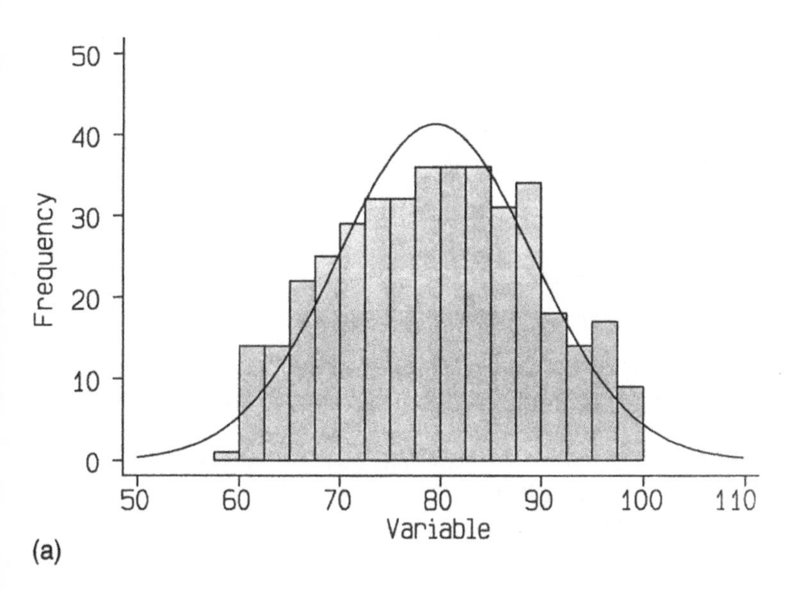


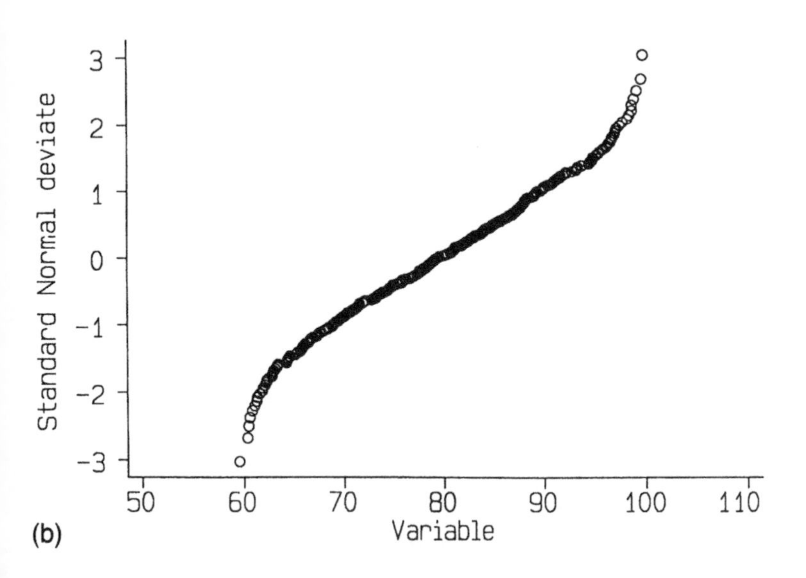


**Figure 7.8** Data with too few values in the tails of the distribution ($n = 400$, mean = 80, SD = 9.7) (a) histogram; (b) Normal plot.

respectively. Normal plots can also reveal a mixture of two distributions in the data. Figure 7.9 shows a Normal plot of birth weights of one litter of piglets, suggesting a normally grown group and a group of three 'runt' piglets with lower weights (Royston *et al.*, 1982). The different slopes indicate different standard deviations in the two putative groups.

### 7.5.4 Constructing a Normal plot

*(This section is more technical and can be omitted without loss of continuity.)*

The scale of the $Y$ axis in the Normal plots such as Figure 7.7 is linear in multiples of the standard deviation of the observations. The Normal plot is constructed by sorting the observations into ascending order and then plotting the data against the corresponding **Normal scores**. The Normal score is the number of standard deviations below or above the mean that we expect to find the observation with a given rank from a sample from a Normal distribution of a given size. Many statistical programs can calculate Normal scores for plotting against the data, and some can produce Normal plots easily. For drawing a Normal plot by hand there is special Normal probability paper with divisions corresponding to the percentage points of the Normal distribution. The observations are sorted and then the $i$th

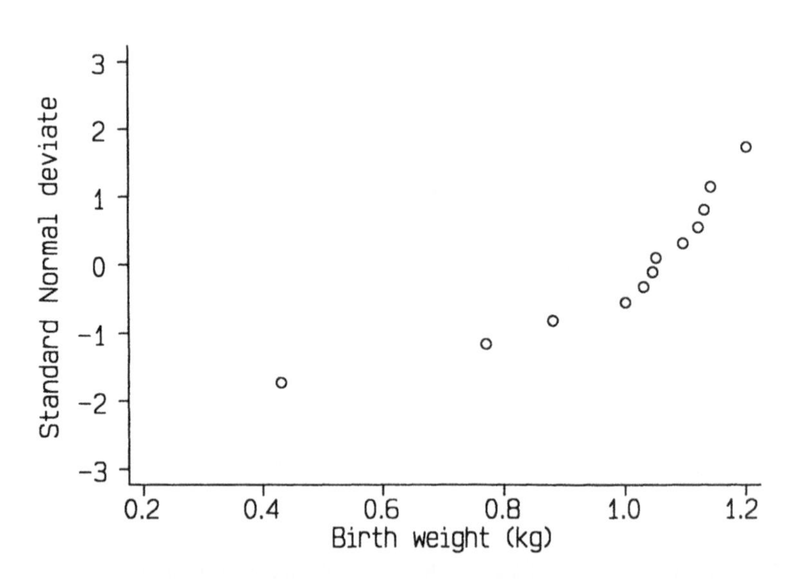


**Figure 7.9** Normal plot of piglet birth weights (Royston *et al.*, 1982).

observation is plotted against the Normal score corresponding to the percentage $P_i$, given by

$$P_i = \frac{i - 3/8}{n + 1/4} \times 100.$$

## 7.6 WHY TRANSFORM DATA?

### 7.6.1 Transforming to Normality

As will be seen in the next few chapters, most statistical methods (**parametric** methods) for analysing continuous data incorporate assumptions about the data in the population from which the sample was drawn. In particular they include an assumption that the data come from a population where the values are Normally distributed. Thus we expect the data to be consistent with that assumption, which is why we need the test of Normality described in section 7.5. We often find that a transformation of the data will yield a distribution that is much nearer to a Normal distribution. By far the most common is the logarithmic or log transformation. The Lognormal distribution was introduced in section 4.6, as the distribution that can be transformed to a Normal distribution by taking logs. The serum bilirubin data shown in Figure 7.6 are an example, as are the $T_4$ cell counts in Figure 7.1.

For some methods the distributional assumption is not too critical, especially if the sample size is large. There are other reasons, however, for wishing data to be near to a Normal distribution. Another important assumption of many parametric methods is that different groups of observations have the same standard deviations. It is often the case that variation in standard deviations accompanies non-Normal data, and both requirements can be met more closely after transforming the data. For example, the $T_4$ data in Table 7.1 for Hodgkin's and non-Hodgkin's disease patients have rather different standard deviations of 566.4 and 397.9, but the standard deviations of $\log_e T_4$ are much more similar, being 0.708 and 0.632, and the distributions are much nearer to Normal (Figure 7.1). The log transformation is likely to work well if the ratio of the standard deviation to the mean is similar among several groups of observations. This calculation has meaning only for the raw data, and may not be very helpful with just two groups. For the $T_4$ data the ratios are 0.69 and 0.56, which are reasonably similar.

Other transformations sometimes used are the square root and reciprocal transformations. Figure 7.10 shows histograms of the serum bilirubin data before and after different transformations. The square root transformation (Figure 7.10c) is less dramatic than taking logs. It is particularly used when the variable is a count (frequency) and thus would be expected to follow a

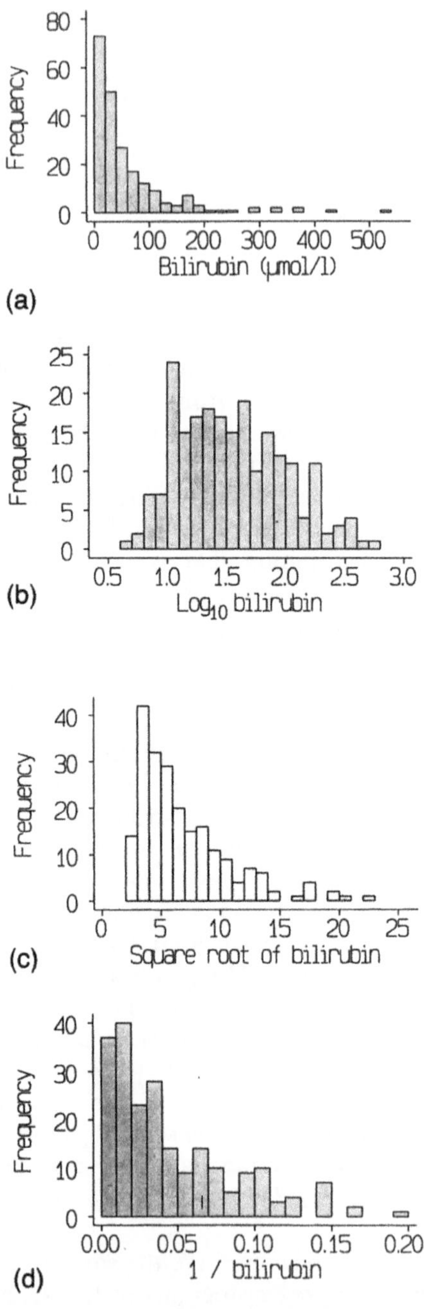


**Figure 7.10** A comparison of different transformations of the serum bilirubin data (a) raw data; (b) after $\log_{10}$ transformation; (c) after square root transformation; (d) after reciprocal transformation.

Poisson distribution. The reciprocal transformation (Figure 7.10d) has a much more drastic effect than taking logs (note that it reverses the order of the observations), and may be useful if the observed data have an extremely skewed distribution. The use of the reciprocal transformation for plasma creatinine values of kidney transplant patients and the square root transformation for tumour size measurements were described by Gore (1982). Their use is not common, however, and there are certain reasons for using the log transformation in preference to any other as long as it yields satisfactory results (see section 9.7). Sometimes there may be a strong logical reason for using a particular transformation. For example, the cube root may be appropriate for data that are volumes and the reciprocal of a recorded time to walk a certain distance will yield the speed.

Another reason for transforming to Normality is to reduce the influence of outlying (and thus atypical) values on the results of analysis, a problem illustrated in Figure 7.2. The overall picture has been well summarized by Armitage and Berry (1987, p. 368): 'It is usually convenient if continuous variables do not depart too drastically from Normal'. When this cannot be achieved we can use rank (non-parametric) methods of analysis (described in subsequent chapters), but these are in general less satisfactory than parametric methods.

Transforming the data is sometimes felt to be a trick used by statisticians, a belief that is based on the idea that the natural scale of measurement is in some way sacrosanct. This is not really the case, and indeed some measurements, such as pH values and titres, are effectively already log transformed values. It is, however, always best to present results in the original scale of measurement. In later chapters I show how this is done.

### 7.6.2 Transforming proportions

The other main use of transformations is in the analysis of proportions. Observed proportions in the range 0.2 to 0.8 have similar uncertainty but very small or large proportions have smaller uncertainty as they are somewhat constrained towards the ends of the scale (zero and one). For statistical analyses we often wish to have equal uncertainty attached to all proportions, and we can achieve this by the **logit** transformation, which is defined by

$$\text{logit}(p) = \log_e\left(\frac{p}{1-p}\right).$$

The logit transformation stretches out proportions in the same way as the percentiles of the Normal distribution are stretched out in the Normal plot, as Table 7.3 shows. The logit transformation is mainly used in regression analysis involving proportions, discussed in Chapter 12, and with the use of odds ratios to compare risks in different groups, described in Chapter 10.

**Table 7.3** Effect of logit transformation of a proportion $p$

| $p$ | logit($p$) |
|---|---|
| 0.01 | −4.60 |
| 0.05 | −2.94 |
| 0.10 | −2.20 |
| 0.25 | −1.10 |
| 0.50 | 0.00 |
| 0.75 | 1.10 |
| 0.90 | 2.20 |
| 0.95 | 2.94 |
| 0.99 | 4.60 |

## 7.7 OTHER FEATURES OF THE DATA

The previous sections of this chapter have discussed the main features to look for when screening data before analysis. This section considers two less obvious aspects of data examination that can shed light on a study.

### 7.7.1 Digit preference

When people measure something they may not do so accurately. The harder the quantity is to measure the greater will be the within-observer variability and also the possibility of subconscious biases. **Digit preference** is the name given to the way individuals can impose their personal (subconscious) prejudice on the way they record observations. We see digit preference in the *final* recorded digit of a measurement. For example, height is usually measured in whole centimetres, and blood pressure to the nearest 2 mm Hg. In a large series of observations we would expect to see equal numbers of height measurements with each terminating digit from 0 to 9, and equal numbers of blood pressure measurements ending in 0, 2, 4, 6 or 8. In practice we often see marked deviations from the expected Uniform distribution. Sometimes this is because the observer does not make the measurements to the precision specified in the study protocol. For example, he or she might measure blood pressure to the nearest 5 mm Hg. Often, however, the distribution varies from expected for no definable reason – it is simply that the person seems to have a preference for numbers ending in, say, 3 or 7. The most common forms of digit preference lead to an excess of

1. zeros
2. zeros and fives
3. even digits.

For (1) there will be a consequent shortage of ones and nines.

Several of these features can be seen in the data in Table 7.4, which shows terminal digits from three sets of blood pressure readings from a case-control study. The cases were measured twice while the controls were measured only once. Two of the three sets of digits show closely similar patterns, indicating that they were made by the same person. However, the third set shows a different pattern, showing that they must have been made by a different person. (I subsequently verified with the study organizer that this had happened.) Notice that both observers had an excess of zeros, but that they were clearly recording blood pressure to different accuracy.

**Table 7.4** Final digits of recorded blood pressures in a case-control study

| | Cases | | Controls |
|---|---|---|---|
| Final digit | First exam | Second exam | |
| 0 | 71 | 23 | 23 |
| 1 | 0 | 0 | 0 |
| 2 | 0 | 15 | 17 |
| 3 | 0 | 0 | 0 |
| 4 | 0 | 18 | 14 |
| 5 | 21 | 1 | 9 |
| 6 | 0 | 10 | 9 |
| 7 | 0 | 1 | 0 |
| 8 | 0 | 24 | 28 |
| 9 | 0 | 0 | 2 |
| Total | 92 | 92 | 102 |

The case of blood pressure is particularly interesting. Blood pressure is a very difficult measurement to take as it involves listening for a change in sound while observing a rapidly falling column of mercury. Because digit preference was such a problem with blood pressure several special machines were designed to get round the problem. The best known is the 'random-zero sphygmomanometer' which incorporates a second, hidden column of mercury of random height which is adjusted before each measurement. The recorded blood pressure is then the sum of the heights of the observed column of mercury and the subsequently measured hidden column. However, even the use of this machine may not remove the strong effect of digit preference (Silman, 1985).

Another example of digit preference is seen in the albumin data in Figure 7.5. The steps in the second and third plots are due to many values having been recorded as a whole number (in g/l) rather than to one decimal place.

A curious feature of digit preference is that even if you know about the phenomenon it is still likely to be present in your measurements. Digit preference will rarely have an important influence on the data analysis, but it is another useful product of data screening that you may see how the measurements were made.

### 7.7.2 Hidden time effects

Many studies are carried out over a period of time. It is usually implicitly assumed that the data collected at different times are comparable, but this will not always be the case. Two main types of hidden time effect may exist. The better known effect is that of seasonal or circadian (24 hour) changes. For example, incidence rates of many diseases are strongly seasonal, and the levels of many hormone levels display a circadian 'rhythm'. Many effects of this nature are well-known, and it is not difficult to design studies to avoid problems. For example, it is advisable to take repeat measurements of blood pressure from the same subject at the same time of day because blood pressure has a strong circadian rhythm, being highest in the morning. There is further discussion of this type of data in section 14.7.

There is a second type of possible hidden time effect that is not widely recognized. In a study in which subjects are recruited over some months or years it is possible that there may be changes in the characteristics of the subjects or in the measurements made on them. For example, in the study of primary biliary cirrhosis previously discussed (Christensen *et al.*, 1985) it was found that the serum bilirubin values of patients entering the trial steadily declined over the 7 years of patient recruitment (Altman and Royston, 1988). Serum bilirubin is a good indicator of liver function, so patients joining the study towards the end of the trial were rather less ill than those joining at the beginning. As this was a randomized trial, with patients given azathioprine or placebo at random throughout the period, the time trend in patient characteristics was not important. (It indicates, however, one of the reasons for using concurrent controls in clinical trials – see Chapter 15.)

If the date of observations is known (and I recommend that it is recorded) then it is simple to plot the data against time to see if there are any trends. Altman and Royston (1988) discuss this issue further and give other examples.

## 7.8 CONCLUDING REMARKS

This chapter has dealt with ways of checking the consistency and, where possible, the accuracy of a set of data, and of screening the data prior to analysis. These procedures are important for any study, although perhaps particularly relevant to large data sets. They are not terribly practical without a computer, but a computer will also be needed to analyse the data, so it is a relatively simple extension to use the computer first to produce the descriptive tabulations and graphs described above. The possible exception is the Normal plot, which cannot be performed by all statistical programs. Further discussion of these matters, together with other aspects of quality control in large studies, is given by Buyse (1984).

For clarity the various aspects of data checking and screening have been considered separately. In practice, however, it is possible to perform range checks, look for outliers and missing values, and examine the shape of the distribution of a set of data in a single analysis.

Although not always discussed as part of statistical methodology the methods described in this chapter are an essential part of statistical analysis, allowing you to check the correctness of your data. Time spent at the beginning checking the data is time well spent; errors in the data that are not detected until the main analysis is under way will require everything to be redone. Screening the data also allows you to get a feel for the data. This last idea is rather nebulous, but by familiarizing yourself with the data you should be much better equipped to choose appropriate and valid methods of analysis.

## EXERCISES

7.1 The table overleaf shows data from a study of 20 patients with chronic congestive heart failure (Caruana *et al*., 1988). Two measurements are shown – ejection fraction, which is a measure of left ventricular dysfunction, and pulmonary arterial wedge pressure:

| Patient | Ejection fraction (%) | Wedge pressure (mm Hg) |
|---|---|---|
| 1 | 28 | 15 |
| 2 | 26 | 14 |
| 3 | 42 | 15 |
| 4 | 29 | 12 |
| 5 | 16 | 37 |
| 6 | 21 | 30 |
| 7 | 25 | 7 |
| 8 | 35 | 14 |
| 9 | 30 | 28 |
| 10 | 36 | 13 |
| 11 | 37 | 5 |
| 12 | 41 | 13 |
| 13 | 20 | 24 |
| 14 | 26 | 8 |
| 15 | 38 | 13 |
| 16 | 26 | 17 |
| 17 | 10 | 27 |
| 18 | 18 | 29 |
| 19 | 10 | 8 |
| 20 | 31 | 5 |

One value has been mistranscribed from the paper. Which patient's data is most likely to be wrong?

7.2 Use the method described in section 7.5.4 to construct a Normal plot of the $\log_e T_4$ cell counts for 20 Hodgkin's disease patients given in the first column of Table 7.1.

7.3 Comment on the terminal digits of the three variables shown in the table in Exercise 3.1.

7.4 Investigate the possibility of digit preference in the final digits of the following serum progesterone data (also shown as Group 2 in Table 14.13).

| Time | Patient 1 | 2 | 3 | 4 | 5 | 6 |
|---|---|---|---|---|---|---|
| 0 | 1.0 | 1.0 | 1.0 | 3.0 | 8.3 | 6.2 |
| 1 | 1.5 | 1.0 | 1.0 | 2.5 | 7.5 | 5.9 |
| 3 | 5.0 | 6.5 | 7.3 | 2.0 | 9.6 | 6.8 |
| 5 | 11.0 | 20.0 | 7.5 | 2.7 | 11.0 | 7.7 |
| 10 | 16.0 | 22.5 | 18.0 | 3.4 | 11.5 | 9.0 |
| 15 | 23.0 | 27.8 | 20.0 | 3.6 | 15.7 | 9.3 |
| 30 | 15.0 | 19.0 | 18.9 | 14.0 | 15.2 | 12.1 |
| 45 | 9.0 | 9.0 | 12.8 | 7.3 | 15.8 | 12.2 |
| 60 | 6.0 | 8.2 | 6.3 | 7.7 | 14.0 | 11.0 |
| 120 | 5.0 | 8.0 | 4.8 | 4.7 | 11.5 | 9.0 |

# 8

# Principles of statistical analysis

A distinctive function of statistics is this: it enables the scientist to make a numerical evaluation of the uncertainty of his conclusion.

Snedecor (1950)

## 8.1 INTRODUCTION

When we analyse medical data for research purposes the intention is to extrapolate the findings from a sample of individuals to the population of all similar individuals. We see this most clearly in animal and laboratory studies as well as in much epidemiological research, where the data cannot be identified with individual subjects, but it applies equally to case-control studies, clinical trials and indeed to clinical research in general. While we may also be interested in each individual from a clinical point of view, research is usually aimed at summarizing the experience of many individuals to draw general conclusions. Thus one of the main ideas of statistics is this – the aim of statistical analysis is to use the information gained from a sample of individuals to make inferences about the relevant population.

In most research studies some data are collected for descriptive purposes, for example information about the demographic and clinical characteristics of subjects being studied. The first step in the analysis of a set of data is to describe such basic data, and simple descriptive methods for this purpose were described in Chapter 3. In observational studies most if not all the data will be of this type. Intervention studies, which include clinical trials and laboratory experiments, are explicitly comparisons between different sets of observations. How do we compare sets of data, especially in view of the desire to generalize the findings?

The following seven chapters describe a large number of statistical methods for analysing data of various types for different research designs. The majority of the problems considered involve making comparisons between groups of observations of the same type or relating different observations within one group of individuals. Despite the enormous variety of medical problems and statistical solutions there are two basic approaches to statistical analysis that run through all of these methods – **estimation** and **hypothesis testing**. The next sections will discuss the principles behind each of these methods, and then they will be compared. The ideas in this chapter are fundamental to an appreciation of statistical thinking and thus to an understanding of the subsequent chapters.

## 8.2 SAMPLING DISTRIBUTIONS

The most important idea, already introduced in section 4.3, is that we take the results obtained in the sample and use them as our best **estimate** of what is true for the relevant population. So, for example, if we find that a new treatment for psoriasis relieves the symptoms of patients more often than a standard treatment, or that serum cholesterol is higher in men than women, or that a certain combination of temperature and light optimizes cell growth in a laboratory experiment, then in each case we would expect that the same is likely to be true in the population. For this interpretation to be valid the sample must be representative of the population. The methods described in this chapter show how to quantify the strength of the evidence, or its uncertainty.

As we saw in Chapter 4, small random samples from a Normal distribution may have a distribution that is not at all like a Normal distribution. Similarly, the mean of a random sample may differ from the population mean, just by chance, although naturally we expect the sample mean to be quite close to the population mean. We use the sample mean as an estimate of the population mean, because that is the best information we have, but how good is the mean of a single sample as an estimate of the population value? We need a way of assessing the uncertainty associated with our estimate. One way to approach this problem is to suppose that we could take many samples of a given size from the population. What can we say about the variability of the means of these samples in relation to the population (i.e. true) mean?

In Chapter 3 the standard deviation was introduced as a measure of the variability of a set of observations around their mean. Measuring the variability of hypothetical sample means about the true mean is clearly a similar problem. It turns out that we can make some surprisingly strong statements about the properties of the means of several samples, and that we can use this information to answer the question posed above, namely what we can say about uncertainty when we have taken only one sample.

It is intuitively reasonable that the variability of sample means will have the following properties:

1. it will be less among the means of large samples than small samples;
2. it will be less than the variability of the individual observations in the population;

3. it will increase with greater variability (standard deviation) among the individual values in the population.

All of these are indeed true. It can be shown mathematically that the distribution of the means of random samples has the following properties:

(i) The **expected value** of the mean of the distribution of the sample means is the same as the population mean. In other words, on average the mean of a sample will be the mean of the population. Further, the expected value of the variance of a sample is the variance of the population.

(ii) The expected value of the standard deviation of the means of several samples is $\sigma/\sqrt{n}$ where $\sigma$ is the standard deviation of the variable in the population and $n$ is the size of each sample. The quantity $\sigma/\sqrt{n}$ is known as the **standard error** of the mean, to distinguish it from the standard deviation of the observations. We can estimate the standard error from a single sample using the observed standard deviation in that sample, $s$, in place of $\sigma$. The interpretation and use of the standard error are discussed in section 8.4.

(iii) The distribution of the sample means will be Normal if the distribution of the data in the population is Normal. Further, and somewhat remarkably, **the distribution of the sample means will be nearly Normal whatever the distribution of the variable in the population as long as the samples are large enough**. This important result is known as the **central limit theorem**. It underlies many of the main statistical methods. Sometimes we will be concerned with the sum of a set of values rather than the mean. The two differ only with respect to division by the number of observations, so the central limit theorem applies equally to sums and means.

In practice, the sample size restriction in (iii) is not relevant when the data have a distribution that is unimodal and not particularly asymmetric. Conversely, if the sample size is large enough the distribution of means will be Normal regardless of the distribution of the data. In general, the more Normal the data, the more reasonable will be the assumption that the mean will itself be Normally distributed in repeated sampling. If we can assume a Normal distribution for the mean it is easy to use the methods based on the Normal distribution (introduced in Chapter 4) to indicate the uncertainty of a sample mean as an estimate of the population mean. I shall return to this problem in the next section.

The preceding discussion has related to the mean of a sample from a population, but statements (i) to (iii) also apply to a sample proportion. If we give the values 1 and 0 to indicate the presence or absence of the attribute of interest, for example having had one's tonsils removed, the proportion with the attribute in a sample is the number with the attribute divided by the sample size. In other words, the proportion $p$ with the attribute is the mean of the 1s and 0s in the sample, and so properties (i) to (iii) above apply. However, as the population values are certainly not Normal, being either 1 or 0, property (iii) will apply only to large samples. Another way of looking at proportions is that the number with an attribute (which is equal to the sample size times $p$) will follow a Binomial distribution. As I mentioned in Chapter 4, the Binomial distribution becomes more like a Normal distribution for larger samples. If the observed proportion is $p$ and the sample size is $n$, then it is in fact the magnitude of the product $np$ that determines the closeness to a Normal distribution.

## 8.3 A DEMONSTRATION OF THE DISTRIBUTION OF SAMPLE MEANS

The truth of the above statements about the distribution of means or proportions estimated from several samples can best be appreciated by seeing what actually happens when many samples are taken from a population. It is not easy to find appropriate real data, so to demonstrate what happens I have used computer simulation, a technique mentioned in Chapter 6.

First I shall consider the case where the distribution in the population is Normal. From (i) and (ii) in the previous section we expect that the means of a set of random samples will also have a Normal distribution, and we expect the standard deviation of all the sample means to be the population standard deviation divided by $\sqrt{n}$. As usual, by 'expect' we mean that this will happen on average – a set of several samples is still subject to sampling variation.

I used the study of patients with primary biliary cirrhosis (PBC) discussed in Chapter 4 as the basis for the simulations. I supposed that among all patients with PBC, which is the population of interest here, serum albumin values have a Normal distribution with a mean of 35 g/l and a standard deviation of 6 g/l. I used computer simulation to study the distributions of samples of sizes 10, 25 and 100 drawn at random from this Normal distribution. Figure 8.1 shows the theoretical Normal distribution of serum albumin in the population of patients with PBC together with histograms of the means of 100 random samples of sizes 10, 25, and 100. (Note that as there were 100 samples the histograms show both frequencies and relative frequencies.) The expected standard deviations of the sets of 100 means are $6/\sqrt{10}$, $6/\sqrt{25}$ and $6/\sqrt{100}$ respectively, or 1.90, 1.20 and 0.60. It can be seen that the observed distributions are reasonably Normal,

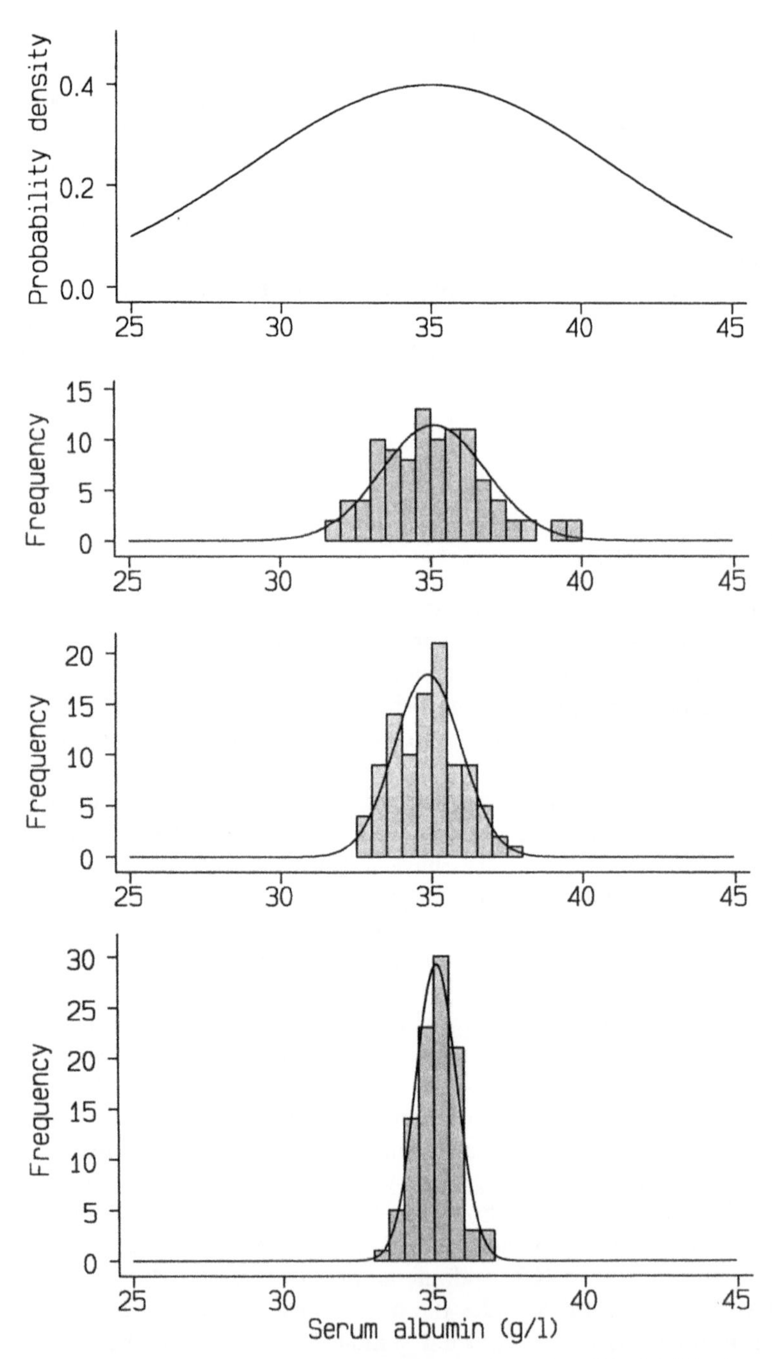


**Figure 8.1** Theoretical Normal distribution (mean 35, SD 6) with observed distributions of means of 100 simulated random samples of sizes 10, 25, and 100.

especially for larger samples, and that their means and standard deviations are close to the expected values. The histograms will get nearer to a Normal distribution as the number of means increases.

Property (iii) in the previous section stated that for samples large enough we should observe a similar phenomenon even when the population values do not have a Normal distribution. We can study this effect using simulation based on the serum bilirubin data in the PBC trial. The actual bilirubin values had a highly skewed distribution with a mean of 60.73 μmol/l and a standard deviation of 77.91 μmol/l, but log serum bilirubin had an approximately Normal distribution, with a mean of 3.55 and standard deviation 1.03. I supposed that in the population of all PBC patients log serum bilirubin has a Normal distribution with a mean of 3.6 log μmol/l and a standard deviation of 1.1 log μmol/l. Figure 8.2 shows the corresponding Lognormal distribution of raw serum bilirubin values and the results of taking random samples of size 10, 25 and 100 from this markedly skewed distribution. We can see that the distribution of the sample means becomes more nearly Normal as the size of the sample increases, but even for samples of 100 the distribution of means is still slightly asymmetric. The more skewed the population values the larger the sample size needed for the means to have a near Normal distribution.

We can study the behaviour of observed proportions in a similar way. On the basis of general practitioner consultations it seems that the prevalence of asthma among women in England is about 0.20 (i.e. 20%) (Fleming and Crombie, 1987). We would expect that the observed proportions of asthma sufferers in a series of random samples of English women would tend to have a Normal distribution as the sample size is increased.

As discussed in Chapter 4, the number of subjects in a sample who have a particular attribute follows a Binomial distribution. The observed proportion can be considered to be a mean, and thus in repeated large samples we expect the distribution of the sample proportions to be approximately Normal. I used computer simulation to study the variation in the sample proportion when the population proportion is 0.2. Figure 8.3 shows the resulting distributions of the proportion of women suffering from asthma in 100 random samples of size 10, 25 and 100. It is clear that the distribution does indeed become more like a Normal distribution as the sample size increases. The speed with which the Binomial distribution resembles a Normal distribution depends upon the proportion and sample size. The nearer the proportion is to 0 or 1 the more asymmetric is the Binomial distribution even for quite large samples.

These simulations have verified empirically the three statements in the previous section. In practice we nearly always have just a single sample, but because we can predict what would happen if many samples *were* taken we can use values from a single sample to make some strong inferences about the population, and can quantify the uncertainty.

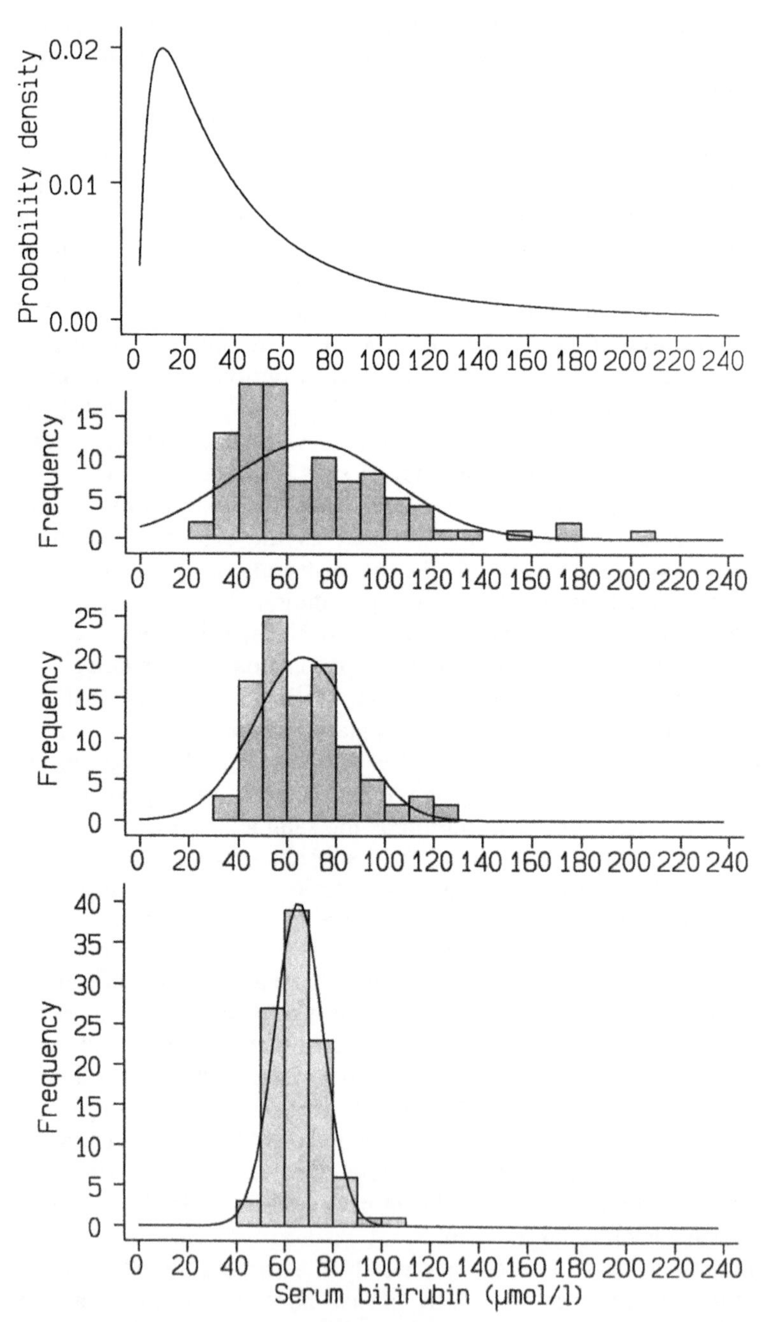


**Figure 8.2** Theoretical Lognormal distribution (antilog of Normal distribution with mean 3.6, SD 1.1) with observed distributions of 100 random samples of sizes 10, 25, and 100.

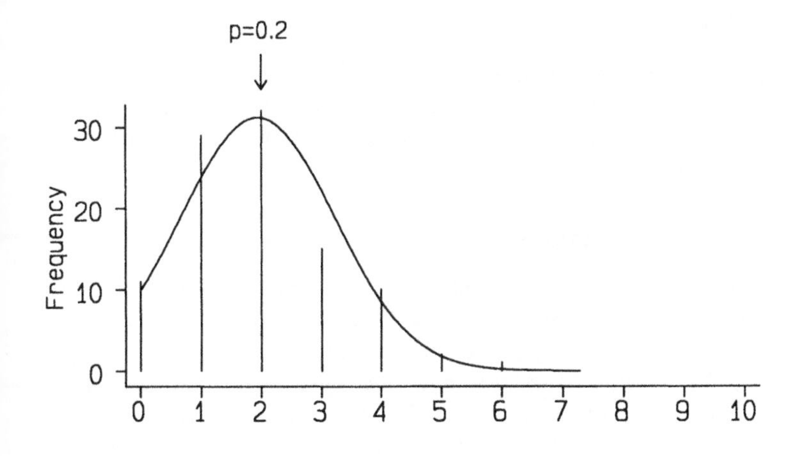


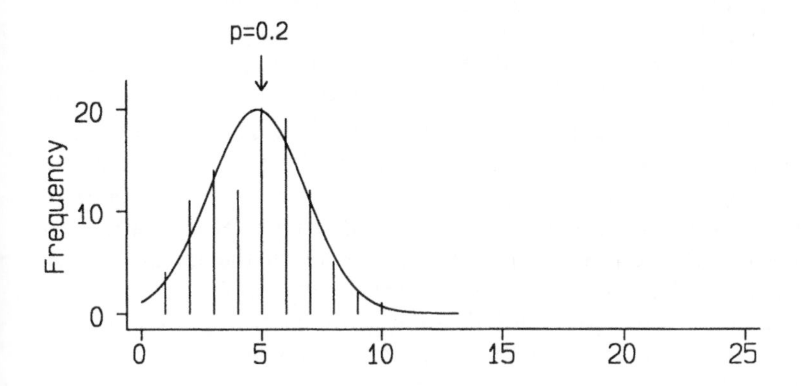


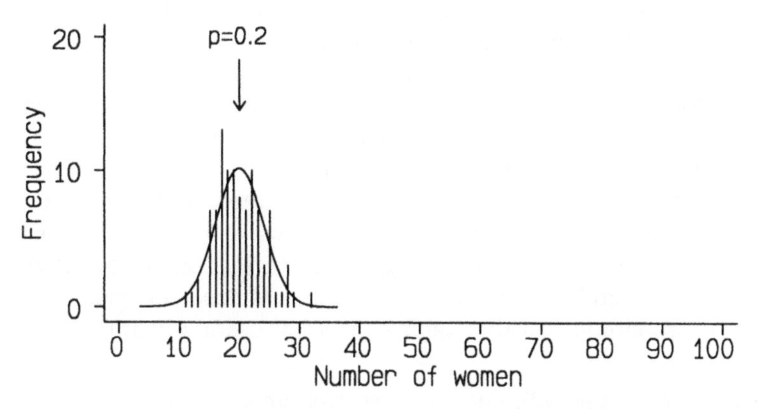


**Figure 8.3** Observed distributions of the number of women with asthma (probability 0.20) in 100 random samples of sizes 10, 25, and 100.

## 8.4 ESTIMATION

I shall first consider the case where we have taken measurements from a sample of people and wish to draw conclusions about the mean of the population, and then consider the same problem relating to a proportion of interest in the population.

### 8.4.1 Standard error of a sample mean

Figure 4.5 showed that the distribution of the observed serum albumin values in 216 patients with PBC was close to a Normal distribution. The mean of these values was 34.46 g/l and the standard deviation was 5.84 g/l. What can we infer about serum albumin values in the population of all patients with PBC from this single sample? Clearly any inference must depend on our sample being representative of the population, and I shall make this assumption for all the examples in this section. From section 8.2 our best estimates of the mean and standard deviation in the population are also 34.46 and 5.84 g/l.

In the previous section I stated that the standard deviation of many sample means will be $\sigma/\sqrt{n}$, where $\sigma$ is the standard deviation in the population, and this was demonstrated by simulation. The standard deviation of sample means is a hypothetical quantity, because in practice we take only a single sample, so we give it the different name of the **standard error of the mean (SEM)**. Although there are other types of standard error associated with other estimates, the standard error of the mean is often abbreviated to standard error (SE) as it is not usually ambiguous to do so. The name standard error gives an indication of the interpretation, because we are interested to quantify in some way how good our estimate of the mean is of the true, and unknown, population mean – how large an error might we be making?

The standard error of the sample mean serum albumin is thus $5.84/\sqrt{216} = 0.397$. We would expect the means of repeated samples of the same size to have a Normal distribution with mean 34.46 g/l and standard deviation 0.397 g/l. Note that the standard error is not an estimate of any quantity in the population, but an indication of the variability among many sample means or, alternatively, a measure of the uncertainty of a single sample mean as an estimate of the population mean. The uncertainty decreases as the sample size increases, as is apparent from the formula and was demonstrated in Figure 8.1. In section 8.4.5 I shall show how to use the standard error to construct a **confidence interval**. The standard error itself, although widely quoted, is a less useful quantity.

### 8.4.2 Standard error of the difference between two sample means

Most medical research is comparative, and so we are more often concerned with two or more samples rather than a single sample. Comparing two samples is particularly common, and for this we need to know the standard error of the difference between the means of two samples.

In a single sample from a population with a standard deviation of $\sigma$ the variance of the sampling distribution of the mean is $\sigma^2/n$, and so the standard error of the mean is $\sigma/\sqrt{n}$. If we have two independent samples the variance of the difference between their means is the *sum* of the separate variances, so the standard error of the difference in means is the square root of the sum of the separate variances. In mathematical notation, if the two means are $\bar{x}_1$ and $\bar{x}_2$, then

$$\begin{aligned} se(\bar{x}_1 - \bar{x}_2) &= \sqrt{var(\bar{x}_1) + var(\bar{x}_2)} \\ &= \sqrt{\{se(\bar{x}_1)\}^2 + \{se(\bar{x}_2)\}^2} \\ &= \sqrt{\frac{s_1^2}{n_1} + \frac{s_2^2}{n_2}}. \end{aligned}$$

For example, a large study of acute myocardial function found that 1551 men had a mean blood urea nitrogen of 23 mg/dl (SD 13) while among 538 women the mean was 25 mg/dl (SD 15) (Dittrich *et al*., 1988). The difference is 2 mg/dl, and its standard error is

$$\sqrt{\frac{13^2}{1551} + \frac{15^2}{538}} = 0.726 \text{ mg/dl}.$$

The standard error can be used to construct a confidence interval for the difference in the means of two independent samples of values of a continuous variable if the samples are large (see section 8.4.5). For small samples a slightly different approach is used, as will be described in Chapter 9.

### 8.4.3 Standard error of a sample proportion

I showed that a sample proportion will have an approximately Normal distribution in large samples. We can thus make an approximation by calculating the standard error of a sample proportion under the assumption that the sample size is large enough. As we have seen, for $p = 0.20$ the approximation is quite good even for fairly small samples. It is reasonable to use this approximation when $p$ and $1 - p$ are greater than $5/n$. For example, the approximation is good for proportions in the range 0.1 and 0.9 for samples greater than about 50, but for values of $p$ outside this range a larger sample is required.

The standard error of the Binomial proportion $p$ in a sample of size $n$ was given in Chapter 4 as $\sqrt{p(1-p)/n}$. Using the Normal approximation we thus expect that if the population proportion is $p$ then in repeated samples of the same size the observed proportions will have a Normal distribution with mean $p$ and standard deviation $\sqrt{p(1-p)/n}$. Returning to the earlier example, if we observe that 13 of a random sample of 80 women have asthma, then from that sample we would estimate that the proportion of women in the population with asthma is $13/80 = 0.16$, with a standard error of $\sqrt{0.16 \times 0.84/80} = 0.041$.

### 8.4.4 Standard error of the difference between two proportions

We can calculate the standard error of the difference between two proportions in the same manner as that of the difference between two means given in section 8.4.2. If we have two observed proportions, $p_1$ and $p_2$, from two independent samples, then the standard error of their difference, $p_1 - p_2$, is given by

$$\begin{aligned} se(p_1 - p_2) &= \sqrt{var(p_1) + var(p_2)} \\ &= \sqrt{\{se(p_1)\}^2 + \{se(p_2)\}^2} \\ &= \sqrt{\frac{p_1(1-p_1)}{n_1} + \frac{p_2(1-p_2)}{n_2}}. \end{aligned}$$

For example, in a large study of adolescents 165 of 712 boys reported that they always used a seat belt compared with 91 of 641 girls (Maron *et al.*, 1986). The two proportions are 0.232 and 0.142, so the difference in proportions is 0.090. The standard error of the difference is

$$\sqrt{\frac{0.232(1-0.232)}{712} + \frac{0.142(1-0.142)}{641}} = 0.0210$$

### 8.4.5 Confidence intervals

I observed in section 8.2 that the mean or proportion observed in a sample is the best estimate of the 'true' value in the population, and that the distribution of the values obtained in several samples would be approximately Normal for large samples. We can combine these features of estimates from a sample with the known properties of the Normal distribution to get an idea of the uncertainty associated with a single sample estimate of the population value. We do this by constructing a **confidence interval**, which is a range of values which we can be confident includes the true value. The basic idea is that the confidence interval covers a large proportion of the sampling distribution of the statistic of interest.

A confidence interval for the estimated mean extends either side of the mean by a multiple of the standard error. For example, the interval between mean − 3SE and mean + 3SE will be a 99.7% confidence interval, because the probability of getting a value from a Normal distribution three or more standard deviations from the mean is 0.3% (as shown in section 4.5 and Table B2). It is most common to calculate a 95% confidence interval, which is the range of values from mean − 1.96SE to mean + 1.96SE. However, there is no particular reason for choosing 95% other than convention, and levels of 80%, 90% and 99% are sometimes used.

We expect that the 95% confidence interval will not include the true population value 5% of the time. We can improve the probability of including the population mean by using, say, a 99% confidence interval, but at the cost of having a wider interval and thus greater uncertainty. The important point is that there is a small chance that the confidence interval constructed from a single sample will not include the true population mean, whatever the sample size.

The 95% confidence interval for the sample mean is usually interpreted as a range of values which contains the true population mean with probability 0.95. We thus expect that if we calculate a 95% confidence interval for the mean serum albumin using each of the 100 random samples shown in Figure 8.1 we would find that about 5% of them would not include the value of 35 g/l. Figure 8.4 shows all 100 confidence intervals based on samples of size 100 of which seven do not include 35 g/l. Figure 8.5 shows the confidence intervals sorted by the size of the sample mean and we can see that seven sample means fall outside the range within which we expect 95% of sample means. This range is calculated using the

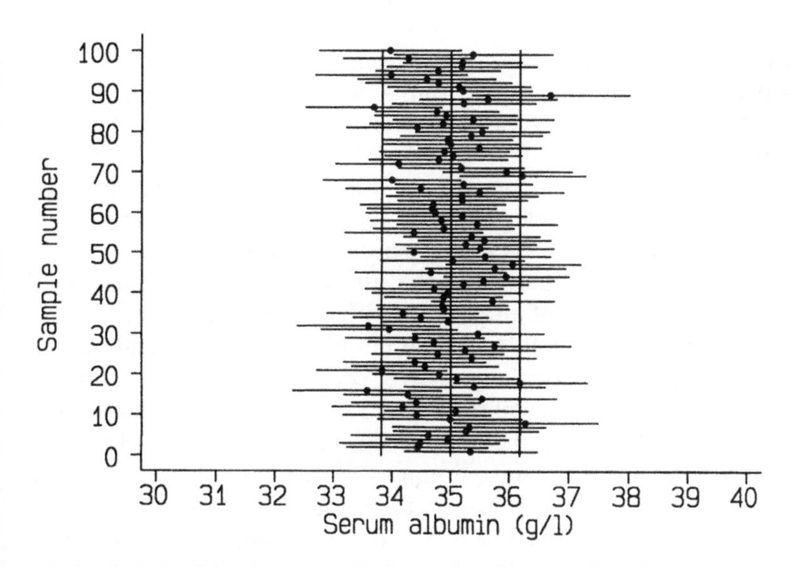


**Figure 8.4** Confidence intervals for mean serum albumin constructed from 100 random samples of size 100. The vertical lines show the range within which 95% of sample means are expected to fall.

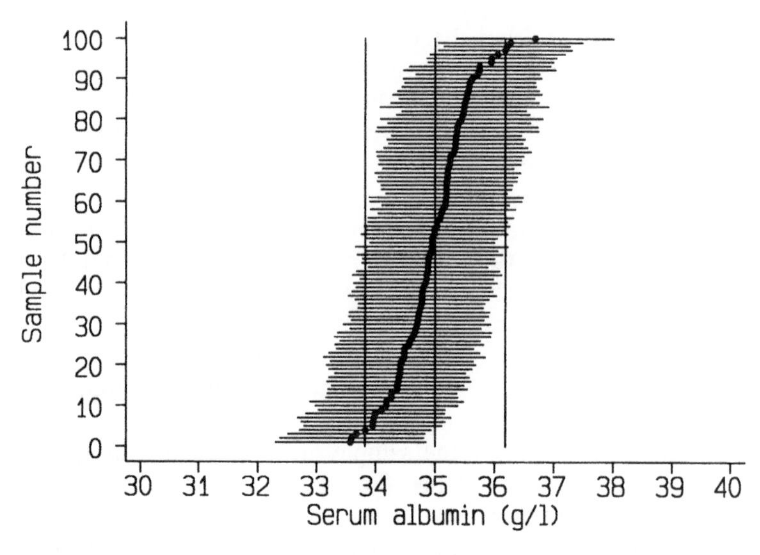


**Figure 8.5** Confidence intervals from Figure 8.4 ordered by the magnitude of the mean of the random sample.

population mean and standard deviation to get mean $\pm$ 1.96SD/$\sqrt{n}$; that is $35 \pm 1.96 \times 6/\sqrt{100}$ or 33.8 to 36.2. The difference between the observed 7% and the expected 5% is of no importance – we would not expect to observe exactly 5%.

In the PBC trial we actually observed a mean serum albumin of 34.46 g/l with a standard error of 0.397 g/l from a sample of 216 patients with primary biliary cirrhosis. The 95% confidence interval is thus given by the range of values from $34.46 - 1.96 \times 0.397$ to $34.46 + 1.96 \times 0.397$, or from 33.68 to 35.24 g/l. We can thus be 95% confident from this study that the true mean serum albumin among all such patients lies somewhere in the range 33.68 to 35.24 g/l, with 34.46 as our best estimate. As mentioned earlier, this interpretation depends on the assumption that the sample of 216 patients is representative of all patients with the disease.

The same 216 patients with PBC had serum bilirubin values that had an approximately Lognormal distribution. We could calculate a confidence interval for the mean serum bilirubin by relying on the central limit theorem and using the same method as for serum albumin. However, because the distribution of serum bilirubin is highly skewed we would be more interested in the median rather than the mean. A more useful confidence interval would therefore be for the median, or we could calculate a confidence interval for the mean of the log serum bilirubin values and back-transform these to give a confidence interval for the geometric mean. These methods are described in the next chapter.

Similarly, we can construct a 95% confidence interval for our sample of 80 women among whom the observed proportion with asthma was 0.16 with a standard error of 0.039. A 95% confidence interval for the sample proportion is from $0.16 - 1.96 \times 0.039$ to $0.16 + 1.96 \times 0.039$, or from 0.08 to 0.24. We are thus 95% confident that on the basis of this sample the proportion of English women with asthma lies in the range 0.08 to 0.24. The confidence interval is wide because the sample size of 80 is rather small for estimating a proportion. In contrast, a 95% confidence interval for the difference in the proportions of boys and girls always using seat belts is narrower because the study was large. The difference in proportions was 0.090 and its standard error was 0.0210, so the 95% confidence interval is from $0.090 - 1.96 \times 0.0210$ to $0.090 + 1.96 \times 0.0210$, or from 0.05 to 0.13.

These examples illustrating the construction of confidence intervals have made use of Normal distribution theory applied to large samples. In later chapters we will use the *t* distribution rather than the Normal distribution for analysis of continuous data, but use the Normal distribution for proportions. The general principle of constructing a confidence interval by adding to or subtracting from an estimate a multiple of its standard error applies in nearly all cases.

Much statistical analysis aims to estimate one or more quantities of interest. Means and proportions have been discussed in this chapter, but the same ideas apply to estimates of other quantities. The standard error of the estimate of interest is calculated, from which one obtains a confidence interval.

## 8.5 HYPOTHESIS TESTING

The approach outlined in the preceding sections seems so straightforward that it may come as some surprise that most statistical analysis in medicine is not of this form, but is based on a different and less intuitive approach called **hypothesis testing**. The majority of statistical analyses involve comparison, most obviously between treatments or procedures or between groups of subjects. The numerical value corresponding to the comparison of interest is often called the **effect**. We can state a hypothesis called the **null hypothesis** that the effect of interest is zero, for example that serum cholesterol is the same on average for men and women or that two treatments for headache are equally effective. This statistical null hypothesis is often the negation of the research hypothesis that generated the data. In the first example, the research hypothesis might be that there was a difference between men and women with respect to their serum cholesterol levels. We also have an **alternative hypothesis**, which is usually simply that the effect of interest is not zero.

Having set up the null hypothesis, we then evaluate the probability that we could have obtained the observed data (or data that were more extreme) **if the null hypothesis were true**. This probability is usually called the **P value**; the smaller it is the more untenable is the null hypothesis. The method is called **testing** because of the aspect of deciding whether or not we can **reject** the null hypothesis. We might find, for example, that in a study comparing serum cholesterol levels of men and women, there was a tendency for higher levels in men, and the P value was 0.10. Notice that there is no direct reference in this method to the *magnitude* of the effect of interest: the analysis is summarized by a probability value. For this and other reasons the approach based on estimation and confidence intervals is widely considered superior, but hypothesis testing remains an important statistical method, and it is essential to understand the underlying principles and interpretation. The Shapiro-Wilk test for non-Normality, described in section 7.5.3, is an example of a hypothesis test.

How do we evaluate the probability of obtaining our data if the null hypothesis is true? For most of the problems discussed in this book the answer lies in calculating a **test statistic** – a value which we can compare with the known distribution of what we expect when the null hypothesis is true. The general form of the test statistic can be expressed in relation to the observed value of the quantity of interest and the value expected if the null hypothesis were true. The observed value is the estimate of interest, such as the difference in mean serum cholesterol between men and women. For the situations so far described the test statistic is given by

$$\text{test statistic} = \frac{\text{observed value} - \text{hypothesized value}}{\text{standard error of observed value}}.$$

In many cases the hypothesized value is zero, so that the test statistic becomes the ratio of the observed quantity of interest to its standard error. The idea that the magnitude of the quantity of interest is evaluated as a multiple of its standard error is common in the main methods of statistical analysis. However, there are several situations discussed in later chapters where the test statistic is not of the above form.

In some circumstances discussed in later chapters we will see that when the null hypothesis is true the test statistic can be considered to have a Normal distribution. In other cases, notably when studying means, we need to use the slightly different $t$ distribution, but the principle is the same.

We evaluate a test statistic by calculating the probability that we could have observed that value, or one that is more extreme (i.e. more unlikely), if the null hypothesis is true. The probability of interest, or P value, is thus the tail area of the distribution. As an example, I shall consider the case where the test statistic has a Normal distribution when the null hypothesis is true. Suppose we wish to use the sample of 216 PBC patients to evaluate the null hypothesis that the mean serum albumin in all PBC patients is 33.5 g/l. As shown earlier, the mean serum albumin in the sample was

34.46 g/l and its standard error was 0.397 g/l. This is a situation where we can use the formula given above, so we calculate the test statistic as (34.46 – 33.5)/0.397, which is 2.42. From Table B1 the tail area of the Normal distribution corresponding to this value of the test statistic is 0.0078, or 0.78%. However, the test statistic could be negative, and the equivalent values in the other tail of the distribution are just as extreme, or unlikely, when the null hypothesis is true so we double the area to get a P value of 0.0155. This value can be obtained directly from Table B2. In other words, a test statistic of 2.42 or more would arise with a probability of only 0.0155 if the null hypothesis is true. We call this a two-tailed test, for obvious reasons. The question of whether to use a two-tailed or a one-tailed test is discussed in section 8.5.6.

We can carry out a hypothesis test for all the situations described in section 8.4 where we can calculate a confidence interval, and this is true in general. In later chapters, however, we will see that there are some circumstances where we can perform a hypothesis test but cannot obtain a confidence interval.

### 8.5.1 Interpretation of P values

P values abound in medical research papers, so it is essential to understand precisely what they mean, and also what they do not mean. The P value is the **probability of having observed our data (or more extreme data) when the null hypothesis is true**. For example, in a clinical trial this statement refers to the observed difference between the treatment groups. We are therefore relating our data to the likely variation in a sample due to chance when the null hypothesis is true in the population.

We have seen that samples give results that differ from what is true in the population, and that the variability among samples decreases as the sample size increases. It will be seen in subsequent chapters that these facts are taken into account when test statistics, and hence P values, are calculated.

The interpretation of a P value is problematic. If we carry out a clinical trial to compare two treatments and get a 'large' value of P, say greater than 0.2, then we can say that data such as ours could occur often when the null hypothesis is really true. We thus cannot rule out the possibility that the null hypothesis *is* true – that is, that the two treatments are equally effective. Conversely if P is very small, say less than 0.001, then the null hypothesis appears implausible because our data could hardly ever arise purely by chance when the null hypothesis is true. We can therefore feel confident that the null hypothesis *is not* true and one treatment is superior. Between these two extremes lies a grey area, but conventionally a cut-off is chosen and if P is smaller than the cut-off value the null hypothesis is rejected. The **test** of the null hypothesis is therefore whether or not P lies below the chosen cut-off point.

Although the choice of cut-off is arbitrary, in practice in most cases we use 0.05. In other words, an outcome that could occur less than one time in 20 when the null hypothesis is true would lead to the rejection of the null hypothesis. In this formulation, when we reject the null hypothesis we accept a complementary alternative hypothesis, which in the clinical trial example is that the two treatments are not equally effective. If the P value exceeds the critical value we do not reject the null hypothesis. However, we cannot say that we believe the null hypothesis is true, but only that there is not enough evidence to reject it. This is a subtle but important distinction.

When P is below the cut-off, say 0.05, the result is called **statistically significant** (and below some lower level, such as 0.01, it may be called **highly significant**); when above 0.05 it is called **not significant**. For this reason hypothesis tests are often called significance tests. The use of the word significant leads to much confusion between statistical and clinical significance. Because of the widespread use of hypothesis tests some medical journals restrict the use of the word significant to its statistical meaning. However, it is common practice to take a statistically significant result as a real effect, and often, by implication, as a clinically important effect too. Neither interpretation is necessarily justified. For example, in the study to compare blood pressure in the left and right arms described in section 5.4, a small difference of about 1 mm Hg (both systolic and diastolic) was found (Gould *et al.*, 1985). This difference was highly statistically significant but of no importance clinically. Similarly it is not reasonable to take a non-significant result as indicating no effect, just because we cannot rule out the null hypothesis.

### 8.5.2 P as a significance level

The cut-off level for statistical significance is usually taken at 0.05, but sometimes at 0.01. **These cut-offs are arbitrary and have no specific importance**. It is ridiculous to interpret the results of a study differently according to whether the P value obtained was, say, 0.055 or 0.045. These P values should lead to very similar conclusions, not diametrically opposed ones. A minor change to the data can easily shift the P value by this amount or more.

In recent years there has been a welcome move away from regarding the P value as significant or not significant, according to which side of the arbitrary 0.05 value it is, towards quoting the actual P value. It is increasingly common to see expressions such as $P = 0.02$ or $P = 0.15$ rather than $P < 0.05$ or $P > 0.05$. One reason for this is that many statistical computer programs give the exact P value, whereas it used to be necessary to evaluate a P value from tables in which test statistics were given corresponding to certain P values only, such as 0.1, 0.05, 0.01 and 0.001. (Table B3 is of this type.) Quoting the actual P value allows the reader to make his or her own interpretation.

But how does one interpret P values if not in relation to the 0.05 level? There is no really satisfactory answer to this question, because P values are an unnatural way of expressing results. In section 8.8 I contrast hypothesis testing and estimation via confidence intervals, and explain why the latter are greatly preferred.

### 8.5.3 Type I and Type II errors

The use of a cut-off for P leads to treating the analysis as a process for making a decision. Within this framework it is customary (but unwise) to consider that a statistically significant effect is a real one, and conversely that a non-significant result indicates that there is no effect. Forcing a choice between significant and non-significant obscures the uncertainty present whenever we draw inferences from a sample. When we construct a confidence interval the uncertainty is shown explicitly, but with a hypothesis test it is implicit, and may easily be overlooked.

Two possible errors can be made when using P to make a decision. Firstly, we can obtain a significant result, and thus reject the null hypothesis, when the null hypothesis is in fact true. This is called a Type I error, and may be thought of as a 'false positive' result. Alternatively, we may obtain a non significant result when the null hypothesis is not true, in which case we make a Type II error. This can be thought of as a 'false negative' finding.

The probabilities of Type I and Type II errors are sometimes called **alpha** ($\alpha$) and **beta** ($\beta$). For any hypothesis test the value of alpha is determined in advance, usually as 5%. The value of beta depends upon the size of effect that one is interested in, and also the sample size. More often we talk about the **power** of a study to detect an effect of a specified size, where the power is $1 - \beta$, or $100(1 - \beta)\%$. A wide confidence interval is an indication of low power.

We can also fix beta in advance by choosing an appropriate sample size. In other words, we can calculate the necessary sample size for a study to have a high probability of finding a true effect of a given magnitude. Chapter 15 shows how to perform the calculations for studies comparing two groups. For more complicated designs it is advisable to get advice on sample size from a statistician.

### 8.5.4 Over-reliance on P values

The formulation of statistical analysis as a test with two possible outcomes – significant or not significant – has had harmful effects on the medical literature. There is increasing evidence of publication bias in favour of papers reporting significant findings. If several identical studies are performed their results will vary because of sampling variation. Those studies that show larger effects will be more likely to be statistically significant and thus more likely to be published. The same applies even when the null hypothesis is true, as we know that one study in 20 will give a result significant at the 5% level. The consequence is that published studies are a biased selection of all studies carried out (see section 15.5.2).

The achievement of statistical significance is often seen as success and a non-significant result as failure. This is exemplified by the use of the terms 'positive' and 'negative' to describe studies with significant or non-significant results, a usage that should be abandoned. The same attitude is also seen in the ugly phrase 'failed to reach statistical significance' which is seen in many papers.

Freiman *et al.* (1978) looked at 71 published trials with 'negative' results, defined as having P values greater than 0.1, and constructed confidence intervals for each study. They found that for nearly half the trials the results were compatible with a 50% therapeutic improvement, which we may reasonably take as clinically valuable for any trial. In other words, the confidence intervals were wide enough to include the possibility that one treatment was 50% better than the other. In none of the original papers had the authors constructed a confidence interval. Other ways of looking at these trials are that they had low power and that the sample size was too small. Because the standard error is related to sample size, a small study may fail to detect (as significant) a difference that is real. These trials demonstrate the non-equivalence of statistical significance and clinical importance.

### 8.5.5 Misinterpretation of P values

A common misinterpretation of the P value is that it is the probability of the data having arisen by chance or, equivalently, that P is the probability that the observed effect is not a real one. The distinction between this incorrect definition and the true definition given earlier is the absence of the phrase **when the null hypothesis is true**. The omission leads to the incorrect belief that it is possible to evaluate the probability of the observed effect being a real one. The observed effect in the sample is genuine, but we do not know what is true in the population. All we can do with this approach to statistical analysis is to calculate the probability of observing our data (or more unlikely data) when the null hypothesis is true.

### 8.5.6 Two-sided or one-sided P values?

To reiterate, the P value is the probability of obtaining a result at least as extreme as the observed result when the null hypothesis is true. I pointed out earlier that extreme results can occur by chance equally often in either direction, which we allow for by calculating a **two-sided** P value. In the vast majority of cases this is the correct procedure. In rare cases it is reasonable to consider that a real difference can occur in only one direction, so that an observed difference in the opposite direction must be due to chance. Here the alternative hypothesis is restricted to an effect in one direction only, and it is reasonable to calculate a **one-sided** P value by considering only one tail of the distribution of the test statistic. For a test statistic with a Normal distribution the usual two-sided 5% cut-off point is 1.96, whereas a one-sided 5% cut-off is given by 1.64. The difference is not particularly large but can lead to a different interpretation in relation to fixed levels of statistical significance.

One-sided tests are rarely appropriate. Even when we have strong prior expectations, for example that a new treatment cannot be worse than an old one, we cannot be sure that we are right. If we could be sure we would not need to do an experiment! If it is felt that a one-sided test really is appropriate, then this decision must be made **before the data are analysed**; it must not depend on what the results were. The small number of one-sided tests that I have seen reported in published papers have usually yielded P values between 0.025 and 0.05, so that the result would have been non-significant with a two-sided test. I doubt that most of these were pre-planned one-sided tests.

The estimation and hypothesis testing approaches will be compared in section 8.8. There is a close relation between the two, but only for a two-sided hypothesis test. Two-sided P values will be used throughout this book, and I recommend that they are used routinely. In some places I quote more exact values than can be obtained from the tables in Appendix B. Many computer programs give exact P values.

## 8.6 NON-PARAMETRIC METHODS

Although confidence intervals and hypothesis testing are rather different approaches to statistical analysis, they have a close mathematical link for the majority of statistical methods, because they are both based on the same statistical model and the same assumptions about sampling distributions. Theoretical distributions are described by quantities called parameters, notably the mean and standard deviation, so methods that use distributional assumptions are called **parametric methods**. There is another class of statistical methods which do not involve distributional assumptions which are called **distribution-free** or **non-parametric methods**. Because these methods are based on analysis of ranks rather than actual data, they are sometimes called **rank methods**. Unfortunately none of these three terms accurately describes all the methods usually considered to fall into this category. In this book I shall usually refer to these methods as non-parametric as this is the term in most frequent use. Note that 'non-parametric' applies to the statistical method used to analyse data, and is not a property of the data.

As they do not usually involve any distributional assumptions, non-parametric methods are most often used to analyse data which do not meet the distributional requirements of parametric methods – usually that the data have a Normal distribution. Skewed data are commonly analysed by non-parametric methods, and methods using ranks are especially suitable for data which are scores rather than measurements. These could have many possible values, such as data from visual analogue scales, or only a few values, such as Apgar scores or stage of disease.

Table 8.1 shows fasting blood glucose data from a study of Type 1 diabetics (Thuesen *et al.*, 1985) together with the ranks of the observations. When there are two or more identical values the average rank is

**Table 8.1** Fasting blood glucose levels in 24 Type 1 diabetics (Thuesen *et al.*, 1985)

| Blood glucose (mmol/l) | Rank order |
|---|---|
| 4.2 | 1 |
| 4.9 | 2 |
| 5.2 | 3 |
| 5.3 | 4 |
| 6.7 | 5.5 |
| 6.7 | 5.5 |
| 7.2 | 7 |
| 7.5 | 8 |
| 8.1 | 9 |
| 8.6 | 10 |
| 8.8 | 11 |
| 9.3 | 12 |
| 9.5 | 13 |
| 10.3 | 14 |
| 10.8 | 15 |
| 11.1 | 16 |
| 12.2 | 17 |
| 12.5 | 18 |
| 13.3 | 19 |
| 15.1 | 20 |
| 15.3 | 21 |
| 16.1 | 22 |
| 19.0 | 23 |
| 19.5 | 24 |

given to each of the 'tied' observations concerned, as is shown for the two values of 6.7 mmol/l. Instead of analysing the actual observations using parametric methods we could analyse the ranks using non-parametric methods. For example, we might wish to compare the blood glucose data for two subgroups of the diabetics, for which the analysis would be based on the sums of the ranks for all subjects within each subgroup. The appropriate methods are discussed in the next chapter.

To compensate for the important advantage of being free of assumptions about the distribution of the data there is the disadvantage that rank methods tend to be more suited to hypothesis testing than estimation. Non-parametric estimates can be calculated, however, the best known example being the median, and it is also possible in some cases to calculate non-parametric confidence intervals. Estimation becomes difficult or impossible for more complex data structures and many problems cannot be handled at all using rank methods.

For simple problems, such as comparing one variable in two groups of subjects or relating two variables within one group the distribution free approach has definite advantages, and its use will be contrasted to the parametric approach in later chapters.

Non-parametric methods are mostly based on comparing sums of ranks. The sum of a set of observations is a simple multiple of their average, so the central limit theorem also applies to these rank sums. Thus unless the samples are small it is often possible to use a Normal approximation when carrying out a non-parametric test, making it easier to apply the method. It seems strange to use the Normal distribution in this way when the methods explicitly avoid having to make any assumptions about the specific nature of the distribution of the observations. It is important to distinguish the two uses of the Normal distribution in statistics: to describe the distribution of a set of observations and to describe (or approximate) the sampling distribution of some quantity of interest.

## 8.7 STATISTICAL MODELLING

Behind the ideas of estimation and hypothesis testing lies a general strategy for statistical analysis called **modelling**. A statistical model is a mathematical relationship between two or more variables that gives an approximate description of the observed data. We do not usually believe that the model describes the underlying *mechanism* of a relation between variables, but it is a simplification which is compatible with the data.

Most of the parametric methods described in this book fall into a unified theoretical framework known as **linear models**, where 'linear' means 'additive'. The idea is that the observed data can be explained by a model in which the effects of different influences are added. To return to the example of blood pressure given at the start of Chapter 3, a statistical model for blood pressure might include contributions relating to age, sex, race, smoking, time of day, and so on.

For most analyses described in this book the underlying statistical model is very simple and will not usually be described, but I shall introduce models explicitly in Chapters 11 and 12. However, two key ideas associated with statistical models will be apparent throughout. First, certain assumptions are made when we fit a model, and it is important to try to verify that these are reasonable. An obvious common example is the assumption that the data have an approximately Normal distribution, some form of which appears in nearly all of the models described in this book. Second, it is also important to consider two aspects of how well the model 'fits' the data. We need to check that there are no systematic discrepancies, and we must also consider how useful the model is at predicting a value for an individual. For example, many researchers have fitted models to try to predict birthweight from maternal characteristics and fetal measurements. Although many variables are known to be related to birthweight, models that include all known influences do not allow us to predict birthweight at all accurately for an individual baby. In a sense to be defined in Chapter 11, the models account for only 25–30% of the variability in birthweight. Here we see again the distinction between estimation and hypothesis testing. The variables in the model are significantly associated with birthweight, both individually and collectively, but the estimates of birthweight derived from the model are too imprecise to be clinically useful (although they may be epidemiologically useful).

## 8.8 ESTIMATION OR HYPOTHESIS TESTING?

Over the last 40 years there has been a dramatic surge in the use of statistical methods in medical research, with widespread use of hypothesis tests and a trend towards more complex methods of analysis. Nowadays few research papers do not include hypothesis tests, but unfortunately their use is often at the expense of any other interpretation of the data. In particular it is common to see the results of some comparison expressed solely as a P value, or even just as 'significant' or 'not significant'. While P values are informative they tell only part of the story, and need to be accompanied by more direct information about what was actually observed.

Some research is purely exploratory, for example looking for possible associations worthy of more detailed study, but for most research the results cannot be meaningfully interpreted from a pronouncement of 'statistically significant'. As discussed above, it is not necessarily true that such a result is clinically significant, nor is a non-significant finding necessarily ignorable. Quantification of the results by simple estimates is an essential part of the analysis of data. Whether a clinician will use a new treatment that reduces blood pressure or the frequency of migraines will depend on the *amount* of the reduction. It may also depend on how consistent the effect is. A drug that reduces everybody's incidence of migraines by 30% may be better than one which reduces the incidence by 50% for some patients but does nothing for others. A single number (the P value) cannot convey all the necessary information; the appropriate estimates and confidence intervals are needed too.

Most published research does include estimates of the effects of interest, and it has become standard practice to include P values, but until recently the use of confidence intervals was rare. Lately, however, there has been a welcome move by several leading medical journals towards encouraging or even requiring authors to present confidence intervals in conjunction with their main findings (see Gardner and Altman, 1989a).

### 8.8.1 Relation between confidence intervals and statistical significance

Different though hypothesis testing and confidence intervals may appear there is in fact a close relation between them. The P value will be less than 0.05 (i.e. 'significant') only when the 95% confidence interval does not include zero (or, more generally, the value specified in the null hypothesis). The reason for this relation is that both methods are based on similar aspects of the theoretical distribution of the test statistic. The same relation applies between the 99% confidence interval and the related significance test at the 1% level, and so on.

The confidence interval shows the uncertainty, or lack of precision, in the estimate of interest, and thus conveys more useful information than the P value. Because of the relation described above, by presenting a confidence interval we also indicate whether P is above or below the cut-off level of 5%. The presentation of both the actual P value and the confidence interval is desirable, but if only one is given the P value may be omitted – it is less important, and in any case can be gauged roughly from the confidence interval.

The issues discussed in this section are considered at greater length by Cox (1982) and Gardner and Altman (1989b).

## 8.9 STRATEGY FOR ANALYSING DATA

I strongly recommend that a computer, or at least a programmable calculator, is used for statistical analysis. Chapter 6 presented various advantages, but also some drawbacks, of using a computer. Section 6.6 gave a strategy for analysing data using a computer, although the principles are not specific to analysis by computer.

One aspect not covered in Chapter 6 was how to tell which is the appropriate method of analysing a set of data. Chapters 9 to 12 describe a large number of different methods of analysis. The titles of these chapters are descriptive of the problems tackled rather than the names of the methods:

| Chapter | Title |
|---|---|
| 9 | Comparing groups – continuous data |
| 10 | Comparing groups – categorical data |
| 11 | Relation between two continuous variables |
| 12 | Relation between several variables |

Chapters 9 and 10 cover analyses where you have a single variable of interest for one, two or more groups. Within these chapters the distinction is made between observations made on different groups of individuals and observations made on more than one occasion on the same individuals – 'paired data'. Chapters 11 and 12, in contrast, cover analyses where we are interested in the inter-relationship between two or more variables for a single group of individuals. Note that in most studies information on a large number of variables is collected, but the variables are analysed separately using the simpler techniques of Chapters 9 and 10. Chapter 12 gives guidance on when this is or is not a sensible approach.

Chapter 13 considers the analysis of survival times, which is a special case of the problems considered in Chapter 9, and requires special methods of analysis, and more general problems in the analysis of time-related data. Chapter 14 discusses some specific common problems in the analysis of medical data. For many of the methods described in these chapters both confidence intervals and hypothesis tests are presented.

## 8.10 PRESENTATION OF RESULTS

The methods introduced in this chapter recur in several subsequent chapters so some general comments on presentation of results may be helpful.

Estimates and confidence intervals should be treated in the same way as means and standard deviations (see section 3.7). The percentage coverage of confidence intervals should be stated.

Where possible give actual P values rather than ranges such as $P<0.05$. No more than two significant figures need be quoted, as in $P=0.14$, $P=0.012$, $P=0.001$. It is not usually necessary to specify P below, say, 0.0001. If you obtain P from tables then you will end up with a value between two limits, according to the values that are tabulated. We used the signs '<' (less than) and '>' (greater than) in expressions such as $P<0.05$ or $0.05>P>0.01$. It is conventional to use the shorter form $P<0.05$ when P is between 0.01 and 0.05, as it is assumed that if P was less than 0.01 you would have used $P<0.01$. For values of P greater than 0.05 it is useful to be more specific than $P>0.05$, for example by $P=0.15$

or $P > 0.2$. Do not use the abbreviation NS for not significant without defining the term (usually $P > 0.05$) and please do not use the appalling '$P = NS$'. It is generally assumed that P values are two-sided unless stated otherwise. The use of one-sided tests should always be noted (and justified).

## 8.11 SUMMARY

Analysing your own data and being able to evaluate the medical literature depend upon understanding the basic ideas behind statistical analysis as well as being familiar with the statistical methods used.

In this chapter I have discussed in detail the idea of a sampling distribution relating to a parameter of interest, such as a mean or a proportion. A major topic covered was the central limit theorem, by which the sampling distribution of the mean of a sample approaches a Normal distribution as the sample size increases, regardless of the shape of the distribution of the data in the population. This result underlies many of the methods described in subsequent chapters.

I have also introduced the two main approaches to statistical inference – estimation and hypothesis testing. The general principles outlined are fundamental to an appreciation of the remaining chapters of this book, and to understanding what statistical analysis and interpretation is all about. Published papers tend to present results in a shorthand way that can be opaque – for example as means and standard errors. It is important to know what can and cannot be inferred from these quantities, especially by constructing confidence intervals. Likewise, most published papers contain P values but the interpretation of them is often faulty. It is important to understand the true meaning of the P value, and to realize that statistical significance and clinical importance are not the same thing.

It may be helpful to re-read parts of this chapter after the next few chapters describing particular statistical methods.

## EXERCISES

8.1 There are two hospitals in a town. On average 45 babies are born each day in the larger hospital, and 15 in the smaller. The probability of a baby being a boy is about 0.52, and the probability of twins is about 0.012. On any day which hospital is more likely

(a) to have a set of twins delivered,
(b) to have more than 60% of babies being boys?
(No mathematics is required to answer these questions.)
(Based on Kahneman and Tversky, 1982)

8.2 Eight diabetic patients had plasma glucose levels (mmol/l) measured before and one hour after oral administration of 100 g glucose (Feingold *et al.*, 1989), with the following results

| Patient | Plasma glucose (mmol/l) Before | After | Change |
|---|---|---|---|
| 1 | 4.67 | 5.44 | 0.77 |
| 2 | 4.97 | 10.11 | 5.14 |
| 3 | 5.11 | 8.49 | 3.38 |
| 4 | 5.17 | 6.61 | 1.44 |
| 5 | 5.33 | 10.67 | 5.34 |
| 6 | 6.22 | 5.67 | −0.55 |
| 7 | 6.50 | 5.78 | −0.72 |
| 8 | 7.00 | 9.89 | 2.89 |

(a) Calculate the standard error of the mean change in plasma glucose.
(b) On the basis of these data, how many diabetic patients would need to be studied so that the width of the 95% confidence interval for the mean change in plasma glucose level was 0.5 mmol/l? (Assume that the Normal distribution is the appropriate sampling distribution for the change in plasma glucose.)

8.3 In a clinical trial in which a total of 100 patients are allocated to two treatments by simple randomization, show that the probability that the difference between the numbers of patients in the two treatment groups exceeds 20 is about 5%. (Hint: consider the distribution of the number of patients allocated to one of the groups.)

8.4 A controlled trial was performed to compare the corticosteroid prednisolone and placebo in patients with chronic active hepatitis positive for hepatitis B surface antigen (Lam *et al.*, 1981). In response to a letter criticizing the analysis the author wrote: 'The one-tailed test was used in the calculations, since in a previous analysis major complications were encountered significantly more frequently in the steroid-treated group' (Ng *et al.*, 1981). (This information had not been given in the original paper.)

Is this a valid justification for performing one-tailed tests? If not, why not?

# 9

# Comparing groups – continuous data

Good answers come from good questions not from esoteric analysis.
Schoolman *et al.*, (1968)

## 9.1 INTRODUCTION

We can now build on the ideas of the previous chapters to consider the main methods of data analysis. In particular we will use the ideas introduced in the previous chapter – estimation and hypothesis testing. Other important ideas are the relation between the analysis and the research design (Chapter 5) and the nature of the observations (Chapter 2).

This chapter deals with comparing groups of observations with respect to continuous data, starting with the simplest case where we wish to compare a single group of observations with some prespecified value, and moving through to the case where we have several sets of observations on each of a group of individuals. Both parametric and non-parametric approaches to analysis are introduced. Chapter 10 considers the same situations when the data are categorical.

## 9.2 CHOOSING AN APPROPRIATE METHOD OF ANALYSIS

When choosing an appropriate method of analysis there are several aspects of the data that we must consider, relating to the design of the study, the nature of the data, and the purpose of the analysis.

### 9.2.1 The number of groups of observations

Although methods of dealing with several groups of observations can be used for just one or two groups it is convenient to consider the one and two group cases separately, as the methods can be simplified, and there are fewer problems of interpretation. The two group case is the most common type of statistical analysis.

### 9.2.2 Independent or dependent groups of observations

When there are two or more sets of observations there are two types of design that must be distinguished:

1. The observations relate to **independent** groups of individuals. For example, we may have birthweights of boys and girls or groups of patients with different diseases. The sample size may vary from group to group.
2. Each set of observations is made on the same group of individuals. For example, we may have antenatal and postnatal blood pressure measurements from one group of women. We call such data **paired** to indicate that the observations are on the same individuals rather than from independent samples. Clearly we must have the same number of observations in each set of data.

Sometimes two different groups of subjects are studied where each person is **individually matched** with a member of the other group. Here the data are clearly linked and should be treated as if they are paired observations on one group.

### 9.2.3 The type of data

The distinction between continuous and categorical data was discussed in Chapter 2. There are several types of continuous data, however, and the nature of the observations has implications for statistical analysis. Specifically, parametric methods are based on calculating means and standard deviations, so they are inappropriate for ordered categorical data such as the Apgar score described in Chapter 2.

### 9.2.4 The distribution of data

For independent groups, parametric methods require the observations within each group to have an approximately Normal distribution, and the standard deviations in each group should be similar. If the raw data do not satisfy these conditions, a transformation may be successful (see Chapter 7). Otherwise a non-parametric method should be used.

For paired data relating to two or more observations on the same people there is no assumption that each set of observations should be Normally distributed, but there is a different assumption of Normality, discussed below.

### 9.2.5 The objective of the analysis

Both estimation and hypothesis testing are considered throughout this chapter. However, with three or more groups of data there are several possible comparisons between groups. The choice of which to investigate should follow directly from the objectives of the study.

## 9.3 THE *t* DISTRIBUTION

In the previous chapter I showed how to calculate confidence intervals and perform hypothesis tests based on the assumption that the estimates of interest, either means or proportions, had a Normal distribution. Because of the central limit theorem we know that this is a reasonable assumption for large samples, but not all samples are large (more than 100, say). In the analysis of continuous data the calculation of means plays a prominent part, and so we need to consider the distribution of the mean for smaller samples.

Early in this century it was shown by W. S. Gossett, writing under the name of 'Student', that the mean of a sample from a Normal distribution with unknown variance has a distribution that is similar to, but not quite the same as, a Normal distribution. He called it the ***t* distribution**, and we still refer to it as Student's *t* distribution. As the sample size increases the sampling distribution of the mean becomes closer to the Normal distribution. We use the *t* distribution for estimation and hypothesis testing relating to the means of one or two samples. Although we can use the Normal distribution for large samples there is little point in doing so, since for large samples the methods give virtually identical answers and it is simpler to use the same method regardless of the sample size.

The *t* distribution has one parameter, a quantity called the **degrees of freedom**. The concept of degrees of freedom is one of the more elusive statistical ideas. In general the degrees of freedom are calculated as the sample size minus the number of estimated parameters. The degrees of freedom for the *t* distribution relate to the estimated standard deviation, which is calculated as variation around the estimated mean. Hence for a single sample of $n$ observations we have $n - 1$ degrees of freedom.

Figure 9.1 shows the *t* distributions with 5 and 25 degrees of freedom, together with the Normal distribution. The latter is close to the Normal distribution, and as the sample size increases the *t* distribution becomes ever more Normal. The difference is most marked in the tails of the distributions, which is usually the part that we are interested in.

Nearly all the parametric methods introduced in this chapter, and most that follow, make use of the *t* distribution. In Chapter 8 I showed how we calculate a test statistic using the Normal distribution by taking the ratio of the quantity of interest to its standard error. We use the same method of calculation when using the *t* distribution. The only difference is that we look up the result in a table of the *t* distribution (Table B4) rather than the Normal distribution. Likewise, we use the *t* distribution to calculate confidence intervals.

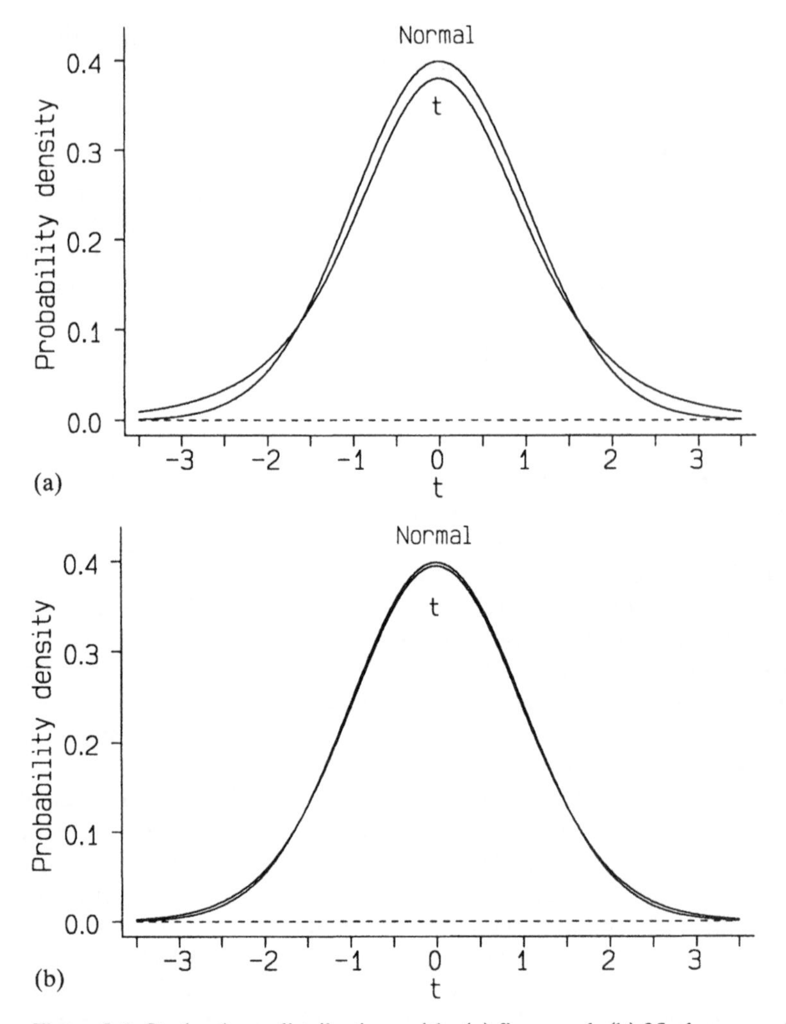


**Figure 9.1** Student's $t$ distribution with (a) five, and (b) 25 degrees of freedom, together with the standard Normal distribution.

This chapter deals first with three situations where we use the $t$ distribution – for one sample, paired samples, and two independent samples. Lastly, for the case with more than two samples we need the method called **analysis of variance**, for which we use the ***F* distribution** (introduced later) rather than the $t$ distribution. All these parametric methods make assumptions about Normality. Section 9.7 describes the analysis of skewed data by taking logarithms. Alternatively, non-parametric methods are available for all the problems discussed in this chapter, and are introduced within each section.

## 9.4 ONE GROUP OF OBSERVATIONS

The simplest case to consider is when we wish to compare the mean of a single group of observations with a specific value. Comparisons like this are not very common, but the methodology for this simple case gives a good introduction to the main methods of statistical inference. Sections 9.4.1 and 9.4.2 describe parametric methods, with the equivalent non-parametric methods described in sections 9.4.3 to 9.4.5.

As an example, suppose we wish to compare the mean dietary intake of a particular group of individuals with the recommended daily intake. Table 9.1 shows the average daily energy intake over ten days in 11 healthy women aged 22–30. Their mean daily intake was 6753.6 kJ. The small sample of observations shows no obvious skewness and may reasonably be taken as approximately Normal. Notice that each observation is itself an average value over several days. It is sometimes a good idea to take several values of a highly variable quantity. What can we say about the energy intake of these women in relation to a recommended daily intake of 7725 kJ?

**Table 9.1** Average daily energy intake (kJ) over 10 days of 11 healthy women (Manocha *et al.*, 1986)

| Subject | Average daily energy intake (kJ) |
|---|---|
| 1 | 5260 |
| 2 | 5470 |
| 3 | 5640 |
| 4 | 6180 |
| 5 | 6390 |
| 6 | 6515 |
| 7 | 6805 |
| 8 | 7515 |
| 9 | 7515 |
| 10 | 8230 |
| 11 | 8770 |
| Mean | 6753.6 |
| SD | 1142.1 |

### 9.4.1 Confidence interval for the mean

On average the 11 women had a daily energy intake below the recommended level of 7725 kJ, the average deficit being 7725 − 6753.6 = 971.4 kJ.

The standard deviation of the eleven daily intakes was 1142.1 kJ, so the standard error of the mean intake is $1142.1/\sqrt{11} = 344.4$ kJ. We use the $t$ distribution to calculate a confidence interval for the mean daily intake, following the principles outlined in section 8.4.5. For a 95% confidence interval we need the value of $t$ corresponding to a tail area of 0.05, denoted $t_{0.975}$, with $11 - 1 = 10$ degrees of freedom. From Table B4 the value of $t$ we need is 2.228. The 95% confidence interval for the mean intake is thus

$$6753.6 - 2.228 \times 344.4 \quad \text{to} \quad 6753.6 + 2.228 \times 344.4$$

or 5986 to 7521 kJ.

This range does not include the recommended level of 7725 kJ. If we assume that the women are a representative sample, then we can infer that for all women of this age average daily energy consumption is less than is recommended. The interpretation would, however, be unwise on the basis of such a small sample, especially without knowledge of how the sample was selected.

Similarly we can calculate a confidence interval for the energy deficit. The mean energy deficit was 971.4 kJ. The standard error of the mean deficit is the same as the standard error of the mean intake because subtracting a constant from each value of a distribution or set of observations does not affect the standard deviation. The 95% confidence interval for the energy deficit is thus obtained by subtracting 7725 from the confidence interval for the mean daily intake. Ignoring the negative sign, we get the 95% confidence interval for the energy deficit as 204 to 1739 kJ.

### 9.4.2 One sample *t* test

We can also carry out a test of the null hypothesis that our data are a sample from a population with a specific 'hypothesized' mean. The test is called the **one sample *t* test**, and the value of $t$ is calculated as

$$t = \frac{\text{sample mean} - \text{hypothesized mean}}{\text{standard error of sample mean}}$$

following the common form of hypothesis tests described in section 8.5. If the hypothetical population mean is some value $k$, we can rewrite the formula as

$$t = \frac{\bar{x} - k}{s/\sqrt{n}}$$

or

$$t = \frac{(\bar{x} - k)\sqrt{n}}{s}$$

where $\bar{x}$ and $s$ are the mean and standard deviation of the sample of size $n$. The magnitude of $t$ is thus the average discrepancy of the sample values from the hypothetical mean, divided by the standard error of the sample mean.

The mean and standard deviation of the dietary intake data were 6753.6 and 1142.1 kJ, and the hypothetical value of interest was the recommended intake of 7725 kJ. We can thus calculate the value of $t$ as

$$t = \frac{6753.6 - 7725}{1142.1/\sqrt{11}}$$
$$= -2.821.$$

We use Table B4 to find the P value associated with an observed value of $t$. We can ignore the sign of $t$ for a two-sided test, and look for the largest tabulated value of $t$ below our observed value, using 10 degrees of freedom. From Table B4 we get $P < 0.02$, so that the dietary intake of these women was significantly less than the recommended level using the usual criterion of $P < 0.05$. Notice that statistical significance gives no information about the magnitude of the energy deficit, nor the uncertainty of that estimate.

Note that we use $t$ to indicate the observed value of the test statistic and also a particular value from the theoretical $t$ distribution. For clarity I always use a subscript in the latter case. For many other statistical methods we use slightly different notation for these two purposes.

### 9.4.3 Confidence interval for the median

The methods using the $t$ distribution to calculate a confidence interval or perform a $t$ test require the data to be approximately Normally distributed. If the data are skewed or have some other non-Normal distribution we can base our inference on the median rather than the mean. The median energy intake in the 11 women was the 6th highest intake, which Table 9.1 shows was 6515 kJ. We can calculate a confidence interval for a sample median without making any assumptions about the distribution of the data. The data are ranked in ascending order, and the ranks of the values defining the confidence interval are found from a table such as that given in Table B11. From that table the 95% confidence interval for the median is given by the data values with ranks 2 and 10; that is, from 5470 to 8230 kJ.

For small samples the confidence interval for the median is rather wide, here being nearly twice as wide as the confidence interval for the mean given earlier. For larger samples of data that have a Normal distribution the mean and median will be very similar as will their confidence intervals (although that for the median will tend to be wider). It is preferable to use the median if the data are not near to Normal.

I shall describe two methods for carrying out a non-parametric hypothesis test for a single sample, the **sign test** and the **Wilcoxon signed rank sum test**.

### 9.4.4 Sign test

If there were no difference on average between the sample values and the hypothesized specific value we would expect an equal number of observations above and below the specific value. We can thus see how likely it would be to have observed our data when the null hypothesis is true by calculating the probability of our observed frequencies above and below the specific value. This is precisely the same type of problem as, for example, calculating the probability of observing given numbers of people in a sample who are in blood group B. We thus use the Binomial distribution, or the Normal approximation to it, to evaluate the probability of the observed frequencies when the true probability of exceeding the expected intake, $p$, is $\frac{1}{2}$.

In our example the hypothesized intake of interest was 7725 kJ. Two women had daily intakes above 7725 and nine were below. We use the general formula for a test statistic given in section 8.5:

$$\text{test statistic} = \frac{\text{observed value} - \text{hypothesized value}}{\text{standard error of observed value}}.$$

Here we are interested in the Binomial distribution with $p = \frac{1}{2}$ and $n = 11$. Our observed count is either $r = 2$ or $r = 9$ – it does not matter which we use because of the symmetry of the distribution when $p = \frac{1}{2}$. The expected count, assuming the null hypothesis is true, is $np = 11 \times \frac{1}{2} = 5.5$. From section 4.9, the standard error of $r$ is

$$\sqrt{np(1-p)} = \sqrt{11 \times \tfrac{1}{2} \times \tfrac{1}{2}} = 1.658.$$

We could use the exact Binomial distribution, but the Normal approximation to the Binomial is reasonable when $p = \frac{1}{2}$ even for small samples, and is simpler to use. We calculate the test statistic, $z$, as

$$\begin{aligned} z &= \frac{r - np}{\sqrt{np(1-p)}} \\ &= \frac{9 - 5.5}{1.658} \\ &= 2.11. \end{aligned}$$

From Table B2 the two-sided tail area of the Normal distribution corresponding to $z = 2.11$ is $P = 0.035$. If we had used $r = 2$, we would have arrived at $z = -2.11$, which would give the same two-sided P value. Thus the difference between the observed data and the recommended value is statistically significant at about the 3% level, and we infer that the average daily intake of these women really is lower than the recommended level.

Two further comments are needed in relation to the sign test. Firstly, it is preferable to incorporate a **continuity correction** into the test. We use the continuity correction in several circumstances when a continuous distribution is used as an approximation to non-continuous data, as is the case here. The adjustment involves reducing the difference between the observed count $r$ and the hypothesized value $np$ by $\frac{1}{2}$. We write this as $|r - np| - \frac{1}{2}$, where the vertical bars indicate that we take the **absolute** value of $r - np$; that is we ignore the sign if $r - np$ is negative. Recalculating our test statistic with the continuity correction gives

$$z = \frac{|r - np| - \frac{1}{2}}{\sqrt{np(1 - p)}}$$

$$= \frac{|9 - 5.5| - 0.5}{1.658}$$

$$= 1.81.$$

Inevitably the use of the continuity correction will reduce $z$ and increase P, but without the correction the calculations are a little too 'optimistic' in favour of rejecting the null hypothesis. Because we have a small sample the corrected value of $z$ is quite a lot smaller, but in large samples the effect is minimal. From Table B2 a $z$ value of 1.81 corresponds to a two-sided P value of 0.07, so that this more correct version of the test gives a result that is not quite significant at the 5% level. The continuity correction should always be used for small samples and can be incorporated routinely.

Secondly, if any of the observations is exactly the same as the hypothesized value then we ignore that observation in the calculation. Thus the sample size for the sign test is the number of observations that differ from the hypothesized value.

The sign test is one of the most basic of hypothesis tests, and occurs in different guises as the solution to other problems, most notably as the McNemar test for comparing paired proportions (section 10.7.5).

### 9.4.5 The Wilcoxon signed rank sum test

The sign test considers only whether each observation is above or below the chosen value of interest. It is preferable to take some account of the *magnitude* of the observations and we can do this by using the **Wilcoxon signed rank sum test**. The method has three steps:

1. calculate the difference between each observation and the value of interest;

2. ignoring the signs of the differences, rank them in order of magnitude;
3. calculate the sum of the ranks of all the negative (or positive) ranks, corresponding to the observations below (or above) the chosen hypothetical value.

Although this method makes no assumptions about the particular form of the distribution of the observations, it does assume that they come from a population with a symmetric distribution. This is not an important consideration for a single sample test (but see section 9.7.2).

For small samples (up to 25) P values can be obtained from Table B9. For larger samples the test statistic has an approximately Normal distribution, with mean $n(n + 1)/4$ and variance $n(n + 1)(2n + 1)/24$. As with the sign test, zero differences are omitted from the calculations, so in this formula $n$ is the number of non-zero differences, and so may be less than the sample size.

Table 9.2 shows the dietary intakes of 11 women from Table 9.1 together with the differences from the recommended intake. Also shown are the ranks of the differences, ignoring their signs. The sum of the ranks of the two observed intakes above the recommended 7725 kJ is $3 + 5 = 8$, so from Table B9 we get $P < 0.05$. We could equally well have used the sum of the ranks of the intakes below the recommended intake, which is $1.5 + 1.5 + 4 + 6 + 7 + 8 + 9 + 10 + 11 = 58$, which from Table B9 also gives $P < 0.05$. It is always worth checking that the ranks have been

**Table 9.2** Daily energy intake of 11 healthy women with rank order of differences (ignoring their signs) from the recommended intake of 7725 kJ

| Subject | Daily energy intake (kJ) | Difference from 7725 kJ | Ranks of differences |
|---|---|---|---|
| 1 | 5260 | 2465 | 11 |
| 2 | 5470 | 2255 | 10 |
| 3 | 5640 | 2085 | 9 |
| 4 | 6180 | 1545 | 8 |
| 5 | 6390 | 1335 | 7 |
| 6 | 6515 | 1210 | 6 |
| 7 | 6805 | 920 | 4 |
| 8 | 7515 | 210 | 1.5 |
| 9 | 7515 | 210 | 1.5 |
| 10 | 8230 | −505 | 3 |
| 11 | 8770 | −1045 | 5 |

calculated correctly, which is easy because the sum of all the ranks is $n(n+1)/2$. Here we have $11 \times 12/2 = 66$ and also $8 + 58 = 66$.

An important general point is that we do not expect different tests to give the same answer when applied to the same data. They do not make the same assumptions and use different aspects of the observations. In general, however, two valid methods will lead to similar answers. In small samples, however, non-parametric methods are rather lacking in power and so, as in the above example, will tend to give a less significant (larger) P value than the equivalent parametric test.

In practice we usually perform only one analysis of a set of data, choosing between parametric or non-parametric alternatives. We usually use a parametric method unless there is some clear indication that it is not valid, that is if the underlying assumptions are not met.

## 9.5 TWO GROUPS OF PAIRED OBSERVATIONS

When we have more than one group of observations it is vital to distinguish the case where the data are paired from that where the groups are independent. Paired data arise when the same individuals are studied more than once, usually in different circumstances. Also, when we have two different groups of subjects who have been *individually matched*, for example in a matched pair case-control study, then we should treat the data as paired.

The dietary intake data analysed in the previous section come from a study in which the 11 women recorded their dietary intake for 60 consecutive days. They were unaware that the purpose of the study was to compare intake on the pre- and post-menstrual days of the menstrual cycle. The data in Table 9.1 already analysed were pre-menstrual dietary intakes. Table 9.3 shows both the pre-menstrual and post-menstrual dietary intakes for one cycle for the same women, from which we see that each woman's post-menstrual average daily intake was lower than her pre-menstrual intake.

With paired data we are interested in the average difference between the observations for each individual and the variability of these differences. We are thus interested in the variability of the within-subject differences rather than between-subject variation. In general we are not particularly interested in variation between subjects, and indeed such variability may obscure the effects that we are interested in. The strength of the paired design is that we can remove between-subject variability by looking only at within-subject differences, and these thus form the basis for the method of analysis to be described. By looking at differences we effectively reduce the analysis to a one sample problem, so that we can use very similar methods to those discussed in the previous section. Because we treat the within-subject differences as a single sample, it is these differences which

**Table 9.3** Mean daily dietary intake over 10 pre-menstrual and 10 post-menstrual days (Manocha *et al.*, 1986)

| | Dietary intake (kJ) | | |
|---|---|---|---|
| Subject | Pre-menstrual | Post-menstrual | Difference |
| 1 | 5260 | 3910 | 1350 |
| 2 | 5470 | 4220 | 1250 |
| 3 | 5640 | 3885 | 1755 |
| 4 | 6180 | 5160 | 1020 |
| 5 | 6390 | 5645 | 745 |
| 6 | 6515 | 4680 | 1835 |
| 7 | 6805 | 5265 | 1540 |
| 8 | 7515 | 5975 | 1540 |
| 9 | 7515 | 6790 | 725 |
| 10 | 8230 | 6900 | 1330 |
| 11 | 8770 | 7335 | 1435 |
| Mean | 6753.6 | 5433.2 | 1320.5 |
| SD | 1142.1 | 1216.8 | 366.7 |

we require to have an approximately Normal distribution. There is no requirement for each set of data to be Normally distributed.

### 9.5.1 Confidence interval for the difference between means

Table 9.3 shows the difference in dietary intake between the pre- and post-menstrual days for each woman, and the mean and standard deviation of the differences. We can treat the differences as if they were a single sample of observations and use the methods introduced in section 9.4 for estimation and hypothesis testing.

Thus, we use the same $t$ value corresponding to a tail area of 0.05 with 10 degrees of freedom, which is $t_{0.975} = 2.228$. The standard deviation of the differences between the pre- and post-menstrual days is 366.7, so the standard error of the mean difference is $366.7/\sqrt{11} = 110.6$ kJ. The 95% confidence interval for the mean difference is thus

$$1320.5 - 2.228 \times 110.6 \quad \text{to} \quad 1320.5 + 2.228 \times 110.6$$

or 1074.2 to 1566.8 kJ. The whole confidence interval is much greater than zero, indicating that we can be reasonably sure that, in general, dietary intake is much lower in the post-menstrual period. Note that this confidence interval is considerably narrower than that for the mean pre-menstrual intake (5986 to 7521 kJ) because we have removed between-subject variability.

### 9.5.2 Paired *t* test

We can use the one sample $t$ test to calculate a P value for the comparison of means. Here we wish to compare the observed mean difference ($\bar{d}$) of 1320.5 kJ with a hypothetical value of zero, i.e. the null hypothesis is that pre- and post-menstrual dietary intake is the same. The $t$ value is then given by

$$t = \frac{\bar{d} - 0}{se(\bar{d})}$$

$$= 1320.5/110.6$$

$$= 11.94$$

on 10 degrees of freedom. From Table B4 we can see that 11.94 is much larger than the $P = 0.001$ value of the $t$ distribution, so that P is considerably less than 0.001. It will usually suffice to write $P < 0.001$. (The actual P value is in fact 0.0000003.)

### 9.5.3 Non-parametric methods

We can also apply the one sample sign test to the differences between paired observations. For the data in Table 9.3 all 11 differences have the same sign, so the test statistic, with the continuity correction, is

$$\frac{|11 - 5.5| - 0.5}{\sqrt{11 \times 0.5 \times 0.5}}$$

$$= 5/1.658$$

$$= 3.02$$

which, from Table B2, corresponds to $P = 0.003$.

We can also apply a Wilcoxon test to paired data, again by working directly on the differences for each individual. In this form the test is called the **Wilcoxon matched pairs signed rank sum test**. Rather than illustrate the test on the same dietary data, for which the result is clear cut, I shall look at the method on some new data in section 9.7.2, where a drawback of the Wilcoxon test is illustrated.

## 9.6 TWO INDEPENDENT GROUPS OF OBSERVATIONS

The most common statistical analyses are probably those used for comparing two independent groups of observations. Most clinical trials yield data of this type, as do observational studies comparing different groups of subjects. For continuous data we can again use either parametric or non-parametric methods, and these will be described in turn.

With paired data we treated the differences between paired observations as a single sample. The standard error of the mean difference, which was used for both the confidence interval and paired $t$ test, was based on the differences within each subject, and was thus unaffected by the variability between subjects.

With independent groups of observations we are again interested in the mean difference between the groups, but the variability between subjects becomes important. Both the confidence interval and the two sample $t$ tests are based on the assumption that each set of observations is sampled from a population with a Normal distribution, and that the variances of the two populations are the same. The assumption of Normality is familiar, and is dealt with in the same way as previously. The assumption of equal variances has not been met before. I shall show later how to examine this assumption formally, and discuss what to do when the sample variances are not similar.

### 9.6.1 Confidence interval for difference between means

The standard error of the mean of one group of observations is derived from the standard deviation of the data and hence from the variance. With two samples we are interested in the variance of the difference between the two means. It can be shown that the standard error we need is based on the average of the two variances, but giving more weight to the larger sample.

The required standard error is obtained from a more complicated formula than for the one sample case, but it involves only the mean, variance and sample size for each group. First we calculate the **pooled variance**, $s^2$, as

$$s^2 = \frac{(n_1 - 1)s_1^2 + (n_2 - 1)s_2^2}{n_1 + n_2 - 2}$$

where $s_1$ and $s_2$ are the standard deviations of the two groups of sizes $n_1$ and $n_2$. Using $\bar{x}_1$ and $\bar{x}_2$ to denote the means of the two samples, and $s$ as the pooled standard deviation, we have

$$se(\bar{x}_1 - \bar{x}_2) = s \times \sqrt{\frac{1}{n_1} + \frac{1}{n_2}}.$$

Each group contributes to the degrees of freedom associated with $s$, to give $n_1 + n_2 - 2$ degrees of freedom. Having acquired the standard error of the difference between the means we can produce a confidence interval. The 95% confidence interval for the difference between the means is given by

$$\bar{x}_1 - \bar{x}_2 \pm t_{0.975} \times se(\bar{x}_1 - \bar{x}_2)$$

where the value of $t$ has $n_1 + n_2 - 2$ degrees of freedom.

**Table 9.4** 24 hour total energy expenditure (MJ/day) in groups of lean and obese women (Prentice *et al.*, 1986)

| | Lean ($n$ = 13) | Obese ($n$ = 9) |
|---|---|---|
| | 6.13 | 8.79 |
| | 7.05 | 9.19 |
| | 7.48 | 9.21 |
| | 7.48 | 9.68 |
| | 7.53 | 9.69 |
| | 7.58 | 9.97 |
| | 7.90 | 11.51 |
| | 8.08 | 11.85 |
| | 8.09 | 12.79 |
| | 8.11 | |
| | 8.40 | |
| | 10.15 | |
| | 10.88 | |
| Mean | 8.066 | 10.298 |
| SD | 1.238 | 1.398 |

Table 9.4 shows the 24 hour energy expenditure of groups of lean and obese women. The obese group had a higher mean energy expenditure of 10.3 compared with 8.1 MJ/day for the lean group and the two standard deviations were very similar. The pooled standard deviation is

$$\sqrt{\frac{12 \times 1.238^2 + 8 \times 1.398^2}{20}}$$

$$= 1.3044 \text{ MJ/day.}$$

The standard error of the difference in mean intakes is given by

$$1.3044 \times \sqrt{\frac{1}{13} + \frac{1}{9}}$$

$$= 0.5656 \text{ MJ/day.}$$

The difference in the mean intakes of the two groups was 2.232 MJ/day. To construct the 95% confidence interval for the mean difference we need the value of $t_{0.975}$ on 20 degrees of freedom, which Table B4 shows is 2.086. The 95% confidence interval for the mean difference in 24 hour energy expenditure between obese and lean women is thus

$$2.232 - 2.086 \times 0.5656 \quad \text{to} \quad 2.232 + 2.086 \times 0.5656$$

or 1.05 to 3.41 MJ/day.

### 9.6.2 Two sample *t* test

There is also a *t* test appropriate for comparing two independent groups of data. The **two sample *t* test** looks much the same as the single sample or paired *t* tests, the statistic being obtained from

$$t = \frac{\bar{x}_1 - \bar{x}_2}{se(\bar{x}_1 - \bar{x}_2)}$$

and compared with the *t* distribution with $n_1 + n_2 - 2$ degrees of freedom. We have already calculated the standard error of the difference in the means as 0.5656 MJ/day, so we have $t = 2.232/0.5656 = 3.95$ on 20 degrees of freedom, giving $P < 0.001$. We can say that the total energy expenditure in the obese women was highly significantly greater than that of the lean women.

Virtually all statistical computer packages include the two sample *t* test, but unfortunately very few will do the calculations if you have already calculated the mean and standard deviation. Thus if you wish to calculate a confidence interval or *t* test using summary statistics from a published paper you will probably have to perform the calculations by hand, using the equations given in the previous section.

### 9.6.3 Confidence interval for difference between medians

There is a non-parametric method for constructing a confidence interval for the difference between the medians of two groups of observations. It requires the restrictive assumption that the samples are from populations with distributions that are identical in shape, and differ only by a shift in location. (It is thus also a non-parametric confidence interval for the difference between two means.) This method is not widely used and is rather complicated to carry out, so details are not given here. The method is described by Campbell and Gardner (1989).

### 9.6.4 Non-parametric comparison of two groups – the Mann-Whitney test

There is a non-parametric alternative to the *t* test for comparing data from two independent groups. There are two derivations of the test, one due to Wilcoxon and the other to Mann and Whitney. It is better to call the method the **Mann-Whitney test** to avoid confusion with the paired test also due to Wilcoxon, although some people refer to the test as the **Mann-Whitney-Wilcoxon test**.

The Mann-Whitney test requires all the observations to be ranked as if they were from a single sample. Then the sum of the ranks in one group is calculated and a P value found from Table B10. Table 9.5 shows the energy expenditure data treated in this way. The sums of the ranks in the

**Table 9.5** Calculations for the Mann-Whitney $U$ test on energy expenditure (EE) data (MJ/day) in Table 9.4

| Lean ($n$ = 13) | | Obese ($n$ = 9) | |
|---|---|---|---|
| Rank | EE | EE | Rank |
| 1 | 6.13 | | |
| 2 | 7.05 | | |
| 3.5 | 7.48 | | |
| 3.5 | 7.48 | | |
| 5 | 7.53 | | |
| 6 | 7.58 | | |
| 7 | 7.90 | | |
| 8 | 8.08 | | |
| 9 | 8.09 | | |
| 10 | 8.11 | | |
| 11 | 8.40 | | |
| | | 8.79 | 12 |
| | | 9.19 | 13 |
| | | 9.21 | 14 |
| | | 9.68 | 15 |
| | | 9.69 | 16 |
| | | 9.97 | 17 |
| 18 | 10.15 | | |
| 19 | 10.88 | | |
| | | 11.51 | 20 |
| | | 11.85 | 21 |
| | | 12.79 | 22 |
| Sum =103 | | | Sum = 150 |

two groups are 103 and 150. (We can check our calculations by noting that the sum of all ranks of $N$ observations must be $N(N + 1)/2$, which here is 253.) We can now use two alternative statistics, $T$ and $U$. The statistic $T$ (due to Wilcoxon) is simply the sum of the ranks in the smaller group, 150 in our example. (Either group can be taken if they are of the same size.) The statistic $U$ (due to Mann and Whitney) is more complicated, being calculated as

$$U = n_1 n_2 + \tfrac{1}{2} n_1(n_1 + 1) - T.$$

The advantage of using $U$ is that it is one of the few non-parametric statistics that has a useful interpretation. $U$ is the number of all possible pairs of observations comprising one from each sample, say $x_i$ and $y_j$, for which $x_i < y_j$. Thus if the sample sizes are $n_1$ and $n_2$ then $U/n_1 n_2$ is the proportion of all such pairs, and so is also the estimated probability that a new observation from the first population will be less than a new observation sampled from the second population. For analysis by computer the Mann-Whitney $U$ statistic is thus preferable because of its interpretation, but for hand calculation the Wilcoxon $T$ statistic is much easier to obtain.

For small samples it is possible to evaluate the observed value of the test statistic by considering the distribution of all the possible sums of ranks with samples of size $n_1$ and $n_2$. To take a simple example, if we have samples of sizes 2 and 5, there are only a small number of possible orderings of the seven observations. The ranks of the two values in the smaller group must be one of the following 21 combinations:

| | | | | | |
|---|---|---|---|---|---|
| 1,2 | 1,3 | 1,4 | 1,5 | 1,6 | 1,7 |
| | 2,3 | 2,4 | 2,5 | 2,6 | 2,7 |
| | | 3,4 | 3,5 | 3,6 | 3,7 |
| | | | 4,5 | 4,6 | 4,7 |
| | | | | 5,6 | 5,7 |
| | | | | | 6,7 |

Each combination yields a sum of ranks as follows

| | | | | | |
|---|---|---|---|---|---|
| 3 | 4 | 5 | 6 | 7 | 8 |
| | 5 | 6 | 7 | 8 | 9 |
| | | 7 | 8 | 9 | 10 |
| | | | 9 | 10 | 11 |
| | | | | 11 | 12 |
| | | | | | 13 |

If the null hypothesis is true, any one of these possibilities is equally likely because there is no difference between the groups. For any pair of sample sizes the same procedure can be used to get the distribution of possible rank sums, from which the probability of obtaining any particular rank sum (or a more extreme one) can be calculated. Thus we can calculate the range of values of the rank sum that is compatible with the null hypothesis at any level of significance. The P values thus obtained are known as *exact* probabilities. In the above example, an observed rank sum of 5 would correspond to an exact one-sided P value of 4/21, or 0.19, so that the two-sided P value is 0.38.

Table B10 gives these critical values of the statistic $T$, showing that with sample sizes of 9 and 13 the rank sum of 150 is outside the $P = 0.01$ range of expected rank sums under the null hypothesis but not outside the $P = 0.001$ range, so we write $P < 0.01$.

For larger samples of about ten or more in each group the statistic $T$ has an approximately Normal distribution with mean $\mu_T = n_S(n_S + n_L + 1)/2$ and standard deviation $\sigma_T = \sqrt{n_L \mu_T / 6}$, where $n_S$ and $n_L$ are the sample sizes in the smaller and larger group respectively. From these we can calculate the test statistic $z$ as $(T - \mu_T)/\sigma_T$ and refer to tables of the Normal distribution (Table B2).

It is reasonable to use the large sample approximation for the above example with sample sizes 9 and 13. The mean and standard deviation of the test statistic under the null hypothesis are given by

$$\mu_T = 9(9 + 13 + 1)/2 = 103.5$$

and

$$\sigma_T = \sqrt{13 \times 103.5/6} = 14.975$$

giving

$$z = \frac{150 - 103.5}{14.975}$$
$$= 3.105,$$

which, from Table B2, corresponds to P = 0.002. There is an equivalent large sample approximation for the statistic $U$; details are given by Bland (1987, p. 223).

The Mann-Whitney test as described is based on the assumption that there are no tied ranks. If there are many identical data values complicated corrections should be applied to the large sample formula. Computer packages ought automatically to adjust for tied ranks, but not all do.

Non-parametric methods in computer programs may use the large sample Normal approximation, even for small samples. For small samples it is advisable to check the calculated statistic (if given) against the appropriate table. However, it is not always clear which statistic is given. For example, in Minitab (release 6.1) $T$ is calculated for the first sample (not necessarily the smaller sample) but it is called $W$.

### 9.6.5 Unequal variances

Sometimes we wish to compare two groups of observations where the assumption of Normality is reasonable, but the variability in the two groups is markedly different. Two questions arise: how different do the variances have to be before we should not use the two sample $t$ test, and what can we do if this happens?

The $t$ test is known to be 'robust' in that it is little affected by moderate failure to meet the assumptions. It is not possible to say how different the variances in the two groups can be before we cannot use the $t$ test. However, the $t$ test is based on the assumption that the two population variances are the same, so we can test the null hypothesis that this is so, using the ***F* test**.

The $F$ test or **variance ratio test** is very simple. Under the null hypothesis that two Normally distributed populations have equal variances we expect the ratio of the two sample variances to have a sampling distribution known as the ***F* distribution**. The variance ratio is the ratio of the sample variances or the square of the ratio of the sample standard deviations. We calculate the variance ratio observed in our sample, by taking the larger standard deviation divided by the smaller, and look up the square of this value in Table B6. The distribution of the $F$ statistic has two values of degrees of freedom, one corresponding to each variance.

Table 9.6 shows serum thyroxine measurements from 16 infants diagnosed as hypothyroid. We wish to compare thyroxine levels in two groups defined by severity of symptoms, but the standard deviations are markedly different. The ratio of variances is $(37.48/14.22)^2 = 6.95$. We use Table B6 to compare 6.95 with the $F$ distribution with 6 and 8 degrees of freedom, the first value relating to the numerator (37.48) and the second to the denominator (14.22), and both being one less than the number of observations. Because we take the ratio of the larger variance to the smaller we consider only the upper tail of the $F$ distribution. We get $P < 0.01$, so it is unlikely that the two samples come from populations with the same variance.

We should not now use the two sample $t$ test to compare the two means. We could instead use the Mann-Whitney test, but we could also use a modification of the $t$ test for the case with unequal variances, known as the Welch test, which is not covered in this book (see Armitage and Berry, 1987, p. 110). If, however, the samples are large we can use the large sample Normal distribution methods described in section 8.4, for which there is no requirement that the groups have the same variance.

**Table 9.6** Serum thyroxine level (nmol/l) in 16 hypothyroid infants by severity of symptoms (Hulse *et al.*, 1979)

| | Slight or no symptoms ($n$ = 9) | Marked symptoms ($n$ = 7) |
|---|---|---|
| | 34 | 5 |
| | 45 | 8 |
| | 49 | 18 |
| | 55 | 24 |
| | 58 | 60 |
| | 59 | 84 |
| | 60 | 96 |
| | 62 | |
| | 86 | |
| Mean | 56.4 | 42.1 |
| SD | 14.22 | 37.48 |

## 9.7 ANALYSIS OF SKEWED DATA

The use of the $t$ test is based on the assumption that the data for each group (with independent samples) or the differences (with paired samples) have an approximately Normal distribution, and for the two sample case we also require the two groups to have similar variances. We sometimes find that at least one requirement is not met. When the data are skewed we can either use a non-parametric method, or try a transformation of the raw data.

The most useful transformation is the logarithmic transformation. It has the special property that it is possible to get a confidence interval for the difference between the groups that relates to the original data. No other transformation has this property. Fortunately taking logs is very often successful in removing skewness and also making variances more equal.

I shall illustrate the paired samples analysis using data from a study of

**Table 9.7** Numbers of $T_4$ and $T_8$ cells/mm$^3$ in blood samples from 20 patients in remission from Hodgkin's disease and 20 patients in remission from disseminated malignancies (Shapiro *et al.*, 1986)

| | Hodgkin's disease | | Non-Hodgkin's disease | |
|---|---|---|---|---|
| | $T_4$ | $T_8$ | $T_4$ | $T_8$ |
| | 396 | 836 | 375 | 340 |
| | 568 | 978 | 375 | 330 |
| | 1212 | 1678 | 752 | 627 |
| | 171 | 212 | 208 | 153 |
| | 554 | 670 | 151 | 101 |
| | 1104 | 1335 | 116 | 72 |
| | 257 | 272 | 736 | 449 |
| | 435 | 446 | 192 | 108 |
| | 295 | 262 | 315 | 177 |
| | 397 | 340 | 1252 | 575 |
| | 288 | 236 | 675 | 318 |
| | 1004 | 786 | 700 | 320 |
| | 431 | 311 | 440 | 200 |
| | 795 | 449 | 771 | 289 |
| | 1621 | 811 | 688 | 263 |
| | 1378 | 686 | 426 | 157 |
| | 902 | 412 | 410 | 140 |
| | 958 | 286 | 979 | 310 |
| | 1283 | 336 | 377 | 108 |
| | 2415 | 936 | 503 | 163 |
| Mean | 823.2 | 613.9 | 522.1 | 260.0 |
| SD | 566.4 | 397.9 | 293.0 | 154.7 |

lymphocyte abnormalities in patients in remission from Hodgkin's disease or diverse, disseminated malignancies (called the non-Hodgkin's disease group). There were 20 patients in each group, but no pairing between the groups. Table 9.7 shows the numbers of $T_4$ and $T_8$ cells per $mm^3$ in their blood. As well as the actual levels of $T_4$ and $T_8$ cells, the authors were particularly interested in the ratio of the numbers of $T_4$ cells (helper cells) to $T_8$ cells (suppressor cells), so the data are tabulated in ascending order of the ratio $T_4/T_8$ within each group. Table 9.7 also shows the mean and standard deviation of each group of observations. The standard deviations are all greater than half the mean, strongly suggesting (for variables where negative values are impossible) that the data are skewed. Also the standard deviations are larger for the larger means, which suggests that a log

| Lower limit of interval | Hodgkin's disease (n=20) $T_4$ | $T_8$ | Non-Hodgkin's disease (n=20) $T_4$ | $T_8$ |
|---|---|---|---|---|
| 0 | * | | *** | ********* |
| 200 | ***** | ******** | ***** | ******** |
| 400 | **** | *** | **** | ** |
| 600 | * | *** | ****** | * |
| 800 | ** | **** | * | |
| 1000 | ** | | | |
| 1200 | *** | * | * | |
| 1400 | | | | |
| 1600 | * | * | | |
| 1800 | | | | |
| 2000 | | | | |
| 2200 | | | | |
| 2400 | * | | | |
| Mean | 823.2 | 613.9 | 522.1 | 260.0 |
| SD | 566.4 | 397.9 | 293.0 | 154.7 |

**Figure 9.2** Histograms of $T_4$ and $T_8$ (cells/$mm^3$) in 20 patients in remission from Hodgkin's disease and 20 patients in remission from disseminated malignancies (non-Hodgkin's disease).

| Lower limit of interval | Hodgkin's disease (n=20) log $T_4$ | log $T_8$ | Non-Hodgkin's disease (n=20) log $T_4$ | log $T_8$ |
|---|---|---|---|---|
| 4.0 | | | | * |
| 4.5 | | | * | **** |
| 5.0 | * | * | *** | ***** |
| 5.5 | ***** | ****** | **** | ******* |
| 6.0 | **** | *** | **** | *** |
| 6.5 | **** | ******* | ******* | |
| 7.0 | ***** | ** | * | |
| 7.5 | * | | | |
| Mean | 6.49 | 6.24 | 6.09 | 5.39 |
| SD | 0.708 | 0.613 | 0.632 | 0.600 |

**Figure 9.3** Histograms of $\log_e T_4$ and $\log_e T_8$.

transformation may be successful both in removing skewness and making the variability more similar.

Figure 9.2 shows histograms of the raw data, clearly showing the skewness and unequal scatter. Figure 9.3 shows the success of the log transformation in producing data that are plausibly Normal and have similar standard deviations. Some of these data were shown graphically in Figure 7.1. Figure 9.4 shows that log transformation has also made the $T_4 - T_8$ differences more Normal, especially in the non-Hodgkin's disease group.

(a) Raw data

| Lower limit of interval | Hodgkin's disease (n=20) $T_4$-$T_8$ | Non-Hodgkin's disease (n=20) $T_4$-$T_8$ |
|---|---|---|
| -600 | *** | |
| -400 | * | |
| -200 | **** | |
| 0 | **** | ******** |
| 200 | ** | ******** |
| 400 | * | ** |
| 600 | ** | ** |
| 800 | ** | |
| 1000 | | |
| 1200 | | |
| 1400 | * | |
| Mean | 209.0 | 262.0 |
| SD | 506.0 | 197.7 |

(b) Log data

| Lower limit of interval | Hodgkin's disease | Non-Hodgkin's disease |
|---|---|---|
| -0.75 | ** | |
| -0.50 | * | |
| -0.25 | ***** | |
| 0.00 | **** | *** |
| 0.25 | * | **** |
| 0.50 | *** | ** |
| 0.75 | ** | ******* |
| 1.00 | * | *** |
| 1.25 | * | * |
| Mean | 0.25 | 0.69 |
| SD | 0.569 | 0.356 |

**Figure 9.4** Histograms of (a) $T_4 - T_8$ and (b) $\log_e T_4 - \log_e T_8$.

### 9.7.1 Parametric analysis

*(a) Confidence Interval*

We can use the paired $t$ test to compare the logs of the numbers of $T_4$ and $T_8$ cells in the Hodgkin's disease group and calculate a confidence interval, using the methods given earlier. From Figure 9.4 the mean and standard deviation of the differences between the $\log_e T_4$ and $\log_e T_8$ counts are 0.25 and 0.569, so the standard error of the mean is $0.569/\sqrt{20} = 0.127$. The value of $t_{0.975}$ on 19 degrees of freedom is 2.093, so the 95% confidence interval for the mean difference between $\log T_4$ and $\log T_8$ cell counts in patients with Hodgkin's disease is given by

$$0.25 - 2.093 \times 0.127 \quad \text{to} \quad 0.25 + 2.093 \times 0.127$$

or $-0.016$ to 0.516.

This confidence interval is for $\log T_4 - \log T_8$, but we are usually more interested in a confidence interval relating to the scale of the original data. We can do this because the difference between the logarithms of two values is exactly the same as the logarithm of their ratio, i.e. $\log X - \log Y = \log(X/Y)$. It follows that the antilog of the mean of the log differences will be an estimate of the geometric mean of the ratio of the variables. The mean value of $\log T_4 - \log T_8$ was 0.25, so that the geometric mean of $T_4/T_8$ is given by $e^{0.25} = 1.28$. Further, we can 'back-transform' our confidence interval for the mean log difference to get a confidence interval for the geometric mean of the ratio $T_4/T_8$. The 95% confidence interval becomes $e^{-0.016}$ to $e^{0.516}$, or 0.98 to 1.67. Thus we can be 95% sure that on average the ratio of $T_4$ to $T_8$ blood cell counts in patients in remission from Hodgkin's disease is between 0.98 to 1.67, with 1.28 as our best estimate.

It is very reasonable to express results for skewed data in terms of ratios. Indeed, it was the $T_4/T_8$ ratio that the researchers (Shapiro *et al.*, 1986) were interested in. Although not in the original units, the back-transformed confidence interval for the ratio is directly related to the original data in an easily interpretable way. No other transformation of data other than taking logs allows back-transformation. Confidence intervals in transformed units are not easily interpretable, so it is a major disadvantage of other transformations, such as taking square roots, that it is not possible to obtain meaningful confidence intervals.

*(b) Paired t test*

The paired $t$ test of the log $T_4$ and $T_8$ data gives $t = 0.25/0.127 = 1.97$ for which we have $P = 0.07$. The data thus suggest that $T_8$ cell counts are lower than $T_4$ among patients in remission from Hodgkin's disease, although the difference is not quite significant at the 5% level.

*(c) Comment*

A similar approach is used for comparing independent groups. For example, $T_4$ counts in the two groups of patients are compared using the confidence interval and two sample $t$ test described in sections 9.6.1 and 9.6.2. The principle of analysing skewed data by taking logs applies equally to more complex analyses described later in this chapter and in subsequent chapters. It will not be illustrated for each method.

### 9.7.2 Non-parametric analysis

The non-parametric equivalent of the paired $t$ test is the **Wilcoxon matched pairs signed rank sum test**, which we can use to perform a non-parametric analysis of the raw $T_4$ and $T_8$ data given in Table 9.7. This test is identical to the one-sample Wilcoxon signed rank sum test described in section 9.4.5, where we treat the differences between the paired values as our sample for calculating the ranks. The calculations are shown in Table 9.8. We can look up either the sum of the ranks of negative differences (63) or positive differences (147) in Table B9, giving $P > 0.10$.

**Table 9.8** Calculations for Wilcoxon matched pairs signed rank sum test to compare $T_4$ and $T_8$ cell counts in the Hodgkin's disease group

| Difference $T_4 - T_8$ (cells/mm$^3$) | Absolute difference $T_4 - T_8$ | Rank |
|---|---|---|
| −440 | 440 | 13 |
| −410 | 410 | 12 |
| −466 | 466 | 14 |
| −41 | 41 | 4 |
| −116 | 116 | 7 |
| −231 | 231 | 10 |
| −15 | 15 | 2 |
| −11 | 11 | 1 |
| 33 | 33 | 3 |
| 57 | 57 | 6 |
| 52 | 52 | 5 |
| 218 | 218 | 9 |
| 120 | 120 | 8 |
| 346 | 346 | 11 |
| 810 | 810 | 18 |
| 692 | 692 | 17 |
| 490 | 490 | 15 |
| 1479 | 1479 | 20 |
| 672 | 672 | 16 |
| 947 | 947 | 19 |

Sum of ranks of negative differences = 63
Sum of ranks of positive differences = 147

**Table 9.9** Calculations for Wilcoxon matched pairs test to compare $\log T_4$ and $\log T_8$

| Difference $\log T_4 - \log T_8$ | Absolute difference | Rank | Rank of raw data |
|---|---|---|---|
| −0.747 | 0.747 | 16 | 13 |
| −0.543 | 0.543 | 12 | 12 |
| −0.325 | 0.325 | 10 | 14 |
| −0.215 | 0.215 | 8 | 4 |
| −0.190 | 0.190 | 5.5 | 7 |
| −0.190 | 0.190 | 5.5 | 10 |
| −0.057 | 0.057 | 2 | 2 |
| −0.025 | 0.025 | 1 | 1 |
| 0.119 | 0.119 | 3 | 3 |
| 0.155 | 0.155 | 4 | 6 |
| 0.199 | 0.199 | 7 | 5 |
| 0.245 | 0.245 | 9 | 9 |
| 0.326 | 0.326 | 11 | 8 |
| 0.571 | 0.571 | 13 | 11 |
| 0.693 | 0.693 | 14 | 18 |
| 0.698 | 0.698 | 15 | 17 |
| 0.784 | 0.784 | 17 | 15 |
| 0.948 | 0.948 | 18 | 20 |
| 1.209 | 1.209 | 19 | 16 |
| 1.340 | 1.340 | 20 | 19 |

Sum of ranks of negative differences = 60
Sum of ranks of positive differences = 150

It is a peculiarity of the Wilcoxon matched pairs test that, alone among the commonly used non-parametric methods, the result can be affected by transforming the data. If we take logs of $T_4$ and $T_8$ before calculating the ranks of the differences we may get a different result. Because of this possibility some statisticians reject this test in favour of the sign test, while others suggest that the data *should* be transformed if the raw data show larger differences for larger data values, as shown by a plot of $X - Y$ against $(X + Y)/2$. In fact, as noted for the single sample test (section 9.4.5), the method is based on the assumption that the differences have a symmetric distribution. A transformation should therefore be used only if it makes the distribution of the differences more symmetric.

Figure 9.4 showed that the distributions of the differences $T_4 - T_8$ are skewed, while those for $\log T_4 - \log T_8$ are more symmetric. Table 9.9 shows the differences between the log values and the Wilcoxon test applied to $\log T_4$ and $\log T_8$. The rank sums are slightly different from those obtained before, but the P value of 0.10 is a similar result in this case. However, comparison of the ranks obtained from the log data and from the raw data (in Table 9.9) shows that there are some quite substantial differences in the rankings for individual patients. Because the Wilcoxon test is based on the assumption of symmetry of the differences between pairs of observations, it is preferable for these data to use the log transformation.

The use of transformations in conjunction with non-parametric methods is unappealing to some people, who feel that the sign test is probably the preferable non-parametric method for analysing paired data. Not all non-parametric or distribution-free methods are completely free of assumptions about the distribution, however, and the Wilcoxon paired test is preferable to the sign test when the assumption of symmetry is plausible.

## 9.8 THREE OR MORE INDEPENDENT GROUPS OF OBSERVATIONS

Most of this chapter so far has related to the analysis of two sets of observations, either paired data for a single sample of individuals or data from two independent samples. These ideas extend to situations where we have three or more sets of observations, either from a single sample or from independent samples. In this section I shall consider only independent groups. The case where several measurements are taken on each individual in a single sample is considered in Chapter 12.

With several groups of observations it is obviously possible to compare each pair of groups using $t$ tests, but this is not a good approach. It is far better to use a single analysis that enables us to look at all the data in one go, and the method we use is called **one way analysis of variance** (sometimes abbreviated to **anova**). The methods introduced in this section, both parametric and non-parametric, can all be used when there are only two groups of observations and will give identical results to the two sample methods already described. The two sample $t$ test is, for example, a special case of one way analysis of variance. As its name implies, one way analysis of variance is the simplest type which is used when there is a single way of classifying individuals. When there are two factors classifying the observations we need two way analysis of variance, and so on. Some more complicated analyses are described in section 12.3.

The analyses covered in this section are better done by computer – we are reaching the limit of what is practicable for 'hand calculation'. Although the formulae will be given for the methods described in this section and in some subsequent chapters, the mathematical details will mostly be in separate sections, and I shall assume that a computer is used for the main analysis.

### 9.8.1 One way analysis of variance

The principle behind analysis of variance is to partition the total variability of a set of data into components due to different sources of variation. For example, the variability of the energy expenditure data in Table 9.4 could be partitioned into that due to variation between individuals *within each group*, and that due to any systematic difference *between the groups*. Indeed, because our null hypothesis is that there is no difference between the groups, the test is based on a comparison of the observed variation between the groups (i.e. between their means) with that expected from the observed variability between subjects. The comparison takes the general form of an $F$ test to compare variances, but for two groups the $t$ test leads to exactly the same answer. The samples do not all have to be the same size.

Analysis of variance should preferably be performed using a statistical computer package, but the method of calculation is given in section 9.9. A statistical package will produce the numerical results, but it is important to understand the principles involved.

1. The analysis is based on the assumption that the samples come from Normally distributed populations with the same standard deviation (or variance). Normality and equal variance should not be assumed, but should be verified, as described in (5) below.
2. Because we assume that the samples are from populations with the same variance, the variance within each group is an estimate of the population variance. We thus pool the sample variances (in the same way as we did for the two sample $t$ test) to get an estimate of the population variance.
3. We can use the pooled estimate of variance to calculate a confidence interval for the difference between any pair of means.
4. We can perform a hypothesis test based on the null hypothesis that the samples are from populations with the same mean and variance. We can thus compare the variation among the observed sample means with what we would expect from random samples if the null hypothesis was true. In other words, we can calculate the probability of observing such variability among means of samples drawn at random from the same population. The comparison takes the form of the ratio of the variance estimated from the means of the groups (the *between* group variation) and the variance between the individuals *within* the groups. As we saw earlier, we use tables of the $F$ distribution to test the equality of two variances.
5. After carrying out the analysis of variance we should examine the variation of the individual observations around the mean of their sample. For each individual the mean of their group is the value fitted by the model, and the difference between the observed and fitted values

is called a **residual**. It is the variance of these residuals that we use as our estimate of between subject variability, against which we evaluate the between group variance. We can construct a Normal plot of the residuals to assess the assumption of Normality. If the Normal plot is unsatisfactory, we must reanalyse the data, perhaps after transforming the data or by using a non-parametric alternative.

Another way of viewing the hypothesis test associated with analysis of variance is that we are comparing two alternative statistical models. In one the mean and standard deviation are the same in each population, while in the other the means are different (and equal to the observed sample means) but the standard deviations are again the same. The $F$ test assesses the plausibility of the first model. If the between group variability is greater than expected (with, say, $P < 0.05$) we will prefer the second model, in which the means of the groups differ.

If we have only two groups the analysis of variance is exactly equivalent to the $t$ test for two independent groups. Thus the $F$ test yields the same P value as the $t$ test. The numerator in the variance ratio has just one degree of freedom and we have the relation $F = t^2$, as can be seen from Tables B4 and B6.

### 9.8.2 Example

Twenty-two patients undergoing cardiac bypass surgery were randomized to one of three ventilation groups:

Group I Patients received a 50% nitrous oxide and 50% oxygen mixture continuously for 24 hours;

Group II Patients received a 50% nitrous oxide and 50% oxygen mixture only during the operation;

Group III Patients received no nitrous oxide but received 35–50% oxygen for 24 hours.

Table 9.10 shows red cell folate levels for the three groups after 24 hours' ventilation. We wish to compare the three groups, and test the null hypothesis that the three groups have the same red cell folate levels.

Examination of the data does not reveal any obvious outliers and the data in each group look plausible samples from a Normal distribution. These attributes are more easily seen from Figure 9.5 than Table 9.10. The standard deviation in group I is rather higher than those in the other groups, but moderate variability is not a problem, especially when the samples are small. In general, however, the assumption that the groups come from populations with the same variance is important. **Bartlett's test** is an extension of the $F$ test (described in section 9.6.5) for assessing the null hypothesis that more than two samples come from populations with

**Table 9.10** Red cell folate levels ($\mu$g/l) in three groups of cardiac bypass patients given different levels of nitrous oxide ventilation (Amess *et al.*, 1978)

| | Group I ($n$ = 8) | Group II ($n$ = 9) | Group III ($n$ = 5) |
|---|---|---|---|
| | 243 | 206 | 241 |
| | 251 | 210 | 258 |
| | 275 | 226 | 270 |
| | 291 | 249 | 293 |
| | 347 | 255 | 328 |
| | 354 | 273 | |
| | 380 | 285 | |
| | 392 | 295 | |
| | | 309 | |
| Mean | 316.6 | 256.4 | 278.0 |
| SD | 58.7 | 37.1 | 33.8 |

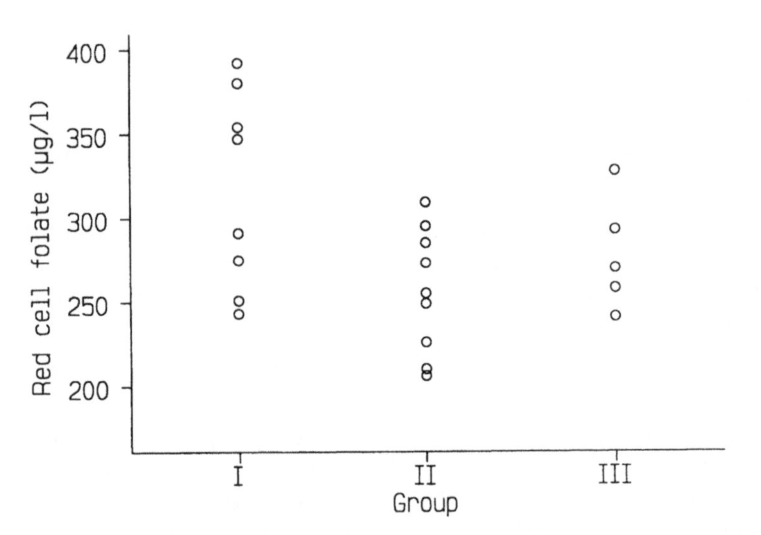


**Figure 9.5** Red cell folate levels in three groups of cardiac bypass patients (data in Table 9.10).

the same variance. Some computer programs incorporate this test, although it is not very powerful (see Armitage and Berry (1987, p. 209) for details).

The analysis of variance calculations are shown in Table 9.11. The total variability of the data set is measured by the **total sum of squares**, which is

**Table 9.11** Analysis of variance table for data in Table 9.10

| Source of variation | Degrees of freedom | Sums of squares | Mean squares | $F$ | P |
|---|---|---|---|---|---|
| Between groups | 2 | 15 515.88 | 7757.9 | 3.71 | 0.04 |
| Within groups | 19 | 39 716.09 | 2090.3 | | |
| Total | 21 | 55 231.97 | | | |

based on the sum of the squares of the differences of each of the 22 observations from the overall mean. This total is partitioned into (a) the **within groups** sum of squares, calculated as the sum of squares of the difference between each observation and the mean of its relevant group, and (b) the **between groups** sum of squares, which is based on the sum of squares of the difference between the mean of each group and the overall mean. Each sum of squares is converted into an estimated variance (known as a **mean square**) by dividing by its degrees of freedom. Following the usual principle that the degrees of freedom for a variance are one less than the number of observations, there are $3-1=2$ degrees of freedom between groups and $7+8+4=19$ degrees of freedom within groups. As Table 9.11 shows, the sums of squares and degrees of freedom add up to the values that are obtained if we consider the data as a single sample.

Under the null hypothesis that all the groups have the same mean and variance we expect the between groups variance and the within groups variance to be the same, so we expect the ratio of the variances to be 1. We can use the $F$ distribution to compare the variances and so evaluate the null hypothesis. The two variances are 7757.9 and 2090.3, and their ratio is 3.71. In other words, the observed variance among the groups is 3.71 times what we would expect if the null hypothesis were true. Comparing 3.71 with the $F$ distribution with 2 and 19 degrees of freedom given in Table B6, we find $P < 0.05$. (A more exact value is $P = 0.04$.)

A last point to note from Table 9.11 is that the square root of the within group mean square is called the residual standard deviation ($s_{res}$) because it is the standard deviation of the residuals. The residual standard deviation is also the pooled within groups standard deviation (analogous to that calculated for the two sample $t$ test) from which we can derive confidence intervals.

### 9.8.3 Confidence intervals

A confidence interval can be constructed for the mean of any group in the usual way, except that the standard error we use is based on the residual standard deviation. Thus, if there are $n_1$ observations in the group of interest with a mean of $\bar{x}_1$, the standard error of the mean is given by

$$se(\bar{x}_1) = s_{res}/\sqrt{n_1}\,.$$

The 95% confidence interval is given by

$$\bar{x}_1 - t_{0.975} \times se(\bar{x}_1) \quad \text{to} \quad \bar{x}_1 + t_{0.975} \times se(\bar{x}_1)$$

where the $t$ value has the number of degrees of freedom associated with the residual in the analysis of variance table.

Similarly, a confidence interval for the difference between any two means, say $\bar{x}_1$ and $\bar{x}_2$, requires the standard error of $\bar{x}_1 - \bar{x}_2$, which is given by

$$se(\bar{x}_1 - \bar{x}_2) = s_{res} \times \sqrt{\frac{1}{n_1} + \frac{1}{n_2}}.$$

The 95% confidence interval for the difference between the two means is thus given by

$$(\bar{x}_1 - \bar{x}_2) - t_{0.975} \times se(\bar{x}_1 - \bar{x}_2) \quad \text{to} \quad (\bar{x}_1 - \bar{x}_2) + t_{0.975} \times se(\bar{x}_1 - \bar{x}_2)$$

where the $t$ value again has the residual degrees of freedom.

For example, we can produce a confidence interval for the difference between groups I and II in Table 9.10. The difference in mean red cell folate levels was $316.6 - 256.4 = 60.2$ μg/l. The residual standard deviation is $\sqrt{2090.3} = 45.72$, so the standard error of the difference in means is $45.72 \times \sqrt{\frac{1}{8} + \frac{1}{9}} = 22.22$. The value of $t_{0.975}$ with 19 degrees of freedom is found (from Table B4) to be 2.093, so the 95% confidence interval for the difference in means is

$$60.2 - 2.093 \times 22.22 \quad \text{to} \quad 60.2 + 2.093 \times 22.22$$

or 13.7 to 106.7 μg/l.

### 9.8.4 Multiple comparisons

With two groups the interpretation of a significant difference is reasonably straightforward, but how do we interpret significant variation among the means of three or more groups? Further analysis is required to find out how the means differ, for example whether one group differs from all the others. If the groups have a clear ordering, for example when different doses of a drug are compared, there is a straightforward approach which will be described in the next section. When the groups are not ordered, however, there is no clearly best approach to investigate variation among the groups. Note that you should only investigate differences between individual groups when the overall comparison of groups in the analysis of variance is significant unless certain comparisons were intended in advance of the analysis.

One possibility is to compare each pair of means in turn, or perhaps just those pairs of interest. The difficulty here is that multiple significance testing gives a high probability of finding a significant difference just by chance. Each test has a 5% chance of a false positive result when there is no real difference (a Type I error) so if we have, say, four groups and perform all six paired tests the probability of at least one false positive result is very much greater than 5%. Several methods have been proposed to deal with this problem, with strange names such as Bonferroni, Newman-Keuls, Duncan and Scheffé. Each method is aimed at controlling the overall Type I error rate at no more than 5% (or some other specified level).

The disadvantage of all of these methods is that they are 'conservative', in that they err on the side of safety (non-significance). It can be disconcerting to find that, although the $F$ test in the analysis of variance is statistically significant, no pair of means is significantly different.

There is no simple nor totally satisfactory solution to these problems, but I recommend the following strategy when the groups do not have any natural order:

1. Decide in advance of the analysis which groups you are particularly interested in comparing (the fewer the better);
2. Perform modified $t$ tests to compare the pairs of groups of interest, using the Bonferroni (or some other) method to adjust the P values.

The modified $t$ test is based on the pooled estimate of variance from *all* the groups (which is the residual variance in the anova table), not just the pair being considered. So $t$ is calculated as

$$t = \frac{\bar{x}_1 - \bar{x}_2}{se(\bar{x}_1 - \bar{x}_2)}$$

where $se(\bar{x}_1 - \bar{x}_2)$ is as given in the previous section.

If we perform $k$ paired comparisons, then we should multiply the P value obtained from each test by $k$; that is, we calculate $P' = kP$ with the restriction that $P'$ cannot exceed 1. This simple adjustment is known as the **Bonferroni method**. For small numbers of comparisons (say up to five) its use is reasonable, but for large numbers it is highly conservative. However, I do not recommend that large numbers of comparisons are performed, which would suggest poorly specified research objectives. Statistical packages may offer different multiple comparison procedures, such as **Duncan's multiple range test**. These all work in a similar way, but are less conservative than the Bonferroni method.

Returning to the red cell folate data in Tables 9.10 and 9.11, the residual standard deviation was $\sqrt{2090.3} = 45.72$. A modified $t$ test to compare groups I and II is performed by calculating

$$t = \frac{316.6 - 256.4}{45.72 \times \sqrt{\frac{1}{8} + \frac{1}{9}}}$$
$$= 2.71 \text{ on 19 degrees of freedom.}$$

If we are comparing each pair of groups we will make three comparisons. The above $t$ value of 2.71 corresponds to $P < 0.02$ (Table B4), with an exact value of $P = 0.014$. The corrected P value is $P' = 0.014 \times 3 = 0.042$ so it is just significant at the 5% level after adjustment. Neither of the other comparisons is significant. The main explanation for the difference between the groups that was identified in the analysis of variance (Table 9.11) is thus the difference between groups I and II.

### 9.8.5 Ordered groups

When the groups are ordered it is not reasonable to compare each pair of groups, but rather we should study the possibility that there is a trend across groups. For many purposes it will suffice to consider whether there is a *linear* trend.

Table 9.12 shows the mean and standard deviation of serum trypsin levels in healthy volunteers divided into six age groups. We can carry out one way analysis of variance from these summary statistics without having the raw observations, using the formulae given in section 9.9, to get the results shown in Table 9.13. (Unfortunately, very few statistical packages

**Table 9.12** Serum levels of immunoreactive trypsin in healthy volunteers divided into six age groups (based on data given by Koehn and Mostbeck, 1981)

| | Age | | | | | |
|---|---|---|---|---|---|---|
| | 10–19 | 20–29 | 30–39 | 40–49 | 50–59 | 60–69 |
| Number of subjects | 32 | 137 | 38 | 44 | 16 | 4 |
| Mean (ng/ml) | 128 | 152 | 194 | 207 | 215 | 218 |
| Standard deviation (ng/ml) | 50.9 | 58.5 | 49.3 | 66.3 | 60.0 | 14.0 |

**Table 9.13** One way analysis of variance of data in Table 9.12

| Source of variation | df | Sums of squares | Mean squares | $F$ | P |
|---|---|---|---|---|---|
| Between groups | 5 | 224 103 | 44 820.6 | 13.5 | < 0.0001 |
| Within groups | 265 | 879 272 | 3 318.0 | | |
| Total | 270 | 1 103 375 | | | |

will perform analysis of variance using means and standard deviations that are already calculated.) Clearly there is highly significant variation among the six age groups. However, we can go further by 'partitioning' the variability between groups into components. Here we would be more interested in whether there was a linear trend, that is whether serum trypsin values tend to rise at a constant rate with increasing age.

Using the formula given in section 9.9 we find that the sum of squares associated with a linear trend is 55 147 on one degree of freedom, so the analysis of variance table can be rewritten as shown in Table 9.14. There is a highly significant linear trend, showing that mean serum trypsin level rises with age. However, the non-linear variation between the age groups is also highly significant, indicating that the linear trend only explains some of the age effect. Fitting a linear trend in one way analysis of variance is equivalent to linear regression analysis, which is described in Chapter 11.

**Table 9.14** Analysis of variance table showing test for linear trend

| Source of variation | df | Sums of squares | Mean squares | $F$ | P |
|---|---|---|---|---|---|
| Between groups: | 5 | 224 103 | 44 820.6 | | |
| (a) linear | 1 | 55 147 | 55 147.0 | 16.6 | < 0.0001 |
| (b) non-linear | 4 | 168 956 | 42 239.0 | 12.7 | < 0.0001 |
| Within groups: | 265 | 879 272 | 3 318.0 | | |
| Total | 270 | 1 103 375 | | | |

### 9.8.6 Non-parametric one way analysis of variance – the Kruskal-Wallis test

Just as analysis of variance is a more general form of $t$ test, so there is a more general form of the non-parametric Mann-Whitney test. The **Kruskal-Wallis test** is an obvious mathematical extension of the Mann-Whitney test, with the same problems of interpretation as were just discussed for one way analysis of variance.

The calculation of the test statistic is simple. The complete set of $N$ observations are ranked from 1 to $N$ regardless of which group they are in, and for each group the sum of the ranks is calculated. If the sum of the ranks of $n_i$ observations in the $i$th group is $R_i$, then the average rank in each group is given by $\bar{R}_i$. We calculate the statistic $H$ defined by

$$H = \frac{12\Sigma n_i(\bar{R}_i - \bar{R})^2}{N(N + 1)}$$

where $\bar{R}$ is the average of all the ranks, and is always equal to $(N + 1)/2$. The summation term in this formula is very similar to the between group sum of squares calculated in parametric one way analysis of variance (shown mathematically in section 9.9). While this formula for $H$ shows the way the test works, there is an equivalent but simpler version for calculation, with $H$ given by

$$H = \frac{12}{N(N+1)} \sum \frac{R_i^2}{n_i} - 3(N+1).$$

The Kruskal-Wallis test statistic has a different distribution from the other methods described in this chapter. When the null hypothesis is true the test statistic follows the **Chi squared distribution**, where Chi is the Greek letter $\chi$ which is pronounced as 'ky' in 'sky'. The Chi squared distribution is mainly used for the analysis of categorical data, and so will be considered in more detail in the next chapter (section 10.6.3). For the moment it should be sufficient to note that any variation among the groups will increase the test statistic $H$. We therefore are concerned with only the upper tail of the Chi squared distribution. The idea of one- and two-sided tests does not apply with three or more groups.

If there are $k$ groups of observations, the statistic $H$ is compared with a Chi squared distribution with $k-1$ degrees of freedom. A statistically significant result means that we reject the hypothesis that the groups come from populations with the same median, and conclude that there are differences among the groups.

Two sample Mann–Whitney tests can be used to try to identify where the differences are, making due allowance for multiple testing. If the groups are ordered it is possible to test for a trend, in a similar way as described above for one way analysis of variance (see section 9.8.7).

Fentress *et al*. (1986) reported the results of a randomized comparison of three groups of six children suffering from frequent and severe migraine. The active treatments given were relaxation response, either with or without biofeedback, and a third group of children was not treated. The frequency and duration of headaches were recorded before and after the study period, and the difference between these measurements was used as a measure of weekly headache activity.

Table 9.15 shows the reduction in headache activity for each child, expressed as a percentage. Note that a negative value indicates an increase in headache activity. Three children had a complete absence of headaches at the end of the study period and thus a reduction of 100%. These observations are clearly unsuited for analysis of variance, but we can apply the Kruskal-Wallis test. Table 9.15 also shows the ranks of the data and the mean rank for each group. Using the equation given above we can calculate the statistic $H$ as

$$H = \frac{12}{18 \times 19}\left(\frac{55^2}{6} + \frac{36^2}{6} + \frac{80^2}{6}\right) - 3 \times 19$$

$$= 5.69.$$

**Table 9.15** Reduction in weekly headache activity for three treatment groups, expressed as a percentage of baseline data (Fentress *et al.*, 1986). Ranks are shown in brackets.

| | Relaxation response and biofeedback | Relaxation response alone | Untreated |
|---|---|---|---|
| | 62 (11) | 69 (10) | 50 (12) |
| | 74 (8.5) | 43 (13) | −120 (17) |
| | 86 (7) | 100 (2) | 100 (2) |
| | 74 (8.5) | 94 (5) | −288 (18) |
| | 91 (6) | 100 (2) | 4 (15) |
| | 37 (14) | 98 (4) | −76 (16) |
| Rank sum | 55 | 36 | 80 |
| Mean rank | 9.17 | 6.00 | 13.33 |

From Table B5 we find that a $\chi^2$ value of 5.69 on 2 degrees of freedom gives P between 0.1 and 0.05, and is much nearer to $P = 0.05$. (It is actually 0.058.)

Because the groups are small, comparison of each pair of groups with Mann-Whitney tests is not very powerful, and in fact all three P values are greater than 0.05 even without allowing for multiple comparisons. However, it is reasonable to consider whether the two actively treated groups together did better than the untreated controls, and a Mann-Whitney test gives $P = 0.03$, supporting the suggestion that both treatments are beneficial but that the study is too small to be able to distinguish them.

If we apply the Kruskal-Wallis test to just two groups of observations we obtain exactly the same result as that from the Mann-Whitney test. The test statistic $H$ from the former is the square of the $z$ statistic from the latter.

### 9.8.7 Non-parametric test for ordered groups

*(This section can be omitted without loss of continuity.)*

There are several non-parametric methods to test for trend across ordered groups. The method described below is due to Cuzick (1985). It is not necessary to perform the Kruskal-Wallis test if the trend is the only aspect of interest.

We have $k$ groups of sample sizes $n_i$ $(i = 1, \ldots, k)$, where $N = \Sigma n_i$. The groups are given scores, $l_i$, which reflect their ordering, such as 1, 2 and 3. The scores do not have to be equally spaced, but they usually are. The total set of $N$ observations are ranked from 1 to $N$, and the sums of the ranks in each group, $R_i$, are obtained. We calculate a weighted sum of all the group scores, $L$, as

$$L = \sum_{i=1}^{k} l_i n_i.$$

The statistic $T$ is calculated as

$$T = \sum_{i=1}^{k} l_i R_i.$$

Under the null hypothesis the expected value of $T$ is $E(T) = \frac{1}{2}(N + 1)L$, and its standard error is

$$se(T) = \sqrt{\frac{N+1}{12}\left(N\sum_{i=1}^{k} l_i^2 n_i - L^2\right)}$$

so that the test statistic, $z$, is given by

$$z = \frac{T - E(T)}{se(T)}$$

which has an approximately standard Normal distribution when the null hypothesis of no trend is true.

Table 9.16 shows ocular exposure to ultraviolet radiation for 32 pairs of sunglasses classified into three groups according to the amount of visible light transmitted. We can use the method just described to test for a trend for increasing exposure across the three groups.

The groups are given scores $-1$, 0 and 1 (which simplifies the arithmetic in comparison with scores of 1, 2 and 3). Some of the calculations, including that of $T$, are shown in Table 9.16. We have

$$E(T) = 33 \times 2/2 = 33$$

and

$$se(T) = \sqrt{\frac{33}{12}(32 \times 14 - 4)} = 34.94$$

so that the test statistic is given by

$$z = \frac{86 - 33}{34.94}$$

$$= 1.52 \ (\mathrm{P} = 0.13).$$

There is thus little evidence to support the suggestion that ocular exposure to ultraviolet radiation is related to the amount of visible light transmitted.

**Table 9.16** The effect of sunglasses on ocular exposure to ultraviolet radiation in relation to amount of visible light transmitted (Rosenthal *et al.*, 1988). Ocular exposure is expressed as the percentage of exposure without sunglasses. The ranks of the observations are shown in brackets

| | Transmission of visible light | | | | | | |
|---|---|---|---|---|---|---|---|
| | < 25% | | 25 to 35% | | > 35% | | |
| | 1.4 | (9) | 0.9 | (2) | 0.8 | (1) | |
| | 1.4 | (9) | 1.0 | (3) | 1.7 | (14) | |
| | 1.4 | (9) | 1.1 | (4.5) | 1.7 | (14) | |
| | 1.6 | (12) | 1.1 | (4.5) | 1.7 | (14) | |
| | 2.3 | (18) | 1.2 | (6.5) | 3.4 | (26) | |
| | 2.5 | (19) | 1.2 | (6.5) | 7.1 | (30) | |
| | | | 1.5 | (11) | 8.9 | (31) | |
| | | | 1.9 | (16) | 13.5 | (32) | |
| | | | 2.2 | (17) | | | |
| | | | 2.6 | (21) | | | |
| | | | 2.6 | (21) | | | |
| | | | 2.6 | (21) | | | |
| | | | 2.8 | (23.5) | | | |
| | | | 2.8 | (23.5) | | | |
| | | | 3.2 | (25) | | | |
| | | | 3.5 | (27) | | | |
| | | | 4.3 | (28) | | | |
| | | | 5.1 | (29) | | | |
| | | | | | | | Total |
| $n_i$ | | 6 | | 18 | | 8 | 32(=$N$) |
| $R_i$ | | 76 | | 290 | | 162 | |
| $l_i$ | | −1 | | 0 | | 1 | |
| $l_in_i$ | | −6 | | 0 | | 8 | 2(=$L$) |
| $R_il_i$ | | −76 | | 0 | | 162 | 86(=$T$) |
| $l_i^2n_i$ | | 6 | | 0 | | 8 | 14 |

### 9.8.8 Replicated observations

The methods described in this section apply only when a single measurement is made for each individual. If two or more *replicated* measurements are taken for each person, then more complex methods must be used, some of which are described in section 12.3. For designs not covered in Chapter 12 it is advisable to consult a statistician. In some cases it may be reasonable to analyse the average of replicate observations but this may throw away valuable information. It is never valid to treat multiple observations from each individual as if they were independent.

## 9.9 ONE WAY ANALYSIS OF VARIANCE – MATHEMATICS AND WORKED EXAMPLE

*(This section gives the mathematical formulae for the calculations described in section 9.8. It can be omitted without loss of continuity.)*

### 9.9.1 One way analysis of variance

Most statistical packages include one way analysis of variance using the raw data, so it should not be necessary to use the formulae in (a) below. However, the method given in (b) will probably be needed when only means and standard deviations are available, as in the worked example in section 9.9.3.

*(a) Raw data available*

The calculations for one way analysis of variance are expressed in relation to the sum of the observations in each sample. Suppose we have $k$ samples of observations, with $n_i$ observations in the $i^{\text{th}}$ sample, then we calculate

$$M_i = \text{mean of observations in } i^{\text{th}} \text{ group},$$

$$S_i = \text{sum of squares of observations in } i^{\text{th}} \text{ group},$$

$$T = \text{sum of all observations} = \sum_{i=1}^{k} n_i M_i,$$

$$S = \text{sum of squares of all observations} = \sum_{i=1}^{k} S_i,$$

$$N = \text{total number of observations} = \sum_{i=1}^{k} n_i.$$

The sums of squares for the one way analysis of variance are as follows:

| Source of variation | Sum of squares |
|---|---|
| Between groups: | $B = \sum_{i=1}^{k} n_i M_i^2 - T^2/N$ |
| Within groups: | $W = S - \sum_{i=1}^{k} n_i M_i^2$ |
| Total | $S - T^2/N \; (= B + W)$ |

There are $k - 1$ degrees of freedom between groups and $n - k$ within groups. The mean squares are the sums of squares divided by the degrees of freedom. The square root of the within groups mean square is the residual standard deviation, $s_{res}$.

*(b) Means and standard deviations available*

If we already have the mean ($M_i$) and standard deviation ($s_i$) for each group of size $n_i$ we can use the above formulae for $T$ and $B$ together with a simpler method of calculating the within groups sum of squares, $W$, as

$$W = \sum_{i=1}^{k} (n_i - 1)s_i^2.$$

### 9.9.2 Linear trend

If there is a natural ordering of the groups, the between groups sum of squares can be partitioned into a component due to a linear trend, and the remaining (non-linear) component. We give scores $l_i$ to the groups, where the values of the $l_i$ are equally spaced and chosen so that their sum is zero. We then calculate

$$L = \sum l_i \bar{y}_i$$

and its standard error

$$se(L) = s_{res}\sqrt{\Sigma(l_i^2/n_i)}.$$

A one sample $t$ test can be performed by comparing $L/se(L)$ to the $t$ distribution with the number of degrees of freedom within groups.

Alternatively, the sum of squares due to $L$ can be calculated as

$$SS(L) = L^2/\sum(l_i^2/n_i)$$

and the analysis of variance table recalculated by partitioning the between group sum of squares into linear and non-linear components. The $F$ test for the linear contrast is exactly equivalent to the above $t$ test.

(This method is equivalent to performing a regression analysis with the $l_i$ as explanatory variable – see sections 11.10 and 11.15.1.)

### 9.9.3 Worked example

For the serum trypsin data in Table 9.12 the sum of the 271 observations is given by

$$T = 32 \times 128 + 137 \times 152 + 38 \times 194 + 44 \times 207 + 16 \times 215 + 4 \times 218$$

$$= 45\,712.$$

The within groups sum of squares is obtained from the formula based on standard deviations as

$$W = 31 \times 50.9^2 + 136 \times 58.5^2 + \ldots + 3 \times 14.0^2 = 879\,271.9$$

and the quantity $\Sigma n_i M_i^2$ is

$$32 \times 128^2 + 137 \times 152^2 + \ldots + 4 \times 218^2 = 7\,934\,756.$$

The between groups sum of squares is thus

$$B = 7\,934\,756 - 45\,712^2/271$$
$$= 224\,103.1.$$

The complete analysis of variance table is shown in Table 9.13. The residual standard deviation is $\sqrt{3318} = 57.602$. To evaluate a possible linear trend we give the groups scores $l_i$ which are equally spaced and add to zero, such as −5, −3, −1, 1, 3, and 5. The value of the linear contrast is then

$$L = -5 \times 128 - 3 \times 152 - 1 \times 194 + 1 \times 207 + 3 \times 215 + 5 \times 218$$
$$= 652$$

and its standard error is

$$se(L) = 57.602 \times \sqrt{\frac{(-5)^2}{32} + \frac{(-3)^2}{137} + \frac{(-1)^2}{38} + \frac{1^2}{44} + \frac{3^2}{16} + \frac{5^2}{4}}$$
$$= 159.93.$$

The calculations for fitting a linear trend across age groups are shown in Table 9.17. The $t$ test for the linear contrast gives $t = 652/159.93 = 4.08$ (P = 0.00006).

Alternatively, the sum of squares for $L$ is $652.0^2/7.7085 = 55\,147$, as shown in Table 9.14. The $F$ test is exactly equivalent to the $t$ test above, as is shown by the value of $F$ (16.6) being equal to the square of the value of $t$ (4.08).

**Table 9.17** Calculating the sum of squares for linear trend in serum trypsin data from Table 9.12

| Group | $n$ | $\bar{y}_i$ | $l_i$ | $l_i\bar{y}_i$ | $l_i^2/n_i$ |
|---|---|---|---|---|---|
| 1 | 32 | 128 | −5 | −640.0 | 0.78125 |
| 2 | 137 | 152 | −3 | −456.0 | 0.06569 |
| 3 | 38 | 194 | −1 | −194.0 | 0.02632 |
| 4 | 44 | 207 | 1 | 207.0 | 0.02273 |
| 5 | 16 | 215 | 3 | 645.0 | 0.56250 |
| 6 | 4 | 218 | 5 | 1090.0 | 6.25000 |
| Total | | | | 652.0 | 7.70849 |

## 9.10 PRESENTATION OF RESULTS

It is never sufficient to present the results of a statistical analysis solely as a P value, or even as a test statistic and P value. Some actual results should be quoted. This chapter has been concerned with continuous data, for which means or medians should be given, along with some measure of variability of the data.

If a $t$ test or analysis of variance has been used then the standard deviation of the data in each group should be given. However, if a paired $t$ test is used the standard deviation of the *differences* between groups should be quoted. For one way analysis of variance it is not necessary to present the analysis of variance table, but it may be helpful. It is valuable to quote the residual standard deviation.

In addition it may be useful to construct one or more confidence intervals for means or differences between means. Confidence intervals are preferable to quoting standard errors, which are not very helpful as they stand (see Chapter 8).

For data analysed by a non-parametric method the median and selected centiles (e.g. 10th and 90th) should be given for each group if the raw data are not shown. For small samples the median and range can be given. For all analyses, it is good practice to quote the test statistic ($t$, $F$ or $\chi^2$) as well as the P value derived from it. It should always be clear what the degrees of freedom are.

Graphical presentation is often by means and standard deviation or standard error 'bars', but it is much more informative to show the raw data where possible. Figure 3.14 showed some data of Lind *et al.* (1984), in which all the raw data and summary statistics are shown. Figure 9.6 shows how comparatively uninformative the means and standard errors are on their own. For data which have a skewed distribution the loss of information is particularly marked. The presentation as, say, mean ±1SD implies a

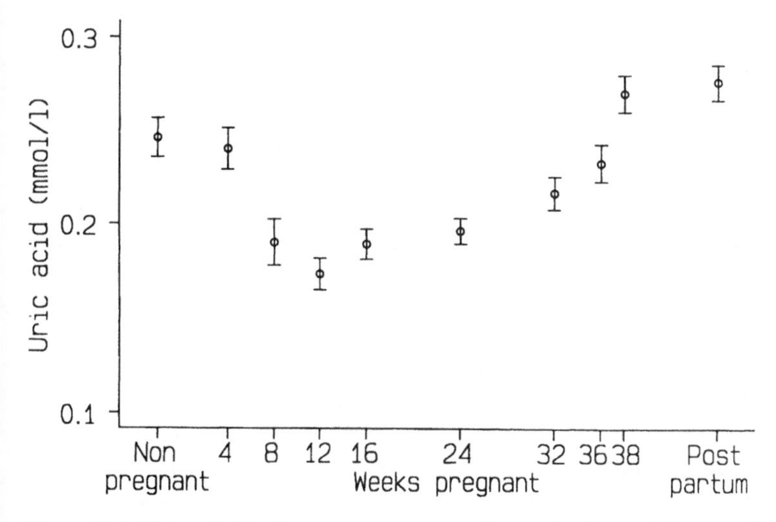


**Figure 9.6** Figure 3.14 shown as means and standard error bars only (data from Lind *et al.*, 1984).

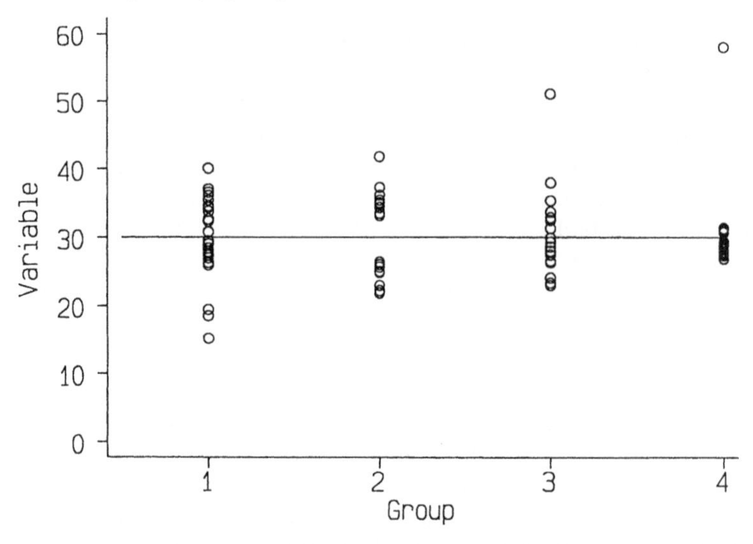


**Figure 9.7** Four groups of 25 observations each having a mean of 30 and standard deviation of 5.9.

symmetry in the data that may not exist. Figure 9.7 shows four groups of 25 observations that all have the same mean (30) and standard deviation (5.9). Where possible it is valuable to show all the data in a figure, with relevant means and standard errors or confidence intervals given in the text or a table.

## 9.11 SUMMARY

This chapter has described various methods for analysing continuous data from one, two, or several independent groups of individuals, and also two sets of paired observations. These methods cover a large proportion of practical problems in the analysis of continuous data. However, there are many circumstances which require a more complicated analysis. For example, when there are two or more classifications for each individual (considered in Chapter 12), or where we are interested in relations between two or more continuous variables (Chapter 11).

I have emphasized the dependence of the methods of analysis on the underlying assumptions about the data. We can carry out any analysis on data that do not meet the assumptions, but the results would not be interpretable. For example, the calculated 95% confidence interval for the difference between two means would not in fact be a 95% confidence interval but an interval with some other, unknown level of confidence. Likewise, the P value associated with a two sample $t$ test will be wrong to an unknown degree if the data do not meet the assumptions. The extent to which data may depart from the assumptions of, for example, having a Normal distribution, with minimal effect on the validity of the results is unclear – it is not possible to give any general rule. Of course no sample of data has an exactly Normal distribution; the assumption is not that it does, but rather that the sample comes from a population which does. Samples from Normal distributions, especially small ones, may look quite unlike the expected symmetric distribution. Although formal methods exist for testing assumptions, this is an area where experience gives a feel for what is or is not reasonable. We would usually carry out either a parametric or a non-parametric test of a set of data, not both. However, sometimes when there are doubts about the validity of the assumptions for the parametric method, a non-parametric analysis is carried out too. If the assumptions are met the two methods should give very similar answers, so if the answers differ (again this is a subjective assessment) then the non-parametric method is likely to be the more reliable.

In summary, both parametric and non-parametric methods can be used for continuous data, and the alternative approaches have been described. If the assumptions are met I favour the use of parametric methods because they are more amenable to estimation and confidence intervals, and also because they are readily extended to the more complicated data structures described in later chapters. With a few exceptions, non-parametric methods do not extend to more complex situations.

## EXERCISES

9.1 A study was made of all 26 astronauts on the first eight space shuttle flights (Bungo *et al.*, 1985). On a voluntary basis 17 astronauts consumed large quantities of salt and fluid prior to landing as a countermeasure to space deconditioning, while nine did not. The table below shows supine heart rates (beats/minute) before and after flights in the space shuttle.

(a) Compare the pre- and post-flight measurements in the countermeasure group using both a parametric and a non-parametric method. Which analysis is preferable?

(b) In the light of the answer to (a), perform a suitable analysis to compare the changes in heart rate in the two groups. What conclusion can be made about the effectiveness of the countermeasure?

(c) Two astronauts each flew on two missions and are thus represented twice in the data set. Does this matter?

(d) Comment on the voluntary aspect of the study, and how it might affect the interpretation of the results.

| | Countermeasure taken | | | Countermeasure not taken | | |
|---|---|---|---|---|---|---|
| | Pre | Post | Change | Pre | Post | Change |
| | 71 | 61 | −10 | 61 | 61 | 0 |
| | 65 | 59 | −6 | 59 | 66 | 7 |
| | 52 | 47 | −5 | 52 | 61 | 9 |
| | 68 | 65 | −3 | 54 | 68 | 14 |
| | 69 | 69 | 0 | 53 | 77 | 24 |
| | 49 | 50 | 1 | 78 | 103 | 25 |
| | 49 | 51 | 2 | 52 | 77 | 25 |
| | 57 | 60 | 3 | 54 | 80 | 26 |
| | 51 | 57 | 6 | 52 | 79 | 27 |
| | 55 | 64 | 9 | | | |
| | 58 | 67 | 9 | | | |
| | 57 | 69 | 12 | | | |
| | 59 | 72 | 13 | | | |
| | 53 | 69 | 16 | | | |
| | 53 | 72 | 19 | | | |
| | 53 | 75 | 22 | | | |
| | 48 | 77 | 29 | | | |
| Mean | 56.88 | 63.76 | 6.88 | 57.22 | 74.67 | 17.44 |
| SD | 7.30 | 8.86 | 10.70 | 8.44 | 13.01 | 10.11 |

9.2 The table below shows concentrations of antibody to Type III Group B Streptococcus (GBS) in 20 volunteers before and after immunization (Baker *et al*., 1980).

| | Antibodyconcentration to Type III GBS | |
|---|---|---|
| | Before immunization | 4 weeks after immunization |
| 1 | 0.4 | 0.4 |
| 2 | 0.4 | 0.5 |
| 3 | 0.4 | 0.5 |
| 4 | 0.4 | 0.9 |
| 5 | 0.5 | 0.5 |
| 6 | 0.5 | 0.5 |
| 7 | 0.5 | 0.5 |
| 8 | 0.5 | 0.5 |
| 9 | 0.5 | 0.5 |

*cont'd*

| | Antibodyconcentration to Type III GBS | |
|---|---|---|
| | Before immunization | 4 weeks after immunization |
| 10 | 0.6 | 0.6 |
| 11 | 0.6 | 12.2 |
| 12 | 0.7 | 1.1 |
| 13 | 0.7 | 1.2 |
| 14 | 0.8 | 0.8 |
| 15 | 0.9 | 1.2 |
| 16 | 0.9 | 1.9 |
| 17 | 1.0 | 0.9 |
| 18 | 1.0 | 2.0 |
| 19 | 1.6 | 8.1 |
| 20 | 2.0 | 3.7 |

(a) The comparison of the antibody levels was summarized in the report of this study as '$t = 1.8$; $P > 0.05$'. Comment on this result.

(b) What method would be more appropriate to analyse these data? Analyse the data with the appropriate method and comment on the result.

9.3 Using the data in Table 9.7 calculate a 90% confidence interval for the comparison of numbers of $T_4$ cells in Hodgkin's disease and non-Hodgkin's disease patients.

9.4 Patients receiving chemotherapy as outpatients were randomized to receive either an active antiemetic treatment or placebo (Williams *et al.*, 1989). The following table shows measurements (in mm) on a 100 mm linear analogue self-assessment scale for nausea.

| Treatment group | |
|---|---|
| Active ($n$ = 20) | Placebo ($n$ = 20) |
| 0 | 0 |
| 0 | 10 |
| 0 | 12 |
| 0 | 15 |
| 0 | 15 |
| 2 | 30 |
| 7 | 35 |
| 8 | 38 |
| 10 | 42 |
| 13 | 45 |

| Treatment group | |
|---|---|
| Active ($n$ = 20) | Placebo ($n$ = 20) |
| 15 | 50 |
| 18 | 50 |
| 20 | 60 |
| 20 | 64 |
| 21 | 68 |
| 22 | 71 |
| 25 | 74 |
| 30 | 82 |
| 52 | 86 |
| 76 | 95 |

Identify and carry out an appropriate analysis to compare the values in the two groups.

9.5 Urinary cotinine excretion was measured in nonsmokers who lived with smokers. The following table shows the summary of findings given in the paper (Matsukura *et al.*, 1984).

| Cigarettes smoked per day by smoker | $n$ | Urinary cotinine excretion ($\mu$g/mg of creatinine) mean (se) |
|---|---|---|
| 1–9 | 25 | 0.31 (0.08) |
| 10–19 | 57 | 0.42 (0.10) |
| 20–29 | 99 | 0.87 (0.19) |
| 30–39 | 38 | 1.03 (0.25) |
| $>40$ | 28 | 1.56 (0.57) |
| Unspecified | 25 | 0.56 (0.16) |

(a) What can you say about the shape of the distribution of urinary cotinine in these nonsmokers?

(b) What would be an appropriate analysis to see if there was a systematic relation between number of cigarettes and urinary cotinine levels?

(c) Does it matter that the standard errors vary greatly among the groups?

(d) The authors used multiple $t$ tests to compare pairs of groups with a correction for multiple testing. Comment on the appropriateness of their analysis.

9.6 Patients with chronic renal failure undergoing haemodialysis were divided into groups with low or normal plasma heparin cofactor II

(HC II) levels (Toulon *et al*., 1987). Five months later the acute effects of haemodialysis were studied by analysing plasma samples taken before and after haemodialysis. As dialysis increases total protein concentration in plasma, the ratio of HC II to protein was calculated, with the results shown in the following table:

| Group 1 (low) | | Group 2 (normal) | |
|---|---|---|---|
| before | after | before | after |
| 1.41 | 1.47 | 2.11 | 2.15 |
| 1.37 | 1.45 | 1.85 | 2.11 |
| 1.33 | 1.50 | 1.82 | 1.93 |
| 1.13 | 1.25 | 1.75 | 1.83 |
| 1.09 | 1.01 | 1.54 | 1.90 |
| 1.03 | 1.14 | 1.52 | 1.56 |
| 0.89 | 0.98 | 1.49 | 1.44 |
| 0.86 | 0.89 | 1.44 | 1.43 |
| 0.75 | 0.95 | 1.38 | 1.28 |
| 0.75 | 0.83 | 1.30 | 1.30 |
| 0.70 | 0.75 | 1.20 | 1.21 |
| 0.69 | 0.71 | 1.19 | 1.30 |

The data were analysed by separate paired Wilcoxon tests on the data for each group, giving $P < 0.01$ for group 1 and $P > 0.05$ for group 2. Why is it wrong to conclude, as the authors did, that HC II activity increased in group 1 but not in group 2? Carry out a better analysis of these data.

9.7 The effect of gestrinone on patients with asymptomatic endometriosis was evaluated in a randomized double-blind placebo controlled trial (Thomas and Cooke, 1987). Before treatment each patient was given a score on a scale derived by the American Fertility Society, and this was repeated after 24 weeks' treatment, with the following results (high scores indicate more serious disease):

(a) Identify and carry out a suitable comparison of the scores after treatment.

(b) The pre-treatment scores were somewhat different in the two groups, with five of the six highest scores being in the placebo group. A simple way to allow for this difference is to consider the change in scores over the period of the trial. Identify and carry out a suitable comparison of the changes in scores in the two groups.

| | Placebo group | | | Gestrinone group | |
|---|---|---|---|---|---|
| | Before treatment | After treatment | | Before treatment | After treatment |
| 1 | 1 | 0 | 1 | 1 | 0 |
| 2 | 1 | 1 | 2 | 1 | 0 |
| 3 | 1 | 2 | 3 | 1 | 0 |
| 4 | 2 | 0 | 4 | 1 | 0 |
| 5 | 2 | 0 | 5 | 1 | 0 |
| 6 | 2 | 2 | 6 | 1 | 1 |
| 7 | 2 | 3 | 7 | 1 | 1 |
| 8 | 3 | 3 | 8 | 2 | 0 |
| 9 | 3 | 5 | 9 | 2 | 0 |
| 10 | 3 | 5 | 10 | 2 | 0 |
| 11 | 3 | 5 | 11 | 2 | 0 |
| 12 | 3 | 9 | 12 | 2 | 1 |
| 13 | 5 | 1 | 13 | 2 | 2 |
| 14 | 5 | 5 | 14 | 3 | 1 |
| 15 | 6 | 4 | 15 | 3 | 2 |
| 16 | 6 | 10 | 16 | 3 | 2 |
| 17 | 6 | 12 | 17 | 4 | 1 |
| | | | 18 | 5 | 1 |

9.8 What test could be used to compare the SI values in the two groups of patients shown in Exercise 3.1?

# 10

# Comparing groups – categorical data

## 10.1 INTRODUCTION

Categorical data are very common in medical research, arising when individuals are categorized into one of two or more mutually exclusive groups. In a sample of individuals the number falling into a particular group is called the **frequency**, so the analysis of categorical data is the analysis of frequencies. When two or more groups are compared the data are often shown in the form of a **frequency table**. Table 10.1 shows an example of a frequency table – these data will be used to illustrate one form of analysis later in the chapter. A frequency table can also be considered as a **cross-tabulation** of two categorical variables, either or both of which can be ordinal.

When there are only two categories for one of the variables, for example whether a patient has a particular symptom or not, the data can be summarized as the proportion of the total number of individuals in one of the categories. The data in Table 10.1 can be expressed as the proportion of women having a Caesarean section in each of the six shoe size groups. For this type of data I shall describe the analysis of categorical data expressed either as proportions or as frequency tables. As the analyses relate to alternative ways of expressing the same information, the two methods yield the same answers. Both are described because they are in

**Table 10.1** Relation between frequency of Caesarean section and maternal shoe size

| | Shoe size | | | | | | |
|---|---|---|---|---|---|---|---|
| Caesarean section | < 4 | 4 | $4\frac{1}{2}$ | 5 | $5\frac{1}{2}$ | 6+ | Total |
| Yes | 5 | 7 | 6 | 7 | 8 | 10 | 43 |
| No | 17 | 28 | 36 | 41 | 46 | 140 | 308 |
| Total | 22 | 35 | 42 | 48 | 54 | 150 | 351 |

common use. The frequency table approach is more common, but the comparison of proportions is preferable because it readily yields estimates and confidence intervals. For larger tables where both variables have at least three categories there is no simple alternative, and we use methods suitable for analysing frequency tables.

Throughout the chapter, except where explicitly stated otherwise, it is assumed that there is only one observation per individual – that is, we have independent observations.

## 10.2 ONE PROPORTION

The simplest case to consider is when we have a single group of individuals, and have observed that a certain proportion have a particular characteristic. What can we say about the proportion with that characteristic in the population?

### 10.2.1 Confidence interval

Suppose a general practitioner chooses a random sample of 215 women from the patient register for her general practice, and finds that 39 of them have a history of suffering from asthma. I shall use $r$ to denote the number of cases with the characteristic out of a sample size of $n$, and $p$ as the proportion of cases, so $p = r/n = 0.18$ in this example. As described in Chapter 8, the relevant sampling distribution for a proportion is the Binomial distribution. However, we can usually use the Normal approximation to the Binomial distribution to obtain the standard error of the observed proportion, and so can obtain a confidence interval for the proportion in the population. It is reasonable to use the Normal approximation when both $np$ and $n(1 - p)$ exceed 5; in other words, both $r$ and $n - r$ should exceed 5. This will usually be the case.

As we saw in section 8.4.3, the standard error of a proportion $p$ is $se(p) = \sqrt{p(1 - p)/n}$. So the standard error of the observed proportion of women with asthma is $\sqrt{0.18 \times 0.82/215} = 0.0262$. The 95% confidence interval for the proportion of women with asthma in the population is thus from

$$0.18 - 1.96 \times 0.0262 \quad \text{to} \quad 0.18 + 1.96 \times 0.0262$$

that is from 0.13 to 0.23. If we can assume that the women in this general practice are representative of all women in the country then we can be reasonably sure on the basis of this sample that the national prevalence of asthma in women is between 13 and 23%.

### 10.2.2 Hypothesis test

We can test the null hypothesis that the population proportion is some pre-specified value. To do this we use the general test statistic given in section 8.5, namely

$$\frac{\text{observed value} - \text{expected value}}{\text{standard error of observed value}}$$

which will have an approximately Normal distribution under the null hypothesis (with the same sample size requirement as in the previous section). We thus calculate

$$z = \frac{p - p_{\text{exp}}}{se(p)}$$

where $p_{\text{exp}}$ is the pre-specified or 'expected' proportion. Note that because we are testing the null hypothesis, we use the standard error of the proportion expected if the null hypothesis is true. In other words, we have

$$se(p) = \sqrt{\frac{p_{\text{exp}}(1 - p_{\text{exp}})}{n}}$$

which will be slightly different from the standard error used to obtain a confidence interval. If we wish to test the pre-specified hypothesis that the national prevalence of asthma in women is 15%, we calculate

$$se(p) = \sqrt{\frac{0.15 \times 0.85}{215}}$$

and so

$$z = \frac{0.18 - 0.15}{0.0244}$$

$$= 1.23$$

which, from Table B2, corresponds to $P = 0.22$. We cannot reject the null hypothesis that the prevalence of asthma in women is 15%, and use the confidence interval given above to give a range likely to include the true prevalence.

### 10.2.3 Continuity correction

The method just described uses the continuous Normal distribution as an approximation to the discrete Binomial distribution. Figure 10.1 shows these two distributions for the example just examined, with $n = 215$ and $p = 0.15$. The hypothesis test is based on calculating the tail area of the Normal distribution beyond the observed value, here 39. The Normal distribution corresponds better to the Binomial distribution when we make a small correction of $\frac{1}{2}$ to the observed frequency to allow for the fact that the variable can only take integer values.

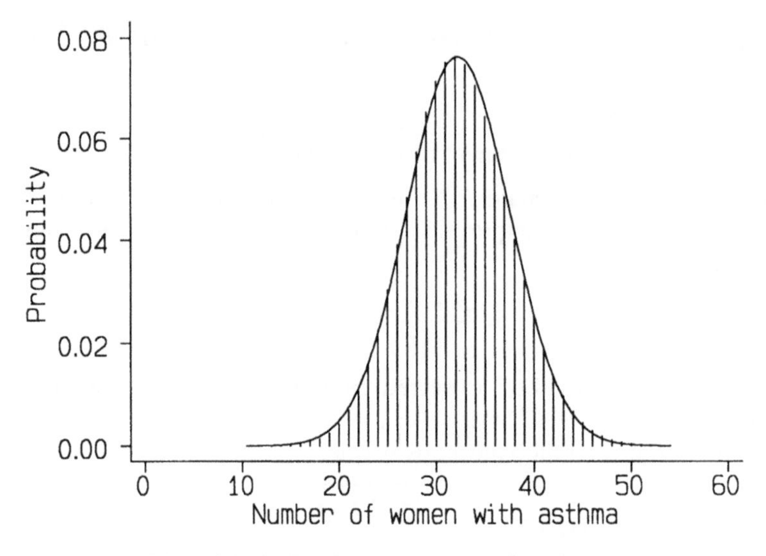


**Figure 10.1** Binomial distribution with $p = 0.15$ and $n = 215$ with the approximating Normal distribution.

The test statistic with the continuity correction is

$$z_c = \frac{|p - p_{\text{exp}}| - \dfrac{1}{2n}}{se(p)}$$

where the symbols $|\ldots|$ indicate that the sign of the difference between the proportions is ignored and $se(p)$ is unchanged. The continuity correction thus consists of reducing the difference between the observed and expected proportions. Clearly the effect of the correction diminishes as the sample size increases.

For the asthma data, the test statistic with the continuity correction is

$$z_c = \frac{|0.18 - 0.15| - \dfrac{1}{2 \times 215}}{0.0244}$$

$$= 1.14$$

which is only slightly lower than before because the sample size is quite large.

## 10.3 PROPORTIONS IN TWO INDEPENDENT GROUPS

Probably the most common question in medical research involves the comparison of observed proportions in two independent groups. Such questions can arise in all types of study, whether observational or experimental.

As an example I will consider data from a randomized clinical trial comparing infra-red stimulation (IRS) with a placebo on the pain caused by cervical osteoarthrosis (Lewith and Machin, 1981). The placebo treatment was mock transcutaneous electrical stimulation and the patients were blind to the treatment given. Twenty-six patients were entered into the trial, but one dropped out before the end. Nine of the 12 patients in the IRS group reported an improvement in pain compared with four of the 13 receiving the placebo treatment. The observed proportions improving were thus 0.75 and 0.31, with a difference of 0.44. In order to calculate a confidence interval for the difference in the population or perform a hypothesis test, we need to consider the sampling distribution of the difference between two proportions.

### 10.3.1 Confidence interval

As shown in section 8.4.4, the standard error of the difference between the observed proportions, $p_1 - p_2$, is given by

$$se(p_1 - p_2) = \sqrt{var(p_1) + var(p_2)}$$
$$= \sqrt{\frac{p_1(1 - p_1)}{n_1} + \frac{p_2(1 - p_2)}{n_2}}.$$

The sampling distribution of $p_1 - p_2$ will be approximately Normal as long as the sample size and proportions are not very small. We can thus calculate the 95% confidence interval very simply as

$$p_1 - p_2 - 1.96 \times se(p_1 - p_2) \quad \text{to} \quad p_1 - p_2 + 1.96 \times se(p_1 - p_2).$$

In the example, the difference in observed proportions is

$$p_1 - p_2 = 0.7500 - 0.3077 = 0.4423$$

and the standard error is

$$se(p_1 - p_2) = \sqrt{\frac{0.75 \times 0.25}{12} + \frac{0.3077 \times 0.6923}{13}}$$
$$= 0.1789.$$

The 95% confidence interval for the difference in proportions with pain relief is thus

$$0.4423 - 1.96 \times 0.1789 \quad \text{to} \quad 0.4423 + 1.96 \times 0.1789$$

or 0.09 to 0.79.

### 10.3.2 Hypothesis test

A similar approach is adopted when performing a hypothesis test to compare two proportions. The standard error of the difference in proportions is again calculated, but because we are evaluating the probability of the data on the assumption that the null hypothesis is true we calculate a slightly different standard error. If the null hypothesis is true, the two samples come from populations having the same true proportion of individuals with the characteristic of interest, say $p$. We do not know $p$, but both $p_1$ and $p_2$ are estimates of $p$. Our *best* estimate of $p$ is given by calculating the proportion with the characteristic using all the data in the two samples combined, which is

$$\hat{p} = \frac{r_1 + r_2}{n_1 + n_2}.$$

The standard error of $p_1 - p_2$ under the null hypothesis is thus calculated on the assumption that the proportion in each group is $\hat{p}$, so that we have

$$se(p_1 - p_2) = \sqrt{\frac{\hat{p}(1-\hat{p})}{n_1} + \frac{\hat{p}(1-\hat{p})}{n_2}}$$

$$= \sqrt{\hat{p}(1-\hat{p})\left(\frac{1}{n_1} + \frac{1}{n_2}\right)}.$$

As noted above, this standard error is not quite the same as that calculated in the previous section.

The sampling distribution of $p_1 - p_2$ is Normal, so we calculate a standard Normal deviate, $z$, as

$$z = \frac{p_1 - p_2}{se(p_1 - p_2)}.$$

In the example, the difference in observed proportions is $p_1 - p_2 = 0.4423$ as before. The two proportions were 9/12 and 4/13, so the pooled estimate of the population proportion under the null hypothesis is

$$\hat{p} = \frac{9 + 4}{12 + 13} = 0.52,$$

and the standard error of the difference in proportions is

$$\sqrt{0.52 \times 0.48 \times (\tfrac{1}{12} + \tfrac{1}{13})} = 0.2000.$$

The test statistic is thus $z = 0.4423/0.2000 = 2.21$, which from Table B2 gives $P = 0.027$. Thus there is evidence of a difference between the treatments. As shown earlier, however, the confidence interval for the difference is wide because the samples are small.

### 10.3.3 Continuity correction

As with the single sample case, it is advisable to use a continuity correction when comparing two proportions, especially when the samples are small. The effect is to reduce slightly the observed difference between the two proportions. The modified formula for $z$ is

$$z_c = \frac{|p_1 - p_2| - \frac{1}{2}\left(\frac{1}{n_1} + \frac{1}{n_2}\right)}{se(p_1 - p_2)}$$

where $se(p_1 - p_2)$ is unchanged. It can be seen that the extra term in the numerator (on the top) is based on a quantity already calculated in the denominator (on the bottom). In our example the continuity corrected test statistic is

$$z_c = \frac{0.4423 - \frac{1}{2}(\frac{1}{12} + \frac{1}{13})}{\sqrt{0.52 \times 0.48 \times (\frac{1}{12} + \frac{1}{13})}}$$
$$= 0.3622/0.2000$$
$$= 1.811$$

which corresponds to P = 0.07.

The continuity correction has made quite a large impact on the test statistic because the samples were small. It is clear from the extra term in the formula that the impact of the correction diminishes as the sample sizes increase.

It is advisable to use the continuity correction routinely for both one and two sample tests. Without it results tend to be slightly optimistic, so that the P values are too small. In the example, the use of the correction gives a rather larger P value which is now above the 5% level. We can still report that there is evidence to suggest a difference in effectiveness of the two treatments, but it is not as strong as was suggested by the uncorrected analysis.

Because the standard error used for calculating the confidence interval differs from that used in the hypothesis test it can occasionally happen, as here, that the confidence interval excludes the value specified under the null hypothesis when the hypothesis test gives a non-significant result. The difference in interpretation will not be important. Note that no continuity correction is necessary for constructing a confidence interval as we are not calculating probabilities based on the tail area of a distribution.

## 10.4 TWO PAIRED PROPORTIONS

There are several circumstances in which we may observe two proportions on the same individuals. We may wish to compare the pain relief by two different analgesics in the same subjects or to compare the proportion of subjects with a particular symptom before and after treatment. A statistically identical problem arises when we wish to compare one characteristic in two pair-matched groups.

As an example, Karacan *et al.* (1976) compared a group of 32 marijuana users with 32 matched controls with respect to their sleeping difficulties. Seven of the marijuana users (22%) reported sleep difficulties sometimes or always compared with 13 (41%) of the controls. Because the groups were individually matched we should not treat the observations as independent and thus need different methods from those described in the previous section. We will see that we cannot perform the appropriate analyses if we know only the two proportions.

### 10.4.1 Confidence interval

We want to calculate a confidence interval for the difference between two proportions $p_1$ and $p_2$ where the two groups of observations are not independent. The standard error of the difference is not, therefore, based simply on the variances of each proportion but must take account of the paired results in some way.

We can divide the paired observations into four groups, according to whether the characteristic is present or not in each member of the pair, as shown in Table 10.2. The two proportions we wish to compare are $p_1 = (a + b)/n$ and $p_2 = (a + c)/n$. These proportions are not independent as they both contain $a$, the number of Yes-Yes pairs. The difference in proportions is, however, given by

$$p_1 - p_2 = \frac{a + b}{n} - \frac{a + c}{n}$$

$$= \frac{b - c}{n}$$

so that the number $a$ disappears, which is rather surprising. Nevertheless,

**Table 10.2** Frequency of each combination of paired characteristics

| Observation | | Number of pairs |
|---|---|---|
| 1 | 2 | |
| Yes | Yes | $a$ |
| Yes | No | $b$ |
| No | Yes | $c$ |
| No | No | $d$ |
| Total | | $n$ |

we are still comparing non-independent proportions. The standard error of the difference in proportions is given by

$$se(p_1 - p_2) = \frac{1}{n}\sqrt{b + c - \frac{(b - c)^2}{n}}.$$

(The derivation of this formula will not be given here.) The 95% confidence interval for $p_1 - p_2$ is thus obtained as

$$p_1 - p_2 - 1.96 \times se(p_1 - p_2) \quad \text{to} \quad p_1 - p_2 + 1.96 \times se(p_1 - p_2).$$

In our example, we need to know the values $a$, $b$, $c$ and $d$ which are shown in Table 10.3. We have $p_m = (a + b)/n = 7/32$ and $p_c = (a + c)/n = 13/32$, so the observed difference in proportions is

$$\begin{aligned} p_c - p_m &= \frac{13 - 7}{32} \\ &= 0.1875 \end{aligned}$$

and its standard error is

$$\begin{aligned} se(p_c - p_m) &= \frac{1}{32}\sqrt{3 + 9 - \frac{6^2}{32}} \\ &= 0.1031. \end{aligned}$$

**Table 10.3** Numbers of marijuana users and matched controls reporting sleeping difficulties (Karacan *et al.*, 1976)

| Sleep difficulties | | |
|---|---|---|
| Marijuana group | Control group | Number of pairs |
| Yes | Yes | $a = 4$ |
| Yes | No | $b = 3$ |
| No | Yes | $c = 9$ |
| No | No | $d = 16$ |
| Total | | $n = 32$ |

So the 95% confidence interval for the difference in the proportions experiencing sleep difficulties is

$$0.1875 - 1.96 \times 0.1031 \quad \text{to} \quad 0.1875 + 1.96 \times 0.1031$$

or -0.01 to 0.39. There is thus some weak evidence that marijuana users experience fewer sleeping difficulties than controls, but the confidence interval for the difference is very wide.

### 10.4.2 Hypothesis test

We can also perform a significance test of the null hypothesis that there is no difference between the paired proportions. As with two independent samples, we need to evaluate the standard error of the difference on the assumption that the null hypothesis is true, which means that we replace both $b$ and $c$ by $(b + c)/2$. The formula for the standard error given in the previous section thus simplifies to

$$se(p_1 - p_2) = \frac{1}{n}\sqrt{\frac{b+c}{2} + \frac{b+c}{2} + 0}$$
$$= \frac{1}{n}\sqrt{b+c}$$

and we calculate our test statistic as

$$z = \frac{p_1 - p_2}{se(p_1 - p_2)}$$
$$= \frac{(b - c)/n}{\sqrt{b + c}/n}$$
$$= \frac{b - c}{\sqrt{b + c}}$$

which is one of the simplest formulae in statistics. An alternative derivation of this formula is given in section 10.4.4.

In the example we get

$$z = \frac{3 - 9}{\sqrt{3 + 9}}$$
$$= -1.73$$

giving $P = 0.08$. We cannot reject the null hypothesis at the 5% level. Note that it does not matter whether we take $b - c$ or $c - b$ in the equation, as $z = +1.73$ would give the same two-sided P value.

### 10.4.3 Continuity correction

We ought to use a continuity correction when comparing paired proportions, especially in small samples. As with the unpaired case we use the formula

$$z_c = \frac{|p_1 - p_2| - \frac{1}{2}\left(\frac{1}{n_1} + \frac{1}{n_2}\right)}{se(p_1 - p_2)}$$

but here the two samples are the same size, so we get

$$z_c = \frac{\frac{1}{n}|b - c| - \frac{1}{2}\left(\frac{1}{n} + \frac{1}{n}\right)}{(\sqrt{b + c})/n}$$

$$= \frac{|b - c| - 1}{\sqrt{b + c}}.$$

In other words, to use the continuity correction we subtract 1 from the absolute difference between $b$ and $c$ before dividing by $\sqrt{b + c}$.

In our example we have

$$z_c = \frac{|3 - 9| - 1}{\sqrt{3 + 9}}$$

$$= 5/\sqrt{12} = 1.44$$

corresponding to P = 0.15. As we saw in the previous section, the effect of the continuity correction is quite marked in small samples. Its use will always increase the P value.

### 10.4.4 An alternative derivation based on the Binomial distribution

As shown above, the hypothesis test for comparing paired proportions is based only on the numbers of pairs showing disagreement, $b$ and $c$. Those showing agreement, $a$ and $d$, do not appear in the formula.

Another way of considering the problem, therefore, is to look at the total number of disagreements, $b + c$. Under the null hypothesis we expect the numbers of 'Yes-No' and 'No-Yes' pairs to be the same so we can evaluate the probability of observing $b$ out of $b + c$ to be in one of these groups (or, equivalently, $c$ out of $b + c$). The number $b$ will follow a Binomial distribution with $p = 0.5$. Because $p$ is 0.5 the Normal approximation to the Binomial distribution is very good even for quite small samples. The standard error of $b$ is

$$se(b) = \sqrt{np(1 - p)} = \sqrt{(b + c) \times \tfrac{1}{2} \times \tfrac{1}{2}} = \frac{\sqrt{b + c}}{2}.$$

The statistic $z$ is calculated as

$$z = \frac{b - \frac{(b + c)}{2}}{se(b)}$$

$$= \frac{(b - c)/2}{\sqrt{b + c}/2}$$

$$= \frac{b - c}{\sqrt{b + c}}$$

as before. This test is identical to the sign test which was introduced in section 9.4.4. Here the comparison is expressed in terms of the proportions whereas in the earlier description it was in terms of the actual frequencies, but the two are exactly equivalent. We will meet other tests which reduce to a simple Binomial test of a single proportion. When the data are expressed as a frequency table the test is usually called the **McNemar test**, under which name it is discussed in section 10.7.5.

### 10.4.5 Are *a* and *d* really ignored?

All of the formulae for analysing paired proportions seem to be based on only those pairs showing disagreement – 'Yes-No' ($b$) or 'No-Yes' ($c$) in Tables 10.2 and 10.3. While it is true that the result of the hypothesis test comparing the two classifications depends only on $b$ and $c$, the confidence interval depends on the sample size too. We expect the confidence interval and hypothesis testing approaches to give closely corresponding results (with some small discrepancies due to the use of different standard errors) and an example will show that this does indeed happen.

Consider the two sets of data in Table 10.4 showing presence or absence of a symptom before and after treatment. In both tables (i) and (ii) $b = 15$ and $c = 6$, so for both of them a test of the null hypothesis that there is no difference between the two features is given by

$$z = \frac{15 - 6}{\sqrt{15 + 6}}$$

$$= 1.96 \ (P = 0.05).$$

(I shall ignore the continuity correction for this illustrative example.) We would expect the confidence interval for the difference between the two proportions to have one end very close to zero because the P value is almost exactly 0.05 – does this happen regardless of the size of $a$ and $d$?

**Table 10.4** Two sets of paired data showing the same numbers of Yes–No and No–Yes pairs

| (i) Presence of symptom Time 1 | Time 2 | | (ii) Presence of symptom Time 1 | Time 2 | |
|---|---|---|---|---|---|
| Yes | Yes | $a = 10$ | Yes | Yes | $a = 51$ |
| Yes | No | $b = 15$ | Yes | No | $b = 15$ |
| No | Yes | $c = 6$ | No | Yes | $c = 6$ |
| No | No | $d = 5$ | No | No | $d = 33$ |
| Total | | $n = 36$ | Total | | $n = 105$ |

The two sets of calculations are shown below in parallel:

| (i) | (ii) |
|---|---|
| $p_1 = (10 + 15)/36 = 0.694$ | $p_1 = (51 + 15)/105 = 0.629$ |
| $p_2 = (10 + 6)/36 = 0.444$ | $p_2 = (51 + 6)/105 = 0.543$ |
| $p_1 - p_2 = 0.250$ | $p_1 - p_2 = 0.086$ |
| $se(p_1 - p_2) = \frac{1}{36}\sqrt{21 - 9^2/36}$ | $se(p_1 - p_2) = \frac{1}{105}\sqrt{21 - 9^2/105}$ |
| $= 0.1203$ | $= 0.0428$ |
| 95% CI is $0.250 \pm 1.96 \times 0.1203$ i.e. 0.014 to 0.486. | 95% CI is $0.086 \pm 1.96 \times 0.0428$ i.e. 0.002 to 0.170. |

Both confidence intervals behave as expected, with the lower limit close to zero. The 95% confidence interval for the difference in proportions is much narrower for the larger sample, as we would expect. Note that the difference between data sets (i) and (ii) is the change in $p_1$ and $p_2$ and thus $p_1 - p_2$, none of which is seen when only testing the hypothesis that $b = c$.

## 10.5 COMPARING SEVERAL PROPORTIONS

When comparing several proportions relating to different groups of subjects two alternative cases must be considered, according to whether the groups are ordered or not. These problems are discusssed in section 10.8, as they are more easily considered in the framework of frequency tables.

The comparison of more than two paired proportions is beyond the scope of this book. The analysis is described by Fleiss (1981, p. 126).

## 10.6 THE ANALYSIS OF FREQUENCY TABLES

Proportions are a way of expressing counts or frequencies when there are only two possible outcomes, such as the presence or absence of a symptom. A more general way of showing frequencies is in a table, where each cell of the table corresponds to a particular combination of characteristics relating to two or more classifications. Here I will deal only with 'two way' tables, which relate to two categorical variables. Frequency tables are sometimes called **contingency tables**.

There is a single, general approach to the analysis of all frequency tables, but in practice the method of analysis varies according to

1. the number of categories
2. whether the categories are ordered or not
3. the number of independent groups of subjects, and

4. the nature of the question being asked.

I will first consider the general approach, and then several special cases.

### 10.6.1 The general case – the $r \times c$ table

An example of a two way frequency table is given in Table 10.5, which shows caffeine consumption by marital status in a sample of 3888 antenatal patients. Although the methods we use to analyse data of this type are based on the observed frequencies, it is easier to see what is going on by expressing the frequencies as percentages of either the row or column totals, especially when there are large variations among the row or column totals. Table 10.6 shows the data from Table 10.5 expressed as row percentages. In this section I shall describe the general approach to frequency tables with $r$ rows and $c$ columns – the $r \times c$ table. Although this method can be used for tables of any size, if either $r$ or $c$ is equal to 2, the method can be simplified (see section 10.7 for $2 \times 2$ tables and section 10.8 for $2 \times k$ tables).

**Table 10.5** Caffeine consumption and marital status in antenatal patients (from Martin and Bracken, 1987)

| | Caffeine consumption (mg/day) | | | | |
|---|---|---|---|---|---|
| Marital status | 0 | 1–150 | 151–300 | > 300 | Total |
| Married | 652 | 1537 | 598 | 242 | 3029 |
| Divorced, separated or widowed | 36 | 46 | 38 | 21 | 141 |
| Single | 218 | 327 | 106 | 67 | 718 |
| Total | 906 | 1910 | 742 | 330 | 3888 |

**Table 10.6** Caffeine consumption and marital status data from Table 10.5 expressed as row percentages

| | Caffeine consumption (mg/day) | | | | |
|---|---|---|---|---|---|
| Marital status | 0 | 1–150 | 151–300 | > 300 | Total |
| Married | 22% | 51% | 20% | 8% | 3029 (100%) |
| Divorced, separated or widowed | 26% | 33% | 27% | 15% | 141 (100%) |
| Single | 30% | 46% | 15% | 9% | 718 (100%) |
| Total | 23% | 49% | 19% | 8% | 3888 (100%) |

The analysis of frequency tables is largely based on hypothesis testing. The null hypothesis is that the two classifications (caffeine consumption and marital status) are unrelated in the relevant population (antenatal patients). We compare the observed frequencies with what we would expect if the null hypothesis were true. We base our calculation of the expected frequencies on the distribution of the variables in the whole sample, as indicated by the row and column totals. The combinations of row and column categories are known as **cells**.

For reasons that will be explained in section 10.6.4 it turns out that the appropriate test statistic is obtained from the observed and expected frequencies, $O$ and $E$ respectively, by calculating the sum of the quantities $(O - E)^2/E$ for all the cells in the table. The further the observed values are away from the expected values, the less likely is it that the null hypothesis is true. Thus a large value of $\Sigma(O - E)^2/E$ is evidence that the row and column variables are not independent.

### 10.6.2 Expected frequencies

If the null hypothesis is true and the two variables are unrelated (i.e. independent) then the probability of an individual being in a particular row is independent of which column they are in. The probability of being in a particular cell of the table is thus simply the product of the probabilities of being in the row and the column containing that cell. These probabilities are estimated using the observed proportions. For example, there were 3029 married women in the sample of 3888, so that the proportion of married women was 3029/3888. Likewise the proportion of women consuming no caffeine was 906/3888. Thus if marital status and caffeine consumption are independent the expected proportion of the whole sample who are married and consume no caffeine is the product of these proportions:

$$\frac{3029}{3888} \times \frac{906}{3888} = 0.182.$$

To get the expected frequency in that cell of the table we multiply by the sample size, to get

$$3888 \times \frac{3029}{3888} \times \frac{906}{3888} = \frac{3029 \times 906}{3888} = 705.8.$$

The expected frequency in each cell is thus the product of the relevant row and column totals divided by the sum of all the observed frequencies in the table (i.e. the sample size). Table 10.7 shows the expected frequencies for the whole table. The hypothesis test is based on the difference between the frequencies in Tables 10.5 and 10.7. As explained in section 10.6.4, the appropriate test statistic is obtained by calculating the

**Table 10.7** Expected frequencies corresponding to Table 10.5

| Marital status | Caffeine consumption (mg/day) 0 | 1–150 | 151–300 | > 300 | Total |
|---|---|---|---|---|---|
| Married | 705.8 | 1488.0 | 578.1 | 257.1 | 3029 |
| Divorced, separated or widowed | 32.9 | 69.3 | 26.9 | 12.0 | 141 |
| Single | 167.3 | 352.7 | 137.0 | 60.9 | 718 |
| Total | 906 | 1910 | 742 | 330 | 3888 |

sum of the quantities $(O - E)^2/E$ for all the cells in the table, where $O$ and $E$ denote the observed and expected frequencies. The test statistic $X^2$ is thus

$$X^2 = \sum_{i=1}^{r} \sum_{j=1}^{c} \frac{(O_{ij} - E_{ij})^2}{E_{ij}},$$

where $i$ indicates the row number and $j$ the column number. This formula is often written simply as

$$X^2 = \sum \frac{(O - E)^2}{E}.$$

Note that the sum of all the differences $O_{ij} - E_{ij}$ is zero because the observed and expected frequencies both add up to the sample size. We square the differences before adding them, as we do when calculating the standard deviation of a set of observations around their mean.

When the null hypothesis is true the statistic $X^2$ has a Chi squared distribution; this was briefly introduced in section 9.8.6. For this reason the test is usually called the **Chi squared test**. The test statistic is often written $\chi^2$, but it is better to call the test statistic $X^2$ to distinguish it from the theoretical distribution.

### 10.6.3 The Chi squared distribution

The definition of the Chi squared distribution is simple. If we have a quantity (variable) $X$ which has a standard Normal distribution, then $X^2$ has a Chi squared distribution. Clearly $X^2$ can have only positive values, and its distribution is highly skewed. This distribution of $X^2$ has one degree of freedom, and is the simplest case of a more general 'family' of Chi squared distributions. If we have several independent variables, each of which has a standard Normal distribution, say $X_1$, $X_2$, $X_3$, ..., $X_k$, then the sum of the squares of all the $X$s, $\Sigma X_i^2$, has a Chi squared

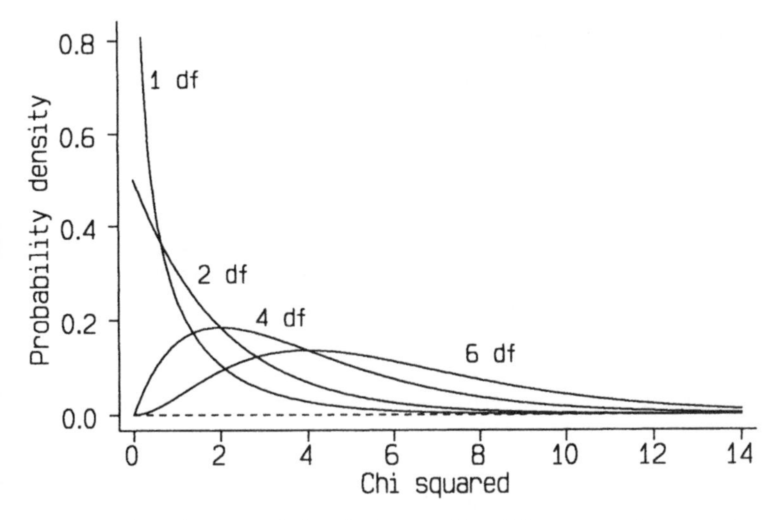


**Figure 10.2** Chi squared distributions with different numbers of degrees of freedom.

distribution with $k$ degrees of freedom. Figure 10.2 shows theoretical Chi squared distributions with different degrees of freedom.

The Chi squared distribution with one degree of freedom is the square of a standard Normal distribution, so the 5% cut-off point for $X^2$ is the square of the 5% cut-off for the Normal distribution, that is, $1.96^2$ or 3.84. Note that the upper tail of the Chi squared distribution with one degree of freedom corresponds to *both* tails of the standard Normal distribution. In other words, for a hypothesis test we compare $X^2$ with $\chi^2_{0.95}$.

The number of degrees of freedom when using the Chi squared test for a two way frequency table is the product $(r-1)(c-1)$, where $r$ is the number of rows and $c$ the number of columns. For a $2 \times 2$ table, therefore, we compare our test statistic $X^2$ with the Chi squared distribution with one degree of freedom. Table 10.5 has 3 rows and 4 columns so we must refer $X^2$ to the Chi squared distribution with $(3-1)(4-1) = 6$ degrees of freedom. The expected value of the Chi squared distribution when the null hypothesis is true is the number of degrees of freedom. Because any differences between observed and expected frequencies are squared, non-independence of the row and column variables is indicated by high values of $X^2$. Table B5 gives upper tail areas for Chi squared distributions with different degrees of freedom. It is simple to verify that the entries for one degree of freedom are the squares of the corresponding two-tailed areas of the Normal distribution in Table B2. The next two sections explain why we use the Chi squared distribution for analysing frequency tables, and also why the degrees of freedom are $(r-1)(c-1)$.

### 10.6.4 Why we use the Chi squared distribution

*(This short section is more theoretical although not highly mathematical. It explains the rationale behind the use of the Chi squared distribution, the most common method for analysing frequency tables. It can be omitted without loss of continuity.)*

Why is the Chi squared distribution appropriate for the analysis of categorical data? Strangely, the answer to this question involves both the Poisson and Normal distributions. If we observe a number of independent individuals, and categorize them into mutually exclusive groups in relation to two classifications, such as in Table 10.5, then the number in any cell of that table will follow a Poisson distribution if the null hypothesis is true. For the purpose of a hypothesis test we wish to compare the observed number, $O$, in each cell with the number expected, $E$, if the null hypothesis is true. The Poisson distribution can be approximated by a Normal distribution with mean $E$ and standard deviation $\sqrt{E}$, when $E$ is not too small. Thus $X = (O - E)/\sqrt{E}$ has approximately a standard Normal distribution, and $X^2 = (O - E)^2/E$ has approximately a Chi squared distribution with one degree of freedom. If we have $k$ independent observed frequencies we can add together the quantities $(O - E)^2/E$ for each to get a Chi squared distribution with $k$ degrees of freedom. When analysing frequency tables not all of the frequencies are independent, however, so we must modify the degrees of freedom.

### 10.6.5 Degrees of freedom

As shown in section 10.6.2, the expected frequency in any cell is the product of the relevant row and column totals divided by the total sample size. The expected frequencies are calculated from the observed row and column totals, and so the Chi squared test is 'conditional' on these totals. Because of the use of observed totals the expected frequencies are not all independent. Consider the first row of Table 10.5. The expected frequencies are 705.8, 1488.0, 578.1 and 257.1, as shown in Table 10.7. We know, however, that the sum of the expected frequencies in the first row is the same as the sum of the observed frequencies, that is 3029. Any of the expected values can therefore be obtained if we already know all the others in that row. The same applies to every row. There are thus only $c - 1$ independent columns in the table. Likewise there are only $r - 1$ independent rows, and consequently $(r - 1)(c - 1)$ independent frequencies. The test statistic $X^2$ thus follows the Chi squared distribution with $(r - 1)(c - 1)$ degrees of freedom under the null hypothesis.

We can see the above process very simply in the $2 \times 2$ table, for which all four expected frequencies can be obtained once we have one of them.

There is thus only one degree of freedom, agreeing with the general formula of $(r - 1)(c - 1) = (2 - 1)(2 - 1) = 1$.

### 10.6.6 The Chi squared test for an $r \times c$ table

In section 10.6.2 I introduced the test statistic $X^2$ for evaluating the null hypothesis that the categorical variables denoting the rows and columns are independent. We can calculate expected frequencies in each cell of the table on the assumption that the null hypothesis is true, and then calculate $X^2$ as

$$X^2 = \sum_{i=1}^{r} \sum_{j=1}^{c} \frac{(O_{ij} - E_{ij})^2}{E_{ij}}$$

where $i$ and $j$ indicate the row and column numbers. Table 10.8 shows the contribution of each cell of Table 10.5 to the test statistic, which is $X^2 = 51.61$. From Table B5 the value of the Chi-squared distribution with 6 degrees of freedom which cuts off 0.1% in the upper tail is 22.46, so there is a highly significant association ($P < 0.001$) between marital status and caffeine consumption in this sample of women. In section 10.9.1 there is further discussion of this data set that takes account of the fact that one of the variables has ordered categories.

**Table 10.8** Contributions of each cell in Table 10.5 to $X^2 = \Sigma(O - E)^2/E$

| Marital status | Caffeine consumption (mg/day) 0 | 1–150 | 151–300 | > 300 | Total |
|---|---|---|---|---|---|
| Married | 4.11 | 1.61 | 0.69 | 0.89 | 7.30 |
| Divorced, separated or widowed | 0.30 | 7.82 | 4.57 | 6.82 | 19.51 |
| Single | 15.36 | 1.88 | 7.02 | 0.60 | 24.86 |
| Total | 19.77 | 11.31 | 12.28 | 8.31 | 51.66 |

### 10.6.7 Interpretation

Many statistical analyses involve evaluation of possible associations between variables, notably the Chi squared test and the equivalent method for relating two continuous variables, correlation (see Chapter 11). It is essential to realize that an observed association does not necessarily indicate a causal relation between variables. We should not infer that marital status influences caffeine consumption, nor indeed that caffeine consumption influences marital status, without external evidence. Very often, as in this example, there will be other factors that influence both variables. Further discussion of the interpretation of association is given in section 11.8.

A different problem is the interpretation of an observed association between two variables each of which has several categories, as in the caffeine example. Just saying that the two variables are associated is often not very informative. We might wish to know, for example, if one of the three marital status groups differs from the other two groups. Here we have a multiple comparison problem comparable to that for continuous variables discussed in section 9.8.4. One way to proceed is to make comparisons between each pair of groups, or if there is some prior hypothesis that one group might differ then that group could be compared with the combined data from the other groups. These procedures are not ideal because they involve some *ad hoc* or subjective analyses. The further testing of subsets of a large table should only be carried out if the overall analysis shows some evidence of departure from the null hypothesis (perhaps $P < 0.1$) or where some specific prior hypothesis exists. Fortunately, as noted below, we do not often have to deal with this type of analysis. In particular, the analysis of tables with only two rows (or columns) is discussed in sections 10.7 and 10.8.

One last important comment on interpretation is the reminder that the size of $X^2$ (or P) does not indicate the strength of the association, but rather the strength of the evidence against the null hypothesis of no association.

### 10.6.8 Sample size

As described in section 10.6.4, the use of Chi squared distribution for the test statistic $X^2$ is based on a 'large sample' approximation. In the context of frequency tables there are some fairly clear guidelines on how large the frequencies need to be for the method to be valid. The guidelines, attributed to the statistician W. G. Cochran, are that 80% of the cells in the table should have expected frequencies greater than 5, and all cells should have expected frequencies greater than 1. Notice that the observed frequencies are not involved here, only the expected frequencies.

If any cell had a very small expected frequency it would contribute enormously to the value of $X^2$. For example, if we observe one subject in a cell with an expected frequency of 0.1, the contribution of that cell to $X^2$ would be $(1.0 - 0.1)^2/0.1 = 8.1$, enough to give a significant result in a $4 \times 2$ table regardless of the other frequencies.

If we have a table with too many small expected frequencies we should find some sensible way to combine some of the categories in the row and/or column variables. There is a special method for $2 \times 2$ tables with small frequencies (section 10.7.2).

### 10.6.9 Particular types of frequency table

The Chi squared test for the $r \times c$ frequency table has been discussed and illustrated in its most general form. There are two considerations that determine special types of table and lead to different analyses: firstly if the categories of one variable (or both) are ordered, and secondly if one variable (or both) has only two categories. In practice large tables are rare where neither variable has ordered categories. Indeed the caffeine data used to illustrate the method had one variable ordered, and I shall return to that data set later.

The importance of ordered categories was discussed in section 9.8, and the same argument applies to categorical variables. If we are analysing data for an ordinal variable we will usually wish to know if there is some trend across the ordered groups rather than just whether the groups differ. This more specific possibility allows for a more sensitive (powerful) statistical analysis.

The case when one variable has only two categories is important because the data can also be considered as proportions; the analyses turn out to be precisely equivalent to the methods for comparing proportions described in sections 10.3 and 10.5. Also, although we still use the same general formula of $X^2 = \Sigma[(O - E)^2/E]$, it can be simplified for easier calculation. The simplest frequency table, the $2 \times 2$ table, turns out to have certain problems all of its own, especially for small samples. The various types of table to consider are listed in Table 10.9 with the numbers of the sections in which the analysis is described.

**Table 10.9** Different types of frequency table, according to number of categories (2 or 3+) and whether categories are ordered

| Number of categories | | Section of book |
|---|---|---|
| Variable 1 | Variable 2 | |
| 2 | 2 | 10.7 |
| 2 | 3+ not ordered | 10.8.1 |
| 2 | 3+ ordered | 10.8.2 |
| 3+ not ordered | 3+ not ordered | 10.6.6 |
| 3+ ordered | 3+ not ordered | 10.9.1 |
| 3+ ordered | 3+ ordered | 10.9.2 |

The analysis of $2 \times 2$ tables is one of the most common in medical research, so I shall consider it first.

## 10.7 2 × 2 FREQUENCY TABLES – COMPARISON OF TWO PROPORTIONS

The analysis of 2 × 2 tables follows the same basic method as used for larger tables, but there are some particular features to note. Table 10.10 shows data from a case-control study carried out among swimmers to investigate the possible association between exposure to chlorinated swimming pool water and erosion of dental enamel. Among 49 swimmers with enamel erosion (the cases) 32 reported swimming six or more hours per week, compared with 118 of 245 swimmers without enamel erosion (the controls). We can see that, although the data are displayed as a 2 × 2 frequency table, the comparison of the groups is in fact a comparison of two proportions. I shall show in section 10.7.4 that the Chi squared test is exactly equivalent to the hypothesis test for comparing two proportions given in section 10.3.

**Table 10.10** Comparison of number of hours' swimming by swimmers with or without erosion of dental enamel (Centerwall *et al.*, 1986)

| Amount of swimming per week | Erosion of dental enamel | | |
|---|---|---|---|
| | Yes (cases) | No (controls) | Total |
| $\geq$ 6 hours | 32 | 118 | 150 |
| $<$ 6 hours | 17 | 127 | 144 |
| Total | 49 | 245 | 294 |

The null hypothesis is that enamel erosion is unrelated to amounts of swimming (and hence exposure to chlorinated water). To perform a Chi squared test we need to calculate the expected frequencies if the null hypothesis is true. It will help in the calculations if we use $a$, $b$, $c$ and $d$ to denote the four observed frequencies, as in Table 10.11.

**Table 10.11** General 2 × 2 frequency table

| | Column 1 | Column 2 | Total |
|---|---|---|---|
| Row 1 | $a$ | $b$ | $a + b$ |
| Row 2 | $c$ | $d$ | $c + d$ |
| Total | $a + c$ | $b + d$ | $N$ |

As we saw in section 10.6.2 the expected frequency in a cell is the product of the relevant row and column totals divided by the sample size. For the cell with observed frequency $a$, for example, the expected value is $(a + b)(a + c)/N$. For the data in Table 10.10 the expected frequencies and contributions to $X^2$ are shown in Table 10.12. The difference $O - E$ is the same, apart from its sign, for all four cells, and this is true for all $2 \times 2$ tables. This demonstrates that we have only one independent observation rather than four and so just one degree of freedom.

**Table 10.12** Expected frequencies and contributions to $X^2$ for the data in Table 10.10

| Observed frequency ($O$) | Expected frequency ($E$) | $O - E$ | $\frac{(O-E)^2}{E}$ |
|---|---|---|---|
| $a = 32$ | $E(a) = 25$ | 7 | 1.960 |
| $b = 118$ | $E(b) = 125$ | −7 | 0.392 |
| $c = 17$ | $E(c) = 24$ | −7 | 2.042 |
| $d = 127$ | $E(d) = 120$ | 7 | 0.408 |
| Total 294 | 294 | 0 | $X^2 = 4.802$ |

For a $2 \times 2$ table the formula for $X^2$ can be simplified. The contribution from the first cell in the table to $X^2 = \Sigma[(O - E)^2/E]$ can be expressed as

$$\frac{\left[a - \frac{(a+b)(a+c)}{N}\right]^2}{\frac{(a+b)(a+c)}{N}}$$

and we can produce similar expressions for the other three cells. The sum of the four terms, after much tedious manipulation, can be turned into

$$X^2 = \frac{N(ad - bc)^2}{(a+b)(a+c)(b+d)(c+d)}.$$

This version of the formula for $X^2$ is often used for $2 \times 2$ tables, because it avoids the need to calculate the expected values explicitly. It is important to appreciate that this formula for $X^2$ from a $2 \times 2$ table is mathematically identical to the general formula $X^2 = \Sigma[(O - E)^2/E]$.

For the data in Table 10.10 we get

$$X^2 = \frac{294 \times (32 \times 127 - 118 \times 17)^2}{150 \times 49 \times 245 \times 144}$$

$$= 4.802$$

which agrees with Table 10.12. From Table B5 we get $P < 0.05$, suggesting that there is evidence in support of an association between amount of swimming and erosion of dental enamel.

The Chi squared test is a hypothesis test. It is an exactly equivalent test to the comparison of two proportions described in section 10.3.3, but no estimate of the difference between the groups (or a confidence interval) is obtained when the data are analysed in this way. The approach based on comparing proportions is therefore preferable. There is a third way of comparing proportions, which involves calculating the ratio of proportions in two groups rather than their difference. This approach is particularly suitable for case-control studies and is described in section 10.11.

### 10.7.1 Continuity correction

When the sample sizes are small the use of the continuous Chi squared distribution to approximate frequencies introduces some bias into the calculation, so that the value of $X^2$ tends to be a little too large. We use a continuity correction to remove the bias, in the same way as when comparing two proportions (section 10.3.3). In the context of $2 \times 2$ tables the correction is known as **Yates' correction** after the statistician who devised it.

The correction consists of moving each $O - E$ nearer to zero by $\frac{1}{2}$. In other words we replace $O - E$ by $|O - E| - \frac{1}{2}$. The short cut formula with Yates' correction becomes

$$X_Y^2 = \frac{N\left(|ad - bc| - \dfrac{N}{2}\right)^2}{(a+b)(a+c)(b+d)(c+d)}.$$

I recommend that this formula is used for all Chi squared tests on $2 \times 2$ tables, although for large samples the effect of the correction will be small.

For the dental erosion data the use of the continuity correction gives

$$X_Y^2 = \frac{294 \times (|32 \times 127 - 118 \times 17| - \frac{294}{2})^2}{150 \times 49 \times 245 \times 144}$$

$$= 4.140$$

and we still have $P < 0.05$.

For small samples, however, the difference between $X^2$ and $X_Y^2$ is more marked. The data from the previously discussed trial of IRS *v* placebo in patients with cervical osteoarthrosis will illustrate the effect; the results are shown as a frequency table in Table 10.13. The uncorrected Chi squared test gives

$$X^2 = \frac{25 \times (9 \times 9 - 4 \times 3)^2}{13 \times 12 \times 12 \times 13}$$

$$= 4.891 \qquad (P < 0.05)$$

**Table 10.13** Results of a clinical trial comparing IRS *v* placebo (Lewith and Machin, 1981)

| | | IRS | Placebo | Total |
|---|---|---|---|---|
| Improvement in pain | Yes | 9 | 4 | 13 |
| | No | 3 | 9 | 12 |
| | Total | 12 | 13 | 25 |

whereas the use of Yates' correction gives

$$X_Y^2 = \frac{25 \times (|9 \times 9 - 4 \times 3| - \frac{25}{2})^2}{13 \times 12 \times 12 \times 13}$$

$$= 3.279 \qquad (P > 0.05).$$

This example shows the advantage of giving more exact P values, rather than imprecise ones obtained from a table. Many computer programs give the precise P values for Chi squared tests, which for $X^2$ and $X_Y^2$ in this example are P = 0.027 and P = 0.070 respectively. As discussed in section 8.5, we should not make a radical adjustment to our interpretation just because the P value has moved the other side of 0.05, but the evidence of an association is weaker when we use the more appropriate version of the test with Yates' correction.

These results are exactly the same as when the proportions in the two groups were compared in section 10.3. As noted, the Chi squared method yields only a P value, whereas the comparison of proportions also yields the difference in proportions and its confidence interval. The mathematical equivalence of the two methods is demonstrated in section 10.7.4. It follows that the Chi squared test is equivalent to a comparison of the proportions in the columns and also a comparison of the proportions in the rows.

### 10.7.2 Small samples – Fisher's exact test

The use of Yates' correction does not remove the requirement concerning the size of the expected frequencies. Using the earlier rule that 80% of cells should have expected values of at least 5 we would require all cells of a 2 × 2 table to have this property, although in practice this rule can be relaxed to allow one cell to have an expected value slightly lower than 5. Note that all the expected frequencies in Table 10.13 are greater than 5 even though two of the observed frequencies are less than 5.

There is an alternative approach for tables with very small expected frequencies, known as **Fisher's exact test** after the famous statistician R. A.

Fisher. Although the method is different in principle from any other described in this chapter, it is also based on the observed row and column totals. The method consists of evaluating the probability associated with all possible 2 × 2 tables which have the same row and column totals as the observed data, making the assumption that the null hypothesis is true. As before, the null hypothesis here is that the row and column variables are unrelated. Like the Chi squared test, the method is purely a hypothesis test.

Table 10.14 shows data from a study comparing the health of juvenile delinquent boys and a control group. For each group, the number of boys with vision defects is shown, together with the numbers who did or did not wear spectacles (glasses). We can test the null hypothesis that the proportions wearing glasses in the population are the same; that is, that juvenile delinquents are equally likely to be aware of poor eyesight as other boys. The expected numbers in three of the four cells are below 5, so we should not use a Chi squared test, but we can use Fisher's exact test for which there is no sample size restriction.

**Table 10.14** Spectacle wearing among juvenile delinquents and non-delinquents who failed a vision test (Weindling *et al.*, 1986)

| | | Juvenile delinquents | Non-delinquents | Total |
|---|---|---|---|---|
| Spectacle | Yes | 1 | 5 | 6 |
| wearers | No | 8 | 2 | 10 |
| | Total | 9 | 7 | 16 |

Table 10.15 shows all the possible sets of frequencies which add up to the observed row and column totals, one of which (table (ii)) corresponds to the observed data. For each table we can calculate the probability of such data arising if the null hypothesis is true. We then use these probabilities to calculate the overall probability of getting the observed data, or a less likely result, when the null hypothesis is true.

The mathematical formula to calculate each probability is rather complicated, so the calculation is much better done by a computer. Unfortunately, many statistical packages do not include Fisher's exact test, so the calculations are described in section 10.7.3.

Table 10.16 shows the probabilities associated with all seven sets of frequencies shown in Table 10.15. The overall probability of obtaining a difference between the groups at least as large as the observed difference

**Table 10.15** All tables of frequencies which have the same row and column totals as Table 10.14

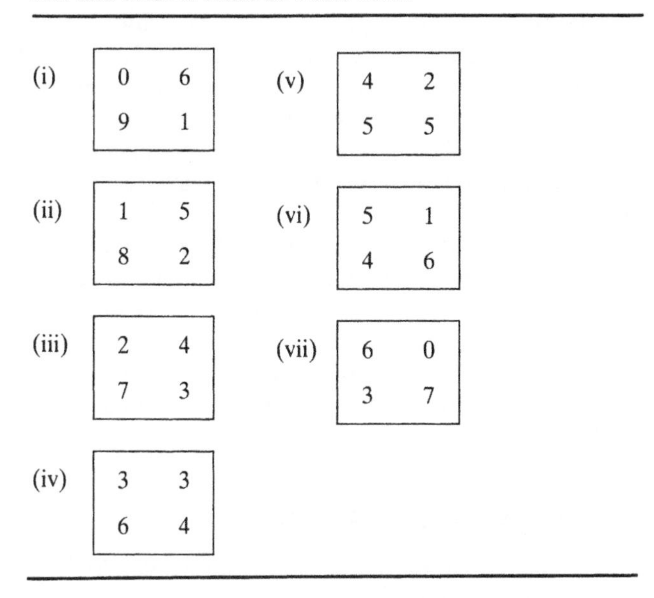

(i)

| | |
|---|---|
| 0 | 6 |
| 9 | 1 |

(ii)

| | |
|---|---|
| 1 | 5 |
| 8 | 2 |

(iii)

| | |
|---|---|
| 2 | 4 |
| 7 | 3 |

(iv)

| | |
|---|---|
| 3 | 3 |
| 6 | 4 |

(v)

| | |
|---|---|
| 4 | 2 |
| 5 | 5 |

(vi)

| | |
|---|---|
| 5 | 1 |
| 4 | 6 |

(vii)

| | |
|---|---|
| 6 | 0 |
| 3 | 7 |

**Table 10.16** Probability associated with each set of frequencies in Table 10.15

| | *a* | *b* | *c* | *d* | P |
|---|---|---|---|---|---|
| (i) | 0 | 6 | 9 | 1 | 0.00087 |
| **(ii)** | **1** | **5** | **8** | **2** | **0.02360** |
| (iii) | 2 | 4 | 7 | 3 | 0.15734 |
| (iv) | 3 | 3 | 6 | 4 | 0.36713 |
| (v) | 4 | 2 | 5 | 5 | 0.33042 |
| (vi) | 5 | 1 | 4 | 6 | 0.11014 |
| (vii) | 6 | 0 | 3 | 7 | 0.01049 |
| | | | | | Total 0.99999 |

when the null hypothesis is true can be calculated in two ways. The first is to evaluate the probabilities in the 'tail' of the distribution in which the observed data fall and then double this value to get a two-tailed test. From Table 10.16 we use the probabilities for tables (i) and (ii) to get $P = (0.00087 + 0.02360) \times 2 = 0.049$. Alternatively, we can add up the probabilities of all tables that have probabilities less than or equal to that corresponding to the observed data. For the example we use the probabilities for tables (i), (ii) and (vii) to get $P = 0.00087 + 0.02360 + 0.01049 = 0.035$. I feel that the second approach is more reasonable, but many statisticians recommend doubling the P value obtained for one tail. In most cases the difference will not be marked (but occasionally it can be). The second approach will always give a value of P less than or equal to that obtained by the first method. In this example we can conclude that there is some evidence that juvenile delinquents are less aware of eyesight problems than non-delinquents.

Lastly, it should be noted that Fisher's exact test usually gives a value for P that is much the same as that from a Chi squared test with Yates' correction even when the expected frequencies are too small for the latter approach, suggesting that the rule relating to expected frequencies is probably too restrictive. Fisher's exact test is purely a hypothesis test – there is no equivalent method of estimation for comparing proportions from very small samples.

### 10.7.3 Fisher's exact test – mathematics and worked example

*(This section is more theoretical although not highly mathematical. It can be omitted without loss of continuity.)*

The probability of obtaining the cell frequencies $a$, $b$, $c$ and $d$ when the null hypothesis is true and the row and column totals are fixed is given by

$$\frac{(a+b)!(a+c)!(b+d)!(c+d)!}{N!a!b!c!d!}$$

where the symbol $x!$, called '$x$ factorial', means that we multiply together all the integers from 1 up to $x$ (see Appendix A). For example, $4! = 1 \times 2 \times 3 \times 4 = 24$. (Note that we need to define $0! = 1$.) This peculiar formula is derived from calculating the number of different ways (combinations) in which the $N$ individuals can be arranged in a table to give the observed row and column totals. Table 10.15 shows the seven such tables for the eyesight data of Table 10.14.

For the first possibility (i) we have $a = 0$, $b = 6$, $c = 9$ and $d = 1$, so that the probability of this table arising by chance when the null hypothesis is true is

$$\frac{6!9!7!10!}{16!0!6!9!1!}.$$

Evaluating this formula is tedious. In this example there are some 70 numbers in the calculation, and multiplying together all the numbers in the top row first may exceed the storage capability of a calculator or computer. However, the calculation can usually be simplified by cancelling out sequences that appear on the top and bottom of the formula. Here 6! and 9! can be deleted immediately, and we can omit 0! and 1! as they are both equal to 1, so that the probability reduces to

$$\frac{7!10!}{16!} = \frac{1 \times 2 \times 3 \times 4 \times 5 \times 6 \times 7}{11 \times 12 \times 13 \times 14 \times 15 \times 16}$$

$$= \frac{1}{11 \times 13 \times 8}$$

$$= 0.0087.$$

For table (ii), which corresponds to the observed data, we get a probability of

$$\frac{6!9!7!10!}{16!1!5!8!2!}.$$

We can simplify this expression by noting that $9!/8! = 9$, and so on, to get

$$\frac{6 \times 9 \times 2 \times 3 \times 4 \times 5 \times 6 \times 7}{11 \times 12 \times 13 \times 14 \times 15 \times 16 \times 2}$$

$$= 0.02360.$$

To perform Fisher's exact test we carry out the same calculation for all tables, as shown in Table 10.16. We could just calculate the probability for those tables which contribute to the tail(s) of the distribution of probabilities, but it is not easy to identify these in advance. The benefit of a computer program is clearly seen.

### 10.7.4 Equivalence of the comparison of proportions and the Chi squared test

*(This section is more theoretical although not highly mathematical. It can be omitted without loss of continuity.)*

I have commented more than once that the method for comparing two independent proportions is identical to the Chi squared test for a $2 \times 2$ table. This can be shown mathematically, by expressing the comparison of two proportions in the notation of Table 10.11. We have $p_1 = a/(a + c)$, $p_2 = b/(b + d)$, and the pooled proportion is $p = (a + b)/N$, so that the value of $z$ for comparing the two observed proportions is

$$z = \frac{p_1 - p_2}{\sqrt{p(1 - p)\left(\frac{1}{n_1} + \frac{1}{n_2}\right)}}$$

$$z = \frac{\dfrac{a}{a+c} - \dfrac{b}{b+d}}{\sqrt{\dfrac{a+b}{N}\dfrac{c+d}{N}\left(\dfrac{1}{a+c} + \dfrac{1}{b+d}\right)}}$$

which, after some manipulation, gives

$$z = \sqrt{\frac{N(ad - bc)^2}{(a+b)(a+c)(b+d)(c+d)}}$$
$$= \sqrt{X^2}.$$

The value of $z$ is thus the square root of the value of $X^2$, and the two tests are equivalent because, as noted in section 10.6.3, the Chi squared distribution with one degree of freedom is the square of the standard Normal distribution.

### 10.7.5 2 × 2 tables – paired samples

Paired proportions may also be shown as a 2 × 2 table. For example, the data in Table 10.3 can be rearranged as in Table 10.17. Although the table closely resembles those relating to the comparison of two independent proportions, such as Tables 10.10, 10.13 and 10.14, it is essential to remember that the proportions are paired and so the usual Chi squared test is inappropriate.

**Table 10.17** Results of Table 10.3 rearranged as a 2 × 2 table, showing numbers with (+) or without (−) sleeping difficulties among marijuana users and matched controls

| | | Marijuana group | | |
|---|---|---|---|---|
| | | + | − | Total |
| Control group | + | 4 | 9 | 13 |
| | − | 3 | 16 | 19 |
| | Total | 7 | 25 | 32 |

The comparison of paired proportions is based on the frequencies of pairs with different outcomes, as we saw in section 10.4 where the confidence interval and hypothesis test were described. In section 10.4.3 the test statistic incorporating the continuity correction was given as

$$z_c = \frac{|b - c| - 1}{\sqrt{b + c}}.$$

Sometimes the test statistic is calculated slightly differently as

$$X^2 = \frac{(|b - c| - 1)^2}{b + c},$$

which is clearly equal to $z_c^2$. The value of $X^2$ is referred to the Chi squared distribution with one degree of freedom. As we have seen for independent proportions these two tests are exactly equivalent.

The test of paired proportions is often known as **McNemar's test**, especially when the data are shown as a 2 × 2 table.

## 10.8 2 × *k* TABLES – COMPARISON OF SEVERAL PROPORTIONS

As indicated earlier, the statistical comparison of proportions derived from more than two groups differs according to whether the categories defining the groups are ordered or not.

Discussing 2 × *k* tables as a special case makes it rather easier to discuss the problems of multiple comparisons, and to consider the special situation of ordered groups. Also there is a 'short-cut' formula available for hand calculations.

### 10.8.1 Unordered categories

Table 10.18 shows reported eye strain for four types of office workers. The data are from a study carried out to assess possible harmful effects of using visual display units (VDUs) (i.e. computer monitors). The null hypothesis is that there is no difference in the proportions reporting eye strain in the four groups.

Analysis of proportions from unordered categories can be based on

**Table 10.18** Eye strain reported by four groups of office workers (Reading and Weale, 1986)

| Type of work | Number in sample | Number with eye strain | Proportion with eye strain |
|---|---|---|---|
| Data entry in VDUs | 53 | 11 | 0.208 |
| Conversational use of VDUs | 109 | 30 | 0.275 |
| Full-time typing | 78 | 14 | 0.179 |
| Traditional office work (clerical) | 55 | 3 | 0.055 |
| Total | 295 | 58 | 0.197 |

calculation of $X^2$ according to the general formula previously given: $X^2 = \Sigma[(O - E)^2/E]$. An alternative formulation is as follows. If there are $n_i$ subjects in group $i$, of whom $r_i$ have the characteristic of interest, we can calculate $X^2$ as

$$X^2 = \frac{\sum_{i=1}^{k}(r_i^2/n_i) - R^2/N}{P(1 - P)}$$

where $R$ is the total number with the characteristic ($R = \Sigma r_i$), $N$ is the total sample size, and $P = R/N$. We compare $X^2$ to the Chi squared distribution with $k - 1$ degrees of freedom. For the data in Table 10.18, we have

$$X^2 = \frac{\frac{11^2}{53} + \frac{30^2}{109} + \frac{14^2}{78} + \frac{3^2}{55} - \frac{58^2}{295}}{\frac{58}{295} \times \frac{237}{295}}$$

$$= \frac{1.8130}{0.1580}$$

$$= 11.48$$

which, from the table of Chi squared with 3 degrees of freedom (Table B5), corresponds to $P < 0.01$ (the exact value is $P = 0.0094$). There is thus strong evidence that eye strain is not equally common in all four groups.

Interpretation of this highly significant variation among the groups depends upon isolating which groups differ from the others. In the absence of any prior hypothesis comparison of each pair of groups requires six further tests, and the risk of a false positive result is high unless we adjust the P values. A better approach is often to combine, or 'collapse', some groups. As this study was carried out to examine the possible adverse health effect of using VDUs, the two VDU groups can reasonably be combined and compared with each of the other two groups. Of the subjects in the two VDU groups combined, 41/162 (0.253) had eye strain.

The results of the three paired comparisons (2 × 2 tables with Yates' correction) are as follows:

| Comparison | $X^2$ | P |
|---|---|---|
| VDU v Typing: | 1.22 | 0.27 |
| VDU v Traditional: | 8.82 | 0.003 |
| Typing v Traditional: | 3.47 | 0.06 |

It seems, therefore, that both typing and using a VDU, especially the latter, are associated with more eye strain than traditional clerical office work. We probably should multiply the P values by three (the Bonferroni correction) to allow for the multiple comparisons. Either way there is no evidence from this study to suggest that use of a VDU is associated with more eye strain than typing.

### 10.8.2 Ordered categories

When we wish to compare frequencies or proportions among groups which have an ordering, we should make use of the ordering to increase the power of the statistical analysis. The method described in the previous section assesses departure of the observed data from the null hypothesis that the groups are the same, but in no particular manner. When the groups are ordered we usually expect any differences among the groups to be related to the ordering. Failure to take account of the ordering of groups is a common statistical error (Moses *et al.*, 1984). Two main possible analyses are described below.

*(a) Chi squared test for trend*

We can subdivide variation among groups into that due to a *trend* in proportions across the groups and the remainder. Although the value of $X^2$ for trend will always be less than $X^2$ for the overall comparison, the **Chi squared test for trend** is a powerful method of analysis because it yields a test statistic from a Chi squared distribution with one degree of freedom rather than $k-1$ degrees of freedom for the usual Chi squared test. If most of the variation is due to a trend across the groups, then the test for trend will yield a much smaller P value.

The test for trend will be illustrated using the data in Table 10.19 (already shown as Table 10.1) relating the frequency of babies delivered by Caesarean section to maternal shoe size. The rationale for this study was that small shoe size is a simple indicator of possible birth difficulty due to a small pelvis. The data for larger shoe sizes have been amalgamated to give adequate expected numbers in all cells. The standard Chi squared test of this $2 \times 6$ table give $X^2 = 9.29$ with 5 degrees of freedom, for which $P = 0.098$.

**Table 10.19** Relation between frequency of Caesarean section and maternal shoe size (Frame *et al.*, 1985)

| | Shoe size | | | | | | |
|---|---|---|---|---|---|---|---|
| Caesarean section | < 4 | 4 | $4\frac{1}{2}$ | 5 | $5\frac{1}{2}$ | 6+ | Total |
| Yes | 5 | 7 | 6 | 7 | 8 | 10 | 43 |
| No | 17 | 28 | 36 | 41 | 46 | 140 | 308 |
| Total | 22 | 35 | 42 | 48 | 54 | 150 | 351 |

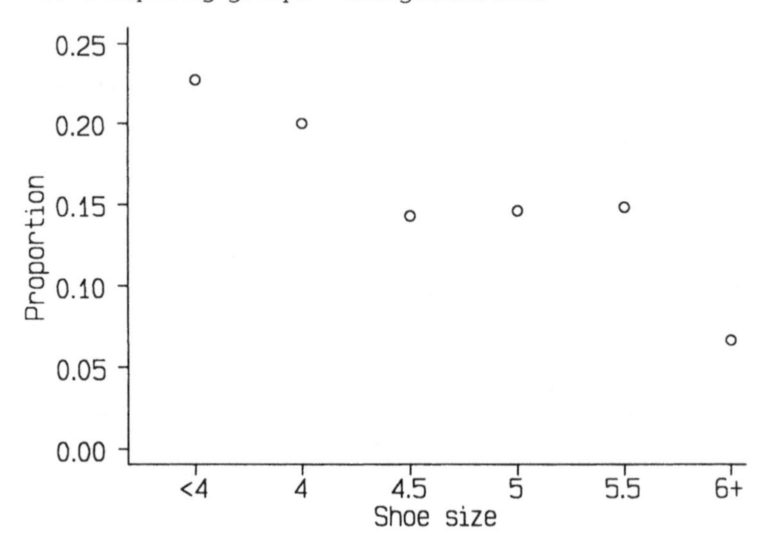


**Figure 10.3** Proportions of women having a baby by Caesarean section in different shoe size groups.

Table 10.19 shows the numbers of women having a baby by Caesarean section in each shoe size group, from which we can obtain the proportions in each group, shown graphically in Figure 10.3. The method for evaluating a trend is effectively to fit a straight line to the proportions, and see if the slope of the line is significantly different from zero (which represents a horizontal line). We need to take account of the fact that each proportion is based on different numbers of women. The method for fitting such a line is called regression analysis, and is not described until section 11.3, but we can obtain the same result by a calculation based on the observed frequencies. From this analysis we get a value of the test statistic $X^2_{trend}$ on one degree of freedom. The calculations are described later.

In order to carry out this test we have to assign scores to each group. If the variable has a clear quantitative interpretation we can derive the scores from the definition of the groups. For example, the shoe size data can be scored 3.5, 4.0, 4.5, 5.0, 5.5 and 6.0 (or, equivalently, 1, 2, 3, 4, 5 and 6). The null hypothesis is now that there is no trend across groups. If the scores are equally spaced we refer to an observed trend as a *linear* trend.

Analysis of the Caesarean section data gives $X^2_{trend} = 8.02$ on 1 degree of freedom ($P = 0.005$). There is thus strong evidence of a linear trend in the proportion of women giving birth by Caesarean section in relation to shoe size. This relation is not directly causal, of course, and no such interpretation should be made. Shoe size is here a convenient indicator of small pelvic size.

The overall value of $X^2$ was 9.29 on 5 degrees of freedom. We can subtract the value of $X^2_{trend}$ (8.02) to get a Chi squared test of the null hypothesis of no variation other than that due to trend. Here we get $X^2 = 1.27$ on 4 degrees of freedom, which is nowhere near to statistical significance. We can conclude that all the observed variation between the groups can be attributed to a linear trend.

Note that, although the linear trend is highly significant, if we tried to use shoe size to predict which women would require a Caesarean section we would be wrong most of the time. This type of problem is considered in section 14.4.

*(b) Method and worked example*

The simplest way to calculate $X^2_{trend}$ is by means of a formula that disguises the nature of the method. Fleiss (1981, p. 144) shows the derivation of the formula using the regression approach (see also section 11.15.2).

For group $i$ we will call the observed frequency with a characteristic $r_i$ and the total number of individuals $n_i$. Further, we let $x_i$ be the score allocated to group $i$. Then we define some simplifying quantities as follows:

$$N = \sum_{i=1}^{k} n_i, \quad R = \sum_{i=1}^{k} r_i, \quad p = R/N, \quad \text{and } \bar{x} = \sum_{i=1}^{k} n_i x_i / N.$$

The test statistic $X^2_{trend}$ is then obtained as

$$X^2_{trend} = \frac{\left[\sum_{i=1}^{k} r_i x_i - R\bar{x}\right]^2}{p(1-p)\left[\sum_{i=1}^{k} n_i x_i^2 - N\bar{x}^2\right]}.$$

**Table 10.20** Calculation of $X^2_{trend}$ for the data in Table 10.19

| | Shoe size | | | | | | |
|---|---|---|---|---|---|---|---|
| | <4 | 4 | $4\frac{1}{2}$ | 5 | $5\frac{1}{2}$ | 6+ | Total |
| Caesarean section ($r_i$) | 5 | 7 | 6 | 7 | 8 | 10 | 43 (= $R$) |
| Total ($n_i$) | 22 | 35 | 42 | 48 | 54 | 150 | 351 (= $N$) |
| Score ($x_i$) | 1 | 2 | 3 | 4 | 5 | 6 | |
| $r_i x_i$ | 5 | 14 | 18 | 28 | 40 | 60 | 165 |
| $n_i x_i$ | 22 | 70 | 126 | 192 | 270 | 900 | 1580 |
| $n_i x_i^2$ | 22 | 140 | 378 | 768 | 1350 | 5400 | 8058 |

$\bar{x} = 1580/351 = 4.5014$; $p = 43/351 = 0.1225$; $1 - p = 0.8775$

Table 10.20 shows the basic calculation for the Caesarean section data. From these elements we get

$$X^2_{trend} = \frac{(165 - 43 \times 4.5014)^2}{0.1225 \times 0.8775 \times (8058 - 351 \times 4.5014^2)}$$

$$= \frac{815.6850}{101.6705}$$

$$= 8.023 \text{ (P} = 0.0046).$$

*(c) Qualitatively ordered groups*

We often have data from groups which are clearly ordered, but where there is either no underlying scale of measurement or such a scale cannot be quantified. Examples of these two types of variable are social class and pain recorded as 'mild', 'moderate' or 'severe'. In the absence of any indication to the contrary it is generally reasonable to give such groups equally spaced scores and evaluate $X^2_{trend}$ as if for a linear trend.

Sometimes, however, it is felt that a different spacing of scores is appropriate. For example, Norton and Dunn (1985) carried out a survey in which they related frequency of snoring to various medical conditions. Subjects were categorized as either non-snorers, occasional snorers, those who snored nearly every night, and those who snored every night, on the basis of their spouses' reports. Table 10.21 shows data relating snoring to heart disease. The authors performed a Chi squared test for trend using scores of 1, 3, 5 and 6 for the four snoring groups. The overall comparison of the groups gives $X^2 = 72.8$ on 3 degrees of freedom while the trend test gives $X^2_{trend} = 72.7$ on 1 degree of freedom. Both of these are very highly significant. It is clear that all of the differences between the groups can be attributed to the trend. That is, there is a strong association between frequency of snoring and prevalence of heart disease.

The scores used in this study were not very different from equal spacing – given the descriptions of the groups perhaps 1, 2, 5 and 6 would have been more reasonable. In practice small differences in scoring are unlikely to have much effect on the test statistic. Of course, the scores should not

**Table 10.21** Snoring behaviour in relation to presence or absence of heart disease (Norton and Dunn, 1985)

| Heart disease | Non-snorers | Occasional snorers | Snore nearly every night | Snore every night | Total |
|---|---|---|---|---|---|
| Yes | 24 (1.7%) | 35 (5.5%) | 21 (9.9%) | 30 (11.8%) | 110 (4.2%) |
| No | 1355 | 603 | 192 | 224 | 2374 |
| Total | 1379 | 638 | 213 | 254 | 2484 |

be decided on the basis of the data but on prior considerations.

*(d) Alternative approach – the Mann-Whitney test*

A different approach to frequency data from ordered groups is to treat the data as two samples of observations on an ordinal scale. For example, in Table 10.19 the two samples are women who had a Caesarean section and those who did not. We can give ranks 1, 2, 3, . . ., etc. to the ordered groups, and then compare the ranks for the subjects with or without the characteristic of interest using the Mann-Whitney test (described in section 9.6.4). There are, of course, vast numbers of tied ranks in data of this type because there are few different values, so it is essential to use the version of the test with a correction for ties. Many statistical packages can perform this test.

In general the Mann-Whitney test gives a very similar answer to the Chi squared test for trend. For example, for the Caesarean section data of Table 10.19 we get $z = 2.91$ ($P = 0.0036$) compared with $P = 0.0046$ from the Chi squared test for trend.

## 10.9 LARGE TABLES WITH ORDERED CATEGORIES

We should always take account of ordering in analysis of $2 \times k$ tables, and we should do likewise for larger tables. There are two cases to consider: where either the row or column variable is ordered and where both are ordered.

### 10.9.1 One ordered variable

With three or more groups of subjects classified by an ordinal variable we can use the Kruskall-Wallis test (section 9.8.6) to compare the groups. If the groups differ significantly we can use the Mann-Whitney test to compare pairs of groups. It is essential to use the versions of the tests that adjust for tied ranks.

Large frequency tables in which neither variable is ordered are rare, which is why the ordered caffeine data (Table 10.5) were used to illustrate the general Chi squared analysis of an $r \times c$ table.

### 10.9.2 Two ordered variables

The simplest way to analyse the relation between two ordered variables is to calculate the rank correlation between them. This method will be described in section 11.7.2. However, the appropriate analysis when we wish to compare two or more *paired* ordinal variables on one sample (or matched samples) is the paired Wilcoxon test, which was described in section 9.7.2.

## 10.10 $k \times k$ TABLES – ANALYSIS OF MATCHED VARIABLES

Sometimes we obtain matched pairs of categorizations of the same subjects. For example, we may wish to compare degrees of pain before and after treatment. The simplest case is when subjects are classified into just two groups; we use the Normal method or the McNemar test to compare the paired proportions, as described in sections 10.4 and 10.7.5. When there are three groups there is an extension of the McNemar test known as the Stuart-Maxwell test (see Fleiss (1981, p. 119) for a description).

With three or more *ordered* categories for paired variables the Wilcoxon matched pairs signed ranks test is appropriate (see section 9.7.2).

A related problem occurs when we wish to assess how well two classifications agree; for example, we may wish to compare the way that two histologists classify stage of disease in a series of biopsy samples. The comparison of observers is described in Chapter 14.

## 10.11 COMPARING RISKS

There is yet another way of analysing two by two tables, which involves the comparison of two groups with respect to the risk of some event. The methods were developed in epidemiology, especially for the analysis of case-control studies, but their use is becoming more widespread. I shall consider only the case where there are two groups of subjects and only two types of outcome, although extensions exist.

### 10.11.1 Prospective study – estimating relative risk

In a prospective study groups of subjects with different characteristics are followed up to see whether an outcome of interest occurs. Many clinical trials are like this, but so too are observational studies where it is not possible to randomize the feature of interest, such as blood group. We can easily calculate the proportions having the outcome in each group, and so the ratio of these two proportions is a measure of the raised risk in one group compared to the other. We term this ratio the **relative risk**. Table 10.22 shows the general layout of the $2 \times 2$ table that arises in this situation. The risks in the two groups are $a/(a + c)$ and $b/(b + d)$, and the relative risk is thus

$$RR = \frac{a/(a + c)}{b/(b + d)}.$$

Under the null hypothesis the expected value of $RR$ is 1.

Table 10.23 shows the results of a study of 107 'small-for-dates' babies, that is, of babies whose birth weight was below the fifth centile for their length of gestation using published standards. The babies were classified as

**Table 10.22** General representation of the results of a prospective study as a $2 \times 2$ table

| | | Group 1 | Group 2 | Total |
|---|---|---|---|---|
| Outcome present | Yes | $a$ | $b$ | $a + b$ |
| | No | $c$ | $d$ | $c + d$ |
| | Total | $a + c$ | $b + d$ | $n$ |

**Table 10.23** Relation between Apgar score < 7 and symmetric or asymmetric fetal growth retardation (Kurjak *et al.*, 1978)

| | | Symmetric | Asymmetric | Total |
|---|---|---|---|---|
| Apgar < 7 | Yes | 2 | 33 | 35 |
| | No | 14 | 58 | 72 |
| | Total | 16 | 91 | 107 |

having either 'symmetric' or 'asymmetric' growth retardation on the basis of the ultrasound examination, and this classification is shown in relation to their Apgar score which is an assessment of their well-being (see section 2.4.4).

The proportions with an Apgar score less than 7 were 2/16 (0.13) in the symmetric group and 33/91 (0.36) in the asymmetric group. The relative risk of a low Apgar score is thus

$$\frac{2/16}{33/91} = 0.345$$

that is, the risk in the symmetric group is about 35% of that in the asymmetric group.

We can construct a confidence interval for the relative risk using the following formula for the standard error of its logarithm:

$$SE(\log_e RR) = \sqrt{\frac{1}{a} - \frac{1}{a + c} + \frac{1}{b} - \frac{1}{b + d}}.$$

The sampling distribution of $\log RR$ is the Normal distribution, so we can construct, say, a 90% confidence interval for the log of the relative risk as

$$\log_e RR - N_{0.95} \times SE(\log_e RR) \quad \text{to} \quad \log_e RR + N_{0.95} \times SE(\log_e RR)$$

where $N_{0.95}$ is the appropriate value from the Normal distribution. The confidence interval for the relative risk is obtained by antilogging these values.

In the example, the relative risk was 0.345 and its logarithm (to base e) is −1.0651. The standard error of this value is

$$SE(\log_e RR) = \sqrt{\tfrac{1}{2} - \tfrac{1}{16} + \tfrac{1}{33} - \tfrac{1}{91}}$$
$$= 0.676.$$

Thus we can obtain the 90% confidence interval for the log of the relative risk in the population of all such babies as

$$-1.0651 - 1.645 \times 0.676 \quad \text{to} \quad -1.0651 + 1.645 \times 0.676$$

or −2.177 to 0.047, giving a 90% confidence interval for the relative risk of 0.11 to 1.05. The confidence interval is wide because the sample size in the symmetric group is small.

This approach to the comparison of two proportions is based on their ratio, whereas the method described in section 10.3 is related to their difference. In general the relative risk is more frequently used in epidemiological work, although it could (and perhaps should) be used more for the analysis of clinical data. A third way of comparing groups is via the **odds ratio** described in the next section.

### 10.11.2 Retrospective study – the odds ratio

*(a) Two samples*

In retrospective case-control studies, we can still arrange the data in a table like Table 10.22, but there is an important difference. The selection of subjects is based on the outcome (the rows) whereas in a prospective study it is based on the characteristic defining the groups (the columns). We cannot evaluate the risk of the outcome in those with and without the characteristic because of the way the subjects were sampled. It is clear that we can get any value we like for the risk by varying the number of cases and controls that we choose to study, and so the relative risk is not a valid estimate. We need a method based on calculations within each group. We can use the ratio $a/c$, which is the **odds** of the outcome in the first group. Thus, for example, if the proportion with the feature in group 1 is 2/20, the odds of the feature in that group are 2 to 18 or 1/9. So the ratio of the odds in the two groups, called the **odds ratio**, is another way of comparing groups.

If the outcome of interest that defines the cases is rare, then $a$ will be small and $a/(a + c)$ will be approximately equal to $a/c$. Similarly $b$ will be small and $b/(b + d)$ will be approximately equal to $b/d$. Thus the relative risk will be approximately equal to $(a/c)/(b/d)$ or $ad/bc$. For case-control studies the outcome of interest is usually rare, so the odds ratio offers a method of getting an approximate relative risk despite the method of sample selection.

The odds ratio is defined as $OR = ad/bc$. A confidence interval can be obtained in a similar manner as for the relative risk. We use the standard error of the logarithm of the odds ratio, given by

$$SE(\log_e OR) = \sqrt{\frac{1}{a} + \frac{1}{b} + \frac{1}{c} + \frac{1}{d}},$$

so that a 95% confidence interval for the log odds ratio is obtained as

$$\log_e OR - N_{0.975} \times SE(\log_e OR) \quad \text{to} \quad \log_e OR + N_{0.975} \times SE(\log_e OR)$$

where $N_{0.975}$ is the appropriate value from the Normal distribution. This method is suitable when none of the four cells in the $2 \times 2$ table is very small; otherwise more advanced methods are needed (see Breslow and Day, 1980, p. 124).

Table 10.10 showed the results of a case-control study of erosion of dental enamel in relation to amount of swimming in a chlorinated pool. The odds ratio for that table is $(32 \times 127)/(118 \times 17) = 2.026$, so $\log_e OR = 0.706$. Also, we have

$$SE(\log_e OR) = \sqrt{\tfrac{1}{32} + \tfrac{1}{127} + \tfrac{1}{118} + \tfrac{1}{17}}$$
$$= 0.326.$$

The 95% confidence interval for the population log odds ratio is thus

$$0.706 - 1.96 \times 0.326 \quad \text{to} \quad 0.706 + 1.96 \times 0.326$$

or from 0.067 to 1.345. Thus the 95% confidence interval for the odds ratio is from $e^{0.067}$ to $e^{1.345}$, or from 1.069 to 3.840. As the whole of the interval is greater than 1, which indicates equal risk (or odds) in the two groups, we can infer that there is a raised risk of erosion in dental enamel among those swimming more than 6 hours per week.

*(b) Paired samples*

With paired samples we need a different approach, which requires us to look at the differences between pairs. Table 10.24 shows the general structure of a matched pair case-control study; a specific example was given in Table 10.17, although the method of analysis was different. As with the earlier methods for analysing paired proportions, it is the numbers of pairs where the exposures differ that are of interest, that is, $b$ and $c$. The odds ratio is derived simply from these frequencies as $b/c$, this being the odds of being a case among the $b + c$ pairs in which only one individual was exposed. A method for calculating a confidence interval is given by Morris and Gardner (1989) and Fleiss (1981, p. 112), as are methods for the situation where there are several controls for each case.

Table 10.25 shows data from a case-control study of stress and relapse of breast cancer. Fifty women developing a first recurrence after treatment

**Table 10.24** General structure of the results from a matched pair case-control study. Presence or absence of exposure to the possible risk are denoted by + or –

| | | Cases | | |
|---|---|---|---|---|
| | | + | – | Total |
| Controls | + | $a$ | $b$ | $a + b$ |
| | – | $c$ | $d$ | $c + d$ |
| | Total | $a + c$ | $b + d$ | $n$ |

**Table 10.25** Results of a matched case-control study of a relapse from breast cancer among women who did (+) or did not (–) experience a stressful life event (Ramirez *et al.*, 1989)

| | | Cases | | |
|---|---|---|---|---|
| | | + | – | Total |
| Controls | + | 9 | 3 | 12 |
| | – | 17 | 21 | 38 |
| | Total | 26 | 24 | 50 |

for operable breast cancer were identified. Using a large database, they were individually matched for several prognostic factors (including type of operation and use of adjuvant chemotherapy) and socio-demographic factors with 50 women who had not had a recurrence. For each woman having a recurrence (the cases) data were collected on stressful life events (such as divorce or the death of their spouse) in the period between their operation and recurrence, while for their matched control the same information was sought for the same period from the time of their own operation. The odds ratio is simply $17/3 = 5.67$, and the 95% confidence interval is from 1.64 to 30.2. Although the odds ratio is large, suggesting that there is an association between stressful events and risk of recurrence of breast cancer, the small sample means that there is a wide confidence interval and thus it is necessary to be cautious about the interpretation of the finding.

### 10.11.3 Combining several 2 × 2 tables

Two common situations arise where we might wish to combine results from several frequency tables, especially 2 × 2 tables. The first is where we wish to examine the relation between two variables in a single study, but making allowance for variation in a third variable. For example, in a case-control study we might have a different age distribution in the two groups and might suspect that age affected the relation between the exposure and the outcome. We could produce a $2 \times 2$ table for each of several age groups, and then combine the tables to get an overall odds ratio that was effectively age-adjusted. The second is where we wish to combine data from several independent studies. This is an increasingly common type of analysis for combining the results from many clinical trials to perform an objective **overview** or **meta-analysis** of all the available data (see section 15.5.2). For both of these circumstances the analysis is by the **Mantel-Haenszel** method, which is described in Fleiss (1981, p. 173).

The odds ratio is approximately the same as the relative risk if the outcome of interest is rare. For common events, however, they can be quite different, so it is best to think of the odds ratio as a measure in its own right. Odds ratios also feature when we relate the presence or absence of a feature to more than one factor. This analysis is described in section 12.5.

## 10.12 PRESENTATION OF RESULTS

Frequency data pose relatively few problems when presenting results. I am in favour of giving all observed frequencies together with summaries as rounded percentages (or proportions). This is because it is often not possible to reconstruct the frequencies from reported percentages. It is useful to give percentages to allow a quick visual appraisal of variation among groups of varying size. Tables 10.18 and 10.21 are examples of this style of presentation. Percentages should be given for all rows when there are more than two rows.

Comparisons of proportions should be accompanied by the test statistic ($z$), the P value, and a confidence interval for the difference. The test statistic $X^2$, the degrees of freedom and the P value should all be quoted when reporting Chi squared tests. The degrees of freedom can be omitted if it is clear that only $2 \times 2$ tables are involved. In this book I have used $X^2$ for the test statistic to distinguish it from $\chi^2$ which is the theoretical distribution. It is common, however, to use $\chi^2$ for the test statistic too, and either is acceptable.

## 10.13 SUMMARY

The approach to frequency data via the comparison of proportions is preferable to the Chi squared approach because it provides estimates of quantities of interest and related confidence intervals. In contrast, Chi squared tests yield only P values. For larger tables, however, there is no simple alternative to using Chi squared tests or sometimes rank methods. Frequency data thus are less amenable than continuous data to statistical methods of estimation rather than hypothesis testing. For this reason alone, it is unwise to categorize a continuous variable to 'simplify' the analysis. While this is often useful when exploring a data set, it is not generally advisable when analysing data as it is throwing away information; an example is given in Table 10.5. There are also statistical methods for modelling frequency data, called **log-linear models**, but they are beyond the scope of this book.

Whatever method of analysis is used, it is important to take any ordering of categories into account. Moses *et al.* (1984) have reviewed the options, and the methods have been described in this chapter.

Frequency tables also arise in other types of analysis, where the aims are rather different. Two such cases are the comparison of observers' assessments, such as of stage of disease, and the use of one variable to predict another in the context of diagnosis. Both of these situations are considered in Chapter 12.

## EXERCISES

10.1 A study was carried out to see if patients whose skin did not respond to dinitrochlorobenzene (DNCB), a contact allergen, would show an equally negative response to croton oil, a skin irritant (Roth *et al.*, 1975). The following table shows the results of simultaneous skin reaction tests to DNCB and croton oil in 173 patients with skin cancer.

| | | DNCB | | |
|---|---|---|---|---|
| | | +ve | −ve | Total |
| Croton oil | +ve | 81 | 48 | 129 |
| | −ve | 23 | 21 | 44 |
| | Total | 104 | 69 | 173 |

(a) The authors reported 'no correlation' between the two tests. Carry out an analysis appropriate to the clinical question posed.

(b) The results of the DNCB test were compared for patients with different stages of cancer, as shown in the following table.

| | | Stage of skin cancer | | | |
|---|---|---|---|---|---|
| | | I | II | III | Total |
| DNCB reaction | +ve | 39 | 39 | 26 | 104 |
| | −ve | 13 | 19 | 37 | 69 |
| | Total | 52 | 58 | 63 | 173 |

Is DNCB reactivity related to stage of cancer in these patients?

10.2 A survey was carried out to test the hypothesis that men with deep singing voices are likely to have higher levels of testosterone than men with higher voices (Lyster, 1984). Professional and student male singers were asked how many brothers and sisters they had. The results for the 195 singers with siblings are shown in the following table:

| Voice group | Brothers | Sisters | Total |
|---|---|---|---|
| Bass | 77 (62%) | 47 | 124 |
| Bass-baritone | 38 (56%) | 30 | 68 |
| Baritone | 75 (56%) | 58 | 133 |
| Tenor-baritone | 5 (56%) | 4 | 9 |
| Tenor | 27 (42%) | 37 | 64 |
| Counter-tenor | 9 (38%) | 15 | 24 |
| Total | 231 (55%) | 191 | 422 |

The author of the report wrote:

> 'A $\chi^2$ test on the frequencies of brothers and sisters in the six voice-groups yields no significance. If, on the other hand, one chooses to look simply at bass, tenor and counter-tenor . . . one obtains $\chi^2 = 11.27$; df = 2; $P < 0.001$. A relationship between the two variables can thus be demonstrated at the extremes, but breaks down in the middle range.'

(a) The $\chi^2$ test ignoring the ordering of the voice groups gives $X^2 = 9.84$ on 5 df, P = 0.08. Comment on the author's interpretation.
(b) Why is this test not appropriate to the aim of the study? Perform an appropriate analysis and interpret the answers.
(c) The author performed a second analysis involving just three groups. Why is this analysis invalid?
(d) Why is his quoted value of $X^2$ of 11.27 clearly wrong?
(e) What feature of the data breaks a fundamental assumption of all Chi squared tests?
(f) How important is this problem, and what can we do about it? (This is rather difficult!)

10.3 A randomized controlled clinical trial was carried out to compare the effects of a single dose of prednisolone and placebo in children with acute asthma (Storr *et al.*, 1987). There were 73 children in the placebo group and 67 in the prednisolone group. The results section of the paper begins with the following statement: '2 patients in the placebo group (3%, 95% confidence interval −1 to 6%) and 20 in the prednisolone group (30%, 19 to 41%) were discharged at first examination ($P < 0.0001$).' The methods section explains that this P value was derived using Fisher's exact test.

(a) Was it reasonable to use Fisher's exact test rather than the Chi squared test?
(b) What is wrong with the confidence intervals, and what would be a better analysis?

10.4 The following table shows the number of hours spent in bed by 14 year old boys and girls (Macgregor and Balding, 1988). Times were rounded up to the next half hour.

(a) Which methods of analysis could be used to compare the distributions for boys and girls?
(b) Is there any difference between boys and girls?

| | Time spent in bed (hours) | | | | | | | | |
|---|---|---|---|---|---|---|---|---|---|
| | ≤ 7.0 | 7.5 | 8.0 | 8.5 | 9.0 | 9.5 | 10.0 | > 10.0 | Total |
| Boys | 88 | 109 | 210 | 324 | 359 | 313 | 182 | 85 | 1670 |
| Girls | 92 | 108 | 217 | 349 | 436 | 334 | 198 | 65 | 1799 |
| Total | 180 | 217 | 427 | 673 | 795 | 647 | 380 | 150 | 3469 |

10.5 A study was made of 65 patients who had received or were receiving sodium aurothiomalate as a treatment for rheumatoid arthritis (Ayesh *et al.*, 1987). The aim was to examine the possibility that toxicity to sodium aurothiomalate (SA) might be linked to sulphoxidation capacity, as assessed by the sulphoxidation index (SI). The data were given in Exercise 3.1. Values of $SI > 6.0$ were taken as indicating impaired sulphoxidation. They obtained the following table:

| | | Major adverse reaction (toxicity) | | |
|---|---|---|---|---|
| | | Yes | No | Total |
| Impaired sulphoxidation | Yes | 30 | 9 | 39 |
| | No | 7 | 19 | 26 |
| | Total | 37 | 28 | 65 |

The authors wrote: 'The incidence of impaired sulphoxidation in patients showing SA toxicity (30/37; 81.0%) was significantly greater than in the group without adverse reaction (9/28; 32.1%) ($\chi^2 = 27.6$, $P < 0.001$). Similarly, the incidence of toxicity was significantly increased in those with impaired sulphoxidation (30/39; 76.9%) compared to those with extensive sulphoxidation (7/26; 26.9%) ($\chi^2 = 36.2$, $P < 0.001$).'

(a) Why can't both of the above Chi squared tests be correct?
(b) Carry out a Chi squared test of the data in the table and compare your answer with the two results in the above paragraph.

10.6 Among patients with oral cancer registered in Kerala, India, between 1982 and 1986, the relation between the site of the cancer and betel chewing, smoking or alcohol consumption was examined (Sankaranarayanan *et al.*, 1989). The data for patients aged > 30 are summarized in the following table:

| | Intra oral subsite | | |
|---|---|---|---|
| Habit | Tongue ($n = 175$) | Buccal mucosa ($n = 300$) | Other ($n = 156$) |
| Chewing | 146 | 267 | 121 |
| Smoking | 71 | 166 | 102 |
| Alcohol | 51 | 71 | 46 |
| None of these | 17 | 12 | 6 |

What sort of test could be performed to relate habit to site of cancer?

10.7 Sixty-five pregnant women at a high risk of pregnancy-induced hypertension participated in a randomized controlled trial comparing 100 mg of aspirin daily and a matching placebo during the third trimester of pregnancy (Schiff *et al.*, 1989). The observed rates of hypertension are shown in the following table:

| | Aspirin treated | Placebo treated | Total |
|---|---|---|---|
| Hypertension | 4 | 11 | 15 |
| No hypertension | 30 | 20 | 50 |
| Total | 34 | 31 | 65 |

Do these data suggest that daily aspirin reduces the risk of hypertension in the last trimester of pregnancy?

10.8 A case-control study was carried out to investigate the aetiology of acoustic neuromas (Preston-Martin *et al.*, 1989). Men aged 25–69 at the time of diagnosis who were resident in Los Angeles County were eligible for inclusion. A total of 118 men were identified who were alive and able to be interviewed. Twenty-eight patients were not interviewed because the physician refused permission (12), the patient chose not to participate (9), or the patient could not be located (7). For 86 of the remaining patients the researchers identified and interviewed a neighbourhood control of the same race and within five years of age.

Both members of each case-control pair were interviewed in the same manner by the same interviewer to obtain information about various life experiences. Exposure to loud noise at work was of particular interest. Overall 58 cases and 46 controls had had some exposure to loud noise at work. There were 20 case-control pairs for which the case but not the control had had such exposure, and 8 pairs where the control but not the case had had some exposure.

(a) Carry out an appropriate analysis to compare the proportions of exposed cases and controls.
(b) Calculate the odds ratio for acoustic neuroma associated with exposure to loud noise at work.

# 11

# Relation between two continuous variables

## 11.1 ASSOCIATION, PREDICTION AND AGREEMENT

A high proportion of statistical analyses are carried out to study the relation between two variables within a group of subjects. Three main purposes of such analyses might be:

1. to assess whether the two variables are associated, that is, if the values of one variable tend to be higher (or, alternatively, lower) for higher values of the other variable;
2. to enable the value of one variable to be predicted from any known value of the other variable;
3. to assess the amount of agreement between the values of the two variables; most commonly this situation arises in the comparison of alternative ways of measuring or assessing the same thing.

In this chapter I shall consider the first two possibilities. The question of agreement is dealt with in section 14.2.

Methods for studying association between categorical variables were introduced in Chapter 10. In this chapter I shall consider comparable methods for assessing the association between continuous variables, using the method known as **correlation**. In contrast, this is the first mention of methods for predicting one variable from another. This chapter considers the prediction of one continuous variable from another, for which the technique of **linear regression** is used. The slightly different technique of **logistic regression**, which is needed when one variable is categorical, will be considered in Chapter 12.

This chapter is devoted to two techniques, correlation and regression, which are so often presented together that it is easy to get the impression that they are inseparable. In fact, they have distinct purposes and it is relatively rare that one is genuinely interested in performing both analyses on the same set of data. The confusion that clearly exists between correlation and regression may well stem from poor differentiation between the techniques in many textbooks, which in turn arises from the very close mathematical relation between the two methods. Clearly the rationale for carrying out a particular analysis is of paramount importance, and this aspect will be particularly stressed in this chapter.

## 11.2 CORRELATION

Correlation is the method of analysis to use when studying the possible association between two continuous variables. Figure 11.1 shows the relation between body fat percentage (%fat) and age among 18 normal adults aged 23 to 61. The data come from a small study investigating a new method of assessing body composition. There appears to be some association between the values of the two variables; we can see that there is a tendency for the older people to have a higher percentage of body fat.

If we want to measure the degree of association, this can be done by calculating the **correlation coefficient**, often loosely just called the **correlation**. The standard method (often ascribed to Pearson) leads to a quantity called $r$ which can take any value from $-1$ to $+1$. This correlation coefficient $r$ measures the degree of 'straight-line' association between the values of the two variables. Thus a value of $+1.0$ or $-1.0$ is obtained if all the points in a scatter diagram lie on a perfect straight line, as shown in Figure 11.2. Also shown are examples of data with intermediate values of $r$. The correlation between two variables is positive if higher values of one variable are associated with higher values of the other and negative if one variable tends to be lower as the other gets higher. A correlation of around zero indicates that there is no linear relation between the values of the two

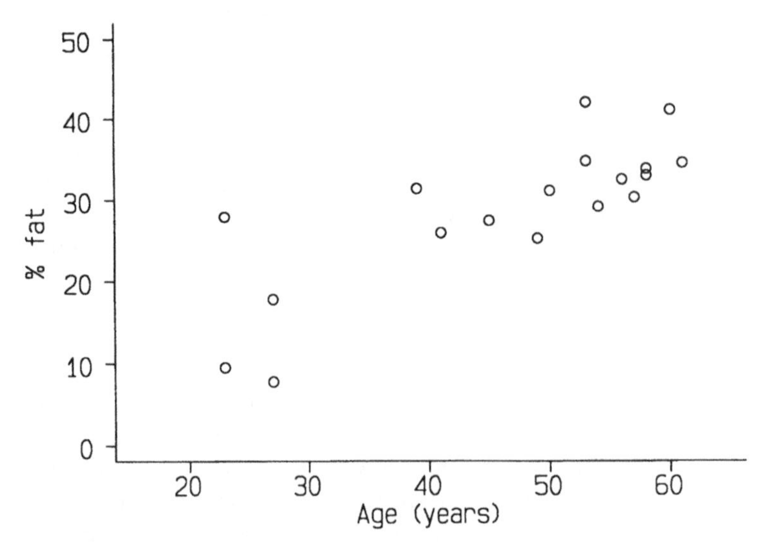


**Figure 11.1** Body fat percentage (%fat) related to age for 18 normal adults (Mazess *et al.*, 1984).

variables (i.e. they are uncorrelated). Clearly the variables in Figure 11.1 are positively correlated; in fact the correlation coefficient can be calculated to be $r = 0.79$.

What are we measuring with $r$? In essence $r$ is a measure of the scatter of the points around an underlying linear trend: the greater the spread of the points the lower the correlation. In the study already referred to, dual-photon absorptiometry was used to derive a measure of body fat as a percentage of total body mass. Figure 11.3 shows %fat plotted against weight for the same 18 subjects. It is clear that there is considerable scatter with no obvious underlying relationship between %fat and weight. The correlation between these two variables is 0.03, confirming the visual impression.

An example of very strong correlation is given by data relating maternal and fetal weight of different species of mammal. Figure 11.4 shows a plot of these data after log transformation. The correlation between the two variables is 0.985, and the relation is clearly remarkably consistent from bats at one extreme through to whales at the other.

### 11.2.1 Data distribution

The correlation coefficient can be calculated for any data set. However, there is a restriction on the validity of the associated hypothesis test, which is that the two variables are observed on a random sample of individuals and that the data for at least one of the variables have a Normal distribution in the population. For the calculation of a valid confidence interval for $r$ both variables should have a Normal distribution.

In practice, therefore, it is preferable for both variables to have approximately Normal distribution for any use of Pearson's $r$. Data of this type will display a roughly elliptical pattern, with the degree of elongation of the ellipse being related to the correlation coefficient. For small samples, or where $r$ is near $+1$ or $-1$, this feature may be hard to detect, however. The easiest way to check the validity of the hypothesis test is by examining a scatter diagram of the data, which ought to be produced as a matter of routine whenever correlation coefficients are calculated. It should be easy to tell whether the data show a reasonably elliptical pattern. Normal plots could be produced, and Normality can be tested formally by the Shapiro-Wilk $W$ test (see Chapter 7), but it is not really necessary because the scatter plot will usually suffice.

If the data do not have a Normal distribution either or both of the variables can be transformed, as for the data shown in Figure 11.4, or a non-parametric correlation coefficient can be calculated, as described in section 11.4.

The mathematical calculations for $r$, its confidence interval, and the associated hypothesis tests are shown in section 11.7.

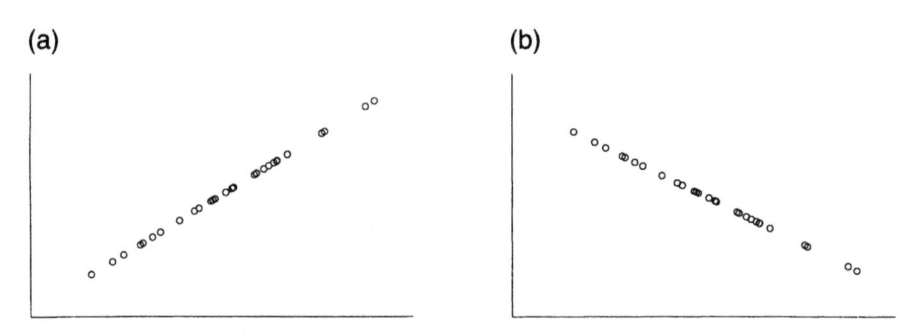


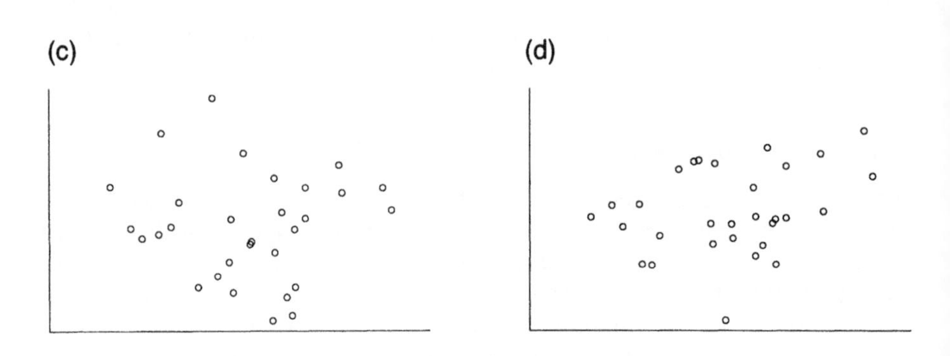


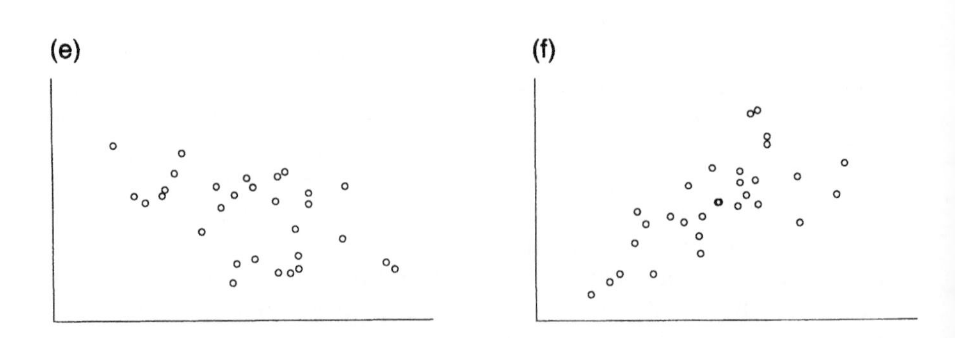


**Figure 11.2** Data with correlation coefficients ($r$) of (a) 1.0; (b) −1.0; (c) 0.0; (d) 0.3; (e) −0.5; (f) 0.7.

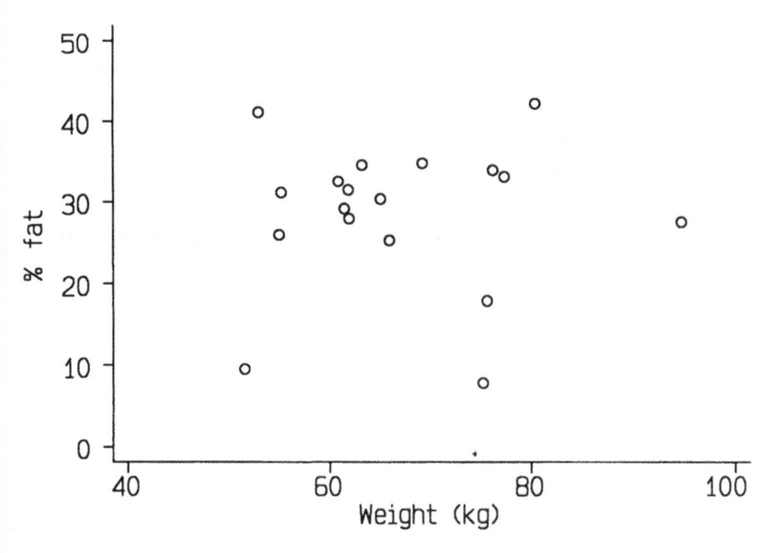


**Figure 11.3** Relation between percentage of fat and bodyweight in 18 normal adults (Mazess *et al.*, 1984).

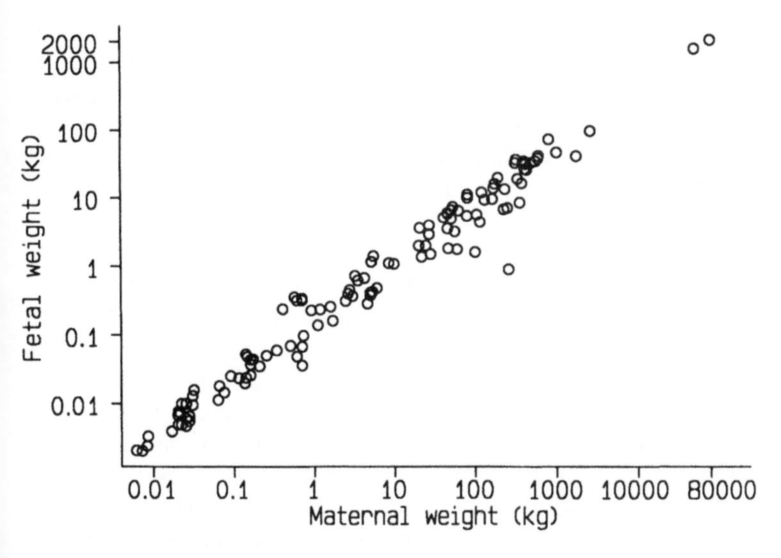


**Figure 11.4** Relation between total fetal weight and non-pregnant maternal weight in 121 species of mammal (Leitch *et al.*, 1959).

### 11.2.2 Confidence interval for *r*

We can obtain a confidence interval for the correlation in the population, on the assumption that the sample is representative. For the data in Figure 11.1 the correlation coefficient is 0.79. Using the method described in section 11.7 we can obtain the 95% confidence interval for the correlation coefficient as being from 0.52 to 0.92. As is usual in small samples, the confidence interval is wide, but it does suggest that there really is quite a strong association between the two variables.

### 11.2.3 Hypothesis test for *r*

There is a simple test of significance of the null hypothesis of no association which is based on the *t* distribution. The method is described in section 11.7. However, Table B7 shows critical values which allow observed values of *r* to be looked up directly; these should suffice for most practical purposes. For example, the correlation between %fat and age in the data shown in Figure 11.1 was 0.79, and from Table B7 we can see that $P < 0.001$.

## 11.3 USE AND MISUSE OF CORRELATION

As well as the distributional assumptions mentioned in section 11.2.1, another restriction is that all the observations should be independent. In practice this means that only one observation of each variable should come from each individual in the study. The analysis is not valid when there is more than one observation for some or all of the subjects. For example, it would not be correct to use correlation to relate, say, blood pressure and oestrogen levels in pregnant women with varying numbers of observations at different gestational ages. In such circumstances a proper analysis can be very complex.

Even when the assumptions just mentioned are not violated the use of correlation is not as simple as it looks. Indeed, misuse of correlation is so common that some statisticians have wished that the method had never been devised. The most obvious general misuse occurs in studies in which large numbers of variables have been recorded. Clearly, with many variables it is possible to calculate hundreds of correlation coefficients and then pick out just those which are statistically significant. While 'data-dredging' is acceptable in a limited way in exploratory analyses, when taken to extremes the scope for over-interpretation is considerable. For example, even with only ten variables 45 correlations between pairs of variables can be calculated. This problem is discussed further in section 11.8.

There are several rather more specific misuses of correlation, each somewhat different in nature but all frequently seen. Six types are discussed below. In each case there is nothing wrong with the mathematical calculations, but the interpretation is flawed.

### 11.3.1 Spurious correlations involving time

The correlation of two variables both of which have been recorded repeatedly over time can be grossly misleading. By such means one may demonstrate relationships between the price of petrol and the divorce rate, consumption of butter and farmers' incomes (a negative relation), and so on. Another example was given in section 5.13.

The same caution applies to studying two variables over time for an individual. Such correlations are often spurious: it is necessary to remove the time trends from such data before correlating them, and this is an area that requires expert assistance. Time-related data are considered futher in section 14.6.

### 11.3.2 Restricted sampling of individuals

As already indicated, there is an implicit assumption that the subjects being studied are a random sample (or nearly so) from some specified population of individuals, such as pregnant women or hypertensive men. Deliberately adding or taking away from our sample some individuals because of their values of one of the variables can have a dramatic effect on the correlation. For example, if we added a few children to the data set shown in Figure 11.1 we would increase the correlation considerably, whereas if we excluded anyone taller than 180 cm we would decrease the correlation (to $r = 0.34$). Neither manoeuvre would allow a valid interpretation of the correlation coefficient because the sample would no longer be a proper random sample. Correlation analysis is especially sensitive to the sample selection because the between subject variation in each variable enters directly into the calculation.

### 11.3.3 Mixed samples

It may be misleading to calculate the correlation when the sample comprises different subgroups. For example, the body fat data in Figure 11.1 relate to 14 women and 4 men. Body fat percentage tends to be lower in men, and it happens that the four men in this study were considerably younger than the women, so mixing the sexes tends to inflate the correlation (see Figure 11.5). It would therefore be better to consider the

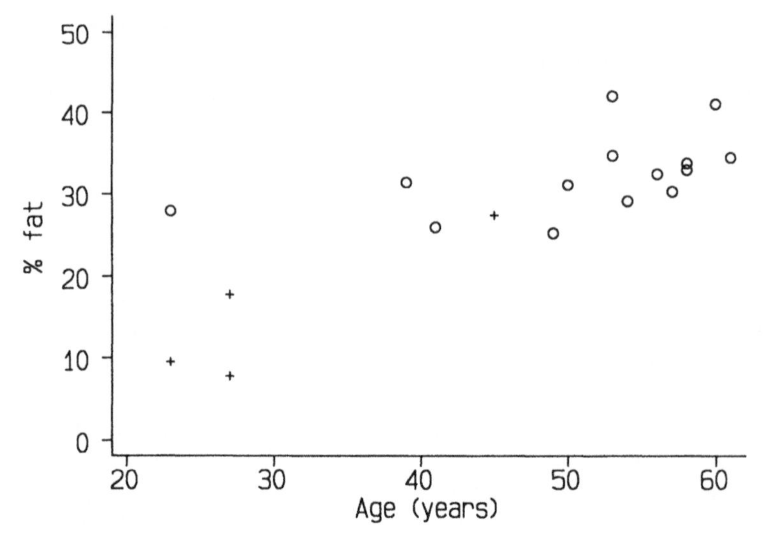


**Figure 11.5** % fat by age showing males (+) and females (O).

women only, for whom we get rather lower $r = 0.51$. Another consequence of the mixing of subgroups is that the data (when mixed) may not be Normally distributed, but the effect cannot be detected unless the groups are very different and the sample is large.

### 11.3.4 Assessing agreement

In medical research there is frequently the need to compare two methods of measuring the same quantity. Laboratory methods throw up many such problems, but they are also common in clinical medicine, particularly where it is not possible to measure directly the quantity of interest. Blood pressure is an obvious example.

The most common method of analysing such data is to calculate the correlation coefficient, but this is a misconceived analysis. As we have seen, the correlation coefficient measures the degree of association between two quantities; it does not measure how closely they agree (Bland and Altman, 1986). Method comparison studies are discussed in detail in section 14.2.

### 11.3.5 Change related to initial value

A rather different problem occurs with the use of correlation to study the relation between an initial measurement and the change in that measurement over time. For example, we may be interested in seeing whether a diet designed to lower serum cholesterol was more effective in people with higher initial values of serum cholesterol. This is a reasonable question, but unfortunately it turns out that the use of correlation here is misleading. This is because for *any* two quantities $X$ and $Y$, $X$ will be correlated with $X - Y$. Indeed, even if $X$ and $Y$ are samples of random numbers we would expect the correlation between $X$ and $X - Y$ to be 0.7. (You can try this with some numbers from the table of random numbers in Table B13.) In other words, we expect to obtain a large correlation between intial serum cholesterol and the change in serum cholesterol even if the diet is ineffective. The name for the phenomenon is **regression to the mean**, giving another confusion between regression and correlation.

The simplest way around this problem is to take the average of the initial and final measurement and calculate the correlation between this quantity and the observed change. In the above notation this means correlating $(X + Y)/2$ with $X - Y$. If this correlation is large it may reasonably be inferred that higher initial levels of the variable are associated with larger falls over time (or smaller rises). However, the best approach to this type of data is complex: further discussion is given by Blomqvist (1986) and Hayes (1988). There is more to this type of problem than is apparent, and statistical advice is recommended.

### 11.3.6 Relating a part to the whole

A similar situation arises if we study the relation between a constituent and the total amount. For example, we would expect to find a correlation between:

1. height at age 5 and adult height;
2. length of the luteal phase and length of the whole menstrual cycle; and
3. intake of protein and intake of calories;

because in each case the second quantity contains the first, although not necessarily explicitly. There may be no relation (or even a negative relation) between the first quantity and its complement within the total. As with the problem discussed in the previous section, expressing the analysis as the correlation between $X$ and $X + Y$ shows that the two quantities are related whatever $X$ and $Y$ are.

## 11.4 RANK CORRELATION

The concept of ranks was introduced in Chapter 2 and applications to the comparison of continuous data from two groups were shown in Chapter 9.

A similar use of ranks is possible when considering the relation between two variables. The idea here is simply to rank a set of subjects for each variable and compare the orderings. For example, Table 11.1 shows the data for age and measurements of %fat from Figure 11.1, together with the ranks of the observations. Where two values are the same the average rank is assigned to both.

To make the relationship clearer, the subjects have been ordered by age. Arranging data like this allows us to get a quick impression about the possibility that the two variables are associated, as it is quite easy to judge whether the values in the second column of ranks are tending to increase or decrease.

There are two commonly used methods of calculating the rank correlation coefficient, one due to Spearman and one to Kendall. It is easier in general to calculate Spearman's $r_s$ (often called Spearman's $\rho$ (rho)) than Kendall's $\tau$ (tau), so it is the Spearman coefficient that is used here. The calculations are shown in section 11.7. In fact, Spearman's rank correlation coefficient $r_s$ is exactly the same as the Pearson correlation coefficient $r$ calculated on the ranks of the observations.

The rank correlation between the age and %fat data shown in Table 11.1 is 0.75, which is close to the value 0.79 obtained as the standard

**Table 11.1** Age and %fat (measured by dual-photon absorptiometry) for 18 normal adults (Mazess *et al.*, 1984)

| Subject | Age | Rank | %Fat | Rank |
|---|---|---|---|---|
| 1 | 23 | 1.5 | 9.5 | 2 |
| 2 | 23 | 1.5 | 27.9 | 7 |
| 3 | 27 | 3.5 | 7.8 | 1 |
| 4 | 27 | 3.5 | 17.8 | 3 |
| 5 | 39 | 5 | 31.4 | 11 |
| 6 | 41 | 6 | 25.9 | 5 |
| 7 | 45 | 7 | 27.4 | 6 |
| 8 | 49 | 8 | 25.2 | 4 |
| 9 | 50 | 9 | 31.1 | 10 |
| 10 | 53 | 10.5 | 34.7 | 16 |
| 11 | 53 | 10.5 | 42.0 | 18 |
| 12 | 54 | 12 | 29.1 | 8 |
| 13 | 56 | 13 | 32.5 | 12 |
| 14 | 57 | 14 | 30.3 | 9 |
| 15 | 58 | 15.5 | 33.0 | 13 |
| 16 | 58 | 15.5 | 33.8 | 14 |
| 17 | 60 | 17 | 41.1 | 17 |
| 18 | 61 | 18 | 34.5 | 15 |

Pearson correlation. This is not always the case, of course. The two methods will tend to differ when the data deviate from an elliptical shape in the scatter diagram. As this is an indication against the calculation of Pearson's $r$, it follows that when $r$ and $r_s$ differ noticeably it is $r_s$ that should be used. In practice we do not calculate both $r$ and $r_s$, but choose the method according to the appearance of the scatter diagram. Rank correlation may be used whatever type of pattern is seen and it has the advantage of not specifically assessing linear association but more general association. This may be seen, for example, from the fact that the value of $r_s$ is unchanged by logarithmic transformation of either of the variables. All my earlier cautions against the use of correlation apply equally to rank correlation, however.

Hughes and Jones (1985) studied the relation between average intake of dietary fibre and the average age of menarche in 46 countries. They quoted a correlation coefficient of $r = 0.84$ ($P < 0.0001$). However, as Figure 11.6 shows, the data tend to cluster in two main groups, corresponding roughly to developed and developing countries, and there is one extreme point. The data are thus not near to a Normal distribution for either variable. We might, therefore, prefer to use rank correlation, which gives $r_s = 0.69$. We can interpret identical values of $r$ and $r_s$ as being roughly equivalent, so from Table B7 the rather weaker rank correlation is also highly significant ($P < 0.0001$).

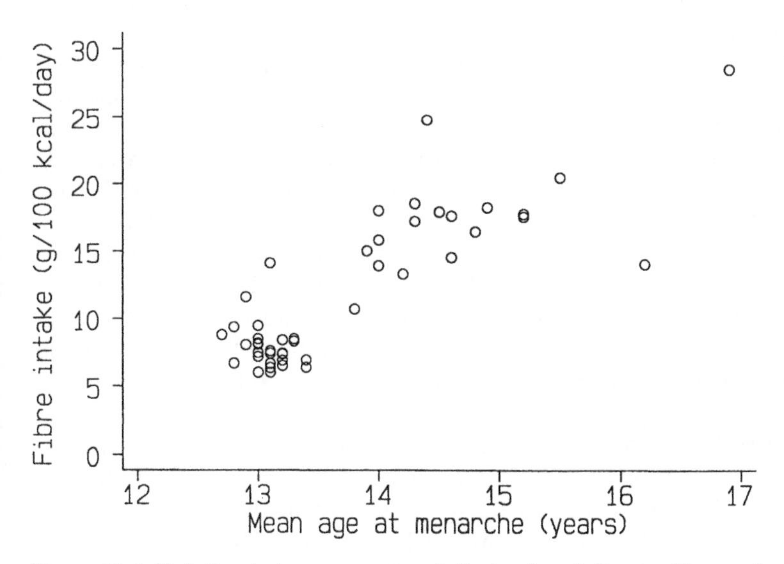


**Figure 11.6** Relation between average daily intake of dietary fibre and mean age of menarche in 46 countries (Hughes and Jones, 1985).

We can calculate a confidence interval for $r_s$ in exactly the same way as for $r$. Following the method given in section 11.7, the 95% confidence interval for the fibre and menarche data is from 0.32 to 0.87. The data are thus compatible with a wide range of possibilities for the population correlation, despite the very small P value.

I mentioned in section 10.9.2 that rank correlation can be used to assess the degree of association between two ordered categorical variables. Clearly there will be huge numbers of ties in this situation so it is essential to use the version of the method that allows for them (see section 11.7.2).

Rank correlation should be used more often. It is the only non-parametric method which gives as much information as its parametric equivalent (rather than just a P value), and it is of wider validity. It is easy to perform using widely available computer programs by ranking the data and performing the usual Pearson correlation analysis.

## 11.5 ADJUSTING A CORRELATION FOR ANOTHER VARIABLE

Sometimes we have data on a third variable that might have influenced the observed relationship between two other variables. We can adjust for the third variable by calculating the **partial correlation coefficient**. We can consider this to be the estimated correlation between two variables among individuals (or countries or whatever) with the same value of the third variable. The same approach can be used for Pearson's or Spearman's correlation coefficient.

Begg and Hearns (1966) were interested in the relative contributions of haematocrit (packed cell volume, PCV), fibrinogen and other proteins (albumin and globulin) to the viscosity of blood. Table 11.2 shows their data from 32 hospital patients. The correlation coefficients between the four variables are shown as a **correlation matrix** in Table 11.3. The correlation between blood viscosity and PCV was 0.88 ($P < 0.001$) and between blood viscosity and fibrinogen was 0.46 ($P < 0.01$). The authors used partial correlation to see if the association of blood viscosity and fibrinogen remained after allowing for the association with PCV. The partial correlation is 0.21 ($P = 0.25$), suggesting that the association between blood viscosity and fibrinogen can be largely explained by variation in PCV.

James (1985) gave data on dizygotic (DZ) twinning rates and average daily milk consumption for 19 European countries in relation to latitude (see Table 11.4). James was especially interested in the relation between DZ twinning rate and latitude, shown in Figure 11.7. The rank correlation is 0.68, which is highly significant ($P < 0.01$). It is clear that the values of all three variables tend to increase together so we might ask whether the observed association could be 'explained' (statistically) by variation in milk consumption. Information on *per capita* consumption of milk was available for 15 countries; for these the correlation between DZ twinning rate and

**Table 11.2** Data on blood viscosity, packed cell volume (PCV), plasma fibrinogen and other proteins from 32 hospital patients (Begg and Hearns, 1966)

| Patient | Blood viscosity (cP) | PCV (%) | Plasma fibrinogen (mg/100 ml) | Plasma protein (g/100 ml) |
|---|---|---|---|---|
| 1 | 3.71 | 40 | 344 | 6.27 |
| 2 | 3.78 | 40 | 330 | 4.86 |
| 3 | 3.85 | 42.5 | 280 | 5.09 |
| 4 | 3.88 | 42 | 418 | 6.79 |
| 5 | 3.98 | 45 | 774 | 6.40 |
| 6 | 4.03 | 42 | 388 | 5.48 |
| 7 | 4.05 | 42.5 | 336 | 6.27 |
| 8 | 4.14 | 47 | 431 | 6.89 |
| 9 | 4.14 | 46.75 | 276 | 5.18 |
| 10 | 4.20 | 48 | 422 | 5.73 |
| 11 | 4.20 | 46 | 280 | 5.89 |
| 12 | 4.27 | 47 | 460 | 6.58 |
| 13 | 4.27 | 43.25 | 412 | 5.67 |
| 14 | 4.37 | 45 | 320 | 6.23 |
| 15 | 4.41 | 50 | 502 | 4.99 |
| 16 | 4.64 | 45 | 550 | 6.37 |
| 17 | 4.68 | 51.25 | 414 | 6.40 |
| 18 | 4.73 | 50.25 | 304 | 6.00 |
| 19 | 4.87 | 49 | 472 | 5.94 |
| 20 | 4.94 | 50 | 728 | 5.16 |
| 21 | 4.95 | 50 | 716 | 6.29 |
| 22 | 4.96 | 49 | 400 | 5.96 |
| 23 | 5.02 | 50.5 | 576 | 5.90 |
| 24 | 5.02 | 51.25 | 354 | 5.81 |
| 25 | 5.12 | 49.5 | 392 | 5.49 |
| 26 | 5.15 | 56 | 352 | 5.41 |
| 27 | 5.17 | 50 | 572 | 6.24 |
| 28 | 5.18 | 47 | 634 | 6.50 |
| 29 | 5.38 | 53.25 | 458 | 6.60 |
| 30 | 5.77 | 57 | 1070 | 4.82 |
| 31 | 5.90 | 54 | 488 | 5.70 |
| 32 | 5.90 | 54 | 488 | 5.70 |

latitude was 0.61. The rank correlation between milk consumption and latitude is 0.92 and between milk consumption and DZ twinning rate it is 0.61. We can calculate the partial correlation between latitude (L) and DZ twinning rate (T) adjusted for milk consumption (M) as $r_s(LT|M) = 0.18$ (see section 11.7.3). This small value suggests that one possible explanation for the observed association between DZ twinning and latitude *might* be milk consumption. Interpretation of such international correlations is

**Table 11.3** Correlation matrix of the data in Table 11.2

| | Viscosity | PCV | Fibrinogen |
|---|---|---|---|
| PCV | 0.8788 | | |
| Fibrinogen | 0.4573 | 0.4155 | |
| Protein | −0.1011 | −0.1575 | −0.0512 |

**Table 11.4** Latitude, age-standardized dizygotic twinning rates and daily *per capita* consumption of milk products (James, 1985). Figures in brackets are ranks

| Country | Latitude (L) | DZ twinning (T) | Milk consumption rate/1000(M) |
|---|---|---|---|
| Portugal | 40 ( 1.5) | 6.5 ( 2) | 3.8 |
| Greece | 40 ( 1.5) | 8.8 (13) | 7.7 |
| Spain | 41 ( 3) | 5.9 ( 1) | 8.2 |
| Bulgaria | 42 ( 4) | 7.0 ( 3) | – |
| Italy | 44 ( 5) | 8.6 (11.5) | 6.5 |
| France | 47 ( 6.5) | 7.1 ( 4) | 10.9 |
| Switzerland | 47 ( 6.5) | 8.1 ( 7.5) | – |
| Austria | 48 ( 8) | 7.5 ( 6) | 15.9 |
| Belgium | 51 ( 9.5) | 7.3 ( 5) | 11.6 |
| FR Germany | 51 ( 9.5) | 8.2 ( 9) | 14.1 |
| Holland | 52 (11.5) | 8.1 ( 7.5) | 18.9 |
| GDR | 52 (11.5) | 9.1 (16) | – |
| England and Wales | 53 (13.5) | 8.9 (14.5) | 17.1 |
| Eire | 53 (13.5) | 11.0 (18) | 24.4 |
| Scotland | 56 (15.5) | 8.9 (14.5) | – |
| Denmark | 56 (15.5) | 9.6 (17) | 16.8 |
| Sweden | 60 (17) | 8.6 (11.5) | 20.9 |
| Norway | 61 (18) | 8.3 (10) | 19.3 |
| Finland | 62 (19) | 12.1 (19) | 30.4 |

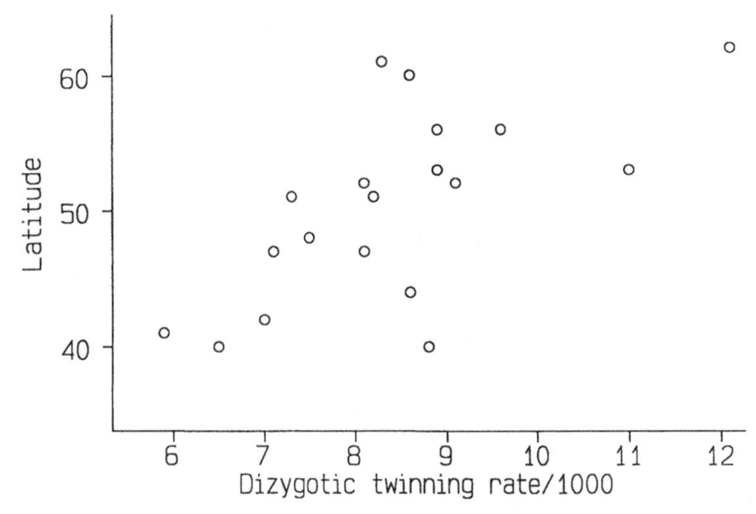


**Figure 11.7** Relation between latitude and dizygotic twinning rate in 19 European countries (James, 1985).

particularly difficult, however. Note that correlation is frequently used for this type of data, although the countries are never randomly sampled as they technically should be. Section 11.8 discusses the general problems of interpreting correlation coefficients.

Partial correlation is not used a great deal in medical studies. The relation between three or more variables is usually investigated using the more informative multiple regression, which will be described in section 12.4. However, the method of calculating the partial correlation is explained in section 11.7.3.

## 11.6 USE OF THE CORRELATION COEFFICIENT IN ASSESSING NON-NORMALITY

In section 7.5.2 I described the use of the Normal plot to get a visual assessment of how compatible a sample of observations is with having been drawn from a population with a Normal distribution. I described the use of the Shapiro-Wilk $W$ test, but this is not available in most statistical packages and is too difficult to perform by hand. A much simpler alternative is to use the similar Shapiro-Francia $W'$ test (Royston, 1983).

The correlation coefficient assesses the degree of straight-line association between the values of two variables. It can thus be used to assess the straightness of a Normal plot, and so whether the data are compatible with the null hypothesis of Normality. The Normal plot is a plot of the observed data against the Normal scores (see section 7.5.4), so we need the Pearson correlation coefficient between these two quantities, which I will call $r_N$.

We cannot use the usual tables for assessing this correlation coefficient, because the null hypothesis here is that the correlation is 1, not 0. It is easier to consider the square of the correlation $r_N$, and it is $r_N^2$ which is termed $W'$. Table B12 shows how to assess an observed value of $W'$.

Table 11.5 shows some blood glucose data that will be used later in this chapter, sorted into ascending order. Also shown are the expected cumulative frequencies ($P_i$), using the formula in section 7.5.2, and the corresponding Normal scores. The correlation coefficient between the raw data and the Normal scores is 0.9772, so the value of $W'$ is $0.9772^2 = 0.955$. From Table B12 we get $P > 0.2$, so that the data are compatible with being a sample from a Normal population.

**Table 11.5** Fasting blood glucose data from 24 type 1 diabetic patients (Thuesen *et al.*, 1985), with calculation of Normal scores

| Patient ($i$) | Blood glucose | $P_i$ | Normal score |
|---|---|---|---|
| 1 | 4.2 | 0.026 | −1.947 |
| 2 | 4.9 | 0.067 | −1.498 |
| 3 | 5.2 | 0.108 | −1.236 |
| 4 | 5.3 | 0.149 | −1.039 |
| 5 | 6.7 | 0.191 | −0.875 |
| 6 | 6.7 | 0.232 | −0.732 |
| 7 | 7.2 | 0.273 | −0.603 |
| 8 | 7.5 | 0.314 | −0.483 |
| 9 | 8.1 | 0.356 | −0.370 |
| 10 | 8.6 | 0.397 | −0.261 |
| 11 | 8.8 | 0.438 | −0.156 |
| 12 | 9.3 | 0.479 | −0.052 |
| 13 | 9.5 | 0.521 | 0.052 |
| 14 | 10.3 | 0.562 | 0.156 |
| 15 | 10.8 | 0.603 | 0.261 |
| 16 | 11.1 | 0.644 | 0.370 |
| 17 | 12.2 | 0.686 | 0.483 |
| 18 | 12.5 | 0.727 | 0.603 |
| 19 | 13.3 | 0.768 | 0.732 |
| 20 | 15.1 | 0.809 | 0.875 |
| 21 | 15.3 | 0.851 | 1.039 |
| 22 | 16.1 | 0.892 | 1.236 |
| 23 | 19.0 | 0.933 | 1.498 |
| 24 | 19.5 | 0.974 | 1.947 |

## 11.7 CORRELATION – MATHEMATICS AND WORKED EXAMPLES

*(This section gives the mathematical formulae for the calculations described in the first part of this chapter, together with a worked example. It can be omitted without loss of continuity.)*

### 11.7.1 Pearson's $r$

The correlation coefficient that is usually calculated is called Pearson's $r$ or the 'product-moment' correlation coefficient. If we have two variables $X$ and $Y$, the correlation between them, denoted by $r(X,Y)$ or usually just $r$, is given by

$$r = \frac{\Sigma(x_i - \bar{x})(y_i - \bar{y})}{\sqrt{\Sigma(x_i - \bar{x})^2\Sigma(y_i - \bar{y})^2}}$$

where $x_i$ and $y_i$ are the values of $X$ and $Y$ for the $i^{th}$ individual. The value of $r$ may loosely speaking be seen as a measure of the elongation of the ellipse that the data approximately fall within. The equation is clearly symmetric in that it does not matter which variable is $X$ and which is $Y$.

For the purposes of calculation a simpler formula to use is

$$r = \frac{\Sigma x_i y_i - (\Sigma x_i)(\Sigma y_i)/n}{\sqrt{[\Sigma x_i^2 - (\Sigma x_i)^2/n][\Sigma y_i^2 - (\Sigma y_i)^2/n]}}$$

for which it is necessary to obtain $\Sigma x_i$, $\Sigma y_i$, $\Sigma x_i^2$, $\Sigma y_i^2$, and $\Sigma x_i y_i$.

If you already have the means ($\bar{x}$ and $\bar{y}$) and standard deviations ($s_x$ and $s_y$) the formula simplifies to

$$r = \frac{\Sigma x_i y_i - n\bar{x}\bar{y}}{(n-1)s_x s_y}$$

so that it is only necessary to calculate the extra term $\Sigma x_i y_i$.

This formula should not be used in a computer program, however, as inaccuracy is occasionally introduced through rounding errors. (The first equation for $r$ should be used.)

*(a) Confidence interval*

The sampling distribution of Pearson's $r$ is not Normal, but we can transform $r$ to get a quantity called $z$ which does have a Normal sampling distribution. The transformation is

$$z = \tfrac{1}{2}\log_e\left(\frac{1+r}{1-r}\right).$$

The standard error of $z$ is approximately $1/\sqrt{n-3}$ where $n$ is the sample size, so we can construct a 95% confidence interval for $z$ as being from

$$z_1 = z - 1.96/\sqrt{n-3} \quad \text{to} \quad z_2 = z + 1.96/\sqrt{n-3}.$$

We back-transform the above values to get a confidence interval for the population correlation coefficient $r$ as

$$\frac{e^{2z_1}-1}{e^{2z_1}+1} \text{ to } \frac{e^{2z_2}-1}{e^{2z_2}+1}.$$

The %fat and age data in Figure 11.1 had a correlation of 0.7921 so we have

$$z = \tfrac{1}{2}\log_e\left(\frac{1+0.7921}{1-0.7921}\right) = 1.0770.$$

We can get a 95% confidence interval for $z$ by calculating

$$z_1 = 1.0770 - 1.96/\sqrt{15}$$

and

$$z_2 = 1.0770 + 1.96/\sqrt{15},$$

giving 0.5710 to 1.5831. We back-transform these values to get a 95% confidence interval for $r$ as

$$\frac{e^{2\times 0.5710}-1}{e^{2\times 0.5710}+1} \text{ to } \frac{e^{2\times 1.5831}-1}{e^{2\times 1.5831}+1},$$

or 0.52 to 0.92. Although the whole confidence interval is much greater than zero, it is very wide.

*(b) Hypothesis test*

The hypothesis test for the correlation coefficient may be performed very easily. Under the null hypothesis that there is no association in the population (i.e. zero correlation) it can be shown that the quantity

$$r\sqrt{\frac{n-2}{1-r^2}}$$

has a $t$ distribution with $n-2$ degrees of freedom. Thus the null hypothesis of no association may be tested by looking this value up in the table of the $t$ distribution (Table B4).

The %fat and age data in Figure 11.1 had a correlation of 0.7921 so we have

$$t = 0.7921\sqrt{\frac{16}{1-0.7921^2}} = 5.19$$

on 16 degrees of freedom ($P < 0.001$).

However, Table B7 shows critical values for $r$ itself, and this is much easier to use. This table will prove sufficient for most practical purposes.

### 11.7.2 Rank correlation

Spearman's rank correlation coefficient $r_s$ is obtained by ranking in order the values of each of the two variables. An example is shown in Table 11.4. The simplest way to get $r_s$ is to calculate Pearson's $r$ on the ranks of the data. For the data on DZ twinning rate and latitude in Table 11.4 this gives $r_s = 0.68$.

There is an alternative approach which is simpler for hand calculation, but it assumes that there are no ties in the data. For each of the $N$ subjects being studied the difference in the ranks, $d_i$, is calculated. Spearman's rank correlation coefficient is then given by

$$r_s = 1 - \frac{6\sum_{i=1}^{n} d_i^2}{N^3 - N}$$

This formula bears no obvious similarity to the formula for Pearson's $r$, but gives the identical answer when there are no ties.

The ranks of the data on latitude and DZ twinning rate are shown in Table 11.4. The sum of the squares of the differences in the ranks is 366.5 so we have

$$r_s = 1 - \frac{6 \times 366.5}{6859 - 19} = 0.68.$$

Although the calculation of $r_s$ should be modified when there are tied ranks in the data, the effect is small unless there are considerable numbers of ties. The latitude and DZ twinning data in Table 11.4 have several tied ranks but the value of $r_s$ is 0.68, to two decimal places, whether the correction is made or not. The advantage of the use of the Pearson correlation coefficient calculated on the ranks is that ties are automatically dealt with. Also, of course, it is easy to perform with standard statistical software.

*(a) Confidence interval*

The distribution of $r_s$ is similar to that of $r$ for samples larger than about 10, so a confidence interval for $r_s$ can be obtained using the method given above for $r$.

*(b) Hypothesis test*

Under the null hypothesis that there is no association in the population (i.e. zero correlation) it can be shown that for large samples ($n > 30$) the quantity

$$r_s\sqrt{\frac{n-2}{1-r_s^2}}$$

has a $t$ distribution with $n-2$ degrees of freedom. Thus the null hypothesis of no association may be tested by looking this value up in the table of the $t$ distribution (Table B4). Equivalently, $r_s$ can be compared with the critical values in Table B7. For smaller samples Table B8 should be used.

### 11.7.3 Partial correlation

We can calculate the correlation between two variables after adjusting for a third if we have the correlation coefficients between each pair of variables, say $r(AB)$, $r(AC)$ and $r(BC)$. To adjust the correlation between variables $A$ and $B$ for the possible effect of variable $C$ we calculate the partial correlation of $A$ and $B$ adjusted for $C$ as

$$r(AB|C) = \frac{r(AB) - r(AC)r(BC)}{\sqrt{[1 - r(AC)^2][1 - r(BC)^2]}}.$$

Similarly the partial rank correlation is calculated as

$$r_s(AB|C) = \frac{r_s(AB) - r_s(AC)r_s(BC)}{\sqrt{[1 - r_s(AC)^2][1 - r_s(BC)^2]}}.$$

The hypothesis test for the partial correlation coefficient is performed in the same way as for the ordinary correlation coefficient, except that there are $N-3$ degrees of freedom. The correlations between pairs of variables in Table 11.4, omitting the four countries without milk consumption rates, were

$$r_s(LT) = 0.6147,\ r_s(LM) = 0.9221, \text{ and } r_s(TM) = 0.6059$$

so that the partial rank correlation coefficient between latitude and DZ twinning rate adjusted for milk consumption is

$$r_s(LT|M) = \frac{0.6147 - 0.9221 \times 0.6059}{\sqrt{(1 - 0.9221^2)(1 - 0.6059^2)}} = 0.18.$$

## 11.8 INTERPRETATION OF CORRELATION

Correlation coefficients lie within the range $-1$ to $+1$, with the midpoint of zero indicating no linear association between the two variables. A very small correlation does not necessarily indicate that two variables are not associated, however. To be sure of this we should study a plot of the data, because it is possible that the two variables display a peculiar (i.e. non-linear) relationship. For example, we would not observe much, if any, correlation between the average midday temperature and calendar month because there is a cyclic pattern. More common is the situation of a curved relationship between two variables, such as between birthweight and length of gestation. In this case Pearson's $r$ will underestimate the association as it is a measure of linear association. The rank correlation coefficient is better here as it assesses in a more general way whether the variables tend to rise together (or move in opposite directions).

It is surprising how unimpressive a correlation of 0.5 or even 0.7 is (Figure 11.2). As Table B7 shows, correlations of this magnitude are significant at the 5% level in samples as small as 16 and 9 respectively. Whether they are important is quite another matter. Feinstein (1985) commented on the lack of clinical relevance of a statistically significant correlation of less than 0.1 found in a sample of over 6000. The problem of clinical relevance is one that must be judged on its merits in each case, and depends on the context. For example, the same small correlation may be important in an epidemiological study but unimportant clinically.

One way of looking at the correlation that helps to modify over-enthusiasm is to calculate $100r^2$, which is the percentage of the variability of the data that is 'explained' by the association between the two variables. So a correlation of 0.7 implies that just about half (49%) of the variability may be put down to the observed association, and so on. This concept ties in with the analysis of variance for regression, discussed in section 11.13.6 and in Chapter 12. It may also be useful to calculate a confidence interval for the correlation coefficient, which for small samples will be wide.

Interpretation of association is often problematic because **causation cannot be directly inferred**. If we observe an association between two variables $A$ and $B$ there are several possible explanations. Excluding the possibility that it is a chance finding, it may be because

1. A influences (or 'causes') $B$;
2. B influences $A$; or
3. both $A$ and $B$ are influenced by one or more other variables.

Where data are available for some suspected common cause $C$, it is possible to see if the observed association between $A$ and $B$ remains when allowing for $C$ by calculating the partial correlation. With this exception, it is not in general possible to distinguish statistically between the three possibilities above, and inferences must be based on other knowledge. **When looking at variables where there is no background knowledge, inferring a causal link is not justified**. This applies regardless of the strength of the observed association.

For example, we are not surprised to see data from many countries that show a relation between consumption of alcohol and deaths from liver cirrhosis (Smith, 1981), because of the large body of scientific knowledge about the effect of alcohol on the liver. But what should we make of international data showing a relationship between pork consumption and cirrhosis mortality? Nanji and French (1985) reported such a correlation of

$r = 0.40$ for 16 countries and a rank correlation of 0.60 for 10 Canadian provinces. In the absence of any scientific reason for such an association one should be sceptical about such a finding. Wherever possible one should try to examine the same variables in a different population. Seely (1985) studied the relation between pork consumption and cirrhosis mortality in 21 European countries, for which the rank correlation was 0.001; there was no association at all.

Interpretation of international correlations is particularly difficult because there are so many differences between countries. We could not safely interpret the data of Figure 11.6 as indicating that a high fibre diet leads to delayed menarche (and certainly not the converse). Other situations are not really any different. We ought not to take *any* correlation as indicating a causal association without collateral evidence, however 'reasonable' the hypothesis may be.

Correlation is often used as an exploratory method for investigating inter-relationships among many variables, for which purpose it is most obvious to use hypothesis tests. Although fine in principle, this approach is often over-done. The problem is that even with a modest number of variables the number of correlation coefficients is large – 10 variables yield 45 $r$ values, and 20 variables yield 190. One in 20 of these will be significant at the 5% level purely by chance, and these cannot be distinguished from genuine associations. Further, the magnitude of correlation that is significant at the 5% level depends upon the sample size. In a large sample, even if there are several significant $r$ values of around 0.2 to 0.3, say, these are unlikely to be very useful. While this way of looking at large numbers of variables can be helpful when one really has no prior hypotheses, significant associations really need to be confirmed in another set of data before credence can be given to them.

Another common problem of interpretation occurs when we know that each of two variables is associated with a third variable. For example, if $A$ is positively correlated with $B$ and $B$ is positively correlated with $C$ it is tempting to infer that $A$ must be positively correlated with $C$. Although this may indeed be true, such an inference is unjustified – we cannot say anything about the correlation between $A$ and $C$. The same is true when one has observed no association. For example, in the data of Mazess *et al.* (1984) the correlation between age and weight was 0.05 and between weight and %fat it was 0.03 (Figure 11.3). This does not imply that the correlation between age and %fat was also near zero. In fact this correlation was 0.79, as we saw earlier (Figure 11.1). These three two-way relations are shown in Figure 11.8. Correlations cannot be inferred from indirect associations.

Correlation is often used when it would be better to use regression methods, discussed in section 11.10 onwards. The two methods are compared in section 11.17.

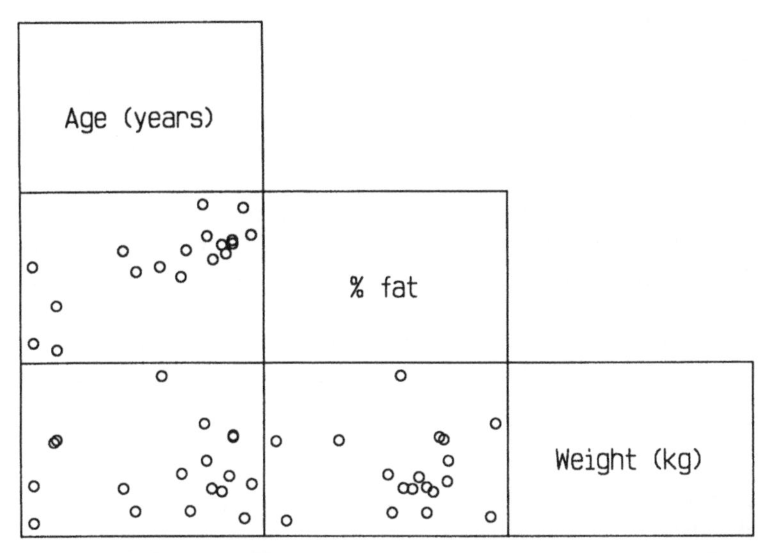


**Figure 11.8** Scatter diagrams showing each two way relation between age, %fat, and weight of 18 normal adults (Mazess *et al.*, 1984) .

## 11.9 PRESENTATION OF CORRELATION

Where possible it is useful to show a scatter diagram of the data. In such a graph it is often helpful to indicate different categories of observations by using different symbols, for example to indicate patients' sex.

The value of $r$ should be given to two decimal places, together with the P value if a test of significance is performed. The number of observations should be stated.

If it is necessary to display the correlations between all pairs of a set of variables this can be done by means of a correlation matrix, as in Table 11.3. In this the correlation coefficients are shown in a triangular display similar to charts in road atlases showing the distances between each pair of towns. The graphical equivalent, shown in Figures 11.8 and 12.2, is even better.

## 11.10 REGRESSION

Other questions may arise when we have a set of data on two continuous variables. In particular we might wish to *describe* the relation between them, and thus be able to predict the value of one variable for an individual when we only know the other variable. Clearly the correlation coefficient does not perform these functions; it just indicates the strength of the association as a single number. We want a way of describing the relation between the values of the two variables, and for this general problem we need the technique called **regression**. In this chapter I shall consider just the simple case where we have two variables; extensions are discussed in Chapters 12 and 14. I shall consider only the common case where we are interested in a linear (straight-line) relationship between two variables.

Table 11.6 and Figure 11.9 show data collected from 24 type 1 diabetic patients. The variables are fasting blood glucose (mmol/l) and mean velocity of circumferential shortening of the left ventricle (Vcf) derived from echocardiography. One patient's Vcf was not recorded. If we are interested in trying to predict Vcf from blood glucose, then, unlike the case for correlation, we do not have a symmetric relation between the two

**Table 11.6** Data from 24 type 1 diabetic patients (Thuesen *et al.*, 1985)

| Patient | Fasting blood glucose (mmol/l) | Mean circumferential shortening velocity (Vcf) (%/sec) |
|---|---|---|
| 1 | 15.3 | 1.76 |
| 2 | 10.8 | 1.34 |
| 3 | 8.1 | 1.27 |
| 4 | 19.5 | 1.47 |
| 5 | 7.2 | 1.27 |
| 6 | 5.3 | 1.49 |
| 7 | 9.3 | 1.31 |
| 8 | 11.1 | 1.09 |
| 9 | 7.5 | 1.18 |
| 10 | 12.2 | 1.22 |
| 11 | 6.7 | 1.25 |
| 12 | 5.2 | 1.19 |
| 13 | 19.0 | 1.95 |
| 14 | 15.1 | 1.28 |
| 15 | 6.7 | 1.52 |
| 16 | 8.6 | — |
| 17 | 4.2 | 1.12 |
| 18 | 10.3 | 1.37 |
| 19 | 12.5 | 1.19 |
| 20 | 16.1 | 1.05 |
| 21 | 13.3 | 1.32 |
| 22 | 4.9 | 1.03 |
| 23 | 8.8 | 1.12 |
| 24 | 9.5 | 1.70 |

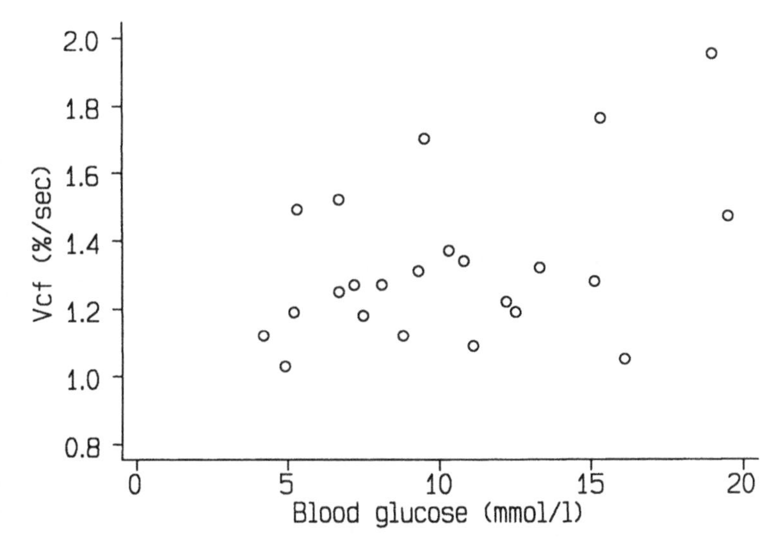


**Figure 11.9** Relation between fasting blood glucose and mean velocity of circumferential shortening of the left ventricle (Vcf). Data from 23 type 1 diabetics (Thuesen *et al.*, 1985).

variables. We may consider these as a **response** (or **outcome**) variable (Vcf) and a **predictor** variable (blood glucose). These are often called **dependent** and **independent** variables respectively, confusing names which indicate which variable is depending on the other. The response variable is always plotted on the vertical, or $Y$, axis and the predictor variable on the horizontal, or $X$, axis, as illustrated in Figure 11.9.

The problem is to fit a straight line to the data that in some sense gives the 'best' prediction of $Y$ for any value of $X$. Intuitively this will be a line that minimizes the distance between the data and the fitted line. There are several possible approaches to this problem, but the standard method is called **least squares** regression. When we use this method to fit a **regression line** we minimize the sum of the squares of the vertical distances of the observations from the line. Figure 11.10 shows the same data with the least squares regression line, together with the vertical distances from the line. Each distance is the difference for an individual between the observed value and the value given by the line, known as the **fitted** value. The technical term for this distance is a **residual**, a term I shall use from now on. Notice that this approach gives a solution that does not depend on the scaling of the graph. If we were to take distances perpendicular to the line (which is an alternative possibility) the solution *would* depend on the way the graph was drawn, which is clearly an undesirable feature.

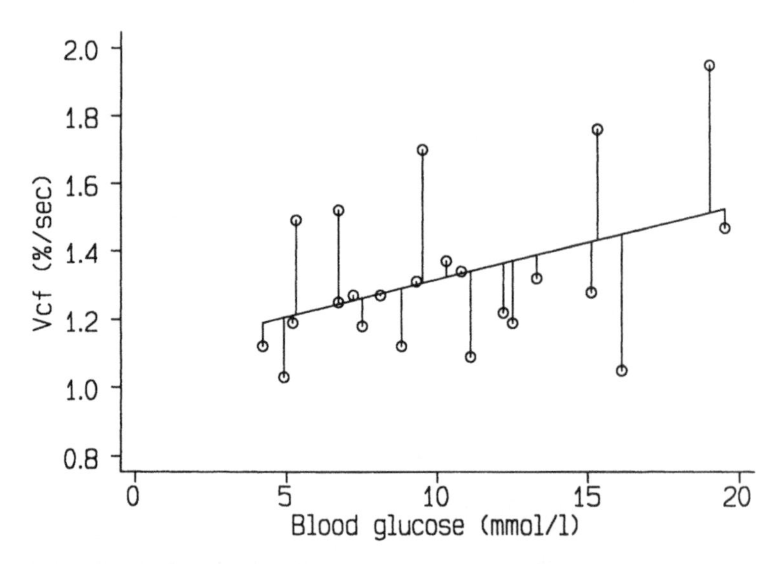


**Figure 11.10** Data of Figure 11.9 with regression line, showing differences between observed and fitted values.

The least squares method produces the line that minimizes the sum of the squares of the residuals, and so it also minimizes the variance of the residuals, which is just the sum of squares divided by the number of observations minus two. This variance, known as the residual variance, is a measure of the 'goodness-of-fit' of the line. The residual variance is very important when assessing the results of a regression analysis.

If we have observed values of two variables, $X$ (blood glucose) and $Y$ (Vcf), we can perform a 'regression of $Y$ on $X$' to derive a straight line that gives a 'fitted' estimated value of $Y$ for any value of the variable $X$. The general equation of a regression line is

$$Y = a + bX.$$

Here $b$ is the **slope** of the line and $a$ is called the **intercept** because it is the fitted value of $Y$ where the line crosses the $Y$ axis, for which $X = 0$. In most medical applications the value of $a$ will have no practical meaning, as the $X$ variable cannot be anywhere near zero; examples are blood pressure and any measurements of body size.

In practice the calculation of $a$ and $b$ for a given set of data is easy (see section 11.13) although it is definitely preferable to use a computer to do the calculations. For the data on diabetics the equation of the regression line shown in Figure 11.10 is

$$\text{Vcf} = 1.10 + 0.0220 \times \text{blood glucose}.$$

What does this equation tell us? For any value of blood glucose the estimate of Vcf derived from the regression equation is the predicted value of Vcf, but we need some measure of the uncertainty of such a prediction. More basically, we would usually wish to consider the possibility that the observed relation between the two variables in these subjects is just a chance finding, and to consider how well the line fits the data. All of these aspects can be studied in relation to the residuals introduced earlier.

### 11.10.1 Assumptions

Before we can consider the use of a regression analysis it is important to consider three assumptions that underlie the method:

1. the values of the outcome variable $Y$ (Vcf in our example) should have a Normal distribution for each value of the predictor variable $X$;
2. the variability of $Y$, as assessed by the variance or standard deviation, should be the same for each value of $X$;
3. the relation between the two variables should be linear.

Unlike for correlation, it is not a requirement that both variables should be random variables: regression analysis is valid if the values of the predictor ($X$) variable have been chosen by the experimenter, as is sometimes the case. Nor do the values of $X$ need to be approximately Normal.

We can usually get a reasonable visual impression of whether the data deviate considerably from the three conditions listed above from a scatter diagram. Fortunately it is possible to assess them in detail after fitting the regression line. Again the residuals contain the relevant information.

If the three above assumptions hold then the residuals should have a Normal distribution (with a mean of zero). If we plot the residuals against the $X$ values the points should be evenly scattered at all $X$ values. I recommend that this plot is produced routinely. Figure 11.11 shows three possibilities for a plot of the residuals where (a) the assumptions are met; (b) the residuals have increasing variability as $X$ increases; (c) there is a curved relation between the residuals and the $X$ values. Plot (b) suggests that the data ($Y$) might need log transformation, and plot (c) indicates a non-linear relation between $X$ and $Y$ (see section 11.12.2). It can happen that different problems occur simultaneously, and that log (or some other) transformation of the $Y$ variable will solve all the problems at once.

The assumption of Normality can be assessed formally by means of a Normal plot of the residuals (see section 7.5.3). Some computer programs incorporate this analysis.

Figure 11.12 shows the residuals plotted against blood glucose, which looks satisfactorily like Figure 11.11(a). Figure 11.13 shows a Normal plot of residuals, which is reasonably straight. However, the Shapiro-Francia

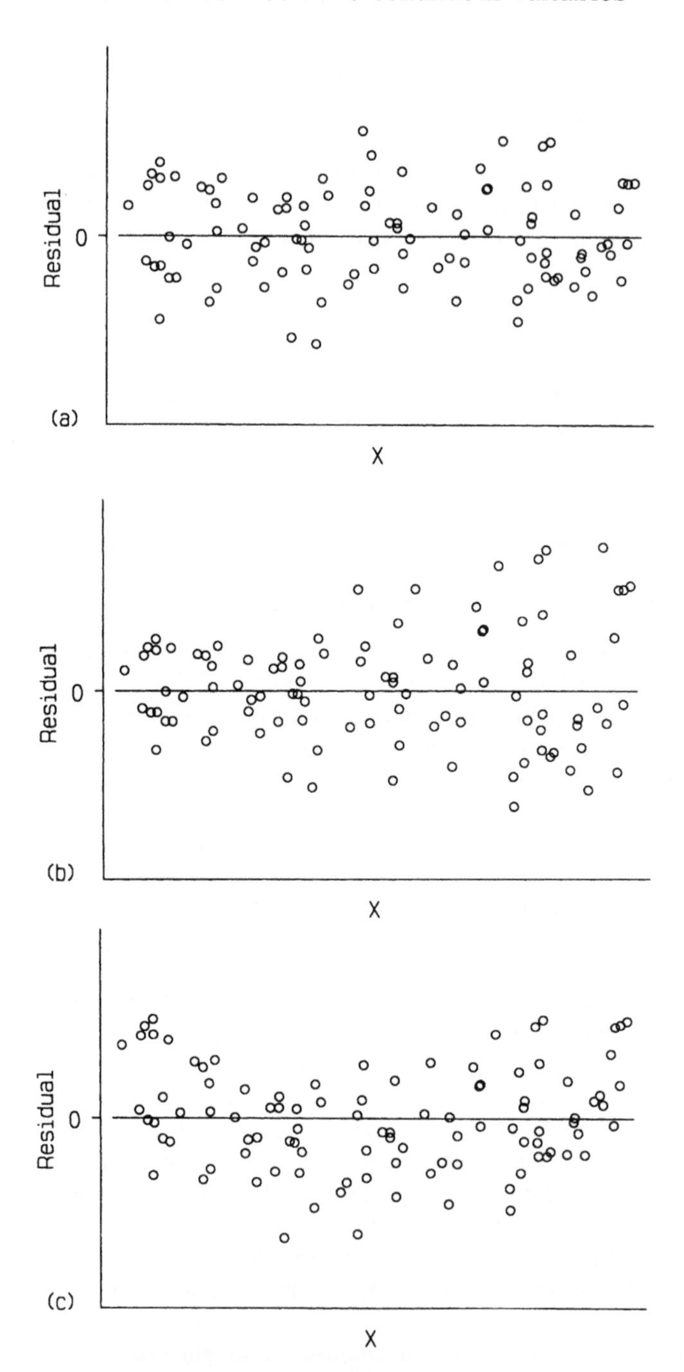


**Figure 11.11** Plots of residuals, showing examples with: (a) the assumptions met; (b) increasing variability; (c) curvature.

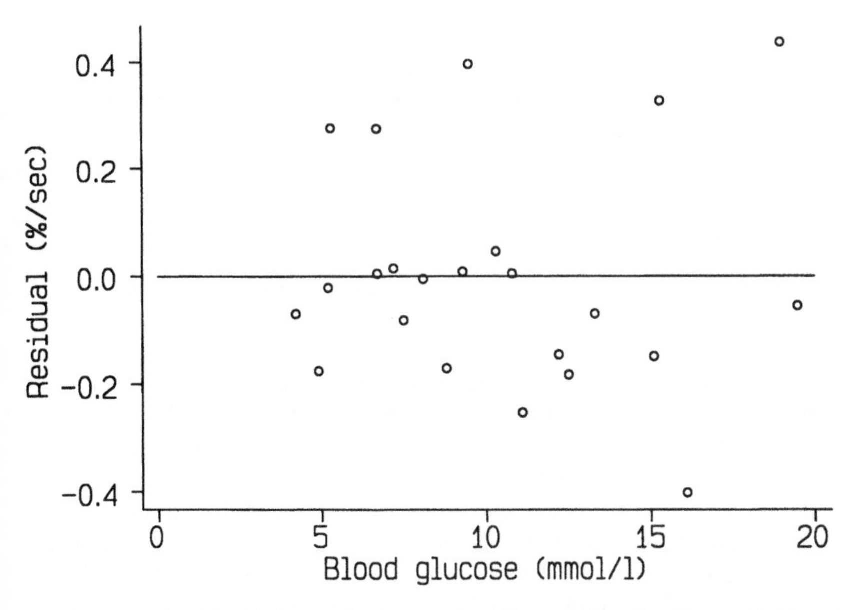


**Figure 11.12** Residuals from the regression line shown in Figure 11.10, plotted against blood glucose.

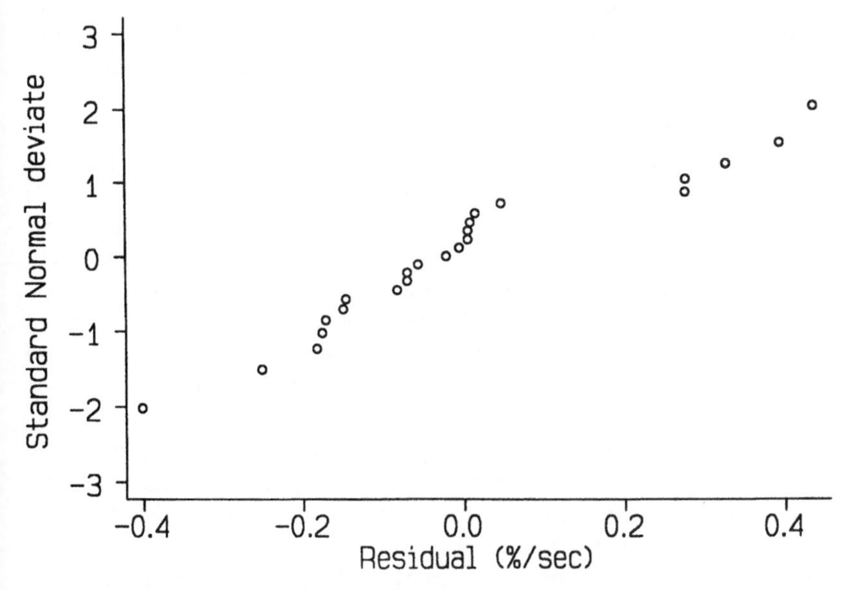


**Figure 11.13** Normal plot of residuals shown in Figure 11.12.

test gives $W' = 0.907$ ($P = 0.03$), indicating some non-Normality. Figure 11.13 suggests that this is not a major problem, but if we were worried we could try log transformation of Vcf. The value of $W'$ for the residuals after regression analysis using $\log_e$ Vcf is $W' = 0.94$ ($P = 0.12$).

## 11.11 USE OF REGRESSION

The least squares regression line shown in Figure 11.10 has the equation

$$Y = 1.10 + 0.0220X.$$

From Figures 11.10 and 11.13 the assumptions of this analysis seem reasonable – the scatter around the regression line is fairly even and symmetric, a linear relation seems plausible, and the residuals have a distribution that is not too far from Normal.

When the assumptions hold, the regression line can be thought of as joining the mean values of $Y$ for each value of $X$. Hence the regression line gives an estimate of the average Vcf for a given blood glucose level. The line fitted to the sample data is an estimate of the relation between these variables in the population, so we should consider the uncertainty of this estimated line. Figure 11.14 shows the regression line together with the 95% confidence interval for the line. We can consider this interval as including the true relation with 95% probability. Alternatively, for any value of blood glucose the confidence interval covers the range of values which we are 95% confident includes the true mean Vcf in the population. The confidence interval is narrowest at the mean blood glucose (10.3 mmol/l) and gets wider with increasing distance from the mean.

The slope is the parameter of main interest in a regression analysis, as it indicates the strength of the relationship between the two variables. The slope of the fitted line is 0.022, which means that we estimate an increase in Vcf of 0.022% per second for every increase of one unit (i.e. 1 mmol/l) in fasting blood glucose. We can calculate the standard error of the slope, which is 0.0105. The estimated slope, $b$, is treated in much the same way as the mean of a sample. We can calculate a confidence interval for the slope, and can test the hypothesis of a zero slope, that is, of no relationship between Vcf and blood glucose. These calculations, which are described in section 11.13, yield a 95% confidence interval for the slope from 0.000 to 0.044; the test statistic is $t = 2.10$, with $P = 0.05$. By conventional criteria the slope is just significantly different from zero. As usual the confidence interval is more informative, showing that the data are compatible with no relation between Vcf and blood glucose or with one that is twice as strong as the observed one.

Implicit in this analysis is the consistency of the relationship, as indicated by the scatter of the observed data around the fitted line. The nearer the points are to the line the narrower will be the confidence interval for the line (Figure 11.14). With the present data there is considerable scatter, and this is more noticeable if we consider the prediction of Vcf for a new subject with a known fasting blood glucose level.

Figure 11.14 showed the 95% confidence interval for the mean Vcf for a given value of fasting blood glucose. We expect greater uncertainty when trying to predict Vcf for an individual, and Figure 11.15 shows that the 95% **prediction interval** is indeed much wider. For any value of blood glucose we would expect 95% of future subjects to have Vcf values between the values shown. There is thus a 95% probability of an individual's Vcf being within this interval, although our best estimate is given by the value on the regression line corresponding to their blood glucose level. The 95% prediction interval also widens with distance from the mean blood glucose level although this is not as easy to see. What is clear is that for a given blood glucose value there is enormous uncertainty attached to the estimated Vcf. A much tighter prediction interval is needed for such a relation to have any clinical value. Note that unlike the confidence interval for the regression line the prediction interval can be made only slightly narrower by increasing the sample size. This is because the prediction interval mainly reflects individual variability about the fitted line, which has nothing to do with sample size. Where the measurements are imprecise (such as blood pressure) the prediction interval can be

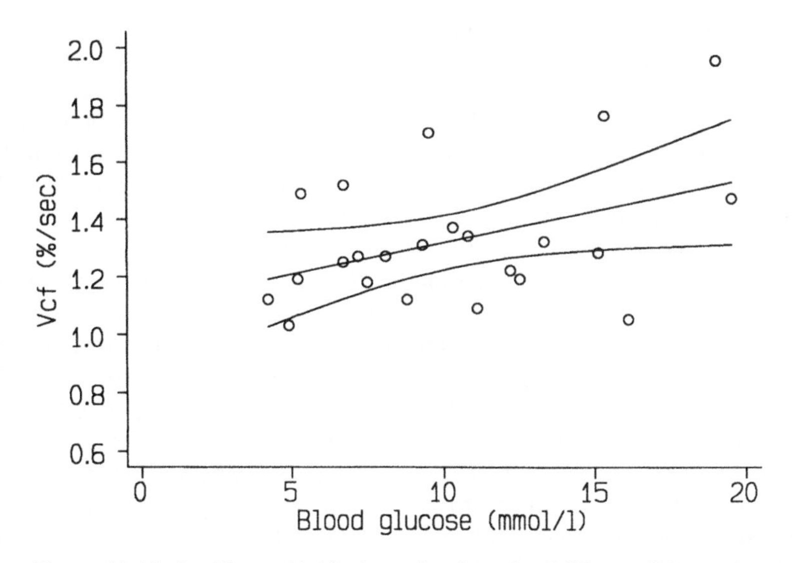


**Figure 11.14** As Figure 11.10, but showing the 95% confidence interval for the regression line.

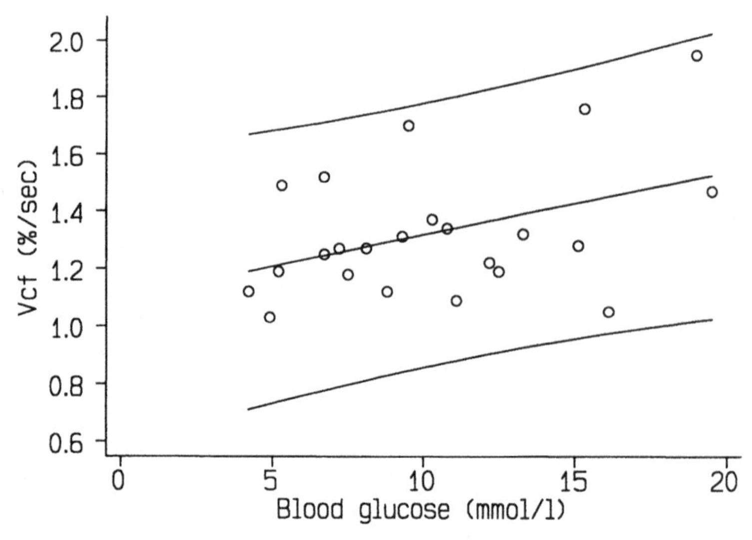


**Figure 11.15** As Figure 11.10, but showing the 95% interval for predicting Vcf from blood glucose for an individual subject.

narrowed by taking the average for each individual of two (or more) readings.

The fitted regression line explains a proportion of the variability in the dependent variable ($Y$), and the residuals indicate the amount of unexplained variability. A regression analysis can thus be displayed as an analysis of variance table which is very similar to those shown in Chapter 9. Table 11.7 shows the analysis of variance table corresponding to the regression of blood glucose on Vcf. The derivation of this table is explained in section 11.13.6. Many software packages present the results in this way. This format for displaying the results of a regression analysis extends easily to complex models, as will be seen in Chapter 12. Two points should be noted. Firstly, as this is an alternative way of displaying the same analysis, the P value is the same as that obtained for the slope. In fact, the $F$ statistic is the square of the $t$ statistic obtained earlier ($4.41 = 2.10^2$). Secondly, the residual mean square (0.0470) is the variance of the residuals, and thus the square of the residual standard deviation.

The residual standard deviation indicates the variation not explained by the regression line so it is a measure of the goodness-of-fit of the line in the units of measurement. A more general way of assessing goodness-of-fit is to consider the proportion of the total variation explained by the model. This is usually done by considering the sum of squares explained by the regression as a percentage of the total sum of squares. From Table 11.7 this value is $0.2073/1.1934 = 0.17$ or 17%. This statistic is called $R^2$, and is

**Table 11.7** Analysis of variance table corresponding to regression of blood glucose on Vcf

| Source of variation | Degrees of freedom | Sums of squares | Mean squares | *F* | P |
|---|---|---|---|---|---|
| Regression | 1 | 0.2073 | 0.2073 | 4.41 | 0.048 |
| Residual | 21 | 0.9861 | 0.0470 | | |
| Total | 22 | 1.1934 | | | |

the square of the correlation coefficient between Vcf and blood glucose. The concept extends to more complex models, and will be discussed again in the next chapter. The low value of $R^2$ here indicates that despite the statistically significant slope the majority of the variability in Vcf is not explained by variation in blood glucose levels.

Section 11.13 gives the mathematical formulae for all the calculations relating to regression.

## 11.12 EXTENSIONS

The previous sections have presented the simplest form of regression analysis, where we wish to describe the linear relation between two continuous variables measured in a single sample. Various extensions are possible, two of which are described below. They are both types of **multiple regression**, whereby we can examine the dependence of one outcome variable on two or more other variables simultaneously. Multiple regression is discussed at more length in Chapter 12.

### 11.12.1 Comparing groups

If we have data from two groups of subjects we can fit regression lines to each, and then compare the slopes of the two lines to see if they are reasonably similar. A confidence interval can be obtained for the difference or a significance test can be carried out. If the two lines can be considered to have the same slope, then it is possible to fit lines to the two sets of data that have the same slope (i.e. they are parallel). The vertical distance between the two lines is then the difference in the means of the $Y$ variable in the two groups adjusted for any difference in the distribution of the $X$ variable. This analysis is known as **analysis of covariance**. Further details are given by Altman and Gardner (1989). Analysis of covariance, which is also discussed in section 12.4.1, can be extended to more than two groups of observations.

### 11.12.2 Non-linear relationships

Sometimes it can be clearly seen from a scatter plot that the relation between two variables is curved. There are several statistical models that can be used to cope with non-linearity. The simplest method, and the only one considered here, is known as **polynomial** regression.

Polynomial regression is a special case of multiple regression when we wish to describe (or 'model') the non-linear relation between an outcome variable and a single predictor variable. A linear relation between variables $X$ and $Y$ leads to a regression equation of the type $Y = a + bX$. This idea can be extended to a non-linear relation by means of the model $Y = a + bX + cX^2$. This model, which is called a **quadratic curve**, considers the outcome variable ($Y$) to be dependent not just on the predictor variable ($X$) but also on its square ($X^2$). By this means we obtain a curved relation between $Y$ and $X$, although (as explained above) this model is a special case of multiple regression, with both $X$ and $X^2$ as predictor variables.

The quadratic model describes a simple curve which rises and then falls (or vice versa) in a symmetric manner about its maximum (or minimum) value. Altman and Coles (1980) fitted such a model to data giving mean birthweight for different lengths of gestation. For example, for female first born babies their fitted model was

$$\text{Birthweight (kg)} = -22.693 + 1.2122 \times \text{age} - 0.014102 \times \text{age}^2$$

where 'age' is the gestational age in weeks. This curve is shown in Figure 11.16.

## 11.13 REGRESSION – MATHEMATICS AND WORKED EXAMPLE

*(This section gives the mathematical formulae for the calculations described in sections 11.10 to 11.12 together with a worked example. It can be omitted without loss of continuity. These formulae can be complicated to use, so it is preferable to perform regression analysis using a computer program if possible.)*

Regression analysis will be illustrated using the data from diabetics shown in Table 11.6. We want the regression line to allow prediction of Vcf (velocity of circumferential shortening) from blood glucose, so the $X$ (predictor) variable is blood glucose and the $Y$ (outcome) variable is Vcf.

### 11.13.1 The regression line

The equation of the least squares linear regression line is $Y = a + bX$ and

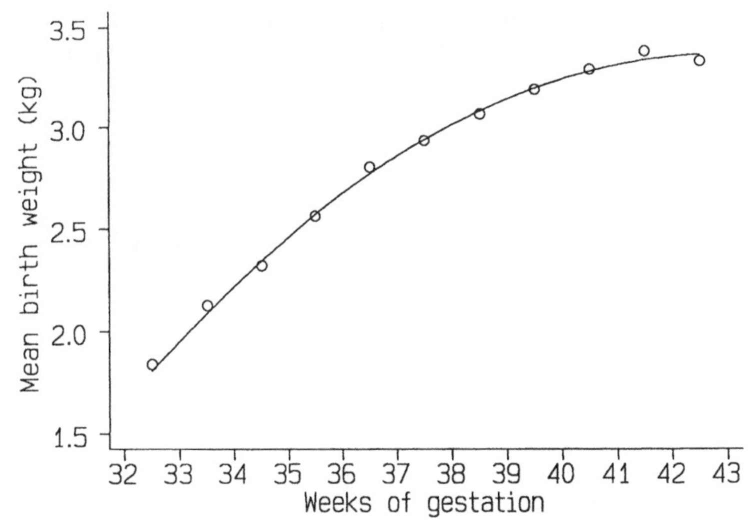


**Figure 11.16** Quadratic curve fitted to mean birth weight by gestational age (Altman and Coles, 1980).

estimates of $a$ and $b$ can be obtained easily. Denoting the observed data as $x_i$ and $y_i$ $(i = 1, \ldots, n)$ it can be shown that the line must pass through the mean of the data $(\bar{x}, \bar{y})$. The estimated slope is given by

$$b = \frac{\Sigma(x_i - \bar{x})(y_i - \bar{y})}{\Sigma(x_i - \bar{x})^2}.$$

Note that, as we should expect from the nature of the analysis, the equation is asymmetric in contrast to that for $r$ given in section 11.7: it *does* matter which variable is $X$ and which is $Y$.

The calculations can be simplified if we first obtain the 'sum of squares' of the $X$ and $Y$ values about their means, and the 'sum of products':

$$S_{xx} = \sum x_i^2 - (\sum x_i)^2/n$$

$$S_{yy} = \sum y_i^2 - (\sum y_i)^2/n$$

$$S_{xy} = \sum x_i y_i - \sum x_i \sum y_i/n.$$

The quantities $S_{xx}$ and $S_{yy}$ are just $n - 1$ times the variances of $X$ and $Y$.

An easier way of calculating $b$ is as

$$b = \frac{S_{xy}}{S_{xx}}.$$

This formula should not be used in a computer program, however, as inaccuracy is occasionally introduced because of rounding errors. Only the first equation given above for $b$ should be used for this purpose.

Because we know that the regression line passes through the mean $(\bar{x}, \bar{y})$, we can estimate $a$ simply as

$$a = \bar{y} - b\bar{x}.$$

So for any value of $X$, say $x_0$, the fitted value of $Y$ predicted by the equation is

$$\begin{aligned} y_{fit} &= a + bx_0 \\ &= (\bar{y} - b\bar{x}) + bx_0 \\ &= \bar{y} + b(x_0 - \bar{x}). \end{aligned}$$

Note that all the results quoted below were obtained using full numeric accuracy, but intermediate calculations have been rounded to clarify the presentation.

For the data on diabetics the mean values of the two variables are $\bar{x} = 10.37$ mmol/l and $\bar{y} = 1.33\%$/sec, and the other quantities we will need are

$$\sum x = 238.60, \sum y = 30.49, \sum x^2 = 2904.92, \sum y^2 = 41.6125$$

$$\text{and } \sum xy = 325.74,$$

$$\begin{aligned} S_{xx} &= 2904.92 - 238.60^2/23 = 429.704, \\ S_{yy} &= 41.61 - 30.49^2/23 = 1.193, \\ S_{xy} &= 325.74 - 238.60 \times 30.49/23 = 9.439. \end{aligned}$$

We estimate the slope $b$ as

$$\begin{aligned} b &= \frac{9.439}{429.704} \\ &= 0.02196. \end{aligned}$$

The intercept $a$ is estimated as

$$\begin{aligned} a &= 1.33 - 0.02196 \times 10.37 \\ &= 1.098\%/\text{sec}. \end{aligned}$$

### 11.13.2 Residual variation

The difference between an observed value $y_0$ and fitted value $y_{fit}$ is thus

$$y_0 - y_{fit} = y_0 - [\bar{y} + b(x_0 - \bar{x})],$$

and the value $y_0 - y_{fit}$ is the **residual** for that individual. It is the sum of the squares of the residuals, $\Sigma(y_i - y_{fit})^2$, that is minimized by the least squares line, but we are more interested in their variance, obtained as

$$s_{res}^2 = \frac{\Sigma(y_i - y_{fit})^2}{n - 2}$$

or, for calculation,

$$s_{res}^2 = \frac{1}{n-2}\left[\sum y_i^2 - \frac{(\Sigma y_i)^2}{n} - b\left(\sum x_i y_i - \frac{\Sigma x_i \Sigma y_i}{n}\right)\right]$$

$$= \frac{1}{n-2}(S_{yy} - bS_{xy}).$$

The square root of this expression, the residual standard deviation, $s_{res}$, is used in subsequent calculations.

We can calculate the residual variance in the example as

$$s_{res}^2 = \frac{1}{21}(1.193 - 0.02196 \times 9.439)$$

$$= 0.04696$$

so that the residual standard deviation is

$$s_{res} = \sqrt{0.04696}$$
$$= 0.2167.$$

### 11.13.3 Confidence intervals

*(a) Slope*

The standard error of the slope, $b$, is strongly related to the residual standard deviation, being

$$se(b) = \frac{s_{res}}{\sqrt{S_{xx}}}$$

so that a 95% confidence interval for $b$ is

$$b \pm t_{0.975}se(b)$$

where $t$ is on $n - 2$ degrees of freedom (the degrees of freedom associated with the residual).

The slope is usually the aspect of most interest. The standard error of $b$ is

$$se(b) = \frac{0.2167}{\sqrt{429.704}}$$

$$= 0.0105.$$

From Table B4 the value of $t_{0.975}$ on 21 degrees of freedom is 2.08, so a 95% confidence interval is given by

$$0.02196 \pm 2.08 \times 0.0105$$

that is, 0.00012 to 0.044. The confidence interval thus extends from zero, representing no relation between the variables, to twice the value observed in the sample.

*(b) Estimated Y for a given X*

The standard error of the estimate $y_{fit}$ for a given value of $X$, say $x_0$, is given by

$$se(y_{fit}) = s_{res}\sqrt{\frac{1}{n} + \frac{(x_0 - \bar{x})^2}{S_{xx}}}$$

and a 95% confidence interval is given by

$$y_{fit} \pm t_{0.975}se(y_{fit})$$

where $t$ is on $n - 2$ degrees of freedom.

We can obtain a 95% confidence interval for the predicted mean value of Vcf for any blood glucose. If $y_{fit}$ is the predicted mean Vcf from the regression equation, then the standard error of $y_{fit}$ is

$$se(y_{fit}) = 0.2167\sqrt{\frac{1}{23} + \frac{(x_0 - 10.37)^2}{429.704}}$$

where $x_0$ is the blood glucose value. So for a blood glucose of 14.5 mmol/l the estimated mean Vcf is given by the regression equation as

$$1.098 + 0.02196 \times 14.5$$
$$= 1.416\%/\text{sec.}$$

The standard error of this estimate is thus

$$se(y_{fit}) = 0.2167\sqrt{\frac{1}{23} + \frac{(14.5 - 10.37)^2}{429.704}}$$
$$= 0.0625\%/\text{sec.}$$

We use the equation above to get a confidence interval for the estimate of 1.419. From Table B4 the value of $t_{0.975}$ with 21 degrees of freedom is 2.080, so that the 95% confidence interval is given by

$$1.416 \pm 2.080 \times 0.0625$$

or 1.29 to 1.55%/sec.

*(c) Intercept*

The intercept is not usually of great interest, but a confidence interval can be obtained for the intercept $a$ using the formula in the previous section to get a confidence interval for $y_{fit}$ when $X = 0$.

### 11.13.4 Prediction interval

The 95% prediction interval is much wider than the 95% confidence interval for the line as the scatter of the individual data about the fitted line becomes more directly relevant.

For any value $x_0$ the predicted value is $y_{fit} = a + bx_0$. To get the prediction interval we do not want the standard error of $y_{fit}$, but the estimated standard deviation of individual values of $Y - y_{fit}$ at that value of $X$. This standard deviation is given by

$$s_{pred} = s_{res}\sqrt{1 + \frac{1}{n} + \frac{(x_0 - \bar{x})^2}{S_{xx}}}$$

and thus the 95% prediction interval is

$$y_{fit} \pm t_{0.975}s_{pred}$$

where $t$ is on $n - 2$ degrees of freedom.

The estimated standard deviation of Vcf values for individuals with a blood glucose of 14.5 mmol/l is

$$s_{pred} = 0.2167\sqrt{1 + \frac{1}{23} + \frac{(14.5 - 10.37)^2}{429.704}}$$

$$= 0.225\%/\text{sec}.$$

The 95% prediction interval is therefore

$$1.416 \pm 2.080 \times 0.225$$

or 0.95 to 1.89%/sec, which is considerably wider than the confidence interval for the mean, as can be seen by comparing Figures 11.14 and 11.15.

### 11.13.5 Hypothesis test for $b$

We have seen that the standard error of the estimated slope, $b$, is $se(b) = s_{res}/\sqrt{S_{xx}}$, so we can perform a test of the hypothesis that $b = 0$ by calculating $b/se(b)$. This ratio is compared with the $t$ distribution with $n - 2$ degrees of freedom.

We can thus test the null hypothesis of no relation between Vcf and blood glucose. We simply divide the estimate of $b$ by its standard error and compare the result with the appropriate value of the $t$ distribution. So we have

$$t = b/se(b) = 0.02196/0.0105$$
$$= 2.10.$$

This value is compared with the $t$ distribution with 21 degrees of freedom, the value of $t_{0.975}$ being 2.08. The slope is thus just significantly different from zero at the 5% level.

### 11.13.6 Analysis of variance table

The results of a regression analysis can be displayed in an analysis of variance table, by partitioning the total variability in the dependent variable into a component explained by the regression line and unexplained or residual variation.

The total sum of squares of the dependent variable $Y$ is $S_{yy}$ (with $n-1$ degrees of freedom) and the sum of squares due to the regression is $(S_{xy})^2/S_{xx}$ with 1 degree of freedom. The residual sum of squares (with $n-2$ degrees of freedom) can be obtained by subtraction.

For the blood glucose data the total sum of squares is 1.1934 and the sum of squares due to regression is $9.439^2/429.704 = 0.2073$. These results are shown in Table 11.7.

## 11.14 INTERPRETATION OF REGRESSION

As discussed in Chapter 8, the variability among a set of observations may be partly attributed to known factors and partly to unknown sources; the latter is often termed 'random variation'. In linear regression we see how much of the variability in the response variable can be attributed to different values of the predictor variable, and the scatter either side of the fitted line shows unexplained variability. Because of this variability, the fitted line is only an estimate of the relation between these variables in the population. As with other estimates (such as a sample mean) there will be uncertainty associated with the estimated slope and intercept, $b$ and $a$. The confidence interval for the slope $b$ will indicate the uncertainty in the estimated strength of the relationship, and confidence intervals for the whole line and prediction intervals for individual subjects show other aspects of variability. The latter are especially useful as regression is often used to make predictions about individuals.

It should be remembered that the regression line should not be used to make predictions for $X$ values outside the range of values in the observed data. Such extrapolation is unjustified as we have no evidence about the relationship beyond the observed data. A statistical model is only an approximation. One rarely believes, for example, that the true relationship is exactly linear, but the linear regression equation is taken as a reasonable approximation for the observed data. Outside the range of the observed data one cannot safely use the same equation. Thus we should not use the regression line shown in Figure 11.14 to predict Vcf for blood glucose values outside the range 4 to 20 mmol/l.

An example of the danger of extrapolation is seen from a quadratic regression model fitted to the world record times to run a mile from 1954 to 1984. Kitson (1984) produced the model

$$\text{time} = 4.777 - 0.02039\text{Year} + 0.0001040\text{Year}^2$$

where 'Year' is the calendar year − 1900. He observed that the 'ultimate mile' will be run in 1998 in a time of 3 min 46.66 sec, and that on the basis of this model 'we may already be within one second of the ultimate mile'. He failed to observe, however, that after 1998 his model indicates that the world record time will start to increase again (see Figure 11.17), which is clearly impossible!

Nor should the regression line be used to predict the $X$ variable from the $Y$ variable. If we wish to predict blood glucose level from Vcf (which is probably not very sensible) we ought first to calculate the regression of

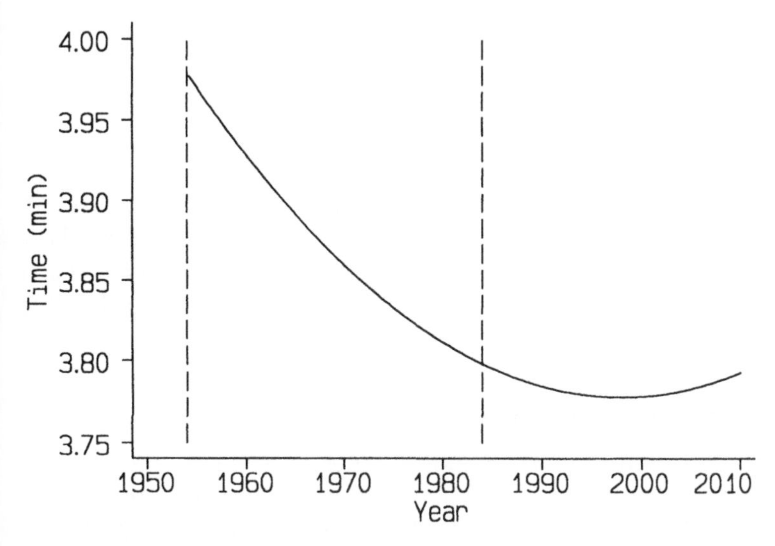


**Figure 11.17** Quadratic curve fitted to world record times to run a mile (Kitson, 1984), showing the range of observations (1954 to 1984).

blood glucose on Vcf. Regression is not a symmetric relation between two variables, so we need the appropriate regression line for our purpose.

Few of the cautions that were made about the interpretation of the correlation coefficient apply to regression analysis. One that does is that relating to the analysis of data from different groups as if they were a single sample. The slope of the regression line may be considerably affected if we pool data from two groups where there is a marked difference in the distribution of the values of either or both variables. An example would be the regression of blood pressure on age for males and females. Such data should either be analysed separately for the different groups or analysis of covariance should be used. Another restriction that is relevant is that the observations should be independent; in practice this means that there should be only one observation per individual.

Regression analysis is valid when values of the predictor variable have been selected by the experimenter, as is common in laboratory experiments. Also, as I have already noted, there is no requirement for the $X$ variable to have a Normal distribution. However, if there is a value of $X$ that is distant from the main body of the data, that observation may exert an undue influence on the position of the regression line especially if the value of the $Y$ variable is also extreme. An example was given in Figure 7.2.

If the distribution of the data or of the residuals leads to concern about the wisdom of using the regression methods described there is a non-parametric form of regression (see Sprent, 1989). Non-parametric regression is very rarely performed, in contrast to non-parametric correlation.

## 11.15 RELATION TO OTHER ANALYSES

(*This section can be omitted without loss of continuity.*)

Two analyses discussed in earlier chapters illustrate specialized uses of regression, although they were not presented as regression analyses. These are the test for linear trend in a one way analysis of variance (section 9.8.5) and the Chi squared test for trend among proportions (section 10.8.2). They are reconsidered briefly below.

### 11.15.1 Trend in one way analysis of variance

The test for trend across three or more groups in a one way analysis of variance was described in sections 9.8.5 and 9.9.2. Scores $l_i$ were given to the groups and the between group sum of squares was partitioned into linear and non-linear components. The test for linear trend is almost equivalent to a regression of the outcome variable on the scores. It is not exactly the same because the analysis of variance also uses one degree of freedom to test for non-linear variation among the groups, but in essence the method is a linear regression analysis. The slope of the regression line is equal to $L/\Sigma l_i^2$, and corresponds to the change in the response variable per unit change in score. This statistic is more useful than the statistic $L$, which depends upon the values of the scores.

When there are only two groups with scores −1 and 1, regression on the group scores is exactly equivalent to the two-sample $t$ test. The slope of the regression line is half the difference between the group means.

### 11.15.2 Trend in a 2 × *k* frequency table

The Chi squared test for trend is used to assess a trend in proportions in a $2 \times k$ frequency table (see section 10.8.2). The method is exactly equivalent to regressing the row variable, coded 0 and 1 say, on the column scores. For the Caesarean section data in Table 10.19, if we give scores 1 to 6 to the six shoe size groups, regression of these scores on the row variable (coded 0 and 1) for the 351 observations gives a slope of −0.0302 (SE 0.0106), giving $t = -2.86$ (P = 0.0045). The P value is thus the same as for the Chi squared test for trend shown in section 10.8.2. However, the regression approach is more informative as it yields an estimate of the change in proportion from one group to the next. Here the estimate is −0.03 (i.e. a reduction of 3%) per increment of $\frac{1}{2}$ in shoe size. We can use the standard error to obtain a confidence interval in the usual way.

## 11.16 PRESENTATION OF REGRESSION

The equation of the regression line should be given, together with the residual standard deviation. Wherever possible the regression line should be shown in a plot together with a scatter diagram of the raw data. The line should not extend beyond the range of the observed values of the predictor variable ($X$). A plot of the regression line alone gives no more information than the equation of the line.

The standard error of the slope is useful, as is the P value for the $t$ test. A confidence interval for the line or, more usefully, prediction intervals for new observations are especially informative and can be shown in the same plot.

The accuracy used for the coefficients should be related to the accuracy of the raw data. It makes no sense, for example, to give an equation that purports to predict birth weight to the nearest $\frac{1}{100000}$ g, which is what is implied by the following quadratic regression equation of birth weight ($y$) on fetal abdominal area ($x$):

$$y = 3518.42829 - 0.26395x + 0.000024x^2$$

(Campogrande *et al.*, 1977). It is common for the estimate of $a$ to be larger than that of $b$, but $a$ and $b$ are frequently reported to the same number of decimal places. However, it is the slope, $b$, that is needed with more precision, not less, when making predictions, so it should be given at least as precisely as $a$, if not more so. Precision here refers to the number of 'significant digits' (i.e. ignoring zeros at the beginning). Thus, in the equation given earlier, Vcf = 1.10 + 0.0220 blood glucose, the intercept and slope are both given to three significant digits. Contrast this with the quadratic equation given above.

Most computer programs for regression analysis give the information necessary to perform all the calculations described in this chapter. Not many will actually calculate and plot confidence intervals and prediction intervals, but they should give the residual standard deviation (perhaps under a different name) to allow these intervals to be calculated.

In output from computer programs the quantity $s_{res}/\sqrt{n}$ is sometimes called the 'standard error of the estimate' (SEE). This is not a good name as it wrongly implies that it is the standard error of any value $y_{fit}$ estimated from the regression line. In fact $s_{res}/\sqrt{n}$ is the standard error of $y_{fit}$ only at the mean value of $X$, i.e. when $X = \bar{x}$ (see section 11.13.3). As we have seen, uncertainty increases as we move away from the mean. This mistake is sometimes seen in published papers where confidence limits are shown parallel to the regression line. Worse, some programs call the residual standard deviation ($s_{res}$) the 'standard error of the estimate', which is highly misleading.

## 11.17 REGRESSION OR CORRELATION?

Regression and correlation have been presented separately in this chapter to clarify the difference between their purposes. Mathematically, however, the two methods are very closely related, as can be seen from the formulae in sections 11.7 and 11.13. In fact the $t$ test of the null hypothesis of zero correlation is exactly equivalent to that for the hypothesis of zero slope in regression analysis – the P values are identical. Many computer programs automatically provide the correlation coefficient when performing a regression analysis, but it helps to remember that regression and correlation are distinct methods which serve different purposes. It is not usually sensible to perform both unless one is genuinely interested in both analyses, which is probably not very common. For example, we would not wish to predict the consumption of pork in Albania if we happened to know the mortality from cirrhosis among Albanians. In contrast, we are not interested in the correlation between Vcf and blood glucose level once we have carried out the much more informative regression analysis.

Correlation is a much over-used technique, with a significant correlation coefficient often wrongly interpreted as important and, even worse, as necessarily indicating a causal relationship. Its use should be mainly for generating hypotheses rather than for testing them. Correlation reduces a set of data to a single number that bears no direct relation to the actual data. Regression is a much more useful method, with results which are clearly related to the measurements obtained. The strength of the relation is explicit, and uncertainty can be seen clearly from confidence intervals or prediction intervals.

> Give a man three weapons – correlation, regression, and a pen – and he will use all three.
>
> (Anon, 1978)

## EXERCISES

11.1 Lactic acidosis, a disorder of acid-base metabolism, is usually rapidly fatal. Dichloroacetate was administered intravenously (50 mg/kg body weight) to 29 paediatric and adult patients (Stacpoole *et al*., 1988). The table below shows the recorded changes in some metabolic and haemodynamic variables, together with the patients' survival times (in hours).

| Patient | Change in arterial level of | | | Survival time |
|---|---|---|---|---|
| | Lactate | Bicarbonate | pH | |
| 1 | 4.1 | −1.2 | −0.05 | 4 |
| 2 | −4.4 | 2.0 | 0.03 | 4 |
| 3 | 0.1 | 2.9 | 0.02 | 14 |
| 4 | 4.4 | −2.5 | 0.07 | 15 |
| 5 | 8.7 | −4.0 | −0.12 | 16 |
| 6 | −30.7 | 4.4 | 0.17 | 24 |
| 7 | 1.7 | −0.9 | 0.01 | 29 |
| 8 | −1.5 | 4.5 | 0.15 | 31 |
| 9 | 7.4 | 1.8 | −0.13 | 32 |
| 10 | 9.9 | −12.9 | −0.28 | 36 |
| 11 | 13.1 | −11.9 | −0.33 | 36 |
| 12 | 3.1 | −6.3 | −0.22 | 36 |
| 13 | 15.2 | −2.0 | −0.16 | 41 |
| 14 | 2.5 | 1.0 | 0.01 | 46 |
| 15 | 7.9 | 2.5 | −0.22 | 48 |
| 16 | 4.2 | −2.2 | −0.03 | 48 |
| 17 | 2.8 | −4.0 | −0.04 | 60 |
| 18 | 14.3 | −2.4 | −0.01 | 60 |

| Patient | Lactate | Change in arterial level of Bicarbonate | pH | Survival time |
|---|---|---|---|---|
| 19 | 16.2 | −12.8 | −0.15 | 72 |
| 20 | 17.5 | −4.4 | −0.09 | 96 |
| 21 | 2.7 | −7.1 | −0.21 | 192 |
| 22 | 4.4 | −4.7 | −0.05 | 336 |
| 23 | 4.8 | −9.8 | −0.05 | 456 |
| 24 | 9.0 | −7.5 | 0.09 | 672 |
| 25 | 14.7 | −7.2 | −0.23 | 768 |
| 26 | 6.2 | −4.2 | −0.13 | 1080 |
| 27 | 18.4 | −12.3 | −0.12 | 2160 |
| 28 | 16.9 | −8.6 | −0.17 | 2160 |
| 29 | 26.0 | −21.3 | −0.32 | 24456* |

*: still alive

(a) The authors used Spearman's rank correlation to look for associations with survival time. Is this a valid analysis, bearing in mind that one of the survival times is censored?
(b) Would the use of Pearson's correlation coefficient be valid?
(c) Which variable has the strongest correlation with survival time?

11.2 The following table shows resting metabolic rate (RMR) (kcal/24 hr) and body weight (kg) of 44 women (Owen *et al.*, 1986).

| | Body weight | RMR | | Body weight | RMR |
|---|---|---|---|---|---|
| 1 | 49.9 | 1079 | 17 | 59.0 | 982 |
| 2 | 50.8 | 1146 | 18 | 59.0 | 1178 |
| 3 | 51.8 | 1115 | 19 | 59.2 | 1342 |
| 4 | 52.6 | 1161 | 20 | 59.5 | 1027 |
| 5 | 57.6 | 1325 | 21 | 60.0 | 1316 |
| 6 | 61.4 | 1351 | 22 | 62.1 | 1574 |
| 7 | 62.3 | 1402 | 23 | 64.9 | 1526 |
| 8 | 64.9 | 1365 | 24 | 66.0 | 1268 |
| 9 | 43.1 | 870 | 25 | 66.4 | 1205 |
| 10 | 48.1 | 1372 | 26 | 72.8 | 1382 |
| 11 | 52.2 | 1132 | 27 | 74.8 | 1273 |
| 12 | 53.5 | 1172 | 28 | 77.1 | 1439 |
| 13 | 55.0 | 1034 | 29 | 82.0 | 1536 |
| 14 | 55.0 | 1155 | 30 | 82.0 | 1151 |
| 15 | 56.0 | 1392 | 31 | 83.4 | 1248 |
| 16 | 57.8 | 1090 | 32 | 86.2 | 1466 |

| | Body weight | RMR | | Body weight | RMR |
|---|---|---|---|---|---|
| 33 | 88.6 | 1323 | 39 | 107.7 | 1473 |
| 34 | 89.3 | 1300 | 40 | 110.2 | 2074 |
| 35 | 91.6 | 1519 | 41 | 122.0 | 1777 |
| 36 | 99.8 | 1639 | 42 | 123.1 | 1640 |
| 37 | 103.0 | 1382 | 43 | 125.2 | 1630 |
| 38 | 104.5 | 1414 | 44 | 143.3 | 1708 |

(a) Perform linear regression analysis of RMR on body weight.
(b) Examine the distribution of residuals. Is the analysis valid?
(c) Obtain a 95% confidence interval for the slope of the line.
(d) Is it possible to use an individual's weight to predict their RMR to within 250 kcal/24hr?

11.3 In the worked example of regression analysis (section 11.10.1) the $W'$ test for non-Normality of the residuals gave $P = 0.03$.

(a) Using the data in Table 11.6, carry out a regression of $\log_e$ Vcf on blood glucose.
(b) Are the residuals from this analysis more nearly Normal?
(c) Compare the predicted Vcf and 95% prediction intervals derived from the two models for a diabetic patient with a fasting blood glucose of 16 mmol/l.

11.4 What is odd about the data in Table 11.2?

11.5 Digoxin is a drug that is largely eliminated unchanged in the urine. Its renal clearance was said to be (a) correlated with creatinine clearance and (b) independent of urine flow. The following table shows measurements of these three variables from 35 consecutive inpatients being treated with digoxin for congestive heart failure (Halkin *et al.*, 1975).

| Patient | Clearances (ml/min/1.73 m²) Creatinine | Digoxin | Urine flow (ml/min) |
|---|---|---|---|
| 1 | 19.5 | 17.5 | 0.74 |
| 2 | 24.7 | 34.8 | 0.43 |
| 3 | 26.5 | 11.4 | 0.11 |
| 4 | 31.1 | 29.3 | 1.48 |
| 5 | 31.3 | 13.9 | 0.97 |
| 6 | 31.8 | 31.6 | 1.12 |

| Patient | Clearances (ml/min/1.73 m²) Creatinine | Digoxin | Urine flow (ml/min) |
|---|---|---|---|
| 7 | 34.1 | 20.7 | 1.77 |
| 8 | 36.6 | 34.1 | 0.70 |
| 9 | 42.4 | 25.0 | 0.93 |
| 10 | 42.8 | 47.4 | 2.50 |
| 11 | 44.2 | 31.8 | 0.89 |
| 12 | 49.7 | 36.1 | 0.52 |
| 13 | 51.3 | 22.7 | 0.33 |
| 14 | 55.0 | 30.7 | 0.80 |
| 15 | 55.9 | 42.5 | 1.02 |
| 16 | 61.2 | 42.4 | 0.56 |
| 17 | 63.1 | 61.1 | 0.93 |
| 18 | 63.7 | 38.2 | 0.44 |
| 19 | 66.8 | 37.5 | 0.50 |
| 20 | 72.4 | 50.1 | 0.97 |
| 21 | 80.9 | 50.2 | 1.02 |
| 22 | 82.0 | 50.0 | 0.95 |
| 23 | 82.7 | 31.8 | 0.76 |
| 24 | 87.9 | 55.4 | 1.06 |
| 25 | 101.5 | 110.6 | 1.38 |
| 26 | 105.0 | 114.4 | 1.85 |
| 27 | 110.5 | 69.3 | 2.25 |
| 28 | 114.2 | 84.8 | 1.76 |
| 29 | 117.8 | 63.9 | 1.60 |
| 30 | 122.6 | 76.1 | 0.88 |
| 31 | 127.9 | 112.8 | 1.70 |
| 32 | 135.6 | 82.2 | 0.98 |
| 33 | 136.0 | 46.8 | 0.94 |
| 34 | 153.5 | 137.7 | 1.76 |
| 35 | 201.1 | 76.1 | 0.87 |

Do these data support statements (a) and (b) above?

# 12

# Relation between several variables

> Exploration of the data set is admirable, but the investigator should know that he is exploring and searching, not reviewing a confirmatory experiment.
>
> Lachenbruch (1977)

## 12.1 INTRODUCTION

Chapters 9, 10 and 11 cover the basic statistical methods used to analyse the large majority of medical data sets. Few research reports do not make use of some of those techniques, and most will not go further. Most studies, however, obtain data on many variables, which are either analysed by a series of simple analyses or by rather more complicated statistical methods. In general it is preferable to use the more advanced methods where these are appropriate, rather than looking separately at several small parts of the data set.

This chapter builds on the methods of Chapters 9 to 11, by extending the ideas in those chapters to more complex data sets. Chapter 13 continues the process, but is devoted to the analysis of survival data, which poses several special problems even in simple comparisons.

## 12.2 ANALYSIS OF VARIANCE AND MULTIPLE REGRESSION

Chapter 9 introduced a variety of methods for comparing two or more groups with respect to a single continuous variable. In section 12.3 I shall show how these methods can be extended to consider data sets with two or more classifying variables, methods given the general name **analysis of variance** whether parametric or non-parametric. If there are two classifying variables the analysis is known as **two way** analysis of variance, and so on. These methods require the same number of observations in each 'cell' of the cross-classification, a condition often, but not always, met in experimental studies but rarely, if ever, true for observational studies. For example, if we wish to compare birth weights of boys and girls with different lengths of gestation we cannot control the numbers of babies in each age-sex group, so we cannot use analysis of variance.

The way round this problem is, perhaps surprisingly, related to the technique of linear regression described in Chapter 11. I showed there how to describe the relation between two variables, or, more specifically, how the value of one variable can be predicted from the value of the other. This method too can be extended, to allow us to predict the value of a variable from the values of **several** other variables. In other words, we have a single dependent (outcome) variable and two or more explanatory (predictor) variables. The method is called **multiple regression**. The explanatory variables can be either continuous or binary (0–1) or categorical. Multiple regression can thus be used to regress birth weight on sex and gestational age. It can be shown that all analysis of variance problems can also be analysed in the framework of multiple regression (see section 12.4), but for balanced data sets (usually from experiments) it is more common to keep to the analysis of variance approach.

The above discussion relates to the case where the outcome variable is continuous. In section 12.5 I shall show how a similar approach can be taken for a binary outcome variable, using **multiple logistic regression**, and in Chapter 13 the same general ideas will be used for the analysis of survival data.

## 12.3 TWO WAY ANALYSIS OF VARIANCE

In Chapter 9 I considered several problems involving the same measurement taken on independent groups of individuals. Often more than one measurement is taken from each person, perhaps under different experimental conditions, and we require a method that may be seen as a generalization of the paired $t$ test. Data of this type can be dealt with by the method known as **two way analysis of variance**, which is used to analyse data which can be displayed within a cross-classification of two categorical variables, called 'factors'.

The general structure of such data sets is shown in Table 12.1 where each 'x' indicates an observation. In this structure, we may have one or more observations for each combination of levels of the two factors A and B. I shall only consider the case where the number of observations in each cell is the same. I shall assume, therefore, that there are no missing observations.

This section deals with two types of study that fall into this framework. The first is where two or more observations of the same variable are taken from the same individuals under different circumstances, for example where each patient receives more than one treatment. Here factor B in the diagram represents different subjects. There may be more than one

**Table 12.1** General structure of a two way cross-classification. Each x represents a single observation, and x . . . x represents a series of observations

| Factor B | Factor A 1 | 2 | 3 | | | *c* |
|---|---|---|---|---|---|---|
| 1 | x . . . x | x . . . x | x . . . x | . | . | x . . . x |
| 2 | x . . . x | x . . . x | x . . . x | . | . | x . . . x |
| 3 | x . . . x | x . . . x | x . . . x | . | . | x . . . x |
| . | . | . | . | . | . | . |
| . | . | . | . | . | . | . |
| . | . | . | . | . | . | . |
| *r* | x . . . x | x . . . x | x . . . x | . | . | x . . . x |

observation per subject on each treatment.

The second case is where there are two factors specifying the nature of the measurements, and each combination is given to one or more patients. For example we may have observations on blood pressure after two or more different treatments for males and females separately. Here factors A and B represent treatment and sex, and there are several different subjects for each combination. I shall consider one example of each in detail, and then discuss other designs.

### 12.3.1 Repeated observation

Table 12.2 shows the heart rate of nine patients with congestive heart

**Table 12.2** Short-term effect of enalaprilat on heart rate (beats per minute) (Maskin *et al.*, 1985)

| | | Time (mins) | | | | |
|---|---|---|---|---|---|---|
| Subject | 0 | 30 | 60 | 120 | Mean | (SD) |
| 1 | 96 | 92 | 86 | 92 | 91.50 | (4.1) |
| 2 | 110 | 106 | 108 | 114 | 109.50 | (3.4) |
| 3 | 89 | 86 | 85 | 83 | 85.75 | (2.5) |
| 4 | 95 | 78 | 78 | 83 | 83.50 | (8.0) |
| 5 | 128 | 124 | 118 | 118 | 122.00 | (4.9) |
| 6 | 100 | 98 | 100 | 94 | 98.00 | (2.8) |
| 7 | 72 | 68 | 67 | 71 | 69.50 | (2.4) |
| 8 | 79 | 75 | 74 | 74 | 75.50 | (2.4) |
| 9 | 100 | 106 | 104 | 102 | 103.00 | (2.6) |
| Mean | 96.56 | 92.56 | 91.11 | 92.33 | 93.14 | |
| (SD) | (16.4) | (17.8) | (17.2) | (16.5) | (16.4) | |

failure before and shortly after administration of enalaprilat, an angiotensin-converting enzyme inhibitor. Measurements were taken before and at 30, 60 and 120 minutes after drug administration. This design appears similar to that analysed by one way analysis of variance in section 9.8, but here the measurements at the different times are on *the same subjects*. Thus this design should more appropriately be seen as a natural extension of the paired *t* test. The strength of this design is that comparisons between the sets of observations are based on *within* subject differences. Variation *between* subjects, which is usually considerable (see Table 12.2), does not affect our ability to distinguish differences between the sets of observations, which here relate to four time points.

In section 9.8 I showed how in one way analysis of variance the total variability is separated into between group and within group components. A similar approach is adopted in two way analysis of variance, but naturally it is a bit more complicated. In the present example, for the heart rate data shown in Table 12.2, we can divide the total variability into components due to variation between times and between subjects, and there is some remaining variation which we refer to as **residual variation**. This term carries the same meaning as in regression analysis, described in Chapter 11.

Table 12.3 shows the analysis of variance table for the heart rate data. The *F* values for testing the between subjects and between times variances (mean squares) are each obtained by dividing by the residual variance. The former is compared with the *F* distribution with 8 and 24 degrees of freedom, and the latter with that with 3 and 24 degrees of freedom. The between subject variation has an extremely small P value, as is often the case with medical data. The null hypothesis that all subjects have the same heart rate is firmly rejected, but this is of no real interest. The purpose of this study was to investigate variation in heart rate over the two hours after administration of enalaprilat, which is examined by considering the 'between times' row of Table 12.3. The P value of 0.018 indicates that we can reasonably reject the null hypothesis that there is no change in heart rate over the two hours. Table 12.2 shows the means for each time point,

**Table 12.3** Analysis of variance of data in Table 12.2

| Source of variation | df | Sums of squares | Mean squares | *F* | P |
|---|---|---|---|---|---|
| Subjects | 8 | 8966.556 | 1120.819 | 90.6 | < 0.0001 |
| Times | 3 | 150.972 | 50.324 | 4.07 | 0.018 |
| Residual | 24 | 296.778 | 12.366 | | |
| Total | 35 | 9414.306 | | | |

indicating that heart rate fell by an average four beats per minute (bpm) after 30 minutes, and remained fairly stable over the next 90 minutes. The average pattern is not obvious from examination of the raw data in the table.

Specific hypotheses relating to the time trend can be examined using the same approach as in one way analysis of variance. We could, for example, compare each pair of times, with a Bonferroni correction to allow for multiple testing, or look for a linear trend over time. We can also construct confidence intervals for the mean at any time or the difference between means. For all of these analyses it is essential that we use the correct variance, after the between subject variation has been removed, which is the residual variance.

The residual variance is 12.366 so the residual standard deviation is $\sqrt{12.366} = 4.516$ bpm. By fitting the model implicit in the analysis of variance we have assumed that the *true* response pattern of heart rate over time is the same for each subject, and (equivalently) that the differences between subjects are the same at each time. Any departures from this model indicate random variation, for example that resulting from measurement error. The mean of all the observations was 93.14 bpm, and we can express the means for each column and row as differences from the overall mean. The value predicted in each cell is then obtained by adding the relevant row and column means, and subtracting the overall mean, as

**Table 12.4** Predicted heart rate based on the two way analysis of variance model

| | Time (mins) | | | | | |
|---|---|---|---|---|---|---|
| Subject | 0 | 30 | 60 | 120 | Mean | Difference from overall mean |
| 1 | 94.92 | 90.92 | 89.47 | 90.69 | 91.50 | −1.64 |
| 2 | 112.92 | 108.92 | 107.47 | 108.69 | 109.50 | +16.36 |
| 3 | 89.17 | 85.17 | 83.72 | 84.94 | 85.75 | −7.39 |
| 4 | 86.92 | 82.92 | 81.47 | 82.69 | 83.50 | −9.64 |
| 5 | 125.42 | 121.42 | 119.97 | 121.19 | 122.00 | +28.86 |
| 6 | 101.42 | 97.42 | 95.97 | 97.19 | 98.00 | +4.86 |
| 7 | 72.92 | 68.92 | 67.47 | 68.69 | 69.50 | −23.64 |
| 8 | 78.92 | 74.92 | 73.47 | 74.69 | 75.50 | −17.64 |
| 9 | 106.42 | 102.42 | 100.97 | 102.19 | 103.00 | +9.86 |
| Mean | 96.56 | 92.56 | 91.11 | 92.33 | 93.14 | |
| Difference from overall mean | 3.42 | −0.58 | −2.03 | −0.81 | | |

**Table 12.5** Residuals from the analysis of variance, calculated as the difference between the entries in Tables 12.2 and 12.4

| | Time (mins) | | | | |
|---|---|---|---|---|---|
| Subject | 0 | 30 | 60 | 120 | Mean |
| 1 | 1.08 | 1.08 | −3.47 | 1.31 | 0.00 |
| 2 | −2.92 | −2.92 | 0.53 | 5.31 | 0.00 |
| 3 | −0.17 | 0.83 | 1.28 | −1.94 | 0.00 |
| 4 | 8.08 | −4.92 | −3.47 | 0.31 | 0.00 |
| 5 | 2.58 | 2.58 | −1.97 | −3.19 | 0.00 |
| 6 | −1.42 | 0.58 | 4.03 | −3.19 | 0.00 |
| 7 | −0.92 | −0.92 | −0.47 | 2.31 | 0.00 |
| 8 | 0.08 | 0.08 | 0.53 | −0.69 | 0.00 |
| 9 | −6.42 | 3.58 | 3.03 | −0.19 | 0.00 |
| Mean | 0.00 | 0.00 | 0.00 | 0.00 | 0.00 |

shown in Table 12.4. Table 12.5 shows the differences between the observed data and the values fitted by the model, called **residuals**. These show the lack of fit of the model, and the variance of the residuals is the residual variance shown in the analysis of variance in Table 12.3. As already noted, these residuals correspond exactly to residuals from the equivalent regression analysis. The residual variance is an estimate of the variance of multiple measurements on a single patient at the same time (even though only one such measurement was made).

### 12.3.2 Assumptions

There is no requirement for the data to be Normally distributed, neither overall nor within a row or column. The residuals, however, are expected to have a Normal distribution, an assumption that can be examined by a Normal plot as in Figure 12.1. The $W'$ test for the heart rate residuals gives $W' = 0.977$ with $P = 0.5$, and so we can be happy that our model is reasonable in this respect.

Even if the distribution of residuals is reasonably Normal it does not necessarily follow that the model is appropriate. Inspection of Table 12.5 shows some large values for subjects 4 and 9 and we might wish to consider the possibility that the response over time is not the same for all individuals. We cannot examine this possibility with these data, because there is only one observation per person at each time. If we had two or more observations for each person–time combination we would carry out a more comprehensive analysis. Specifically, we could examine the possible existence of a significant **interaction** between the two factors subject and time. An example of this more complex analysis is described below. If the

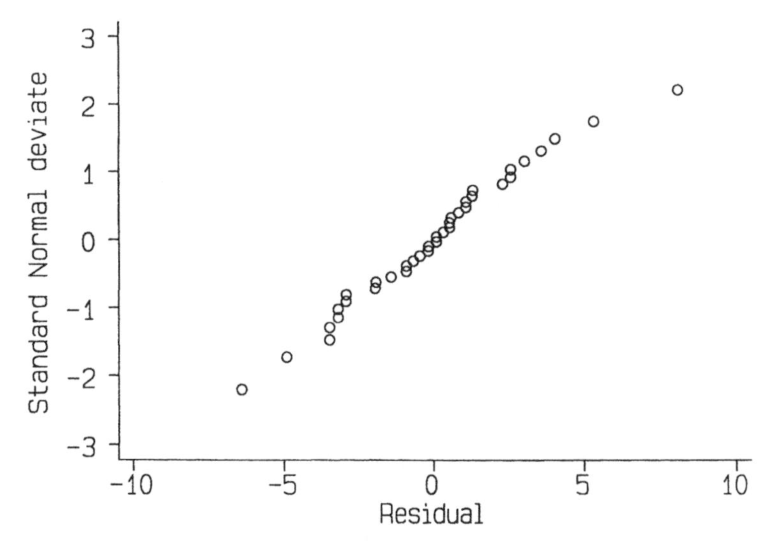


**Figure 12.1** Normal plot of residuals from analysis of variance of the data in Table 12.2.

distributional assumption of the analysis of variance is not met, we can perform a non-parametric analysis, as described in section 12.3.5.

A criticism of the heart rate data used to illustrate two way analysis of variance is that the observations relate to a sequence of repeated measurements in one experiment. Such data are not strictly appropriate for the analysis described. Some programs can perform a 'repeated measures' analysis of variance that is more correct for this type of data. Another way of looking at serial observations is described in section 14.6.

### 12.3.3 Replicated data

Analysis of variance can also be used to study measurement variability. Table 12.6 shows part of a large set of data from a study investigating the reproducibility of ultrasonic fetal head circumference data. Four observers each took three measurements on the same three fetuses. The observers were kept unaware of their previous measurements, in contrast to usual clinical practice. The structural difference between this data set and the heart rate data is the availability of three replicate readings per fetus. These enable us to investigate the possibility of an interaction between observers and fetuses; in other words, we can see if the differences between observers vary from fetus to fetus more than we expect just from chance variation. Interaction is more important when we investigate one or two factors of direct interest, such as treatment and dose. With this data

**Table 12.6** Measurements of fetal head circumference (cm) by four observers

| | Observer 1 | Observer 2 | Observer 3 | Observer 4 |
|---|---|---|---|---|
| Fetus 1 | 14.3 | 13.6 | 13.9 | 13.8 |
| | 14.0 | 13.6 | 13.7 | 14.7 |
| | 14.8 | 13.8 | 13.8 | 13.9 |
| Fetus 2 | 19.7 | 19.8 | 19.5 | 19.8 |
| | 19.9 | 19.3 | 19.8 | 19.6 |
| | 19.8 | 19.8 | 19.5 | 19.8 |
| Fetus 3 | 13.0 | 12.4 | 12.8 | 13.0 |
| | 12.6 | 12.8 | 12.7 | 12.9 |
| | 12.9 | 12.5 | 12.5 | 13.8 |

set we are not especially interested in these particular fetuses or observers, but wish to estimate the reproducibility of the measurements.

Table 12.7 shows the analysis of variance table for the head circumference data. Again the $F$ values for testing each effect are obtained by dividing the mean squares by the residual mean square. The interaction between subjects and observers is not nearly significant ($P = 0.33$). If the interaction is not significant it is best to remove it from the model by pooling its sum of squares with the residual variation to give the simplified analysis shown in Table 12.8. In general, if the interaction is significant the main effects (here 'fetuses' and 'observers') do not have a simple interpretation because the effect of each depends upon the level of the other factor.

Using the residual variance from Table 12.8 we can calculate the residual standard deviation as $\sqrt{0.080} = 0.283$ cm. Thus replicated measurements

**Table 12.7** Results of two way analysis of variance of the head circumference data in Table 12.6

| Source of variation | Degrees of freedom | Sums of squares | Mean squares | $F$ | P |
|---|---|---|---|---|---|
| Fetuses | 2 | 324.009 | 162.004 | 2113 | < 0.001 |
| Observers | 3 | 1.199 | 0.400 | 5.21 | 0.006 |
| Fetuses × Observers (Interaction) | 6 | 0.562 | 0.094 | 1.22 | 0.33 |
| Residual | 24 | 1.840 | 0.077 | | |
| Total | 35 | 327.610 | | | |

**Table 12.8** Analysis of variance of the head circumference data omitting the interaction

| Source of variation | Degrees of freedom | Sums of squares | Mean squares | *F* | P |
|---|---|---|---|---|---|
| Fetuses | 2 | 324.009 | 162.004 | 2023 | < 0.001 |
| Observers | 3 | 1.199 | 0.400 | 4.99 | 0.006 |
| Residual | 30 | 2.402 | 0.080 | | |
| Total | 35 | 327.610 | | | |

of the same fetus by the same observer have an estimated standard deviation of only 0.283 cm, which shows that measurement error is small. Notice that this most interesting aspect of the analysis is an estimation problem – the hypothesis tests are not really of interest.

The evaluation of $F$ values in the analysis of variance differs according to whether the classifying variables are interesting in their own right or whether they are representative of a wider population. The analysis described assumes that we are interested in these particular fetuses and observers, which is probably untrue in this case. However, the analysis described corresponds exactly to multiple regression, and is more widely used.

### 12.3.4 Extensions

Some of the ideas of multi-way analysis of variance have been introduced by means of two simple data sets. As noted, both have features that make them slightly inappropriate for the methods used. The requirements are very strict, and are not often met perfectly by medical research data. An example of a more complex data set was given in section 5.4, where I described a study to investigate the possible difference in blood pressure between the left and right arms. Each subject had 16 measurements made, two for each combination of arm (left or right), observer and cuff. Thus the data were analysed by a four way analysis of variance.

For three way designs and above the same principles are involved. However, further problems may arise which are beyond the scope of this book, especially when the variables are not fully cross-classified. For example, if we measure a group of subjects' metabolic rates before and after each of two types of diet, we could analyse the data by a three way analysis of variance (with factors time, diet and subject). But if the two diets were given to different groups of subjects, as in a clinical trial, we cannot use that analysis, nor can we use a two way analysis. (We could, however, perform a one way analysis of variance – or a two sample $t$ test –

on the changes in metabolic rate in the two groups.) Some of the issues arising in more complex designs are discussed by Armitage and Berry (1987, Chapter 8). As with many of the more advanced methods introduced in this chapter, the advice of a statistician would be valuable.

More often, data from a multiple classification arise in an unstructured way, in which case we can analyse the data by multiple regression, described in section 12.4.

### 12.3.5 Non-parametric two way analysis of variance

The assumption that the residuals have a Normal distribution cannot be assessed before fitting the model. Sometimes, however, it can be seen from the raw data that the model will not fit well. In particular, wide variation in the standard deviations for each row or column will suggest problems with the parametric analysis of variance just described.

There is a non-parametric form of two way analysis of variance that can be used for data sets which do not fulfil the assumptions of the parametric method. The method, which is sometimes known as **Friedman's two way analysis of variance**, is purely a hypothesis test.

Table 12.9 shows some data from an experiment to compare the leakage from four different types of immersion suit during simulated underwater helicopter escapes. The wide variability of the SDs for the four suits suggests that a rank analysis would be advisable.

The values for the four suits are ranked for each subject as shown in Table 12.10. There are no ties in this data set, but if there are any ties we calculate average ranks in the usual way.

**Table 12.9** Immersion suit leakage (g) during simulated helicopter underwater escape (Light *et al.*, 1987)

| | Suit type | | | |
|---|---|---|---|---|
| Subject | A | B | C | D |
| 1 | 308 | 132 | 454 | 64 |
| 2 | 102 | 526 | 0 | 28 |
| 3 | 182 | 134 | 96 | 30 |
| 4 | 268 | 324 | 264 | 90 |
| 5 | 166 | 228 | 134 | 34 |
| 6 | 332 | 296 | 458 | 6 |
| 7 | 198 | 350 | 200 | 90 |
| 8 | 28 | 274 | 16 | 24 |
| Mean | 198 | 283 | 203 | 45.7 |
| SD | 103 | 127 | 179 | 31.6 |

**Table 12.10** Ranks of the data in Table 12.9

| | Suit type | | | |
|---|---|---|---|---|
| Subject | A | B | C | D |
| 1 | 3 | 2 | 4 | 1 |
| 2 | 3 | 4 | 1 | 2 |
| 3 | 4 | 3 | 2 | 1 |
| 4 | 3 | 4 | 2 | 1 |
| 5 | 3 | 4 | 2 | 1 |
| 6 | 3 | 2 | 4 | 1 |
| 7 | 2 | 4 | 3 | 1 |
| 8 | 3 | 4 | 1 | 2 |
| Total ($R$) | 24 | 27 | 19 | 10 |
| Mean rank | 3.00 | 3.38 | 2.38 | 1.25 |

The analysis proceeds in a similar way to the Kruskal-Wallis non-parametric one way analysis of variance (described in section 9.8.6). If $R_i$ is the sum of the ranks in the $i$th group, and we have $k$ groups (here types of suit) and $n$ subjects, then we calculate the statistic $H$ defined by

$$H = \frac{12}{nk(k+1)} \sum_{i=1}^{k} [R_i - n(k+1)/2]^2.$$

The quantity $n(k+1)/2$ is the expected value for $R_i$ if the null hypothesis is true and all groups are the same. The test is thus based on the variation of the observed sums of ranks around the expected values, a common form of hypothesis test. Under the null hypothesis $H$ has a $\chi^2$ distribution with $k-1$ degrees of freedom. Again there is a simpler version of the formula for calculating $H$, which is

$$H = \frac{12}{nk(k+1)} \sum_{i=1}^{k} R_i^2 - 3n(k+1).$$

This method is not suitable for data where there is more than one observation in each cell of the two way table. It assumes that there are no ties in the data for each group, but will be little affected by a few ties.

Table 12.10 shows the sums of the ranks for each type of diving suit. We calculate $H$ as:

$$H = \frac{12}{8 \times 4 \times 5}[24^2 + 27^2 + 19^2 + 10^2] - 3 \times 8 \times 5 = 12.45.$$

Using Table B5 for the Chi squared distribution with three degrees of freedom we find $P < 0.01$. (The exact value is 0.006.)

As with all comparisons of more than two groups, an overall significant P value does not indicate where the differences lie, although in this case inspection of the data shows clearly that suit D is far less leaky. Pairs of groups can be compared by Wilcoxon matched pair tests, making due allowance for multiple testing. Note, however, that the Friedman analysis with two groups is equivalent to an extension of the sign test rather than the Wilcoxon test.

## 12.4 MULTIPLE REGRESSION

None of the methods of statistical analysis discussed in previous chapters allows us to look at more than one or two variables at a time. Frequently, however, data are collected on many variables. In the previous section I showed how analysis of variance can be extended to situations where we have one measurement recorded for combinations of several categorical variables (factors). Analysis of variance can be used only for structured data sets, which arise from designed experiments. In observational studies we are often interested in the way one variable is influenced by several variables, but the data are unstructured. This section introduces the technique of **multiple linear regression**, which we use to analyse that type of data. We often refer to the method as **multiple regression**.

Chapter 11 dealt mainly with simple linear regression, the method we use to describe the linear relation between two continuous variables. As I noted in section 12.2, regression methods can be extended to the case where we wish to predict the value of one variable from values of two or more other variables. Multiple regression analysis yields a regression **model** in which the dependent (or outcome) variable is expressed as a combination of the explanatory variables (sometimes called **predictor variables** or **covariates**). As we will see, it is not necessary for the explanatory variables to be continuous.

For example, suppose we wish to predict an index of respiratory muscle strength PEmax (in cm $H_2O$) from height (in cm) and weight (in kg). We would obtain a regression model like the following:

$$\text{PEmax} = 47.35 + 0.147 \times \text{height} + 1.024 \times \text{weight}.$$

The numbers 0.147 and 1.024 are called the **regression coefficients** for height and weight. They indicate the predicted increase in PEmax for each unit increase in the explanatory variable, here 1 cm and 1 kg respectively. The value of 47.35 is the **constant**, corresponding to PEmax when weight and height are both zero. Like the intercept in linear regression, it is not usually of great interest.

From the analysis we also obtain standard errors for each regression coefficient, from which we can calculate the statistical significance of a variable and a confidence interval for the regression coefficient. As with analysis of variance and linear regression, the residual variance provides a measure of how well the model fits the data.

There are several situations in which we may wish to perform a multiple regression analysis:

1. we may wish to remove the possible effects of other 'nuisance' variables from a study of the relation between just two variables;
2. we may be exploring possible prognostic variables with little or no prior information of which variables are important;
3. we may wish to develop a prognostic index from several explanatory variables for predicting the dependent variable of interest.

In practice it is not always easy to distinguish these possibilities and one analysis may incorporate all three ideas. The method of analysis is the same in each case.

An example of the first of the above possibilities is given by a study of the effect of parental birth weight on infant birth weight. Langhoff-Roos *et al.* (1987) analysed data for 276 Swedish infants with birth weights exceeding 2500 g born at 37–41 weeks of gestation. An initial multiple regression analysis considered just three 'fetal factors' – maternal birth weight, paternal birth weight and fetal sex. The regression coefficients for maternal and paternal birth weights were 0.214 g (SE 0.062 g) and 0.122 g (SE 0.049 g) respectively, both highly statistically significant. They then carried out an analysis incorporating maternal pre-pregnancy weight and height, number of previous children, weight gain during pregnancy and maternal smoking, all of which are known to be associated with birth weight. This larger analysis assessed whether the observed association between infant birth weight and parents' birth weight could be 'explained' by some subtle inter-relationships between parental birth weights and the additional variables. For example, it might be that mothers who had had low birth weights are more likely to smoke.

The regression coefficients for maternal and paternal birth weights in the larger analysis were 0.187 g (SE 0.062 g) and 0.157 g (SE 0.047 g) respectively. Both are still highly significant and the magnitudes of the coefficients are little changed. We can conclude that the relation between parental and infant birth weights cannot be explained by variation in the other variables, and thus can infer that the association is a real one. Given the nature of the data we may reasonably also infer that the association is causal. However, the association is weak, as we shall see below. As with simple linear regression, the regression coefficients are interpreted as the estimated increase in the outcome variable for an increase of one unit in the predictor variable. In this example it is helpful to multiply by 100, so that the regression coefficients are interpreted as indicating an increase of 19 g and 16 g in infant birth weight for every extra 100 g of maternal and paternal birth weight respectively. Notice that to interpret the coefficients we need to know the units of measurement.

Multiple regression is relatively straightforward when we know which variables we wish to have in the model. Difficulties occur when we wish to identify from a large number of variables those which are related to the dependent variable, and also assess how well the model obtained fits the data. We are thus trying to carry out exploratory and confirmatory analyses on the same data. Problems arise particularly from the way in which multiple significance testing is used.

Multiple regression analysis will be illustrated using data from a study of 25 patients with cystic fibrosis (O'Neill *et al.*, 1983), some of which were

**Table 12.11** Data for 25 patients with cystic fibrosis (O'Neill *et al.*, 1983)

| Sub | Age | Sex | Height | Weight | BMP | $FEV_1$ | RV | FRC | TLC | PEmax |
|---|---|---|---|---|---|---|---|---|---|---|
| 1 | 7 | 0 | 109 | 13.1 | 68 | 32 | 258 | 183 | 137 | 95 |
| 2 | 7 | 1 | 112 | 12.9 | 65 | 19 | 449 | 245 | 134 | 85 |
| 3 | 8 | 0 | 124 | 14.1 | 64 | 22 | 441 | 268 | 147 | 100 |
| 4 | 8 | 1 | 125 | 16.2 | 67 | 41 | 234 | 146 | 124 | 85 |
| 5 | 8 | 0 | 127 | 21.5 | 93 | 52 | 202 | 131 | 104 | 95 |
| 6 | 9 | 0 | 130 | 17.5 | 68 | 44 | 308 | 155 | 118 | 80 |
| 7 | 11 | 1 | 139 | 30.7 | 89 | 28 | 305 | 179 | 119 | 65 |
| 8 | 12 | 1 | 150 | 28.4 | 69 | 18 | 369 | 198 | 103 | 110 |
| 9 | 12 | 0 | 146 | 25.1 | 67 | 24 | 312 | 194 | 128 | 70 |
| 10 | 13 | 1 | 155 | 31.5 | 68 | 23 | 413 | 225 | 136 | 95 |
| 11 | 13 | 0 | 156 | 39.9 | 89 | 39 | 206 | 142 | 95 | 110 |
| 12 | 14 | 1 | 153 | 42.1 | 90 | 26 | 253 | 191 | 121 | 90 |
| 13 | 14 | 0 | 160 | 45.6 | 93 | 45 | 174 | 139 | 108 | 100 |
| 14 | 15 | 1 | 158 | 51.2 | 93 | 45 | 158 | 124 | 90 | 80 |
| 15 | 16 | 1 | 160 | 35.9 | 66 | 31 | 302 | 133 | 101 | 134 |
| 16 | 17 | 1 | 153 | 34.8 | 70 | 29 | 204 | 118 | 120 | 134 |
| 17 | 17 | 0 | 174 | 44.7 | 70 | 49 | 187 | 104 | 103 | 165 |
| 18 | 17 | 1 | 176 | 60.1 | 92 | 29 | 188 | 129 | 130 | 120 |
| 19 | 17 | 0 | 171 | 42.6 | 69 | 38 | 172 | 130 | 103 | 130 |
| 20 | 19 | 1 | 156 | 37.2 | 72 | 21 | 216 | 119 | 81 | 85 |
| 21 | 19 | 0 | 174 | 54.6 | 86 | 37 | 184 | 118 | 101 | 85 |
| 22 | 20 | 0 | 178 | 64.0 | 86 | 34 | 225 | 148 | 135 | 160 |
| 23 | 23 | 0 | 180 | 73.8 | 97 | 57 | 171 | 108 | 98 | 165 |
| 24 | 23 | 0 | 175 | 51.1 | 71 | 33 | 224 | 131 | 113 | 95 |
| 25 | 23 | 0 | 179 | 71.5 | 95 | 52 | 225 | 127 | 101 | 195 |

| | |
|---|---|
| Sub | Subject number |
| Sex | 0 = male, 1 = female |
| BMP | Body mass (Weight/Height$^2$) as a percentage of the age-specific median in normal individuals |
| $FEV_1$ | Forced expiratory volume in 1 second |
| RV | Residual volume |
| FRC | Functional residual capacity |
| TLC | Total lung capacity |
| PEmax | Maximal static expiratory pressure (cm $H_2O$) |

shown in Table 3.1. Table 12.11 shows the dependent variable, PEmax, which is a measure of malnutrition in these patients, and various possible explanatory variables, several of which relate to body size or lung function.

### 12.4.1 Categorical variables

If we include in the regression model a binary variable having values 0 or 1 for each individual, for example indicating non-smokers and smokers, the regression coefficient indicates the average difference in the dependent variable between the groups defined by the binary variable, adjusted for any differences between the groups with respect to the other variables in the model. This is because the difference between the codes for the groups is one. If the model contains two explanatory variables, one of which is continuous and the other binary, then we can think of the analysis as fitting two parallel lines representing simple linear regression of the dependent variable on the continuous independent variable for each of the two groups. This analysis is known as **analysis of covariance**; it was also discussed briefly in section 11.12.1.

We can also deal with categorical variables that have more than two categories. For example, if we have a variable for marital status coded 1 for married, 2 for single, and 3 for divorced, widowed or separated, then if we were to put this variable in an analysis as it stands we would be imposing the unreasonable assumption that the relation was linear with the codes 1, 2 and 3. We can get round this by creating two new binary variables (often called dummy variables), for example defined as:

1. 1 if single, 0 otherwise;
2. 1 if divorced, widowed or separated, 0 otherwise.

For a married person both of these variables will be zero. If the variable (1) is significant then the dependent variable is significantly different between those who are married or single, and similarly for (2). In general we need $k - 1$ dummy variables for $k$ categories. It is often best to fit all or none of the dummy variables to get an overall assessment of whether that categorical variable is associated with the dependent variable, but it is sometimes reasonable to consider dummy variables as separate entities.

If the categories are ordered, then we must as usual take note of this in the analysis. The above approach does not meet this requirement, but it may be reasonable to use the variable as it stands, with the codes given. For example, we may have a variable coded 1 to 4 representing progressive stages of disease. This is the same as investigating a linear trend, as was described for one way analysis of variance and the Chi squared test for trend (see section 11.15). We can also use this approach as an alternative way of dealing with continuous variables, especially when the relation with the dependent variable is clearly non-linear. We could, for example, create a new variable with codes from 1 to 5 indicating different age groups. The number of cigarettes smoked per day is often treated in this way.

### 12.4.2 Different approaches to choosing a model

Sometimes we know in advance which variables we wish to include in a multiple regression model. Here it is straightforward to fit a regression model containing all of those variables. The study of parental birth weight was of this type. Variables that are not significant can be omitted and the analysis redone. There is no hard rule about this, however. Sometimes it is desirable to keep a variable in a model because past experience shows that it is important. In large samples the omission of non-significant variables will have little effect on the other regression coefficients. The strategy will also depend upon the purpose of the analysis. If the aim is to identify important predictor variables then it makes sense to omit variables that do not contribute much to the model, which are usually taken to be those for which the P value exceeds 0.05. I discuss these issues further in section 12.4.10.

The statistical significance of each variable in the multiple regression model is obtained simply by calculating the ratio of the regression coefficient to its standard error and relating this value to the $t$ distribution with $n - k - 1$ degrees of freedom, where $n$ is the sample size and $k$ is the number of variables in the model. The $t$ statistic, which is calculated as $b/se(b)$, where $b$ is the regression coefficient, is equal to the square root of the $F$ statistic for the extra variability explained by the present model in comparison with the model excluding that particular variable. The latter approach must be used to assess the combined effect of a set of dummy variables representing a categorical variable.

In medical research it is more common to be faced with several contenders from which we wish to obtain the model which is, in some sense, *best*. By 'best' we refer to the ability of the model to *predict* the dependent variable or, equivalently, to *explain* variation in that variable. There are several ways of trying to find the best model, none of which can be taken as clearly better than the rest. Some subjective assessment may be necessary, especially when different approaches yield different answers. This chapter is intended as an introduction, so that the following exposition should not be taken as a comprehensive discussion of the many issues. Interpretation of multiple regression models will be discussed after the various strategies have been introduced.

### 12.4.3 Forward stepwise regression

The first step in many analyses of multivariate data is to examine the simple relation between each potential explanatory variable and the

**Table 12.12** Results of separately regressing PEmax on each explanatory variable

| Explanatory variable | Regression coefficient | Standard error | *t* | P |
|---|---|---|---|---|
| Age | 4.055 | 1.088 | 3.73 | 0.0011 |
| Sex | −19.045 | 13.176 | −1.45 | 0.16 |
| Height | 0.932 | 0.260 | 3.59 | 0.0016 |
| Weight | 1.187 | 0.301 | 3.94 | 0.0006 |
| BMP | 0.639 | 0.565 | 1.13 | 0.27 |
| $FEV_1$ | 1.354 | 0.555 | 2.44 | 0.023 |
| RV | −0.123 | 0.077 | −1.59 | 0.12 |
| FRC | −0.319 | 0.145 | −2.20 | 0.038 |
| TLC | −0.358 | 0.404 | −0.89 | 0.38 |

outcome variable of interest *ignoring all the other variables*. In other words, we carry out linear regression analyses on each variable in turn. Table 12.12 summarizes these analyses for the data in Table 12.11. Five of the nine variables are significantly associated with PEmax ($P < 0.05$).

Forward stepwise regression analysis uses this analysis as its starting point. The method can be broken down into a few simple steps:

*(a) Find the single variable that has the strongest association with the dependent variable and enter it into the model*

The variable with strongest association is that with the most significant slope (i.e. that with the smallest P value). This is equivalent to finding the variable that is most highly correlated with the dependent variable.

*(b) Find the variable among those not in the model that, when added to the model so far obtained, explains the largest amount of the remaining variability*

The method for carrying out this step is given below. It is equivalent to finding the variable with the largest correlation (ignoring sign) with the *residuals* from the model so far.

*(c) Repeat step (b) until the addition of an extra variable is not statistically significant at some chosen level such as $P = 0.05$*

We need to stop the process at some point otherwise we will end up with all the variables in the model. As well as having an unusable model, we will have 'overfitted' the data, in a sense described in section 12.4.6. Unfortunately, the cut-off of $P = 0.05$ (or any other) is arbitrary and not directly related to how well the model fits the data.

We will see how the stepwise procedure works by finding a model to predict PEmax using the data in Table 12.11. Note first that for the purposes of the first step we do not need to perform nine separate regression analyses (Table 12.12), but can get the same information from looking at the correlation matrix shown in Table 12.13. It is useful to look at the correlation matrix anyway, because it also shows the correlations among the explanatory variables. For this data set, there are many large correlation coefficients: from Table B7 $r = 0.505$ corresponds to $P = 0.01$. Figure 12.2 shows a graphical representation of the correlation matrix, with each small panel showing the relevant scatter diagram. We can see that there are no obvious outliers in the data, but the distribution of body mass

**Table 12.13** Correlation matrix for PEmax and nine potential explanatory variables

| | PEmax | Age | Sex | Height | Weight | BMP | $FEV_1$ | RV | FRC |
|---|---|---|---|---|---|---|---|---|---|
| Age | 0.613 | | | | | | | | |
| Sex | −0.289 | −0.167 | | | | | | | |
| Height | 0.599 | 0.926 | −0.168 | | | | | | |
| Weight | 0.635 | 0.906 | −0.190 | 0.921 | | | | | |
| BMP | 0.230 | 0.378 | −0.138 | 0.441 | 0.673 | | | | |
| $FEV_1$ | 0.453 | 0.294 | −0.528 | 0.317 | 0.449 | 0.546 | | | |
| RV | −0.316 | −0.552 | 0.271 | −0.570 | −0.622 | −0.582 | −0.666 | | |
| FRC | −0.417 | −0.639 | 0.184 | −0.624 | −0.617 | −0.434 | −0.665 | 0.911 | |
| TLC | −0.182 | −0.469 | 0.024 | −0.457 | −0.418 | −0.365 | −0.443 | 0.589 | 0.704 |
| | PEmax | Age | Sex | Height | Weight | BMP | $FEV_1$ | RV | FRC |

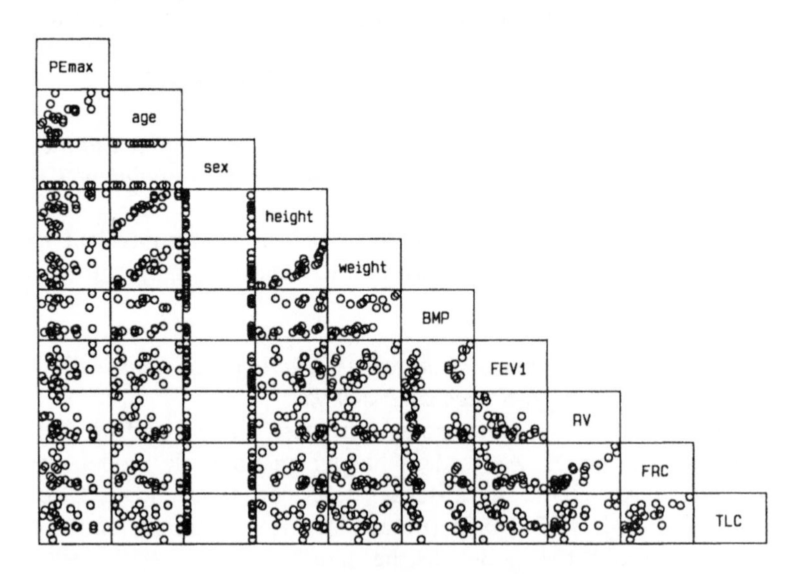


**Figure 12.2** Scatter diagrams corresponding to Table 12.13.

percentage (BMP) is rather odd. Tables 12.12 and 12.13 both show that the most predictive single variable is weight. Table 12.14 shows the analysis of variance table for this linear regression analysis.

The best variable to include with weight turns out to be BMP. The regression model is shown in Table 12.15, in the usual style of presenting a multiple regression model, together with the analysis of variance table. The $t$ test for each variable indicates whether omitting that variable would lead to a significant loss of information. It is equivalent to this square root of the $F$ value associated with the improvement in how well the model fits the data compared with the model without that variable. Thus the $t$ test for BMP in the top half of Table 12.15 is exactly equivalent to the $F$ test

**Table 12.14** Regression analysis of PEmax on weight

| Source of variation | Degrees of freedom | Sum of squares | Mean squares | $F$ | P |
|---|---|---|---|---|---|
| Regression on weight | 1 | 10 827.16 | 10 827.16 | 15.56 | 0.0006 |
| Residual | 23 | 16 005.48 | 695.89 | | |
| Total | 24 | 26 832.64 | | | |

Residual SD = $\sqrt{695.89}$ = 26.38

**Table 12.15** Regression analysis of PEmax on weight and BMP

| Variable | Coefficient $b$ | Standard error $se(b)$ | $t$ | P |
|---|---|---|---|---|
| Constant | 124.830 | 37.479 | | |
| Weight | 1.640 | 0.390 | 4.21 | 0.0004 |
| BMP | −1.005 | 0.581 | −1.73 | 0.10 |

| Source of variation | Degrees of freedom | Sum of squares | Mean squares | $F$ | P |
|---|---|---|---|---|---|
| Regression on weight | 1 | 10 827.16 | 10 827.16 | 15.56 | 0.0006 |
| Addition of BMP | 1 | 1914.94 | 1914.94 | 2.99 | 0.10 |
| Residual | 22 | 14 090.54 | 640.48 | | |
| Total | 24 | 26 832.64 | | | |

Residual SD = $\sqrt{640.48}$ = 25.31

in the lower part. We can see that the additional effect of BMP over that achieved by including only weight in the model is not statistically significant at the 5% level, but is significant at the 10% level. If, as is usual, the 5% or 1% level is used, we would conclude that the 'best' model is that including just weight. If we were using a 10% level for including variables, we would add BMP to the model and continue the analysis. The choice of significance level is discussed below.

Forward stepwise regression is available as an option in some of the larger statistical packages. It can be carried out using any program for multiple regression, most simply by calculating the correlations between the residuals from the model so far obtained and all those variables not so far included in the model.

### 12.4.4 Backward stepwise regression

As its name implies, with the backward stepwise method we approach the problem from the other direction. The argument is put forward that we have collected data on these variables because we believe them to be potentially important explanatory variables. Therefore we should fit the *full model*, including *all* of these variables, and then remove unimportant variables one at a time until all those remaining in the model contribute significantly. We use the same criterion, say $P < 0.05$, to determine significance. At each step we remove the variable with the smallest contribution to the model (or the largest P value) as long as that P value is greater than the chosen level.

**Table 12.16** Backward stepwise regression model to predict PEmax

| Variable | Coefficient $b$ | Standard error $se(b)$ | $t$ | P |
|---|---|---|---|---|
| Constant | 126.334 | 34.720 | | |
| Weight | 1.536 | 0.364 | 4.22 | 0.0004 |
| BMP | −1.465 | 0.579 | 2.53 | 0.019 |
| $FEV_1$ | 1.109 | 0.514 | 2.16 | 0.043 |

Analysis of variance:

| Source of variation | Degrees of freedom | Sum of squares | Mean squares | $F$ | P |
|---|---|---|---|---|---|
| Regression | 3 | 15 294.46 | 5089.15 | 9.28 | 0.0004 |
| Residual | 21 | 11 538.18 | 549.44 | | |

Residual SD = $\sqrt{549.44} = 23.44$

The final backward stepwise model obtained in this way includes weight, BMP and $FEV_1$, as shown in Table 12.16, together with the analysis of variance table for the three variable model.

For this data set, when we use the 5% significance level as the criterion for inclusion of a variable in the model we get different models by the forward and backward stepwise approaches. The two methods often yield the same model, but differences are not uncommon. Neither approach is more correct than the other. In this case, we might choose the larger model as it includes three variables all significant at the 5% level. On the other hand, it is peculiar to include both weight and BMP in the model, and the negative coefficient for BMP (which is positively correlated with PEmax) might suggest a degree of overfitting. This example shows that P values alone cannot choose an appropriate model.

### 12.4.5 All subsets regression

A third approach to selecting the 'best' model is to examine every possible model. It is easy to compare all models including the same number of variables by their $R^2$ statistics (see below), although we may wish to impose a condition that every variable in the model should be statistically significant at some pre-chosen level. Comparing models with different numbers of variables is more difficult, as we expect $R^2$ to increase as we continue to add more variables. One solution is to use a statistic called $C_p$, which incorporates a penalty for each additional variable in the model. Using this method for the illustrative data set yields the same model as the backward stepwise approach, shown in Table 12.16. All subsets regression is not widely used, partly because it requires much more computing.

### 12.4.6 Goodness-of-fit

We can assess how well a model 'fits' the data or, equivalently, how well the model predicts the dependent variable, by considering the proportion of the total sum of squares that can be explained by the regression. For example, in Table 12.16 the sum of squares due to the model is 15 294.46, so that the proportion of the variation explained is 15 294.46/26 832.64 = 0.57. This statistic is called $R^2$, and is often expressed as a percentage, here 57%.

Even when none of the possibly explanatory variables is related to the dependent variable, the expected value of $R^2$ will increase as more variables are added to the model. We thus cannot use $R^2$ as a criterion for deciding which variables should be in the model, as we would end up with all the variables. This full model might fit the observed data almost exactly, yet may be a worse predictor of the relation in the population than a model with fewer variables. Some programs produce an **adjusted $R^2$**, which compensates for the expected chance prediction when the null hypothesis is true, and is thus more appropriate. The adjusted $R^2$ for the model in Table 12.16 is 51%. Unlike $R^2$, adjusted $R^2$ can drop when a variable is added to the model.

When we perform linear regression, $R^2$ is exactly the same as $r^2$, the square of the Pearson correlation coefficient. For multiple regression models, the value of $R$ is called the **multiple correlation coefficient** by analogy, but it must not be interpreted in the same way. The $F$ test is the only way to assess whether a model explains a significant proportion of variability – using tables of $r$ to assess the significance of $R$ is completely invalid and wildly misleading.

$R^2$ assesses crudely how well the model fits the data overall, but we should also examine how well the model predicts values of the dependent variable *for individuals*. In other words we should study the residuals.

### 12.4.7 Analysis of residuals

The residual standard deviation is a measure of the average difference between the observed $y$ values and those predicted or fitted by the model. The multiple regression model can be written

$$y_{fit} = b_0 + b_1x_1 + b_2x_2 + \ldots$$

where $b_0$ is the intercept; $b_1$, $b_2$, etc. are the regression coefficients; $x_1$, $x_2$, etc. are the individual's values of the variables in the model; and $y_{fit}$ is the fitted or predicted value. The residuals are given by $y_{obs} - y_{fit}$, where $y_{obs}$ is the observed value of the dependent variable. We cannot plot the original multi-dimensional data, but we can examine plots of the residuals to see if the model is reasonable. Specifically, we ought to check that the residuals have a Normal distribution and that the model is an equally good fit throughout the range of values of the dependent variable.

As with linear regression (section 11.10) several plots are possible:

1. We can produce a Normal plot of the residuals, to check the overall fit and verify that the residuals have an approximately Normal distribution. The Normal plot may identify outliers for further investigation. Such observations may have unremarkable values of all the variables, but a peculiar combination of them.
2. We can plot the residuals against each of the explanatory variables in turn. We expect to see no association if the true relation is linear. As with simple linear regression, a curved pattern indicates that transformation or a non-linear term may be required.
3. We can plot the residuals against the observed values of $y$, but this plot will show a strong negative correlation and will not be very helpful. The correlation does not indicate lack of fit.

4. More usefully, we can plot the residuals against the fitted values. No pattern should be discernible. In particular, the variability of the residuals should be constant across the range of the fitted values.

The Normal plot for the residuals from the three variable model for PEmax is very straight (Figure 12.3), and provides no reason to question the validity of the analysis.

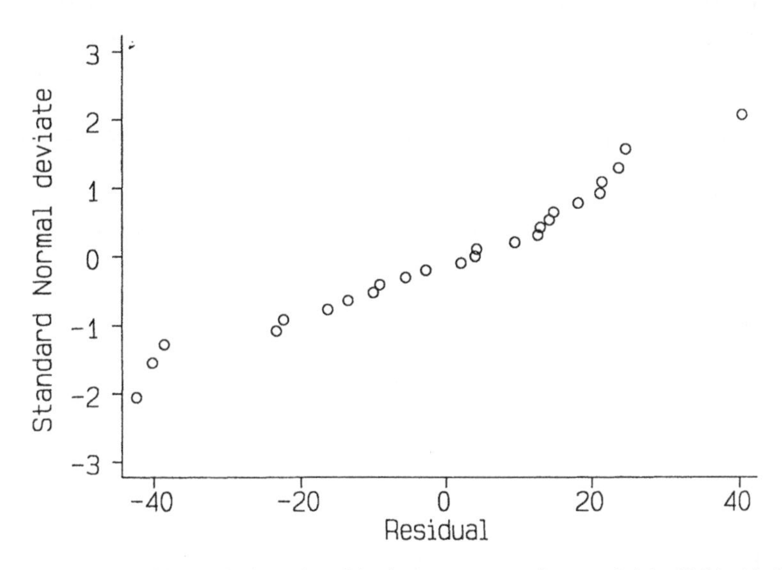


**Figure 12.3** Normal plot of residuals from regression model in Table 12.16.

### 12.4.8 Prognostic index

We can use the multiple regression equation to obtain a predicted value of the dependent ($y$) variable for any individual with cystic fibrosis. For example, using the model in Table 12.16 the predicted PEmax for an individual is:

$$y_{fit} = 126.334 + 1.536 \times \text{weight} - 1.465 \times \text{BMP} + 1.109 \times \text{FEV}_1.$$

Another way of thinking of the predicted value, $y_{fit}$, is as a **prognostic value** or **prognostic index**. If the model explains a high proportion of the variability in the dependent variable, high and low predicted values will indicate widely differing prognoses. This terminology is more commonly used in connection with logistic regression (section 12.5) and regression models for analysing survival data (Chapter 13).

Note that unlike the case for linear regression, it is difficult to calculate the standard error of $y_{fit}$ because it depends upon the distance of each of the predictor variables from its mean and also the interrelations between the variables. Some statistical packages can perform these calculations, however, so that a confidence interval can be obtained.

### 12.4.9 Relation to partial correlation

In section 11.5 I described the calculation of the partial correlation coefficient to examine the relation between two variables after adjusting for the effect of a third variable. I noted that it is more usual to use multiple regression for this type of problem. In fact, the two analyses are exactly equivalent.

The illustrative example was based on data in Table 11.2. The partial correlation between blood viscosity and fibrinogen adjusted for haematocrit (PCV), denoted $r(\mathrm{VF}|\mathrm{P})$, was 0.212. Table 12.17 shows analysis of variance tables for linear regression of blood viscosity on PCV, and multiple regression with fibrinogen added to the model. The proportion of the residual sum of squares from the first model that is explained by adding fibrinogen is

$$\frac{2.7209 - 2.5982}{2.7209}$$
$$= 0.045$$

**Table 12.17** Regression analyses of blood viscosity in Table 11.2
(a) Regression of blood viscosity on haematocrit (PCV)

| Source of variation | Degrees of freedom | Sum of squares | Mean squares | *F* | P |
|---|---|---|---|---|---|
| Regression on PCV | 1 | 9.2295 | 9.2295 | 101.8 | < 0.001 |
| Residual | 30 | 2.7209 | 0.0907 | | |
| Total | 31 | 11.9504 | | | |

(b) Regression of blood viscosity on PCV and fibrinogen

| Source of variation | Degrees of freedom | Sum of squares | Mean squares | *F* | P |
|---|---|---|---|---|---|
| Regression on PCV | 1 | 9.2295 | 9.2295 | 103.0 | < 0.001 |
| Addition of fibrinogen | 1 | 0.1227 | 0.1227 | 1.37 | 0.25 |
| Residual | 29 | 2.5982 | 0.0896 | | |
| Total | 31 | 11.9504 | | | |

which is equal to $0.212^2$ – it is the square of the partial correlation coefficient. The hypothesis of no relation between fibrinogen and blood viscosity after adjusting for PCV gives P = 0.25 by either approach. The multiple regression approach is more informative as we have an estimated regression coefficient and can examine the residuals.

### 12.4.10 Comments

It is not possible here to discuss in detail many of the important issues that affect multiple regression analysis and its interpretation, but the following brief comments indicate areas of interest or difficulty.

When there is a large number of potential explanatory variables we expect some of them to be significant just by chance. There is no completely satisfactory way of searching for the most suitable model without incurring the penalty of an over-optimistic answer. With many candidates for inclusion in the model, some researchers use the results of univariate analyses to decide which variables should be explored in the multivariate analysis. This strategy saves nothing with forward stepwise regression, but may dramatically cut computing time (and costs) for backwards stepwise or all subsets regression. I do not recommend pre-selection, but if it is used, selection should be based on a lax criterion, say $P < 0.2$ or even higher, because variables may contribute to a multiple regression model in unforeseen ways due to complex interrelationships among the variables. As an example, the cystic fibrosis data set gave P = 0.27 for BMP on its own, but P = 0.019 for the same variable in the multiple regression model.

Because of the multiple testing at each step, a model derived by stepwise (or all subsets) regression is likely to be over-optimistic with respect to the importance of each variable and the goodness-of-fit, particularly in small samples. Where the number of variables being considered is large and the sample size is small, it is often possible to find a model that appears to fit remarkably well. However, a model containing, say, seven variables fitted to 18 observations will be extremely unreliable. One solution is to suggest that multiple regression should not be applied to small data sets. In addition, it is useful to decide in advance the maximum size of model that is acceptable. I have found the square root of the sample size a useful rule of thumb here, but even that may be over-generous. Alternatively, it is sometimes suggested that the number of variables examined should be restricted. Again there is no rule, but a guideline might be to look at no more than $n/10$ variables, where $n$ is the sample size. With this approach, the illustrative analysis of the data in Table 12.11 would not be acceptable, and nor would many published multiple regression analyses.

When the sample is very large statistical significance can be achieved for tiny effects. For example, Rantakallio and Mäkinen (1984) fitted a model to data from 9795 infants on the number of teeth at one year of age. Six of the 15 variables were statistically significant (P < 0.05), one being the sex of the child (P < 0.001). The regression coefficient was −0.051, indicating a mean difference of one-twentieth of a tooth in favour of boys. The value of $R^2$ for this model was only 3.1%.

Automatic procedures for selecting a model are useful, but a degree of common sense is required. For example, sometimes there is an accumulation of evidence that a particular variable is prognostically important for the outcome being analysed. It is not sensible to omit, say, age or smoking in such circumstances because P was 'only' 0.07.

A definite advantage of using automatic selection can be seen when independent variables are highly correlated. Table 12.12 shows that both height and weight are highly correlated with PEmax. If we put weight and height in the model together, however, something strange happens. Table 12.18 shows the model with just height and weight. Neither variable appears to contribute significantly, yet the model explains 40% of the variability of PEmax. The reason is that height and weight are very highly correlated ($r = 0.92$ in Table 12.13) and thus explain much the same variability in PEmax. The values of $R^2$ are 40.4% for weight, 35.9% for height, and 40.5% for weight and height together. In fact, adding height gains us nothing and obscures the effect of weight by reducing its regression coefficient and increasing its standard error. It is a major advantage of stepwise regression that this type of misleading finding cannot occur.

**Table 12.18** Regression of PEmax on weight and height

| Variable | Coefficient $b$ | Standard error $se(b)$ | $t$ | P |
|---|---|---|---|---|
| Constant | 47.355 | 73.462 | | |
| Weight | 1.024 | 0.787 | 1.30 | 0.21 |
| Height | 0.147 | 0.655 | 0.22 | 0.82 |

The multiple regression model incorporates some subtle unstated assumptions. Firstly, it is assumed that the relation between the dependent variable and each continuous explanatory variable is *linear*. We can examine this assumption for any variable, by plotting the residuals against that variable. Any curvature in the pattern will indicate that a non-linear relation is more appropriate – transformation of the explanatory variable may help here. Secondly, it is assumed that the effects of each variable are *independent*, so that the effect of one variable is the same regardless of the values of the other variables in the model. If we suspect, for example, that the relation between height and lung function may be different for males and females then we need to consider the possibility of adding an interaction term to the model. Note that interaction is a quite different concept from the *correlation* between two variables. The interaction between two variables (continuous or binary) is examined by creating a new variable which is their product and adding this to the model. The effect is tested via the $F$ statistic for the improved fit. The new variable makes the contribution of each variable to the prediction dependent upon the value of the other variable. I do not recommend the investigation of all interactions, which would greatly increase the risk of a spurious finding. Occasionally, however, a particular interaction may be of prior interest.

The question of how well the model fits the data was discussed in section 12.4.6. The statistics $R^2$ and adjusted $R^2$ are one way of assessing goodness of fit, but they are measures of the correlation between the observed and predicted values of the dependent ($y$) variable. We cannot get any idea of the accuracy of prediction for an individual from the significance of variables nor from $R^2$, however large it is. As with ordinary linear regression, the residual standard deviation gives a measure of the discrepancies between the observed and predicted $y$ values, from which a 95% prediction or confidence interval can be obtained.

Lastly, because of the risk that the model may be over-optimistic, it is desirable to assess the predictive capability of a model on a new, independent set of data, but this is not usually possible.

### 12.4.11 Presentation of results

When reporting the results of multiple regression analysis details should be given about the strategy adopted (such as forward stepwise regression) and all the variables which were included in the analysis – not just those in the final model. For categorical variables, especially those featuring in models that are described, it is essential to explain the coding used. For example, there are numerous ways of categorizing the number of cigarettes smoked daily.

For each model described in detail the regression coefficients and their standard errors should be given. The residual standard deviation should be given and $R^2$ or, preferably, adjusted $R^2$ may be useful too.

## 12.5 LOGISTIC REGRESSION

The preceding section dealt with multiple regression with a continuous dependent variable, extending the methods of linear regression introduced in Chapter 11. In many studies the outcome variable of interest is the presence or absence of some condition, such as responding to treatment or having a myocardial infarction. We cannot use ordinary multiple (linear) regression for such data, but instead we can use a similar approach known as **multiple linear logistic regression** or just **logistic regression**.

The basic principle of logistic regression is much the same as for ordinary multiple regression. The main difference is that instead of developing a model that uses a combination of the values of a group of explanatory variables to predict the value of a dependent variable, we instead predict a *transformation* of the dependent variable.

Before explaining the method it is useful to recall that if we have a binary variable and give the categories numerical values of 0 and 1, usually representing 'No' and 'Yes' respectively, then the mean of these values in a sample of individuals is the same as the proportion of individuals with the characteristic. We might expect, therefore, that the appropriate regression model would predict the proportion of subjects with the feature of interest (or, equivalently, the probability of an individual having that characteristic) for any combination of the explanatory variables in the model. In practice a statistically preferable method is to use a transformation of this proportion, as described below. One reason is that otherwise we might predict impossible probabilities outside the range 0 to 1.

The transformation we use is called the **logit** transformation, written $\text{logit}(p)$. Here $p$ is the proportion of individuals with the characteristic. For example, if $p$ is the probability of a subject having a myocardial infarction, then $1 - p$ is the probability that they do not have one. The ratio $p/(1 - p)$ is called the **odds** and thus

$$\text{logit}(p) = \log_e\left(\frac{p}{1 - p}\right)$$

is the **log odds**. If, from our model, we wish to compare predictions for subjects with or without a particular characteristic, such as age greater than 50, we will estimate $l_1 = \text{logit}(p_1)$ for one group of subjects and $l_2 = \text{logit}(p_2)$ for the other. Then we have

$$l_1 - l_2 = \text{logit}(p_1) - \text{logit}(p_2) = \log\left(\frac{p_1}{1 - p_1}\right) - \log\left(\frac{p_2}{1 - p_2}\right)$$

$$= \log\left[\frac{p_1(1 - p_2)}{p_2(1 - p_1)}\right],$$

which is the log of the **odds ratio**. As described in section 10.11.2, the odds ratio is an important method for relating disease to exposure in epidemiological studies. The estimated value of $p$ can be derived from $\text{logit}(p)$, and always lies in the range 0 to 1. If $l = \text{logit}(p)$, then we have $e^l = p/(1 - p)$ and thus $p = e^l/(1 + e^l)$.

Table 12.19 summarizes some data relating hypertension to smoking, obesity and snoring in 433 men aged 40 or over. We can use logistic regression to see which of the factors smoking, obesity and snoring are predictive of hypertension. The full model is shown in Table 12.20(a). The

**Table 12.19** Hypertension in men aged 40+ in relation to smoking, obesity and snoring (Norton and Dunn, 1985)

| Smoking* | Obesity* | Snoring* | Number of men | Number (%) of men with hypertension |
|---|---|---|---|---|
| 0 | 0 | 0 | 60 | 5 (8%) |
| 1 | 0 | 0 | 17 | 2 (11%) |
| 0 | 1 | 0 | 8 | 1 (13%) |
| 1 | 1 | 0 | 2 | 0 (0%) |
| 0 | 0 | 1 | 187 | 35 (19%) |
| 1 | 0 | 1 | 85 | 13 (15%) |
| 0 | 1 | 1 | 51 | 15 (29%) |
| 1 | 1 | 1 | 23 | 8 (35%) |
| | | | Total433 | 79 (18%) |

* Codes are 0 for No, 1 for Yes

**Table 12.20** Logistic regression analysis of the hypertension data in Table 12.19
(a) All variables

| | Regression coefficient $b$ | Standard error $se(b)$ | $z$ | P |
|---|---|---|---|---|
| Constant | −2.378 | 0.380 | | |
| Smoking ($x_1$) | −0.068 | 0.278 | 0.24 | 0.81 |
| Obesity ($x_2$) | 0.695 | 0.285 | 2.44 | 0.015 |
| Snoring ($x_3$) | 0.872 | 0.398 | 2.19 | 0.028 |

(b) Omitting smoking

| | Regression coefficient $b$ | Standard error $se(b)$ | $z$ | P |
|---|---|---|---|---|
| Constant | −2.392 | 0.376 | | |
| Obesity ($x_1$) | 0.695 | 0.285 | 2.44 | 0.015 |
| Snoring ($x_2$) | 0.866 | 0.397 | 2.18 | 0.029 |

significance of each variable can be assessed by treating $z = b/se(b)$ as a standard Normal deviate; the P values are shown in the table. Clearly smoking has no association with hypertension, but both obesity and snoring seem to be independently prognostic. Omission of smoking (Table 12.20b) makes a minimal difference to the other coefficients. The analyses presented relate only to the **main effects** of obesity, smoking and snoring. Ideally we should also investigate the possibility that there may be an important interaction between two of these factors, for example that the effect of smoking is different for snorers and non-snorers. We can do this very simply if we have coded the binary variables as 0 or 1, by creating a new variable that is the product of the two variables that we are interested in. So we can create a new variable by multiplying together the values of smoking and snoring, and add this variable to the model. In fact, in this data set neither this nor any other interaction term is anywhere near to statistical significance.

The regression equation for the model with three variables is

$$\text{logit}(p) = -2.378 - 0.068x_1 + 0.695x_2 + 0.872x_3.$$

The estimated probability of having hypertension can be calculated from any combination of the three variables smoking, obesity and snoring. Specifically, we can compare the predicted probabilities for different groups, such as snorers and non-snorers. Setting $x_3$ first to 1 and then to 0 we have

$$\text{logit}(p_s) = -2.378 - 0.068x_1 + 0.695x_2 + 0.872$$

and

$$\text{logit}(p_{ns}) = -2.378 - 0.068x_1 + 0.695x_2$$

where $x_1$ and $x_2$ are the coded values of smoking and obesity. Thus we have $\text{logit}(p_s) - \text{logit}(p_{ns}) = 0.872$. As noted earlier, this expression is the log odds ratio, so that the odds ratio for hypertension associated with snoring is $e^{0.872} = 2.39$. We can therefore obtain the estimated odds ratio for a variable directly from its regression coefficient. The interpretation of the odds ratio was discussed in section 10.11.2. We can consider it as a measure of the estimated probability, or risk, of hypertension among snorers in relation to the risk among non-snorers.

Clearly for any binary variable the odds ratio can be estimated from the regression coefficient $b$ as $OR = e^b$. We can use the standard error of $b$ to get a confidence interval for $b$ and thus for $e^b$. The standard error of the regression coefficient for snoring was 0.398 (Table 12.20a) and a confidence interval is obtained by taking $b$ to have an approximately Normal sampling distribution. A 95% confidence interval for $b$ is thus given by

$$0.872 - (1.96 \times 0.398) \quad \text{to} \quad 0.872 + (1.96 \times 0.398)$$

that is, from 0.09 to 1.65. The 95% confidence interval for the odds ratio is thus from $e^{0.09}$ to $e^{1.65}$, that is, from 1.10 to 5.22. We are thus 95% sure that the risk of hypertension in snorers compared with non-snorers lies in the range 1.1 to 5.2, which is rather a wide range, but just excludes the value 1.0 that indicates no increased risk.

### 12.5.1 Computing

Logistic regression appears very similar to ordinary multiple regression, but the computing method is different. For each individual the dependent variable (hypertension in the example) is either 0 or 1 by definition, for which $\text{logit}(p) = \log[p/(1 - p)]$ is minus infinity or infinity respectively. The method of analysis uses an iterative procedure whereby the answer is obtained by several repeated cycles of calculation using an approach known as maximum likelihood. Because of this extra complexity, logistic regression is only found in large statistical packages or those primarily intended for the analysis of epidemiological studies. The same stepwise options that were discussed for ordinary multiple regression can be used for multiple logistic regression.

### 12.5.2 Discrimination

A logistic regression model enables us to predict the probability of a particular outcome in relation to several prognostic variables. In other words, it allows us to distinguish those patients likely or unlikely to have the condition, and as such can be a diagnostic aid. The statistical term for this type of analysis is **discriminant analysis**. An alternative method of discriminant analysis, which can be extended to more than two outcomes, is discussed in section 12.6.

As with multiple regression (see section 12.4.8) we can use the logistic regression model as a prognostic or diagnostic index. If we define $L$ as the logit of the probability $p$ that an individual will have the characteristic of interest, then

$$L = \log\left(\frac{p}{1 - p}\right) = b_0 + b_1x_1 + b_2x_2 + \ldots + b_kx_k$$

where there are $k$ variables in the model. We can calculate $L$ for all the subjects in the study and compare the distributions among those with and without the characteristic. From these we can discover how good the separation is between the two groups, and can determine the best cut-off point to maximize the discrimination. If all the explanatory variables are binary, as in the hypertension data, then there are only a few possible values for $L$. For example, the model shown in Table 12.20(b) allows only four groups, defined by presence or absence of obesity and snoring. There are thus only four possible values for $L$, each leading to an estimated probability of hypertension. These are shown in Table 12.21 together with the observed proportions with hypertension in the four groups. The

**Table 12.21** Predicted probability of hypertension ($p$) and observed proportions

| Obesity | Snoring | $L$ | $p$ | Observed proportion |
|---|---|---|---|---|
| No | No | −2.392 | 0.08 | 0.09 (7/77) |
| Yes | No | −1.697 | 0.15 | 0.09 (1/11) |
| No | Yes | −1.526 | 0.18 | 0.18 (48/272) |
| Yes | Yes | −0.831 | 0.30 | 0.31 (23/74) |

agreement is excellent. It is clear, however, that we could not predict hypertension with any accuracy using information about obesity and snoring, even though we can say that hypertension is much more common if both are present than if neither is. To be useful diagnostically, we would need much greater variation in the risk of hypertension among groups.

If one or more of the variables in the model is continuous the values of the score, $L$, will have a continuous distribution. The question that then arises is: How different are the distributions in the groups defined by the outcome variable? If there is little overlap, we can choose a cut-off that will give us good discrimination, but if there is considerable overlap the model will not be clinically useful. We are thus using the model to create a **diagnostic test**; this problem is discussed further in section 14.4.

Peeters *et al.* (1987) examined the predictive values of a positive test result in screening for breast cancer by mammography. Over a ten year period 801 women had positive mammography results and were referred for clinical examination. Breast cancer was histologically confirmed within one year in 302 women, 10 women were excluded for various reasons, and 489 women were classified as having had a false positive mammography result. The researchers compared the 302 true positives with the 489 false positives to see if they could improve the diagnosis by incorporating other information including epidemiological characteristics. Fifteen variables were examined of which five – age at referral, body mass index, menopausal status, breast complaints, and Wolfe classification of the contralateral breast – were significantly related to risk of cancer ($P<0.01$). Multiple logistic regression analysis yielded a model containing just two significant variables, age at referral (in years) and breast complaints (No or Yes; this refers to previous history of pain, skin problems, and so on). Their regression model to predict $p$, the probability of being a true positive, was

$$\text{logit}(p) = 4.005 + 0.0606x_1 + 0.8398x_2$$

where $x_1$ is age and $x_2$ is breast complaints (No $= 0$, Yes $= 1$). For each woman the researchers evaluated $p$, the probability of being diagnosed as having breast cancer predicted by their model. They divided these probabi-

**Table 12.22** Distribution of 787 mammography test results in relation to predicted probability of being a true positive (Peeters *et al.*, 1987). (Four cases with missing data excluded)

| | Probability of a true positive test result | | | | | | | | | |
|---|---|---|---|---|---|---|---|---|---|---|
| Test result | 0.0 −0.1 | 0.1 −0.2 | 0.2 −0.3 | 0.3 −0.4 | 0.4 −0.5 | 0.5 −0.6 | 0.6 −0.7 | 0.7 −0.8 | 0.8 −0.9 | 0.9 −1.0 |
| Negative ($N$ = 487) (False positive) | 0 | 68 | 167 | 99 | 75 | 51 | 22 | 3 | 2 | 0 |
| Positive ($N$ = 300) (True positive) | 0 | 10 | 55 | 56 | 80 | 56 | 28 | 9 | 5 | 1 |
| Observed proportions of true positives | – | 0.13 | 0.25 | 0.36 | 0.52 | 0.52 | 0.56 | 0.75 | 0.75 | |

lities into ten equal intervals and examined the frequencies of positive and negative diagnoses in the ten groups, to get the results shown in Table 12.22. As they observed, the considerable overlap of the distributions means that the model cannot help to distinguish false positives from true positives. A model that is highly significant does not guarantee good discrimination. Indeed, this type of finding is common, and discrimination good enough to aid diagnosis is rare.

A counter-example is given by a study of anti-smoking advice given by general practitioners in Australia (Richmond *et al.*, 1988). They developed a model using six variables to predict which smokers would abstain for six months, with correct prediction for 73/100 patients. This finding suggests that those patients predicted as unlikely to abstain could receive more intensive counselling. It also indicates that the adequacy of a model depends on the clinical situation: 73% accuracy was good in this study, but would be awful in many circumstances (see discussion of diagnostic tests in section 14.4). It is worth noting that we would be right half the time by guessing at random.

It is not always desirable to impose a cut-off between high and low risk groups, but rather it may be better to calculate a risk score. This was the approach used to produce the 'ready reckoner' for identifying men at high risk of heart attack, described in sections 1.1 and 1.4.1. The risk score was calculated by taking

$7 \times$ years of smoking cigarettes

$+ 6.5 \times$ mean blood pressure (mm Hg)

+ 270 if the man recalls a diagnosis of ischaemic heart disease

+ 150 if there was evidence of angina (from a questionnaire)

+ 85 if either parent had died of heart trouble

+ 150 if he was diabetic

(Shaper *et al.*, 1986). Here the numbers used to derive the score were derived from the logistic regression coefficients, with slight modification to make a score of 1000 correspond to the cut-off for 20% of men with the highest risk. The score was calculated for each of the 7506 men included in the analysis. Table 12.23 shows the scores corresponding to selected centiles of the distribution, together with the estimated risk of ischaemic heart disease.

**Table 12.23** Risk scores and estimated risk at selected centiles of the distribution of risk among 7506 men aged 40–59 (Shaper *et al.*, 1986)

| Centile of distribution of risk scores | Risk score | Estimated rate of risk per 1000 men per year |
|---|---|---|
| 10 | 647 | 1.8 |
| 20 | 713 | 2.4 |
| 30 | 766 | 3.1 |
| 40 | 812 | 3.9 |
| 50 | 856 | 4.8 |
| 60 | 898 | 5.8 |
| 70 | 944 | 7.1 |
| 80 | 1000 | 9.2 |
| 90 | 1091 | 13.5 |

### 12.5.3 Comments

With the exception of the method used to derive the regression model and the method for testing the significance of individual variables, fitting a logistic regression model is subject to the same difficulties as discussed in section 12.4.10 for ordinary multiple regression. The other main difference is that we cannot use scatter plots to plot the residuals because all of the observed data values are 0 or 1. The simplest solution is to divide the data into groups, as in Tables 12.21 and 12.22, and compare the observed and predicted proportions. Formal methods exist for assessing goodness-of-fit, but they are beyond the scope of this book.

## 12.6 DISCRIMINANT ANALYSIS

As noted at the beginning of section 12.5, there is another (older) method for using several variables to help distinguish groups, known as **discrimi-**

**nant analysis**. The usual situation is that we wish to be able to find some combination of variables that classifies a large proportion of subjects into the correct group, so that we can have a good chance of allocating (diagnosing) new subjects correctly. Simultaneously we usually wish to choose for the discrimination a subset of useful variables from a larger set of candidates. Discriminant analysis is more complicated than multiple regression, and I do not recommend that it is used without prior experience or expert assistance. In most cases discriminant analysis is used as an exploratory technique, so it is valuable to have an independent data set on which to assess how good the model is.

The basic idea of discriminant analysis is as follows. We first find the combination of variables that maximises the separation between the groups, as with logistic regression. With more than two groups we can further separate the groups by constructing a second combination of the same variables. These combinations are called **canonical variates** or **discriminant functions**. The method is perhaps best understood by considering a graph showing the results of an analysis. The method is based on the strong assumption that all of the variables have a Normal distribution with the same standard deviation *within each group*. It is generally agreed that some departure from this principle is acceptable, for example to include a few binary variables, but as usual it is difficult to say how much flexibility can be granted before the method becomes unreliable.

Thompson *et al.* (1985) carried out a study to try to differentiate diagnoses of ulcerative colitis, Crohn's disease and other forms of inflammatory bowel disease using rectal biopsy measurements. Seventy-five biopsies were studied, comprising 20 patients with normal biopsies, 20 with ulcerative colitis, 20 with Crohn's disease and 15 with culture positive diarrhoea. Stepwise discriminant analysis on 12 variables yielded a model comprising five variables, all highly statistically significant ($P < 0.001$).

Figure 12.4 shows the first two discriminant functions for the 75 observations, with superimposed circles indicating the areas in which we would expect (on the basis of the model) 80% of observations for each group. It is clear that the circle for the Crohn's disease group overlaps those for the other groups, so that we cannot use the model to get a reliable diagnosis. Of the 75 observations, the model correctly predicted 19/20 (95%) of the normal group, 9/20 (45%) with Crohn's disease, 14/20 (70%) with ulcerative colitis, and 12/15 (80%) with infective diarrhoea. We would expect the model to do worse when a completely new set of cases are examined, and Thompson *et al*. found only 14 out of a new series of 24 cases were correctly 'diagnosed' by the model, a 58% success rate compared with 72% on the original set.

Sample size is again an issue, and it has been suggested that there should be at least five times as many subjects per group as variables examined (Lachenbruch, 1977).

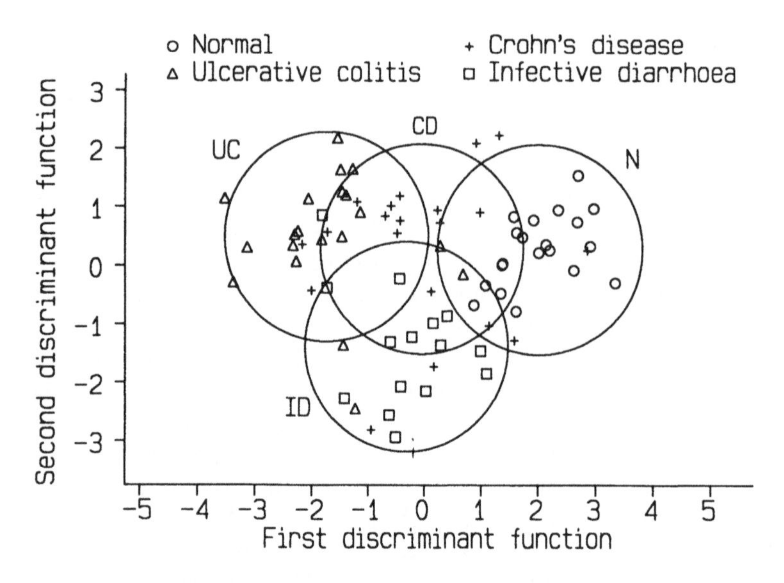


**Figure 12.4** Discriminant functions from data of Thompson *et al*. (1985).

Discriminant analysis is a complex technique, and more detailed discussion is inappropriate in this book. More details can be found in some textbooks, or in the useful papers by Lachenbruch (1977) and Brown (1984). When there are only two groups discriminant analysis usually gives similar answers to logistic regression analysis (see section 12.5.2).

## 12.7 OTHER METHODS

It is important to be aware that there are many other complex statistical methods that are not covered by introductory books. Other multivariate methods exist, such as **cluster analysis** and **factor analysis**. There is a vast **time series** methodology for dealing with long series of observations. There are important methods adapted from industrial quality control for assessing whether there has been a (sudden) change in the level of a variable, with applications in monitoring kidney transplants or detecting the time of ovulation from daily body temperature measurements. There are special methods for dealing with multi-way frequency tables – crosstabulations of three or more categorical variables. And there are many other specialized techniques.

While complicated problems do not necessarily require a complicated statistical analysis, it is unwise to try to force a complex problem to fit into the framework of a more familiar simpler technique. Expert statistical advice should be sought if at all possible.

## EXERCISES

12.1 The table below shows data from an experiment to compare resting metabolic rates (kcal/min) in five volunteers each given two diets, a normal diet and an overfeeding diet which contained 50% more energy (Welle *et al.*, 1986). Data were collected before and after eating a meal.

| Subject | Diet | Before meal | After meal |
|---|---|---|---|
| 1 | N | 1.47 | 1.78 |
| | O | 1.72 | 2.49 |
| 2 | N | 1.42 | 1.68 |
| | O | 1.44 | 1.87 |
| 3 | N | 1.10 | 1.26 |
| | O | 1.11 | 1.36 |
| 4 | N | 0.84 | 1.11 |
| | O | 0.90 | 1.29 |
| 5 | N | 0.91 | 1.09 |
| | O | 1.00 | 1.25 |

N: Normal diet; O: Overfed diet

(a) What methods of analysis could be used to examine the difference between the metabolic rates in relation to diet:
 (i) for the post-prandial data;
 (ii) for the change between pre- and post-prandial resting metabolic rates;

(b) Carry out an analysis to see if there is a significant difference between the two diets in the change between pre- and post-prandial resting metabolic rates.

12.2 Using the data in Table 12.11, find a suitable multiple regression model to predict functional residual capacity (FRC) from age, sex, height, weight and $FEV_1$. Check that the residuals from this model have a nearly Normal distribution.

12.3 Data from 37 patients receiving a non-depleted allogeneic bone marrow transplant were examined to see which variables were associated with the development of acute graft-versus-host disease (GvHD) (Bagot *et al.*, 1988). The table below shows separately for the groups who did not and did develop GvHD, the age of the recipient and donor, the type of leukaemia, whether or not the donor had been pregnant and an index of mixed epidermal cell-lymphocyte reactions. Donor pregnancy (Preg) is coded 0 for No and 1 for Yes. Type of leukaemia is coded 1 (acute myeloid leukaemia – AML), 2 (acute lymphocytic leukaemia – ALL) or 3 (chronic myeloid leukaemia – CML). Each group is ordered by their index values. (Also shown is the survival time, which is not used here.)

| Patient | Recipient age | Donor age | Type | Preg | Index | Survival time (days) |
|---|---|---|---|---|---|---|
| Patients without GvHD | | | | | | |
| 1 | 27 | 23 | 2 | 0 | 0.27 | 95 |
| 2 | 13 | 18 | 2 | 0 | 0.31 | 1385* |
| 3 | 19 | 19 | 1 | 0 | 0.39 | 465 |
| 4 | 21 | 22 | 2 | 0 | 0.48 | 810 |
| 5 | 28 | 38 | 2 | 0 | 0.49 | 1497* |
| 6 | 22 | 20 | 2 | 0 | 0.50 | 1181 |
| 7 | 19 | 19 | 2 | 0 | 0.81 | 993* |
| 8 | 20 | 23 | 2 | 0 | 0.82 | 138 |
| 9 | 33 | 36 | 1 | 0 | 0.86 | 266 |
| 10 | 18 | 19 | 1 | 0 | 0.92 | 579* |
| 11 | 17 | 20 | 2 | 0 | 1.10 | 600* |
| 12 | 31 | 21 | 3 | 0 | 1.52 | 1182* |
| 13 | 23 | 38 | 2 | 0 | 1.88 | 841* |
| 14 | 17 | 15 | 2 | 0 | 2.01 | 1364* |
| 15 | 26 | 16 | 2 | 0 | 2.40 | 695* |
| 16 | 28 | 25 | 1 | 0 | 2.45 | 1378* |
| 17 | 24 | 21 | 1 | 1 | 2.60 | 736* |
| 18 | 18 | 20 | 2 | 0 | 2.64 | 1504* |
| 19 | 24 | 25 | 1 | 1 | 3.78 | 849 |
| 20 | 20 | 24 | 3 | 0 | 4.72 | 1266* |
| Patients with GvHD | | | | | | |
| 21 | 23 | 35 | 1 | 1 | 1.10 | 186 |
| 22 | 21 | 35 | 2 | 1 | 1.16 | 41 |
| 23 | 21 | 23 | 3 | 0 | 1.45 | 667* |
| 24 | 33 | 43 | 3 | 0 | 1.50 | 112 |
| 25 | 29 | 24 | 3 | 1 | 1.85 | 572* |
| 26 | 42 | 35 | 2 | 1 | 2.30 | 45 |
| 27 | 27 | 31 | 3 | 0 | 2.34 | 1019* |
| 28 | 43 | 29 | 2 | 1 | 2.44 | 479 |
| 29 | 22 | 20 | 1 | 0 | 3.70 | 190 |
| 30 | 35 | 39 | 1 | 1 | 3.73 | 100 |
| 31 | 16 | 14 | 1 | 0 | 4.13 | 177 |

| Patient | Recipient age | Donor age | Type | Preg | Index | Survival time (days) |
|---|---|---|---|---|---|---|
| 32 | 39 | 35 | 2 | 1 | 4.52 | 80 |
| 33 | 28 | 25 | 3 | 1 | 4.52 | 142 |
| 34 | 29 | 32 | 3 | 0 | 4.71 | 1105* |
| 35 | 23 | 19 | 3 | 0 | 5.07 | 803* |
| 36 | 33 | 34 | 3 | 0 | 9.00 | 1126* |
| 37 | 19 | 20 | 1 | 0 | 10.11 | 114 |

(a) Use appropriate tests to compare the first five variables in the two groups. Which variables are significantly associated with the development of graft versus host disease ($P < 0.05$)?
(b) Use multiple logistic regression to see which variables are significantly related to GvHD (with $P < 0.05$). (Hint: Create two new 'dummy' variables indicating disease groups 2 and 3, and use log transformed index values.)
(c) Calculate the odds ratio for the risk of GvHD in relation to each binary variable in the model, with a 90% confidence interval.

12.4 Multiple logistic regression was used to construct a prognostic index to predict significant coronary artery disease from data on 348 patients with valvular heart disease who had undergone routine coronary arteriography before valve replacement (Ramsdale *et al.*, 1982). Forward stepwise selection was used, using $P < 0.01$ as the criterion for including variables. The prognostic index obtained was based on a model containing seven variables.

(a) The regression coefficient for a family history of ischaemic heart disease (coded 0 = No, 1 = Yes) was 1.167. What is the estimated odds ratio for having significant coronary artery disease associated with a positive family history?
(b) One of the variables in the model was the estimated total number of cigarettes ever smoked, calculated as the average number smoked annually × the number of years smoking. The regression coefficient was 0.0106 per 1000 cigarettes. What total number of cigarettes ever smoked carries the same risk as a family history of ischaemic heart disease? Convert this figure into years of smoking 20 cigarettes per day.
(c) What is the odds ratio for major coronary artery disease for someone with a family history of ischaemic heart disease who had smoked 20 cigarettes a day for 30 years compared with a non-smoker with no family history?

12.5 For lung transplantation it is desirable for the donor's lungs to be of a similar size as those of the recipient. Total lung capacity (TLC) is difficult to measure, so it is useful to be able to predict TLC from other information. The following table shows the pre-transplant TLC of 32 recipients of heart-lung transplants, obtained by whole-body plethysmography, and their age, sex and height (Otulana *et al.*, 1989).

| | Age | Sex | Height (cm) | TLC (l) | | Age | Sex | Height (cm) | TLC (l) |
|---|---|---|---|---|---|---|---|---|---|
| 1 | 35 | F | 149 | 3.40 | 17 | 30 | F | 172 | 6.30 |
| 2 | 11 | F | 138 | 3.41 | 18 | 21 | F | 163 | 6.55 |
| 3 | 12 | M | 148 | 3.80 | 19 | 21 | F | 164 | 6.60 |
| 4 | 16 | F | 156 | 3.90 | 20 | 20 | M | 189 | 6.62 |
| 5 | 32 | F | 152 | 4.00 | 21 | 34 | M | 182 | 6.89 |
| 6 | 16 | F | 157 | 4.10 | 22 | 43 | M | 184 | 6.90 |
| 7 | 14 | F | 165 | 4.46 | 23 | 35 | M | 174 | 7.00 |
| 8 | 16 | M | 152 | 4.55 | 24 | 39 | M | 177 | 7.20 |
| 9 | 35 | F | 177 | 4.83 | 25 | 43 | M | 183 | 7.30 |
| 10 | 33 | F | 158 | 5.10 | 26 | 37 | M | 175 | 7.65 |
| 11 | 40 | F | 166 | 5.44 | 27 | 32 | M | 173 | 7.80 |
| 12 | 28 | F | 165 | 5.50 | 28 | 24 | M | 173 | 7.90 |
| 13 | 23 | F | 160 | 5.73 | 29 | 20 | F | 162 | 8.05 |
| 14 | 52 | M | 178 | 5.77 | 30 | 25 | M | 180 | 8.10 |
| 15 | 46 | F | 169 | 5.80 | 31 | 22 | M | 173 | 8.70 |
| 16 | 29 | M | 173 | 6.00 | 32 | 25 | M | 171 | 9.45 |

(a) How well can an individual's lung capacity be predicted from a multiple regression model including age, sex and height?
(b) Compare the result just obtained with that derived from linear regression on height alone.
(c) Calculate the 95% prediction interval from the linear regression on height for someone with average height.
(d) How could we investigate whether the relation between lung capacity and height is the same for males and females?

# 13

# Analysis of survival times

## 13.1 INTRODUCTION

In most studies the data are a mixture of measurements and attributes. The preceding four chapters have presented methods for the analysis of both quantitative and qualitative data for various study designs. Another type of data arises when interest is focused on the time taken for some event to occur. One of the most common sources of such data is when we record the time from some fixed starting point, such as surgery, to the death of the subject. For this reason we usually refer to **survival times** or **survival data** and the statistical treatment of survival times is known as **survival analysis**. As we shall see, similar data arise in other situations, but it is customary to stick to the same terminology.

In clinical studies survival times often refer to the time to death, to development of a particular symptom, or to relapse after remission of disease. Although there is usually a clear definition of the end of the time period of interest, the start may be less well defined. It is, for example, rarely possible to know how long somebody has had a disease, so the date of diagnosis is often the best alternative. For some diseases these two dates can be very different.

There is one inherent feature of survival times that makes them unsuitable for analysis by any of the methods described in the preceding chapters, which is that we almost never observe the event of interest in all subjects. For example, in a study to compare the survival of patients having different types of surgery for breast cancer, although the patients will be followed up for several years there will be many who are still alive at the end of the study. For these patients we do not know when they will die, only that they are still alive at the end of the study. Nor, therefore, do we know their survival time from surgery, only that it will be longer than their time in the study. We call such survival times **censored**, to indicate that the period of observation was cut off before the event of interest occurred. Note that as the event of interest is usually something that is undesirable, such as death, the 'interest' is scientific, not clinical.

If all subjects were followed for exactly the same length of time it would perhaps be possible to use the rank methods introduced in Chapter 9 for analysing survival times, giving all censored times the equal highest rank.

However, patients are nearly always followed for varying lengths of time. In any case patients may leave the study before the end, perhaps moving to a different area. Withdrawals thus lead to censored observations of a different type.

Figure 13.1 illustrates the different ways in which patients can proceed through a study. It shows a six month period during which patients are recruited to the study, and a further 12 months of observation. The patients are thus observed for between 12 and 18 months, the most recently accrued patients being observed for the shortest time. Figure 13.1 shows that four patients died and four were still alive at the end of the study. Two other patients withdrew from the study before the end. We thus have four firm survival times and six censored times, as shown in Table 13.1, where the asterisk denotes a censored survival time. We ignore the different starting times when analysing survival data, and it helps to order the observations by survival time. Figure 13.2 shows the effect of these changes.

With data of this type we often wish to estimate the probability of an individual surviving for a given time period such as one year. With two or more groups we will also be interested in comparing their survival experience. This chapter introduces methods to answer these and other questions relating to survival data. For convenience, I shall assume that the data have already been sorted into ascending order of survival times. (Computer programs may require this.)

The analysis of medical survival data has become widespread since the

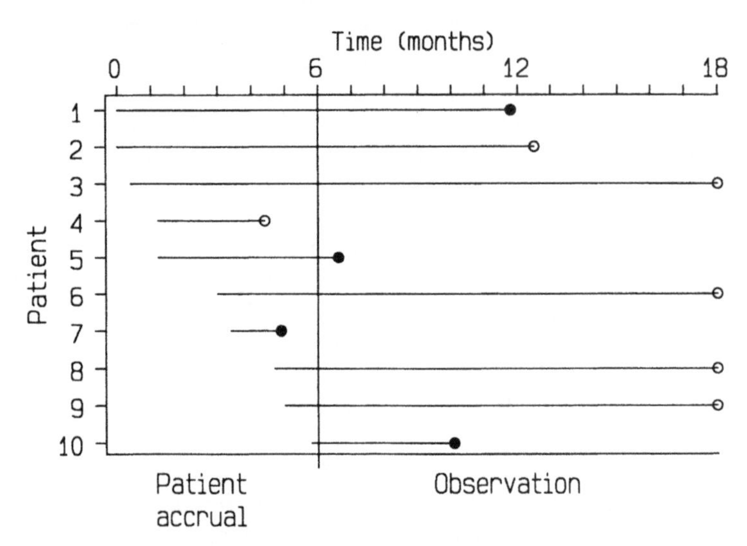


**Figure 13.1** Diagram showing patients entering a study at different times and the observation of known (•) and censored (○) survival times.

**Table 13.1** Survival times for patients shown in Figure 13.1

| Patient | Time at entry (m) | Time at death or censoring (m) | Dead or censored | Survival time |
|---|---|---|---|---|
| 1 | 0.0 | 11.8 | D | 11.8 |
| 2 | 0.0 | 12.5 | C | 12.5* |
| 3 | 0.4 | 18.0 | C | 17.6* |
| 4 | 1.2 | 4.4 | C | 3.2* |
| 5 | 1.2 | 6.6 | D | 5.4 |
| 6 | 3.0 | 18.0 | C | 15.0* |
| 7 | 3.4 | 4.9 | D | 1.5 |
| 8 | 4.7 | 18.0 | C | 13.3* |
| 9 | 5.0 | 18.0 | C | 13.0* |
| 10 | 5.8 | 10.1 | D | 4.3 |

*censored observation

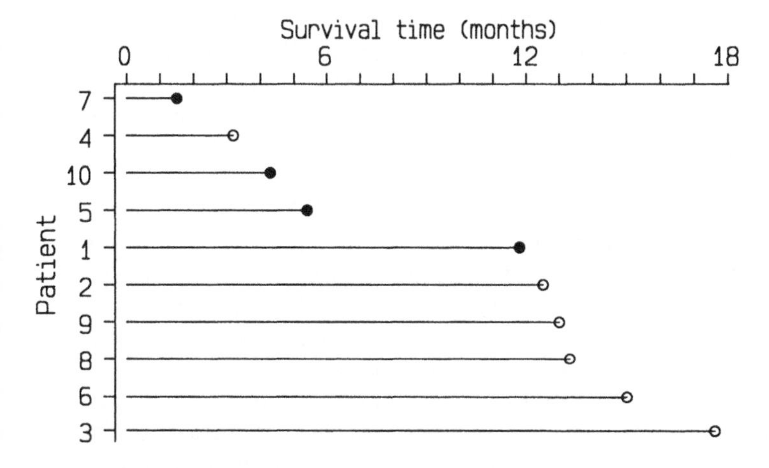


**Figure 13.2** Figure 13.1 reorganized to correspond to method of analysis.

early 1970s when new methods were developed. Most of the methods described in this chapter are discussed in much more detail in two excellent papers by Peto *et al*. (1976 and 1977), especially in the second paper. These papers also contain a wealth of practical advice about the design and execution of studies of survival times.

## 13.2 SURVIVAL PROBABILITIES

From a set of observed survival times (including censored times) from a sample of individuals we can estimate the proportion of the population of such people who would survive a given length of time in the same circumstances. For example, we can use data from a study of patients having liver transplants to estimate the probability of new patients surviving a given length of time after transplantation (with the usual proviso about the representativeness of the original sample). The method is clever in that it not only makes proper allowances for those observations that are censored, but also makes use of the information from these subjects up to the time when they are censored. The method yields a graph or a table, which goes under various names: **life table**, **survival curve**, **Kaplan-Meier curve**.

### 13.2.1 Kaplan-Meier survival curve

The probability of surviving a given length of time can be calculated by considering time in many small intervals. For example, the probability of a patient surviving two days after a liver transplant can be considered to be the probability of surviving one day, multiplied by the probability of surviving the second day given that the patient survived the first day. This second probability is known as a **conditional probability**. If we write $p_{100}$ as the probability of surviving the hundredth day conditional on having already survived the first 99 days, then the overall probability of surviving 100 days after a liver transplant is given by

$$p_1 \times p_2 \times p_3 \times \ldots p_{99} \times p_{100}.$$

The probability of surviving the 100th day is estimated simply as the proportion of the sample surviving that day *of those still known to be alive after 99 days*. The probability $p$ is thus 1 on days when nobody dies, so the calculations are simplified by the fact that it is only necessary to calculate the probabilities for days on which at least one person dies.

The survival curve calculations will be illustrated on a small data set arising from a research programme aimed at the prediction of motion sickness at sea (Burns, 1984). Subjects were placed in a cubical cabin mounted on a hydraulic piston and subjected to vertical motion (known as 'heave'!) for two hours. The endpoint of interest was the time when the subject first vomited (known as 'frank emesis'). Some subjects requested an early stop to the experiment although they had not vomited, yielding censored observations, while others successfully survived two hours. Twenty-one subjects were studied with a frequency of 0.167 Hz and acceleration of 0.111 G, 14 of whom survived two hours without vomiting. The survival times (in minutes) of the other seven subjects were

30, 50, 50*, 51, 66*, 82 and 92

where the two observations marked * were censored. The other 14 observations were censored at 120 minutes.

**Table 13.2** Life table for motion sickness data from an experiment with vertical movement at a frequency of 0.167 Hz and acceleration 0.111 G (Burns, 1984) (Experiment 1)

| Subject number | Survival time (min) | Survival proportion | Standard error |
|---|---|---|---|
| 1 | 30 | 0.952 | 0.045 |
| 2 | 50 | 0.905 | 0.062 |
| 3 | 50* | | |
| 4 | 51 | 0.855 | 0.077 |
| 5 | 66* | | |
| 6 | 82 | 0.801 | 0.089 |
| 7 | 92 | 0.748 | 0.097 |
| 8 | 120* | | |
| 9 | 120* | | |
| . | . | | |
| . | . | | |
| . | . | | |
| 21 | 120* | | |

* censored observation

Table 13.2 shows the life table for these data, giving the survival proportion at each uncensored survival time. Because only five subjects vomited there are only five estimated survival probabilities. Note that the survival probability remains 1 up to the time of the first event (30 minutes), and we cannot estimate survival beyond the last observation of 120 minutes. It is usual to present survival probabilities as a graph, as shown in Figure 13.3.

From the survival curve we can calculate the survival time corresponding to any proportion of the sample. For example, the time when the curve crosses the probability of 0.5 corresponds to the estimated median survival time. In this example, however, we cannot estimate the median as the curve does not fall to 0.5.

The survival curve is drawn as a 'step function': the proportion surviving remains unchanged between events, even if there are some intermediate censored observations. It is incorrect to join the calculated points by sloping lines. The times of censored observations are sometimes indicated by ticks on the survival curve, which shows at a glance the survival times of the surviving subjects.

We can calculate a confidence interval for the survival proportion. If there are no censored values we can use standard methods for deriving a confidence interval for a proportion (see section 10.2), but in general we

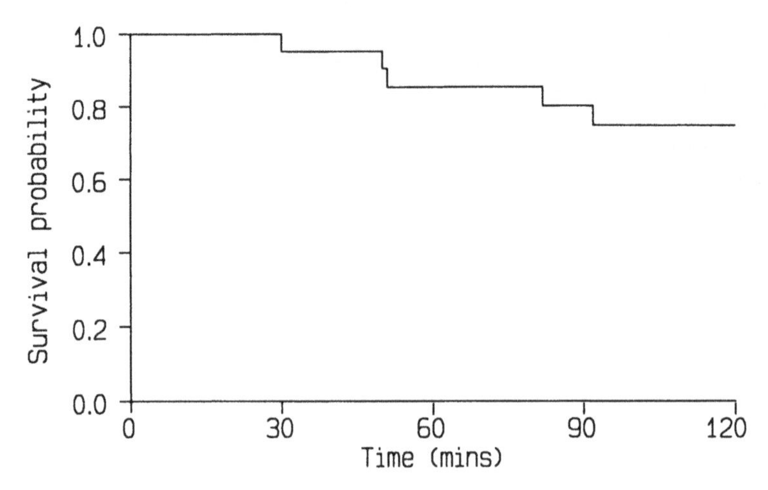


**Figure 13.3** Survival curve corresponding to the motion sickness data in Table 13.2.

will need to make a modification to allow for the censoring. Section 13.4.1 gives a method for calculating the standard error; Table 13.2 shows standard errors for the motion sickness data. Some computer programs will provide standard errors, although these may have been produced by a more complex method than is given in section 13.4.1.

From the standard error we can calculate a confidence interval, assuming a Normal sampling distribution for the survival proportion in large samples. For example, the proportion surviving 90 minutes without vomiting was 0.801 with a standard error of 0.089. The 95% confidence interval is thus

$$0.801 - 1.96 \times 0.089 \quad \text{to} \quad 0.801 + 1.96 \times 0.089$$

or 0.63 to 0.98. As usual, with a small sample the confidence interval is wide. Note that when the proportion surviving is near 1 or 0 the calculated confidence interval may include impossible values above 1 or less than 0. If this happens we can take 1 as the upper limit or 0 as the lower limit. However, this occurrence indicates that the Normal approximation is not really appropriate and some other method may be preferable. Better methods exist for calculating standard errors, but they are also more complicated.

The data used in this example are from an experiment of fixed duration, so that most of the censored observations are at the same time. In observational studies, such as the study of liver transplant patients, it is customary to stop the period of observation on a specific day. Because subjects enter on different days (as shown in Figure 13.1) survivors have widely varying periods of follow up and thus survival times censored at different points. All of the methods described in this chapter apply equally in both circumstances.

### 13.2.2 Life table analysis

Although the Kaplan-Meier survival curve is often called a **life table**, the term life table is also frequently used to describe data where the results are grouped into time intervals, often of equal length. This method is often described as **actuarial**. The method of calculation is similar in principle to the Kaplan-Meier method, but differences arise because of the lack of precision of recording of times. Details are given by Armitage and Berry (1987, p. 424).

Life tables are also used in demography to estimate the survival curve for a cohort of people from birth using current age and sex specific mortality rates. These **cohort** life tables are calculated somewhat differently (Armitage and Berry, 1987, p. 422; Bland, 1987, p. 302).

## 13.3 COMPARING SURVIVAL CURVES IN TWO GROUPS

For studies in which the aim is to compare the survival experience of two groups of subjects we can calculate the Kaplan-Meier curves separately for each group. The standard error of the difference in the proportions surviving at any time can be calculated, and a confidence interval obtained. The weakness of this approach is that it does not provide a comparison of the total survival experience of the two groups, but rather gives a comparison at some arbitrary time point(s). The choice of the time point to make a comparison should really be made in advance of the analysis, not after inspection of the survival curves: the comparison of proportions thus chosen is invalid. The use of multiple time points creates further problems of interpretation, especially if the curves are significantly different at some points but not at others. Comparing survival probabilities can be useful as an adjunct to other analyses, however, and is described later. First I shall consider methods for comparing the complete survival curves for two or more independent sets of observations.

The most common method of comparing independent groups of survival times is the **logrank test**. As its name indicates, the logrank test is a hypothesis test – the null hypothesis is that the groups come from the same population. There is no similarly widely used method of estimation, but some possibilities are considered later in this chapter.

### 13.3.1 The logrank test

The logrank test is a non-parametric method for testing the null hypothesis that the groups being compared are samples from the same population as regards survival experience. The method is based on a simple idea which avoids the arbitrary decisions referred to above.

Table 13.3 shows the data (and the life table) from a second motion sickness experiment using different subjects in which both the frequency and acceleration were doubled in comparison with the first experiment. The logrank test can be used to compare the data from the two experiments.

The principle of the logrank test is to divide the survival time scale into intervals according to the distinct observed survival times, ignoring censored survival times. There were five definite events (vomiting) in the first experiment at 30, 50, 51, 82 and 92 minutes. In the second experiment there were 14 events, one each at 5, 13, 24, 63, 65, 79, 102 and 115 minutes, and 2 each at 11, 69 and 82 minutes. For the two experiments combined there were 15 distinct recorded survival times. Figure 13.4 shows the time scale divided into 15 time intervals, each of which includes the

**Table 13.3** Life table for motion sickness data from an experiment with vertical movement at a frequency of 0.333 Hz and acceleration 0.222 G (Burns, 1984) (Experiment 2)

| Subject number | Survival time (min) | Survival proportion | Standard error |
|---|---|---|---|
| 1 | 5 | 0.964 | 0.034 |
| 2 | 6* | | |
| 3 | 11 | | |
| 4 | 11 | 0.890 | 0.058 |
| 5 | 13 | 0.853 | 0.067 |
| 6 | 24 | 0.816 | 0.073 |
| 7 | 63 | 0.779 | 0.078 |
| 8 | 65 | 0.742 | 0.082 |
| 9 | 69 | | |
| 10 | 69 | 0.668 | 0.086 |
| 11 | 79 | 0.631 | 0.090 |
| 12 | 82 | | |
| 13 | 82 | 0.556 | 0.090 |
| 14 | 102 | 0.519 | 0.093 |
| 15 | 115 | 0.482 | 0.093 |
| 16 | 120* | | |
| 17 | 120* | | |
| . | . | | |
| . | . | | |
| 28 | 120* | | |

* censored observation

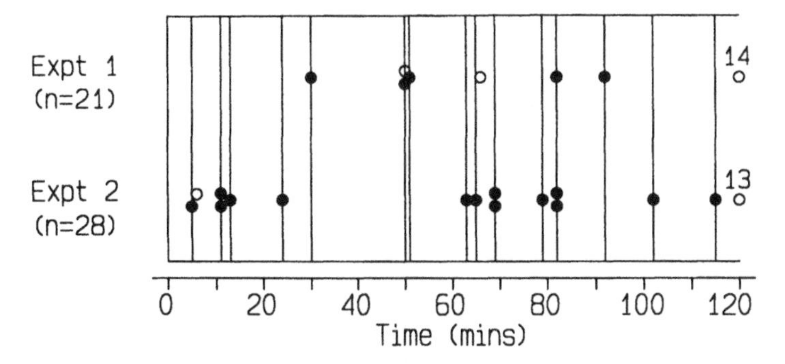


**Figure 13.4** Times of events (•) and censoring (○) for two different motion sickness experiments, showing the time intervals used for calculating the logrank test. Experiment 1 was described in Table 13.2 and Experiment 2 in Table 13.3.

time of an event at the upper limit. The first interval is from 0 to 5 minutes, the second is from 6 to 11 minutes, and so on. For each time period we compare the observed data with what we would expect if the null hypothesis that there is no real difference between the experiments is true.

The logrank test to compare $k$ groups produces for each group an observed ($O$) and an expected ($E$) number of events. These are compared in a familiar way by calculating the sum of $(O - E)^2/E$, called $X^2$, comparing the result to a $\chi^2$ distribution with $k - 1$ degrees of freedom.

The motion sickness data give

$$O_1 = 5, \; E_1 = 8.8607, \; O_2 = 14 \text{ and } E_2 = 10.1393$$

so that the logrank statistic is

$$X^2 = \frac{(5 - 8.8607)^2}{8.8607} + \frac{(14 - 10.1393)^2}{10.1393}$$

$$= 3.152.$$

Comparing this value to a $\chi^2$ distribution with one degree of freedom gives $P = 0.08$, so there is some evidence to suggest a difference between the results of the two experiments. Figure 13.5 shows that the survival without vomiting was better in experiment 1.

Note that the sum of the observed and expected numbers is the same: it is important to check this when performing the calculation by hand. Note too that the quantity $E$ is better thought of as a measure of the extent of exposure of the subjects rather than the expected number of events. The reason is that under some unusual circumstances $E$ can be larger than the sample size.

The logrank test can be used to compare several groups of subjects.

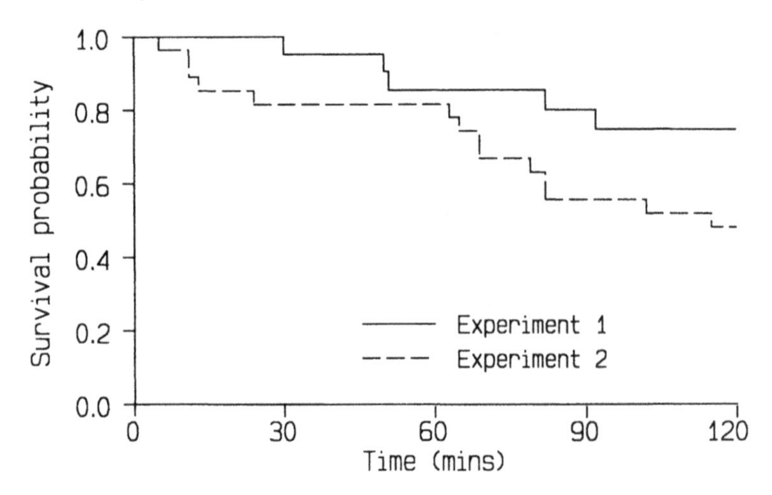


**Figure 13.5** Survival curves for data shown in Table 13.2 and Table 13.3.

Often, however, the categories defining those groups will have a natural ordering, and we should examine the more specific possibility of a trend in survival across the groups. We might, for example, wish to compare survival in several age groups, or in relation to stage of disease, or in relation to amount of exposure of some suspected environmental hazard (such as smoking). The method is a simple extension of the standard logrank test.

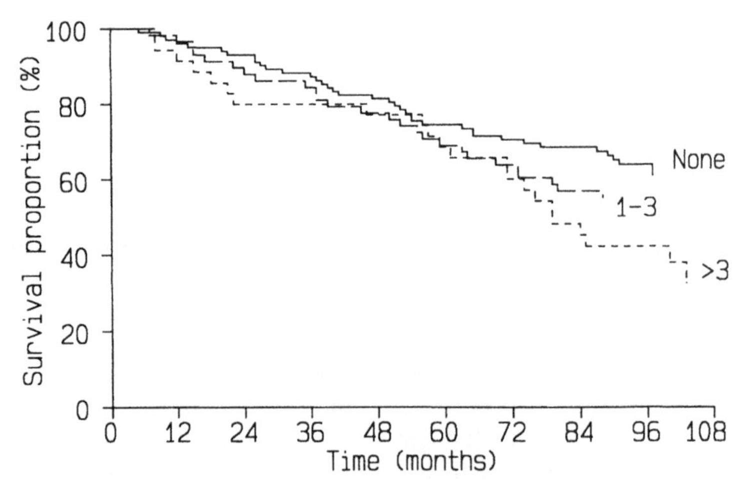


**Figure 13.6** Kaplan-Meier curves for patients with breast cancer with none ($n$ = 102), 1–3 ($n$ = 58), or more than 3 ($n$ = 35) positive nodes (data from Barnes *et al.*, 1988).

Figure 13.6 shows survival curves for three groups of women operated on for breast cancer, classified by the number of positive nodes found. An ordinary logrank test gives $X^2 = 5.59$ on 2 degrees of freedom ($P = 0.06$). Because the groups are ordered, however, the trend test should be used, which gives $X^2_{trend} = 5.26$ on 1 degree of freedom ($P = 0.02$). There is thus a significant (negative) association between survival and number of positive nodes.

The logrank test can also be extended to allow an adjustment to be made for other variables. For example, in a randomized trial to compare survival in groups of breast cancer patients given different types of surgery we may wish to allow for the stage of breast cancer in the analysis, or for some other prognostic variable. In this **stratified** analysis, the subjects are divided into subgroups according to the prognostic variable (stage of cancer) and the values of $O$ and $E$ calculated for each treatment group within each stratum (subgroup). For each treatment group the values of $O$ and $E$ from each stratum are added up and then these sums are compared using the usual logrank formula to get $X^2$. If, by chance, one treatment group includes more subjects with a poor prognosis this stratified analysis will adjust for the imbalance. The same method can be used to combine data from different centres in a multicentre study. There is further discussion of the need to make adjusted comparisons in Chapter 15. The method for performing the logrank test is shown in detail in section 13.4, which also gives a rather more accurate formula for the logrank statistic $X^2$. The test for trend and stratified analysis are also described. Several computer programs can perform the logrank analysis, which is tedious by hand except for very small data sets, but they do not all give enough information in their output of results (see section 13.8). Peto *et al.* (1977) give detailed discussion of all the methods discussed in this section, and much else besides – their paper is essential reading.

### 13.3.2 The hazard ratio

The logrank test is very widely used for comparing survival in two or more groups, but it is solely a hypothesis test. It provides no direct information of *how* different the groups were.

One way to measure the relative survival in two groups is to compare the observed number of events with the expected numbers. The ratio $O_1/E_1$ gives the observed event rate in the first group as a proportion of that expected if the null hypothesis were true, and so the ratio

$$R = \frac{O_1/E_1}{O_2/E_2}$$

gives an estimate of the relative event rates in the two groups. This ratio is also called the **hazard ratio**. For the motion sickness data we have

$$R = \frac{5/8.8607}{14/10.1393} = 0.4087$$

so that the estimated relative risk or hazard of vomiting under the conditions of experiment 1 is 0.41 (41%) of that for experiment 2.

We can calculate an approximate confidence interval for $R$, as described in section 13.4.5. In this case the 95% confidence interval is from 0.18 to 1.08, and thus includes the value of 1 corresponding to equal hazards. As we should expect from this small sample, the confidence interval is very wide. Sample size and power are discussed in section 13.7.

The calculation of the relative hazard in the two groups is based on the complete period studied. It is not necessarily true that the relative hazard stays much the same in the two groups throughout that period. Indeed it is quite likely that it will vary, in which case the hazard ratio will not apply throughout the period studied. The plot of survival curves will give a visual impression of the consistency of the effect and is an essential component of the analysis of survival data. With large samples we can calculate the hazards in each group, and thus the hazard ratio, for each of several time periods, and examine the consistency of the hazard ratio over time.

### 13.3.3 Comparison of survival probabilities

Just as we can obtain a confidence interval for a survival probability calculated from a single group of individuals, so we can calculate a confidence interval for the difference between the survival probabilities calculated from two groups of individuals. The method for calculating such a confidence interval is given in section 13.4.6.

For example, we can calculate the confidence interval for the difference between the estimated probabilities of surviving 60 minutes without being sick for the two experiments already described. The two survival probabilities, as shown in Tables 13.2 and 13.3, are 0.855 and 0.816. The difference is $0.855 - 0.816 = 0.039$, and the 95% confidence interval is from $-0.17$ to 0.25.

The main disadvantage of this method is that the confidence interval applies only to one time point. To be valid, that time point must be chosen in advance of seeing the data – it is wrong to choose the time from an inspection of the survival curves. It is possible to calculate confidence intervals for several (or even all) times, but there is no easy way to interpret the results. Unless there is a prior reason for comparing survival proportions at a particular time point it is probably better to use the hazard ratio to derive an estimate of the difference in survival between two groups. In any case, the hazard ratio is a more natural way of comparing survival. Another option is to calculate the ratio of the median survival times; this method is described in section 13.4.7.

## 13.4 MATHEMATICAL CALCULATIONS AND WORKED EXAMPLE

*(This section can be omitted without loss of continuity.)*

Most statistical computer programs do not include methods for analysing survival times. Further, those that do cannot perform all of the calculations described in sections 13.2 and 13.3, especially those needed to produce confidence intervals. The methods are not mathematically complex, but they can be somewhat fiddly.

### 13.4.1 Survival curve (Kaplan-Meier)

The principle behind the calculation of survival probabilities was outlined in section 13.2. The proportion surviving a given length of time, say 100 days, is calculated by multiplying the probabilities of surviving each day up to that time. We need only consider days on which there is an event or 'failure' (e.g. death). If there is a death at 100 days, then we estimate the proportion surviving 100 days as the proportion surviving 99 days multiplied by the proportion of those surviving 99 days who also survive 100 days. If $p_k$ is the probability of surviving $k$ days, $r_k$ is the number of subjects still *at risk* (i.e. still being followed up) immediately before the $k$th day, and $f_k$ is the number of observed failures on day $k$, then we have

$$p_k = p_{k-1} \times \frac{r_k - f_k}{r_k}.$$

This is a mathematical representation of the statement in the previous sentence.

For the data in Table 13.2 the time unit is minutes, and a 'failure' was vomiting. The proportion surviving without vomiting is 1 up to 29 minutes. We therefore have $p_{29} = 1$, and $r_{30} = 21$ because all subjects are still at risk at 30 minutes. There was one failure at 30 minutes, so $f_{30} = 1$ and we can calculate the proportion surviving 30 minutes as

$$p_{30} = p_{29} \times \frac{(21 - 1)}{21} = 0.952$$

as shown in Table 13.2. The estimated proportion surviving stays the same until the next failure time, which is 50 minutes. We assume that subject 3 who was censored at the same minute was still at risk at the time when subject 2 'failed', so we have

$$p_{50} = p_{30} \times \frac{(20 - 1)}{20} = 0.905$$

because there were only 20 subjects still at risk at 50 minutes. One subject withdrew at 50 minutes so their time was censored, and the number at risk

**Table 13.4** Calculation of survival probabilities (Kaplan–Meier survival curve) for data in Table 13.2

| Subject number ($k$) | Survival time (min) | Number at risk ($r_k$) | Observed failures ($f_k$) | $\frac{r_k - f_k}{r_k}$ | Survival proportion ($p_k$) |
|---|---|---|---|---|---|
| 1 | 30 | 21 | 1 | 0.9524 | 0.9524 |
| 2 | 50 | 20 | 1 | 0.9500 | 0.9048 |
| 3 | 50* | | | | |
| 4 | 51 | 18 | 1 | 0.9444 | 0.8545 |
| 5 | 66* | | | | |
| 6 | 82 | 16 | 1 | 0.9375 | 0.8011 |
| 7 | 92 | 15 | 1 | 0.9333 | 0.7476 |
| 8 | 120* | | | | |
| 9 | 120* | | | | |
| . | . | | | | |
| . | . | | | | |
| . | . | | | | |
| 21 | 120* | | | | |

* censored observation

at 51 minutes was thus only 18. The calculations for the complete set of data are shown in Table 13.4. The column of interest, the survival proportion, is simply the product of all the entries from the top of the table in the previous column. Note that the only effect of the censored observations is to alter the number at risk at the next uncensored survival time.

The standard error of the survival proportion can be calculated in various ways, although the different formulae give very similar results. A simple formula is

$$SE(p_k) = p_k\sqrt{(1 - p_k)/r_k}$$

where $p_k$ is the estimated proportion surviving at time $k$. The standard errors in Tables 13.2 and 13.3 were calculated using this formula. On the assumption that $p_k$ will have an approximately Normal sampling distribution we can calculate a 95% confidence interval for $p_k$ as

$$p_k - 1.96SE(p_k) \quad \text{to} \quad p_k + 1.96SE(p_k).$$

This is not a good approximation for small sample sizes or for very large or small probabilities, say outside the range 0.2 to 0.8, under which circumstances the confidence interval can go outside the range 0 to 1. While the confidence interval can be curtailed at the limit (e.g. change the range

'0.75 to 1.10' to '0.75 to 1.0') this is an indication of an inadequate amount of data. There are many alternative formulae for the standard error of an estimated survival probability, the best known being due to Greenwood:

$$SE(p_k) = p_k \sqrt{\sum_{j=1}^{k} \left[ \frac{f_j}{r_j(r_j - f_j)} \right]}.$$

Computer programs are likely to use a more accurate formulae than the one used in the example. Tables 13.2 and 13.3 show how the standard errors for the motion sickness data increase as the number still at risk falls, as we would expect in general.

### 13.4.2 The logrank test

The logrank test of the null hypothesis of the same survival experience in two or more groups of subjects involves calculating the observed and expected numbers of failures in separate time intervals, and summing these. The method is illustrated using the two groups of observations shown in Table 13.2 and 13.3.

As shown in Figure 13.4, the time span of the study is divided into time intervals ending with one or more failures, although this is equivalent to considering only the minutes of failures, as for the calculation of survival probabilities. For each minute with a failure we calculate the numbers at risk in each group ($r_1$ and $r_2$) and the numbers of observed failures ($f_1$ and $f_2$). From these we calculate the expected number of failures assuming the null hypothesis is true. At each time we have a 2 × 2 table as follows:

| | Group 1 | Group 2 | Total |
|---|---|---|---|
| Failures | $f_1$ | $f_2$ | $f$ |
| Not failures | $r_1 - f_1$ | $r_2 - f_2$ | $r - f$ |
| Total | $r_1$ | $r_2$ | $r$ |

We calculate expected numbers of failures as in Chapter 10, so that $e_1 = r_1 f/r$ and $e_2 = r_2 f/r$. We then sum the observed and expected values for the whole table to get $O_1 = \Sigma f_1$, $E_1 = \Sigma e_1$, etc. Note that $O_1 + O_2 = E_1 + E_2$, an equivalence that should be verified for hand calculations. The simplest way to calculate the logrank test statistic is by

$$X^2 = \frac{(O_1 - E_1)^2}{E_1} + \frac{(O_2 - E_2)^2}{E_2}.$$

However, a slightly better answer can be obtained by calculating the variance of $f_1 - e_1$ at each time as

$$v = \frac{r_1 r_2 f(r - f)}{r^2(r - 1)}$$

and summing these values overall to get $V = \Sigma v$. The alternative form of the test statistic is given by

$$X^2 = \frac{(O_1 - E_1)^2}{V}.$$

In practice the two methods usually give similar answers.

The calculations for the motion sickness data are shown in Table 13.5. There were two failures at 11 and 69 minutes and three at 82 minutes, so we will not get the same answer using the two versions of the logrank test. The first method gives

$$X^2 = \frac{(-3.8607)^2}{8.8607} + \frac{(3.8607)^2}{10.1393} = 3.152$$

**Table 13.5** Calculating the logrank test statistic for the motion sickness data. The subscripts refer to Experiments 1 and 2

| Time (mins) | $r_1$ | $r_2$ | $r$ | $f_1$ | $f_2$ | $f$ | $e_1 = \frac{r_1 f}{r}$ | $f_1 - e_1$ | $v = \frac{r_1 r_2 f(r - f)}{r^2(r - 1)}$ |
|---|---|---|---|---|---|---|---|---|---|
| 5 | 21 | 28 | 49 | 0 | 1 | 1 | 0.4286 | −0.4286 | 0.2449 |
| 6* | 21 | 27 | 48 | | | | | | |
| 11 | 21 | 26 | 47 | 0 | 2 | 2 | 0.8936 | −0.8936 | 0.4836 |
| 13 | 21 | 24 | 45 | 0 | 1 | 1 | 0.4667 | −0.4667 | 0.2489 |
| 24 | 21 | 23 | 44 | 0 | 1 | 1 | 0.4773 | −0.4773 | 0.2495 |
| 30 | 21 | 22 | 43 | 1 | 0 | 1 | 0.4884 | 0.5116 | 0.2499 |
| 50 | 20 | 22 | 42 | 1 | 0 | 1 | 0.4762 | 0.5238 | 0.2494 |
| 50* | 19 | 22 | 41 | | | | | | |
| 51 | 18 | 22 | 40 | 1 | 0 | 1 | 0.4500 | 0.5500 | 0.2475 |
| 63 | 17 | 22 | 39 | 0 | 1 | 1 | 0.4359 | −0.4359 | 0.2459 |
| 65 | 17 | 21 | 38 | 0 | 1 | 1 | 0.4474 | −0.4474 | 0.2472 |
| 66* | 16 | 21 | 37 | | | | | | |
| 69 | 16 | 20 | 36 | 0 | 2 | 2 | 0.8889 | −0.8889 | 0.4797 |
| 79 | 16 | 18 | 34 | 0 | 1 | 1 | 0.4706 | −0.4706 | 0.2491 |
| 82 | 16 | 17 | 33 | 1 | 2 | 3 | 1.4545 | −0.4545 | 0.7025 |
| 92 | 15 | 15 | 30 | 1 | 0 | 1 | 0.5000 | 0.5000 | 0.2500 |
| 102 | 14 | 15 | 29 | 0 | 1 | 1 | 0.4828 | −0.4828 | 0.2497 |
| 115 | 14 | 14 | 28 | 0 | 1 | 1 | 0.5000 | −0.5000 | 0.2500 |
| Total | | | | 5 | 14 | 19 | 8.8607 | −3.8607 | 4.6478 |
| | | | | $O_1$ | $O_2$ | | $E_1$ | $O_1 - E_1$ | $V$ |

NB: $E_2 = O_1 + O_2 - E_1 = 10.1393$

while the second, more precise, method gives

$$X^2 = \frac{(-3.8607)^2}{4.6478} = 3.207.$$

There is clearly a negligible difference here, and in general the first formula for the statistic $X^2$ will be satisfactory. It has the advantage of not requiring the calculation of the rather complicated variances.

Under the null hypothesis the statistic $X^2$ has a $\chi^2$ distribution with $m - 1$ degrees of freedom when there are $m$ groups of observations. Thus for the example we should compare the calculated value of $X^2$ with a $\chi^2$ distribution with 1 degree of freedom, which gives $P = 0.07$.

The logrank test can be carried out with more than two sets of data. The statistic $X^2$ is calculated using an extension of the first equation above with a term for each group. If we have $m$ groups we have

$$X^2 = \sum_{i=1}^{m} \frac{(O_i - E_i)^2}{E_i}.$$

The value of $X^2$ is compared with a $\chi^2$ distribution with $m - 1$ degrees of freedom. If there is a natural ordering of the groups, however, then a test for trend should be performed, as described below.

### 13.4.3 The logrank test for trend

With three or more ordered groups, a more appropriate test is to consider the possibility that there is a trend in survival across the groups. We may, for example, wish to compare age groups, or patients with different stages of cancer. This test is also appropriate for studying the possible effect of continuous variables which have been separated into three or more groups. The analysis is similar in principle to the Chi squared test for trend for a $2 \times k$ frequency table, described in section 10.8.2.

Using the method given in the previous section, we can obtain $O_g$ and $E_g$ for each group where $g$ denotes the group's number ($g = 1, 2, \ldots, m$). If we give a code $h_g$ to each group (not necessarily equally spaced), then we can calculate for each group

$$A_g = h_g(O_g - E_g); \qquad B_g = h_g E_g; \qquad C_g = h_g^2 E_g.$$

The test statistic for trend is obtained as

$$X^2_{trend} = \left(\sum A_g\right)^2 / V_T$$

where

$$V_T = \sum C_g - \left(\sum B_g\right)^2 \Big/ \sum E_g.$$

The test statistic $X^2_{trend}$ is compared with the $\chi^2$ distribution with one degree of freedom, however many groups are being analysed. Note that the statistic $X^2_{trend}$ must lie between zero and the usual logrank statistic $X^2$, which is used to evaluate general heterogeneity among the groups. Again the method is purely a hypothesis test.

An example is given by the survival data from 195 women with breast cancer shown in Figure 13.6. Women were divided into three groups according to whether they had no positive nodes, a few (1–3) or many (more than 3). The values of $O$ and $E$ for each group were as follows:

| Positive nodes | Number of women | Number of deaths ($O_g$) | Expected ($E_g$) | $O_g - E_g$ |
|---|---|---|---|---|
| none | 102 | 38 | 46.41 | −8.41 |
| few (1–3) | 58 | 26 | 25.21 | 0.79 |
| many (> 3) | 35 | 22 | 14.38 | 7.62 |

The usual logrank test on these data yields $X^2 = 5.59$ on 2 degrees of freedom (P = 0.06). However, the groups are ordered so the logrank test for trend should be used. If we give the groups codes of −1, 0 and 1, we get the following:

| Positive nodes | $A_g$ | $B_g$ | $C_g$ |
|---|---|---|---|
| none | 8.41 | −46.41 | 46.41 |
| few | 0.00 | 0.00 | 0.00 |
| many | 7.62 | 14.38 | 14.38 |
| Total | 16.03 | −32.03 | 60.77 |

(Note how the above choice of codes simplifies the arithmetic.)

From these values we can calculate $V_T = 60.77 - (-32.03)^2/86 = 48.84$ and $X^2_{trend} = 5.26$. Thus almost all of the variation among the groups can be attributed to a trend; the statistic $X^2_{trend}$ is compared with the Chi squared distribution with one degree of freedom, giving P = 0.02.

### 13.4.4 Stratified logrank test

We can combine data for subsets of subjects to get a more sensitive comparison of the groups of main interest. For example, if we are interested in comparing two groups given different treatments we may wish to stratify by age or some other prognostic variable, especially if the numbers of high risk subjects differ between the groups. The effect of stratification here is much the same as adjusting for other variables in a multiple regression analysis (see section 12.4). The same method can be used to combine data from independent trials of the same treatments. In either case the stratified analysis will be more reliable than an analysis simply pooling all the data.

The stratified logrank test is very simple. If we have two groups of subjects, then for each subgroup (stratum) of interest we calculate $O_1$, $E_1$, $O_2$ and $E_2$. These are then summed over all strata and the logrank statistic calculated as

$$X^2 = \frac{(\Sigma O_1 - \Sigma E_1)^2}{\Sigma E_1} + \frac{(\Sigma O_2 - \Sigma E_2)^2}{\Sigma E_2}.$$

If the null hypothesis is true the statistic $X^2$ has a $\chi^2$ distribution with $m - 1$ degrees of freedom, where there are $m$ groups.

### 13.4.5 The hazard ratio

As noted in section 13.3.2, the relative survival experience of two groups can be expressed as

$$R = \frac{O_1/E_1}{O_2/E_2}$$

which is termed the **hazard ratio**. We can calculate an approximate confidence interval for $\log_e R$ and so obtain a confidence interval for $R$ (Simon, 1986). We use the variance derived from the second formula given in section 13.4.2 and calculate

$$K = \frac{O_1 - E_1}{V}$$

which is an estimate of the log hazard ratio (and will be similar to the log of the observed hazard ratio). The standard error of this estimate is approximately $1/\sqrt{V}$, so a 95% confidence interval for $\log_e R$ is given by $K - 1.96/\sqrt{V}$ to $K + 1.96/\sqrt{V}$. A 95% confidence interval for $R$ is thus obtained easily by antilogging these values.

For the motion sickness data we had

$$O_1 = 5,\ E_1 = 8.8607,\ O_2 = 14,\ E_2 = 10.1393 \text{ and } V = 4.6478$$

so we have

$$R = \frac{5/8.8607}{14/10.1393} = 0.41;$$

$$K = \frac{5 - 8.8607}{4.6478} = -0.8307;$$

$$K - 1.96/\sqrt{4.6478} = -1.7398;$$
$$K + 1.96/\sqrt{4.6478} = 0.0785.$$

The 95% confidence interval for the hazard ratio $R$ is thus from $e^{-1.7398}$ to $e^{0.0785}$, that is from 0.18 to 1.08.

### 13.4.6 Comparison of survival probabilities

Using the method given in section 13.4.1 we can estimate the survival probability and its standard error at some time point separately for two independent groups of individuals, say $p_1$, $SE(p_1)$, $p_2$ and $SE(p_2)$. The standard error of $p_1 - p_2$ is, as usual, given by

$$SE(p_1 - p_2) = \sqrt{SE(p_1)^2 + SE(p_2)^2}.$$

A 95% confidence interval for the difference in survival proportions is thus given by

$$(p_1 - p_2) - 1.96SE(p_1 - p_2) \quad \text{to} \quad (p_1 - p_2) + 1.96SE(p_1 - p_2).$$

For example, we can compare the survival proportion at 60 minutes in the two motion sickness experiments. We have

$$p_1 = 0.855,\ SE(p_1) = 0.078,\ p_2 = 0.816 \text{ and } SE(p_2) = 0.074$$

so

$$p_1 - p_2 = 0.855 - 0.816 = 0.039$$

and

$$SE(p_1 - p_2) = \sqrt{0.078^2 + 0.074^2} = 0.1075,$$

and thus the 95% confidence interval for $p_1 - p_2$ at 60 minutes is

$$0.039 - 1.96 \times 0.1075 \quad \text{to} \quad 0.039 + 1.96 \times 0.1075,$$

that is, from −0.17 to 0.25. There is little apparent difference between the two sets of data at 60 minutes, although the logrank test showed some evidence of a difference overall.

### 13.4.7 Comparing median survival times

As I observed earlier, it is easy to derive an estimate of the median survival time from the Kaplan-Meier survival curve. Simon (1986) gives a method for calculating a confidence interval for the median survival time.

Simon also gives the following simple method for calculating an approximate confidence interval for the ratio of two independent estimated median survival times.

If $m_1$ and $m_2$ are the median survival times of two independent samples, the approximate 95% confidence interval is

$$\frac{m_1}{m_2} - e^{-1.96s} \quad \text{to} \quad \frac{m_1}{m_2} + e^{-1.96s}$$

where

$$s = \sqrt{\frac{1}{O_1} + \frac{1}{O_2}}.$$

The method assumes that the failure times have an **exponential distribution**; a quick check of this assumption is to see if each calculated median is similar to that expected if the assumption is true, namely the sum of the survival times (whether censored or not) divided by $\sqrt{2}$ times the number of events. For example, the observed median for the data in Table 13.3 is 115 minutes whereas the expected value if the distribution was exponential is $2356/(14\sqrt{2}) = 119$ minutes. We cannot compare the medians for the two motion sickness experiments, however, as we have no estimated median for the data in Table 13.2.

### 13.4.8 Comment

The most important part of survival analysis is to produce a plot of the survival curves for each group of interest, but assessment of possible differences should be based on statistical analysis. The logrank test is the most common form of statistical analysis, but it is a hypothesis test and yields no estimate of relative survival. None of the estimates proposed is without problems, but the hazard ratio is the most appealing as long as the curves suggest that the relative survival rates do not vary greatly over time. This would not be so, for example, for survival curves that crossed. The hazard ratio also gives a link with the more complex regression approach to the analysis of survival data, described in section 13.6, where an important assumption is that the hazard ratio is constant over time.

An assumption of all survival analyses is that there is no information in the times of censored observation. In the motion sickness example, we may question whether those individuals who requested an early stop to the experiments would have been near to being sick. There is a case here for regarding an early stop as a failure rather than as a censored observation.

## 13.5 INCORRECT ANALYSES

Peto *et al*. (1977) describe several incorrect approaches to the analysis of survival data, some of which are discussed below. Some others relate to clinical trials in general and are discussed in Chapter 15. I also explain why it is invalid to compare the survival of those who do or do not respond to treatment.

### 13.5.1 Summarizing survival

A common error is to summarize survival by the proportion of subjects still alive (or whatever) at some suitable time after the start of the study. For example, in a study of a beta-blocking drug given to men who had suffered a myocardial infarction (MI) (heart attack) we could calculate the proportion who had had another MI within a year of being on the drug. Apart from the arbitrary choice of one year, such an analysis ignores information about exactly how long the subjects survived without another attack and it will give a biased answer if, as is likely, not all subjects were followed up for a year. An even worse approach is to calculate the mean survival time, as this cannot provide a sensible answer when some of the survival times are censored.

The calculation of the median survival time is sensible, but it must be derived from the Kaplan-Meier curve, and not from the raw data unless there are no censored observations. The median survival time can easily be read from the plotted survival curve, being the time corresponding to a survival proportion of 0.5. Unfortunately, the sample median cannot be calculated unless the survival curve drops below 0.5, and even if it does it is an imprecise estimate of the median survival time in the population except in large samples.

### 13.5.2 Survival curves

The survival curve should be drawn as a 'step function' as in Figures 13.3 to 13.6; it is incorrect simply to join the estimated survival probabilities at each time of death with sloping lines.

Mistaken interpretation of survival curves often involves over-interpretation of the right-hand part of the curve. It is common for survival curves to flatten out after a while, as events become less frequent. It is unwise to intepret this flattening as meaningful unless there are many subjects still at risk. In contrast, if the last death occurs after the last censored time, not a rare occurrence, the survival curve will plunge to zero. We should not take this as an indication that nobody will survive beyond that time. When two survival curves are compared there is frequently a larger gap between the curves at the end of the period under study than at the beginning. This should not of itself be taken as an indication that the curves diverge. All of these situations often occur simply because the tail of the curve is very unstable due to small numbers at risk. There are two simple remedies: always show the numbers at risk at regular time intervals (e.g. every month or year, as appropriate) and curtail the survival curve when there are, say, only five subjects still at risk. The comparison of two survival curves should be based upon the methods already described, especially the logrank test using all the data, *not upon visual impression*.

This is an appropriate place to repeat the earlier warning about not comparing the proportions surviving a certain period when the time point for the comparison is chosen by inspecting the survival curves. The comparison is only valid if the time was chosen in advance of collecting the data.

### 13.5.3 Comparing responders and non-responders

In many clinical studies it is possible to categorize patients according to whether or not there is some observed response to treatment. For example, in cancer drug trials it is usual to see if the tumour has responded (shrunk) following treatment. It is then natural to wish to compare the survival of responders and non-responders. Unfortunately, this analysis is not valid (Oye and Shapiro, 1984) because the groups are defined by a factor not known at the start of treatment. The analysis is biased because the responders must have survived for a certain period in order to achieve a response. Also, the patients who respond may have been more likely to survive longer even if not treated. The fact that responders survive longer does not mean that the treatment is useful. Some cancer journals have specifically banned this type of analysis.

A better approach is to compare the survival of non-responders from the start of treatment with that of responders from the time of response. This analysis too may give misleading results, however (Simon and Makuch, 1984). Expert statistical advice is strongly recommended if this type of analysis is contemplated.

### 13.5.4 Multiple comparisons

As with other simple analyses (such as the $t$ test and correlation) the logrank test should be used with care when we wish to explore the relation of numerous variables to survival. While it is useful to see which variables seem to be associated with a better prognosis, these variables are likely to be correlated with each other too. Also, one variable in 20 will be significant and thus appear important just by chance. A better approach, therefore, is one that is analogous to multiple regression analysis; such an approach is described in the next section.

## 13.6 MODELLING SURVIVAL – THE COX REGRESSION MODEL

*(This section is more complex than the others in the book.)*

The logrank test is a non-parametric method for comparing the survival experience of two or more groups. It cannot be used to explore the effects of several variables on survival. The regression method introduced by Cox

(1972) is used widely when it is desired to investigate several variables at the same time. It is also known as **proportional hazards regression analysis**.

Cox's method is a 'semi-parametric' approach – no particular type of distribution is assumed for the survival times, but a strong assumption is made that the effects of the different variables on survival are constant over time and are additive in a particular scale. The actual method is too complex for detailed discussion in this book; this section is intended to give an introduction to the ideas of the method, which should help when reading the results of such analyses. There are many potential difficulties when performing Cox regression, and I do not recommend that the method is used by non-statisticians.

The **hazard function** is closely related to the survival curve, representing the risk of dying in a very short time interval after a given time, assuming survival thus far. It can therefore be interpreted as the risk of dying *at* time $t$. Cox's method is equivalent in its capability to multiple regression analysis as described in section 12.4, except that the regression model defines the hazard at a given time. If we have several independent variables of interest, say $X_1$ to $X_p$, we can express the hazard at time $t$, $h(t)$, as

$$h(t) = h_0(t) \times \exp(b_1X_1 + b_2X_2 + \ldots + b_pX_p).$$

The quantity $h_0(t)$ in the equation is estimated from the data, and clearly corresponds to the hazard when all the variables are zero (because $e^0 = 1$). It is called the **baseline** or **underlying hazard function**. The regression coefficients, $b_1$ to $b_p$, also have to be estimated. If we have just one variable of interest, such as age, then we have

$$h(t) = h_0(t) \times \exp(b_{age} \times age).$$

Under this model a proportional change in age, such as a 50% increase from 40 to 60 years, results in a proportional change in the log of the hazard. In practice the proportional hazards regression model is often found very suitable for modelling survival data, but the assumption of proportional hazards can and should be tested.

The hazard gives the risk of dying at time $t$, so we can add all the hazards up to time $t$ to get the risk of dying between time 0 and time $t$; this is called the **cumulative hazard**, $H(t)$. It is defined as

$$H(t) = H_0(t) \times \exp(b_1X_1 + b_2X_2 + \ldots + b_pX_p)$$

where $H_0(t)$ is the cumulative underlying hazard function. Because of the way $H(t)$ is calculated it can be shown that the probability of surviving to time $t$, $S(t)$, can be estimated by $\exp[-H(t)]$. We can thus estimate the survival probability for any individual with specific values of the variables in the model.

### 13.6.1 Interpretation

The Cox model must be fitted using an appropriate computer program. Some allow for stepwise selection of variables. The final model from a Cox regression analysis will yield an equation for the hazard as a function of several covariates. How can we interpret the results?

The selection of variables for inclusion in the model follows exactly the same lines as described in section 12.4. I shall thus assume that we have obtained a model and wish to interpret it, especially in relation to the prognosis of a new patient with certain values of the variables in the model (often called covariates).

Cox regression analysis was performed on the data from a long randomized trial comparing azathioprine and placebo in the treatment of patients with primary biliary cirrhosis (PBC). The chosen model included the six variables shown in Table 13.6, each of which was statistically significant at the 5% level at least. The model is shown in Table 13.7. An approximate

**Table 13.6** Variables included in Cox regression model fitted to data from a clinical trial comparing the effects of azathioprine and placebo on the survival of 216 patients with primary biliary cirrhosis (Christensen *et al.*, 1985). The second column shows the scoring of the variables used in the regression analysis

| Variable | Scoring |
|---|---|
| Serum bilirubin | $\log_{10}$(value in μmol/l) |
| Age | exp[(age in yrs − 20)/10] |
| Cirrhosis | 0 = No; 1 = Yes |
| Serum albumin | value in g/l |
| Central cholestasis | 0 = No; 1 = Yes |
| Therapy | 0 = Azathioprine; 1 = Placebo |

**Table 13.7** Cox regression model fitted to data from PBC trial of azathioprine versus placebo ($n = 216$)

| Variable | Regression coefficient ($b$) | $SE(b)$ | $e^b$ |
|---|---|---|---|
| Serum bilirubin | 2.510 | 0.316 | 12.31 |
| Age | 0.00690 | 0.00162 | 1.01 |
| Cirrhosis | 0.879 | 0.216 | 2.41 |
| Serum albumin | −0.0504 | 0.0181 | 0.95 |
| Central cholestasis | 0.679 | 0.275 | 1.97 |
| Therapy | 0.520 | 0.207 | 1.68 |

test of significance for each variable is obtained by dividing the regression estimate by its standard error and comparing the result with the standard Normal distribution.

The first feature to note in such a table is the sign of the regression coefficients. A positive sign means that the hazard is higher, and thus the prognosis worse, for subjects with higher values of that variable. Thus, from Table 13.7 higher serum bilirubin and age are associated with poorer survival, but higher values of serum albumin are beneficial. The three binary (0-1) variables show better prognosis for subjects without cirrhosis (not necessarily present in PBC) and without central cholestasis, and also for subjects treated with azathioprine rather than placebo.

An individual regression coefficient is interpreted quite easily. The ratio of the estimated hazards for two different values of a covariate $X$, say $x_1$ and $x_2$, with regression coefficient $b$, is given by

$$\frac{h_1(t)}{h_2(t)} = \frac{h_0(t) \times \exp(bx_1)}{h_0(t) \times \exp(bx_2)} = \exp(bx_1 - bx_2) = \exp[b(x_1 - x_2)].$$

Note that because of the assumption in the model this result is not dependent upon the choice of time $t$. Notice too that we do not need to know the value of the baseline hazard function, $h_0(t)$. In the special case where we have a binary variable coded 0 or 1 the hazard ratio is equal to $\exp(b)$ (see Table 13.7). Thus the estimated hazard with placebo is $\exp(0.52) = 1.68$ (or 168%) of that with azathioprine. Equivalently, the effect of azathioprine is to reduce the hazard to $\exp(-0.52) = 0.59$ (or 59%) of that with placebo. The effect on the survival probability, however, cannot be described simply as it depends on the patient's values of the other variables in the model, as described below. For continuous covariates the regression coefficient refers to the increase in log hazard for an increase of 1 in the value of the covariate. Because of the assumption of a linear effect this means that the estimated change in hazard of albumin increasing from 30 to 31 g/l is the same as a change from 40 to 41 g/l, and is equal to $\exp(-0.050) = 0.95$, i.e. a reduction of 5%. For serum bilirubin the value of $\exp(2.51)$ corresponds to the change in hazard for an increase of 1 in the log scale. Thus the estimated hazard increases 12.3 times if bilirubin is higher by a factor of 10. Notice that the estimated hazard ratio $\exp(b)$ is analogous to that described in section 13.3.2. The difference is that this hazard ratio is adjusted for the effects of the other variables in the model.

As with ordinary multiple linear regression and logistic regression (both discussed in Chapter 12), the combination of regression coefficients and values of variables can be used as a prognostic index. The part of the equation for the hazard function within brackets gives a prognostic index (PI) as

$$\text{PI} = b_1X_1 + b_2X_2 + \ldots + b_pX_p.$$

The hazard and the estimated survival probability at any time depend only upon PI, not upon the values of the individual variables. Because the survival probability at time $t$ is $S(t) = \exp[-H(t)]$ we have

$$S(t) = \exp[-H_0(t) \times \exp(\text{PI})].$$

The cumulative underlying hazard function, $H_0(t)$, is a step function over time, and should be given in the output of the computer program. We can thus express $S(t)$ as a step function too. Some programs may instead give the survival function corresponding to $H_0(t)$, i.e. $S_0(t) = \exp[-H_0(t)]$. The survival function for any set of covariates is given by

$$S(t) = S_0(t)^{\exp(\text{PI})}.$$

Figure 13.7 shows estimated survival curves for patients given azathioprine and placebo, based on the model shown in Table 13.7 and setting all other variables to their mean values. The relation between survival probability and prognosis can be examined by fixing $t$ in the last equation, perhaps at a few values of interest. Figure 13.8 shows estimated 2, 5 and 8 year survival probability as a function of PI derived from the PBC trial. For any new patient it is easy to estimate the probability of surviving a given time. Unfortunately, it is difficult to calculate a confidence interval for the estimated survival probability.

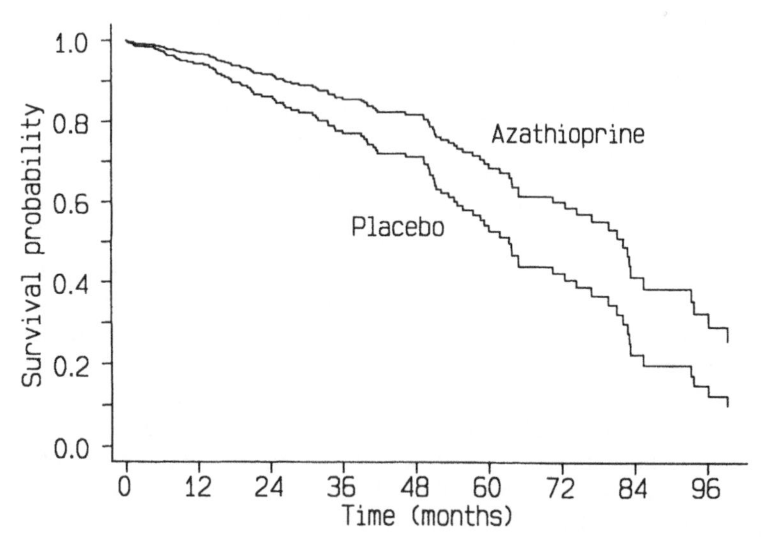


**Figure 13.7** Estimated survival curves for patients treated with azathioprine or placebo based on the Cox model in Table 13.7 (from Christensen *et al.*, 1985).

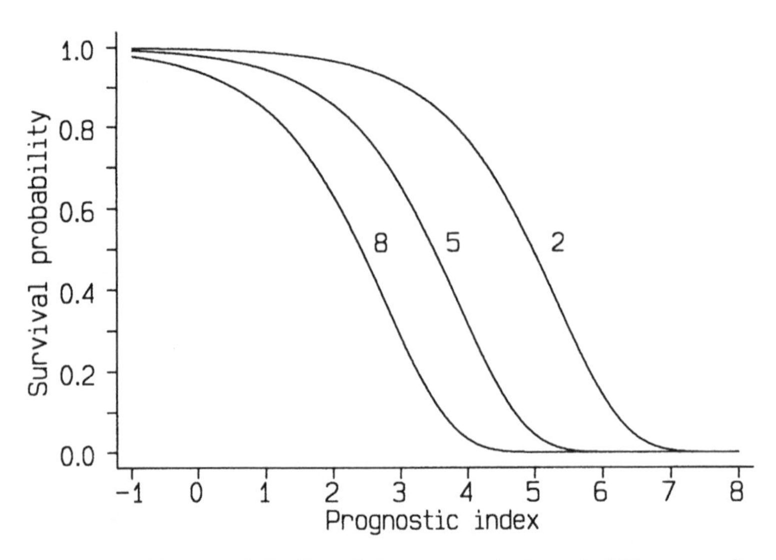


**Figure 13.8** Estimated 2, 5 and 8 year survival probability as a function of the prognostic index (PI) in the trial of azathioprine versus placebo. Note that the therapy given is incorporated in PI (from Christensen *et al.*, 1985).

### 13.6.2 Technical note

With ordinary multiple regression (section 12.4) the assumption of a linear relation between the outcome and predictor variables is easily examined by scatter diagrams. Because of the censoring of some survival times we cannot use the same approach here, nor can we calculate residuals in the usual way. A general discussion of assessing the goodness-of-fit of the Cox model is beyond the scope of this chapter. However, some brief comments can be made regarding the possible transformation of predictor variables (covariates). There are ways to examine the linearity of effect on the hazard function. The transformations of age and bilirubin seen in Table 13.7 were based on such considerations. Where linearity of effect is in doubt it may be preferable to divide the ordered values into three or more equally sized groups. The variable can then be entered into the model as two or more dummy variables or the group codes can be used to test for trend.

Also, if a variable has a highly skewed distribution the extreme values will exert an undue influence on the choice of model. We might therefore wish to take logarithms to reduce the effect of extreme values. The bilirubin data from the PBC trial were shown in Figure 4.10 to have a highly skewed Lognormal distribution. In this study log transformation was indicated for the bilirubin data on both counts.

### 13.6.3 Comment

Non-technical discussion of Cox regression is given by Elashoff (1983) and Tibshirani (1982). A more detailed but fairly non-mathematical explanation is given by Christensen (1987), who also considers the more complicated model in which the values of the covariates may themselves vary over time. Expert statistical advice should be sought for carrying out Cox regression on survival data.

## 13.7 DESIGN OF SURVIVAL STUDIES

When the main outcome of interest is survival time, planning of a study should include some special considerations. It is most important to realize that the power of a test to compare survival in two or more groups is related not to the total sample size but to the number of events of interest such as deaths. When there is a small risk of the event of interest a vast study may be needed. One way to increase the power of a study is therefore to consider taking a more common event as the end-point of the study, such as using either recurrence of the original condition or death rather than death alone. (Many reports of studies of cancer patients give separate analyses relating to both time to recurrence and time to death.) Other ways to increase power are to increase the total sample size and to extend the length of follow-up of each subject. For example, the PBC trial just discussed had a six year period during which patients were recruited to the trial, and a further six years' follow-up. Thus patients were potentially followed for between 6 and 12 years. Even then it was only possible to get adequate numbers by recruiting patients in several countries. Of the 216 patients included in the final analysis only 105 had died, which is not a large number when the power of the study is considered.

Because of the various effects described, it is not simple to calculate the appropriate sample size for survival time studies. Machin and Campbell (1987) give tables and Schoenfeld and Richter (1982) give a nomogram for calculating sample size.

Apart from these considerations the design of studies with survival time as the end-point are subject to the same considerations as other studies. Chapters 5 and 15 discuss design, and Peto *et al*. (1976) is a valuable paper to read in conjunction with their description of the analysis of such studies (Peto *et al*., 1977).

## 13.8 PRESENTATION OF RESULTS

Studies of survival require special consideration with respect to the presentation of the results. Graphical display is especially important for survival data. The suggestions below are in addition to those that may apply more generally, for example for clinical trials, described in other chapters.

### 13.8.1 Numerical presentation

The distribution of the length of follow-up of subjects should be given; the range will probably suffice. It may mislead to quote only the maximum follow-up period. It is also useful to indicate the numbers of failures of each type of interest (e.g. deaths and recurrences of disease), separately for different groups of subjects if this is relevant.

The results of logrank tests should be given as the observed ($O$) and expected ($E$) numbers of failures as well as the test statistic ($X^2$) and P.

### 13.8.2 Graphical display

Graphs of survival curves are enormously valuable. These should be based on the Kaplan-Meier method, or perhaps the life table method for data grouped by time interval. Kaplan-Meier survival curves should be drawn as step functions, as in this chapter. It is helpful to use different line types (e.g., solid, dashed) for different groups of subjects. For small studies it is possible to mark the times of censored observations by ticks on the survival curve. More generally, it is useful to show the numbers still at risk at regular intervals, for example every month or year, as appropriate. These can be shown beneath the time scale or along the top of the graph.

To avoid misinterpretation of the unreliable right-hand part of the survival curve it is advisable to terminate the curves when the number of subjects still at risk is small, say five. This also has the benefit of expanding the left-hand part of the curve which contains the important information.

## EXERCISES

13.1 In view of the comment in section 13.4.8, carry out a logrank test to compare the motion sickness data in Tables 13.2 and 13.3, taking an event (failure) as either vomiting or stopping before 120 minutes. Compare the results with those given in section 13.3.1.

13.2 Exercise 11.1 included survival times of 29 patients with lactic acidosis, together with some possibly prognostic variables.

(a) What problem is there with these data regarding a Kaplan-Meier plot of survival?
(b) How could logrank tests be used to assess the possible relation between the three variables and survival time? Perform such tests.
(c) Compare the results of Cox regression analyses using these

variables as they are or each divided into three roughly equal groups.

13.3 Exercise 12.3 showed data relating various factors to the occurrence of acute graft-versus-host disease (GvHD) in 37 patients having a bone marrow transplant. Backward stepwise Cox regression analysis using diagnosis, recipient's age and sex, donor's age and sex, whether the donor had been pregnant, MECLR/MLR index and GvHD to predict survival yields the following model:

| Variable | Regression coefficient | Standard error |
|---|---|---|
| GvHD (0 = No, 1 = Yes) | 2.306 | 0.5898 |
| CML (0 = No, 1 = Yes) | −2.508 | 0.8095 |

(a) What is the interpretation of the opposite signs for the regression coefficients?
(b) Calculate the relative risks of dying (hazard ratio) for the following patients relative to non-GvHD non-CML patients:
 (i) with GvHD but not CML,
 (ii) CML but without GvHD,
 (iii) CML and GvHD.
(c) Calculate the 95% confidence interval for the hazard ratio associated with GvHD
(d) Comment on the reliability of the Cox regression model in view of the sample size (37) and number of deaths (18).

# 14

# Some common problems in medical research

> Omniscient as statisticians are, their ability to diagnose abnormality is not generally acknowledged by the medical community, and indeed they usually refrain from claiming it.
>
> Oldham (1979)

> A picture may be worth a thousand *t* tests.
>
> Cooper and Zangwill (1989)

## 14.1 INTRODUCTION

The methods of analysis described in Chapters 9 to 13 cover a high proportion of the methods used in medical research. None is specific to medical data, although survival analysis is much more common in medical research than in other fields. There are some types of medical investigation, however, that are not covered by these methods. Epidemiological studies in particular require many statistical techniques that are not used much in other fields. There are many books devoted to epidemiological methods.

This chapter covers a small miscellany of common medical problems that need a special approach – method comparison studies, observer agreement studies, diagnostic tests and the calculation of reference ranges. These methods have in common the absence of any complicated mathematics. Their difficulties lie in requiring a clear understanding of the aim of the analysis, and in the interpretation of the results. Also considered is the analysis of data that comprise a series of measurements on each subject, for which a simple approach is also recommended. Lastly, there is a brief introduction to the investigation of cyclic variation.

## 14.2 METHOD COMPARISON STUDIES

Most clinical measurements are not precise. Either it is not possible to measure directly the quantity of interest, such as heart volume or tumour size, or the measurement, although direct, is difficult to make, such as arm circumference. Further, the variable may change with time, such as peak expiratory flow rate or blood pressure.

Because of these uncertainties there is usually a variety of techniques available and studies comparing two (or more) methods are common. The aim of these studies is usually to see if the methods 'agree' well enough for one method to replace the other, or perhaps for the two methods to be used interchangeably. For example, we may wish to see if a new cheap and/or quick method gives results that agree with those of an existing expensive, slow method. The same considerations apply to studies comparing two observers using one method. Note that we need to define what we mean by agreement. Also, we are concerned with the degree of agreement, so that this problem is one of *estimation* rather than hypothesis testing.

Put simply, the best approach to this type of data is to analyse the differences between the measurements by the two methods on each subject. A fuller discussion of method comparison studies is given by Bland and Altman (1986).

### 14.2.1 Analysis

Table 14.1 shows measurements of transmitral volumetric flow (MF) by Doppler echocardiography and left ventricular stroke volume (SV) by cross-sectional echocardiography in 21 patients without aortic valve disease. The researchers expected these measurements to be the same in such patients, but to differ in patients with aortic regurgitation. They thus first wished to see how well MF and SV agreed in patients without aortic valve disease. Figure 14.1 shows a scatter diagram of the data. If the methods agreed exactly the points would all lie on the line of equality, but of course real data never agree exactly. We can see, however, that all these data points are quite near to the line of equality. An alternative, more informative plot is shown in Figure 14.2. Here the differences between the methods (SV−MF) have been plotted against the average of the two measurements. There are several advantages of this plot. We can see the size of differences much more easily and also their distribution around zero, and we can check visually that the differences are not related to the *size* of the measurement. For this purpose the average acts as our best estimate of the unknown true value. Section 14.2.2 describes what we do when the scatter of the differences gets wider as the mean increases. Figure 14.2 shows no such problem, so we can investigate the differences further. We can construct a histogram, and can calculate the mean and standard deviation, which are $-0.24\ \text{cm}^3$ and $6.96\ \text{cm}^3$. We could use a one sample $t$ test of the differences against zero (or, equivalently, a paired $t$ test on the original data) to see if the mean difference is significantly different

**Table 14.1** Transmitral volumetric flow (MF) and left ventricular stroke volume (SV) in 21 patients without aortic valve disease (Zhang *et al.*, 1986). Data (in $cm^3$) in order of MF values

| Patient | MF | SV |
|---|---|---|
| 1 | 47 | 43 |
| 2 | 66 | 70 |
| 3 | 68 | 72 |
| 4 | 69 | 81 |
| 5 | 70 | 60 |
| 6 | 70 | 67 |
| 7 | 73 | 72 |
| 8 | 75 | 72 |
| 9 | 79 | 92 |
| 10 | 81 | 76 |
| 11 | 85 | 85 |
| 12 | 87 | 82 |
| 13 | 87 | 90 |
| 14 | 87 | 96 |
| 15 | 90 | 82 |
| 16 | 100 | 100 |
| 17 | 104 | 94 |
| 18 | 105 | 98 |
| 19 | 112 | 108 |
| 20 | 120 | 131 |
| 21 | 132 | 131 |
| Mean | 86.0 | 85.8 |
| SD | 20.3 | 21.2 |

from zero, but it is more important to quantify the variability of the individual data points.

The question being asked relates to how well the methods agree, and there are two components to the answer. Firstly, the mean difference is an estimate of the average *bias* of one method relative to the other. Here the mean is negligible and we can say that the methods agree excellently *on average*. Secondly, it is essential to consider also how well the methods are likely to agree *for an individual*, for which purpose we use the standard deviation of the differences. Although we could simply quote the standard deviation of the differences ($s_{diff}$) as a measure of agreement (or disagreement), it is more useful to use the standard deviation to construct a range of values which we expect to cover the agreement between the methods for most subjects.

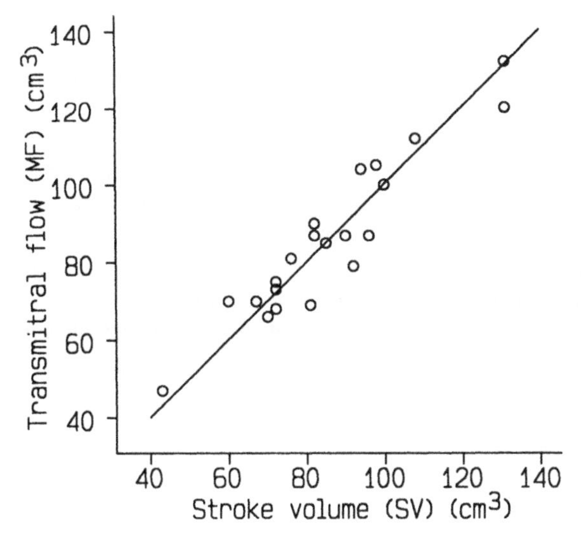


**Figure 14.1** Transmitral volumetric flow (MF) and left ventricular stroke volume (SV). Data from Zhang *et al*. (1986).

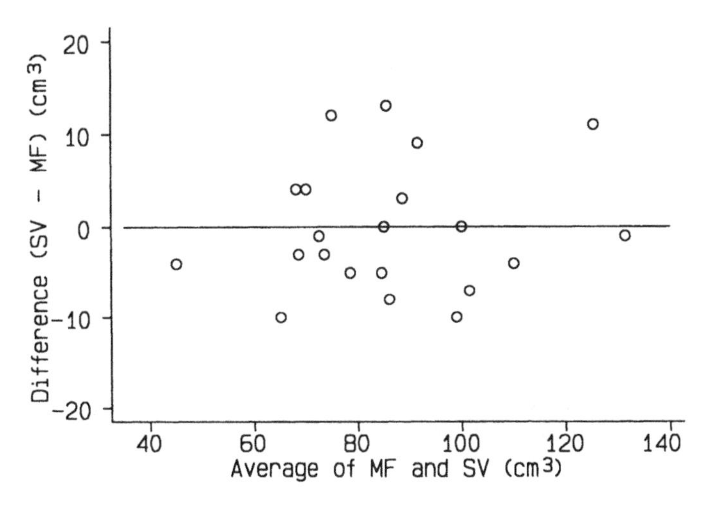


**Figure 14.2** Difference between transmitral volumetric flow and left ventricular stroke volume (SV–MF) plotted against average, (MF + SV)/2.

We saw in section 3.4 that for reasonably symmetric distributions we expect the range mean ±2SD to include about 95% of the observations. For a method comparison study we can therefore take mean $\pm 2s_{diff}$ as a 95% range of agreement for individuals. This range of values defines the 95% **limits of agreement**. For the present data we get a range from

$$-0.24 - 2 \times 6.96 \quad \text{to} \quad -0.24 + 2 \times 6.96$$

which is −14.2 to +13.7 cm$^3$. In other words, for a new subject we expect the two methods to give measurements that differ by less than 14 cm$^3$, with any discrepancy being equally likely in either direction.

The researchers also compared MF and SV in 25 patients with aortic valve disease. Figure 14.3 compares the differences between the methods for patients with or without disease. For only two of the 25 patients with aortic valve disease was SV–MF within the 95% limits of agreement for patients without disease, supporting the researchers' expectations.

The interpretation of the mean and standard deviation of the differences must depend upon the clinical circumstances – it is not possible to use statistics to define acceptable agreement.

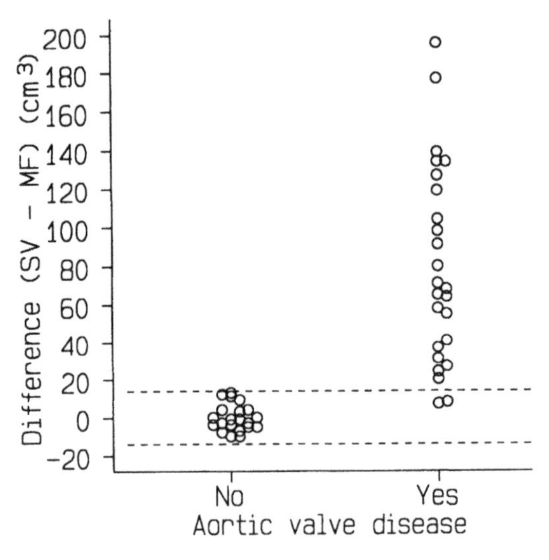


**Figure 14.3** Differences between SV and MF for patients with or without aortic valve disease, showing 95% limits of agreement for patients without disease.

### 14.2.2 Variable agreement (relation between difference and mean)

Sometimes a plot of the differences between two methods against the average shows that there is a wider scatter as the average increases. In other words, the standard deviation of the differences increases. Although the approach given in the previous section may not be unreasonable, a better analysis is often obtained by taking logs of the data before calculating the limits of agreement. Here we are implicitly considering the differences between methods to be an approximately constant *proportion* of the size of the measurement. As with other uses of the log transformation described in previous chapters, we perform the usual analysis on the logs of the data and then back-transform the results. Antilogs of the limits of agreement thus give us a range of *proportional* agreement between the methods. For example, we may conclude that for a new subject method A will be likely to give a value between 80% and 130% of that obtained by Method B. Bland and Altman (1986) discuss this type of analysis, and give a worked example.

### 14.2.3 Repeatability

An important aspect of method comparison is the comparison of the repeatability of each method. If we have two (or more) measurements of the same subjects by each method then we can assess the similarity of the duplicate measurements made using the same technique. For paired observations we simply calculate the standard deviation of the differences between the pairs of measurements using the same method. We can then compare the standard deviations to see which method is more repeatable. Each standard deviation can also be used to calculate limits within which we expect the differences between two measurements by the same method to lie. Bland and Altman (1986) give a worked example.

Replicate measurements are rarely made in method comparison studies, so that an important aspect of comparability is often overlooked. A method with poor repeatability will never agree well with another method.

### 14.2.4 Erroneous analyses

Method comparison studies are frequently mis-analysed. In particular, the correlation between the values by the two methods is often calculated, with a high value of $r$ interpreted as an indication of good agreement. There are several reasons why correlation is an inappropriate analysis. Firstly, the correlation coefficient is a measure of the strength of *linear association* between two variables, which is not the same as a measure of *agreement*. As we have seen, agreement should be assessed in terms directly related to the measurements. It is not possible to interpret, say, $r = 0.92$ in the same way as the limits of agreement. Secondly, we may have a high degree of correlation when the agreement is clinically poor. For example, in a study of the variability of knee circumference measurements Kirwan *et al*. (1979) found that the repeatability of measurements made 15 cm above the patella by two observers was far too poor for the measurement to be clinically valuable. Nevertheless, there was a correlation of 0.99 between the observers' readings. A high value of $r$ can be obtained because, as in their study, there is large variation between subjects. It is clearly not reasonable to assess agreement by a statistical method that is highly sensitive to the choice of the sample of subjects. Similar criticisms can be levelled at the use of regression analysis for assessing agreement.

Another common incorrect analysis is the comparison of means by a hypothesis test, often a paired $t$ test. We cannot deduce that methods agree well because they are not significantly different. Indeed a high scatter of differences may well lead to an important difference in means (bias) being non-significant. Using this approach worse agreement decreases the chance of finding a significant difference and so increases the chance that the methods will appear to agree!

### 14.2.5 Presentation

Comparing methods of measurement is very simple and informative using the approach of section 14.2.1. The mean difference and limits of agreement give an excellent summary of the data. It is useful to have one or two plots as well, especially one showing the difference against the mean, on which the other values can be superimposed as three horizontal lines. A plot of the raw data, such as in Figure 14.1, should be square and should show the line of equality.

### 14.2.6 Discussion

We should remember the limitations of this type of analysis. We cannot tell which method is nearer to the 'truth' because we do not usually know the true values. Nor for unreplicated studies can we compare the repeatability of different methods of measurement. It is important to realize that if one method is either inaccurate or has poor repeatability (or both) comparison with any other method will inevitably show poor agreement, however good the second method is. Thus we should not infer from poor agreement that *both* methods are poor. In contrast, good agreement is most unlikely unless we have two methods that are both accurate and repeatable.

Care should be taken with the design of method comparison studies. The sample size should be large enough to allow the limits of agreement to be estimated well. We can calculate confidence intervals for the limits of agreement, and these will be wide in small samples. Thus a sample size of at least 50, but preferably rather larger, is desirable for a method comparison study. It is definitely valuable to take two measurements on each subject by each method, so that the repeatability of the two methods can be compared. The analysis can then be based on the average of the two replicates, but a correction must then be made to the standard deviation of the differences to allow for this fact (Bland and Altman, 1986). It is most undesirable for the two techniques being compared to be carried out by different observers. Any systematic variation between observers (a common phenomenon) will be inseparable from any difference between methods. This may be necessary, however, when the techniques involve considerable skill and experience.

As indicated by the knee circumference example, we can use the same statistical approach for studies of observer comparability. We cannot, though, use this method when comparing assessments in categories as opposed to measurements. Section 14.3 considers such problems, which usually arise in observer comparisons rather than method comparisons.

## 14.3 INTER-RATER AGREEMENT

Agreement between categorical assessments is usually considered as a problem of comparing the ability of different raters (observers) to classify subjects into one of several groups. The approach outlined below does, however, also apply to studies that compare two alternative categorization schemes, that is, a method comparison study for categorical data. I shall consider an example of each.

Table 14.2 shows the classification by two radiologists of 85 xeromammograms as 'Normal', 'Benign disease', 'Suspicion of cancer' or 'Cancer'. The data come from a larger study of nine radiologists (Boyd *et al.*, 1982). As with the comparison of continuous data discussed in the previous section, we require some measure of agreement rather than association. Thus we do not use the $\chi^2$ test, both because we do not wish to assess association and also because this is not a hypothesis testing problem. (Further, the data are paired).

**Table 14.2** Assessments of 85 xeromammograms by two radiologists (Boyd *et al.*, 1982)

| | Radiologist B | | | | |
|---|---|---|---|---|---|
| Radiologist A | Normal | Benign | Suspected cancer | Cancer | Total |
| Normal | 21 | 12 | 0 | 0 | 33 |
| Benign | 4 | 17 | 1 | 0 | 22 |
| Suspected cancer | 3 | 9 | 15 | 2 | 29 |
| Cancer | 0 | 0 | 0 | 1 | 1 |
| Total | 28 | 38 | 16 | 3 | 85 |

### 14.3.1 Measuring agreement

The simplest approach to assessing agreement is simply to see how many exact agreements were observed, which here is $21 + 17 + 15 + 1 = 54$.

There is thus agreement for 54/85 = 0.64 (64%) of the films. There are two weaknesses of this simple calculation. Firstly, it takes no account of where in the table the agreement was, and secondly, we would expect some agreement between the radiologists by chance even if they were guessing. We can get a more reasonable answer by considering the agreement in excess of the amount of agreement that we would expect by chance.

We saw in section 10.3 that the expected frequency in a cell of a frequency table (under the null hypothesis of no association) is the product of the total of the relevant column and the total of the relevant row divided by the grand total. Thus the expected frequencies along the diagonal in Table 14.2 are

| | | |
|---|---|---|
| Normal | $33 \times 28/85 =$ | 10.87 |
| Benign disease | $22 \times 38/85 =$ | 9.84 |
| Suspected cancer | $29 \times 16/85 =$ | 5.46 |
| Cancer | $1 \times 3/85 =$ | 0.04 |
| Total | | 26.20 |

So the number of agreements expected just by chance is 26.2, which as a proportion of the total is 26.2/85 = 0.31. The question, therefore, is how much better were the radiologists than 0.31. The maximum agreement is 1.00, so we can express the radiologists' agreement as a proportion of the possible scope for doing better than chance, which is 1.00 – 0.31. We thus calculate the agreement as

$$\frac{0.64 - 0.31}{1.00 - 0.31} = 0.47.$$

The name for this measure of agreement is **kappa**, written $\kappa$. It has a maximum of 1.00 when agreement is perfect, a value of zero indicates no agreement better than chance, and negative values show worse than chance agreement, which is unlikely in this context.

How do we interpret values between 0 and 1, such as 0.47? While no absolute definitions are possible the following guidelines (slightly adapted from Landis and Koch, 1977) should help:

| Value of $\kappa$ | Strength of agreement |
|---|---|
| < 0.20 | Poor |
| 0.21–0.40 | Fair |
| 0.41–0.60 | Moderate |
| 0.61–0.80 | Good |
| 0.81–1.00 | Very good |

We can thus say that there was moderate agreement between the radiologists. It is of some interest that these two observers showed the best agreement of any pair of observers in the study.

The reduction of the data to a single number inevitably yields an answer that is not terribly meaningful without examination of the table of frequencies. In practice, any value of $\kappa$ much below 0.5 will indicate poor agreement, although the degree of acceptable agreement must depend upon circumstances. There is no substitute for inspecting the table of frequencies, because many different tables will yield similar values of $\kappa$.

An example of the comparison of alternative methods of categorical assessment is given by the data in Table 14.3. The aim of the study was to compare a radioallergosorbent (RAST) test and a multi-RAST (MAST) test on sera for specific IgE as a test of allergy in subjects for whom prick tests cannot be used. The MAST was a new, simpler and cheaper method.

As Table 14.3 shows, there was considerable disagreement between the methods, with some samples in nearly all the cells of the table. The value of $\kappa$ for Table 14.3 is 0.32, confirming the visual impression.

Section 14.3.4 shows the mathematical expression for calculating $\kappa$.

**Table 14.3** Comparison of RAST and MAST methods of testing serum for allergies (Brostoff *et al.*, 1984)

| | RAST | | | | | |
|---|---|---|---|---|---|---|
| | Negative | Weak | Moderate | High | Very high | Total |
| MAST | 1 | 2 | 3 | 4 | 5 | |
| Negative (1) | 86 | 3 | 14 | 0 | 2 | 105 |
| Weak (2) | 26 | 0 | 10 | 4 | 0 | 40 |
| Moderate (3) | 20 | 2 | 22 | 4 | 1 | 49 |
| High (4) | 11 | 1 | 37 | 16 | 14 | 79 |
| Very high (5) | 3 | 0 | 15 | 24 | 48 | 90 |
| Total | 146 | 6 | 98 | 48 | 65 | 363 |

### 14.3.2 Confidence interval

We can obtain a standard error for $\kappa$, and thus a confidence interval. In general this is not all that useful because unless the sample is small the confidence interval will be narrow and thus will not allow for much variation in interpretation. For the radiologists' assessments we had $\kappa = 0.47$ and can calculate $se(\kappa) = 0.07$, so that a 95% confidence interval for $\kappa$ is given by 0.33 to 0.61. For the rather larger MAST/RAST study $\kappa$ was 0.32 with a 95% confidence interval from 0.26 to 0.38. The method of calculation is given in section 14.3.4.

### 14.3.3 Weighted kappa

A weakness of the kappa statistic is that it takes no account of the degree of disagreement – all disagreements are treated equally. Where the categories are ordered, as is often the case, it may be preferable to give different **weights** to disagreements according to the magnitude of the discrepancy. Here observations near to the diagonal, representing a difference of only one category, are considered less serious than those where the discrepancy is two or three categories.

We can build this idea into the calculation of $\kappa$ to get a quantity called **weighted kappa**. For the MAST-RAST study weighted kappa is $\kappa_w = 0.56$, somewhat better than the unweighted $\kappa = 0.32$. Similarly, weighted kappa for the radiologists' assessments is $\kappa_w = 0.57$ compared with unweighted $\kappa = 0.47$. Weighted kappa is usually higher than unweighted kappa because disagreements are more likely to be by only one category than by several categories.

### 14.3.4 Mathematics for kappa

*(This section can be omitted without loss of continuity.)*

Kappa is calculated from the observed and expected frequencies on the diagonal of a square table of frequencies. If there are $n$ observations in $g$ categories, then the observed proportional agreement is

$$p_o = \sum_{i=1}^{g} f_{ii}/n$$

where $f_{ii}$ is the number of agreements for category $i$. The expected proportion of agreements by chance is given by

$$p_e = \sum_{i=1}^{g} r_i c_i/n^2$$

where $r_i$ and $c_i$ are the row and column totals for the $i$th category. The index of agreement, kappa, is given by

$$\kappa = \frac{p_o - p_e}{1 - p_e}.$$

The approximate standard error of $\kappa$ is

$$se(\kappa) = \sqrt{\frac{p_o(1 - p_o)}{n(1 - p_e)^2}}$$

so that a 95% confidence interval for the population value of $\kappa$ is given by

$$\kappa - 1.96\, se(\kappa) \quad \text{to} \quad \kappa + 1.96\, se(\kappa).$$

**Weighted kappa** is obtained by giving weights to the frequencies in each cell of the table according to their distance from the diagonal that indicates agreement. For the cell in row $i$ and column $j$, with observed frequency $f_{ij}$, a weight is calculated as

$$w_{ij} = 1 - \frac{|i - j|}{g - 1}.$$

Thus we give cells on the diagonal a weight of 1, while those where the difference is by one category get a weight of $1 - 1/(g - 1)$. For the MAST-RAST data weights for discrepancies of 0, 1, 2, 3 and 4 are thus 1, 0.75, 0.5, 0.25 and 0 respectively.

The weighted observed and expected proportional agreement are obtained as

$$p_{o(w)} = \frac{1}{n} \sum_{i=1}^{g} \sum_{j=1}^{g} w_{ij} f_{ij}$$

and

$$p_{e(w)} = \frac{1}{n^2} \sum_{i=1}^{g} \sum_{j=1}^{g} w_{ij} r_i c_j$$

and weighted kappa is given by

$$\kappa_w = \frac{p_{o(w)} - p_{e(w)}}{1 - p_{e(w)}}.$$

Fleiss (1981, p. 223) shows how to calculate the standard error of weighted kappa.

### 14.3.5 Discussion

As with other methods of looking at small, square frequency tables, there are difficulties associated with the use and interpretation of kappa. The most often cited problem is that the value of kappa depends upon the proportion of subjects (prevalence) in each category. This can be seen most clearly using a simple artificial example, where we have only two categories. Table 14.4 shows two tables with the same proportional agreement of 0.8, but with different proportions in the two categories (+ and −) and with markedly different values of $\kappa$. The reason for the difference is that the chance expected frequencies are very different, as shown in Table 14.5. The consequence of this property of $\kappa$ is that it is misleading to compare values of $\kappa$ from different studies where the prevalences of the categories differ. For larger tables the same is true, but it is even more complicated to judge comparability.

**Table 14.4** Comparison of two observers' diagnoses with different prevalences in the two categories

(a)

| | | Observer 1 + | − | Total |
|---|---|---|---|---|
| Observer 2 | + | 70 | 10 | 80 |
| | − | 10 | 10 | 20 |
| | Total | 80 | 20 | 100 |

$\kappa = 0.38$

(b)

| | | Observer 1 + | − | Total |
|---|---|---|---|---|
| Observer 2 | + | 40 | 10 | 50 |
| | − | 10 | 40 | 50 |
| | Total | 50 | 50 | 100 |

$\kappa = 0.60$

**Table 14.5** Expected frequencies corresponding to the data in Table 14.4

(a)

| | | Observer 1 + | − | Total |
|---|---|---|---|---|
| Observer 2 | + | 64 | 16 | 80 |
| | − | 16 | 4 | 20 |
| | Total | 80 | 20 | 100 |

(b)

| | | Observer 1 + | − | Total |
|---|---|---|---|---|
| Observer 2 | + | 25 | 25 | 50 |
| | − | 25 | 25 | 50 |
| | Total | 50 | 50 | 100 |

Another problem is that $\kappa$ depends on the *number* of categories. The data in Table 14.3 can be grouped into three rather than five categories; 0, 1 or 2, 3 or 4. For the resulting $3 \times 3$ table we find $\kappa = 0.42$, compared with $\kappa = 0.32$ for the full $5 \times 5$ table. If we consider that the methods are really only going to be used to categorize samples as negative (0) or positive (1, 2, 3 or 4) we can collapse the data into a $2 \times 2$ table, for which $\kappa = 0.53$, not wonderful but better than $\kappa = 0.32$.

Despite these shortcomings, the use of kappa is becoming common for data like the examples discussed. It is undoubtedly the right type of approach. Incorrect analyses of such data are still common, however. The MAST-RAST data were analysed by calculating the correlation coefficient (Brostoff *et al.*, 1984). The authors concluded from the value of $r = 0.72$ that the methods gave similar results and recommended the use of the simpler and cheaper MAST methods. Not only is Pearson's correlation coefficient unsuitable for ordinal data but, as we saw in section 14.2.4, it is an inappropriate approach to judge agreement. Nor is their conclusion compatible with the data shown in Table 14.3. Similarly, it would be incorrect to judge agreement by a $\chi^2$ test, which is also a test of association. The kappa statistic, which may be interpreted as the *chance-corrected proportional agreement*, is the best approach to this type of problem, but it is important to show the raw data if at all possible. Acceptable agreement depends upon the circumstances. There is no value of kappa that can be regarded universally as indicating good agreement – statistics cannot provide a simple substitute for clinical judgement.

## 14.4 DIAGNOSTIC TESTS

Diagnosis is an essential part of clinical practice, and much medical research is carried out to try to improve methods of diagnosis. The statistical analysis of these studies is fairly simple, but causes difficulty because of unfamiliar and confusing terminology.

The simplest case to consider is that where patients can be classified into two groups according to the results of an investigation, perhaps an X-ray or biopsy, or the presence or absence of a symptom or sign. An example is given in Table 14.6, which shows the relation between the results of liver scans and diagnosis based on either autopsy, biopsy or surgical inspection. The question of interest here is how good is the liver scan at diagnosis of abnormal pathology. While we could simply calculate the agreement between the two classifications using the methods described in section 14.3, this problem is different because of the asymmetry of the relation between the two classifications. We wish to describe the ability of the scan to diagnose the true patient status. In practice we rarely know the truth, and so evaluate the test in relation to the diagnosis. This distinction is considered further in section 14.4.7.

**Table 14.6** Relation between results of liver scan and diagnosis in 344 patients (Drum and Christacapoulos, 1972)

| | Pathology | | |
|---|---|---|---|
| | Abnormal | Normal | Total |
| Liver scan | (+) | (−) | |
| Abnormal (+) | 231 | 32 | 263 |
| Normal (−) | 27 | 54 | 81 |
| Total | 258 | 86 | 344 |

### 14.4.1 Sensitivity and specificity

One approach is to calculate the proportions of patients with normal and abnormal liver scans who are likewise 'diagnosed' by the scan. The terms **positive** and **negative** refer to the presence or absence of the condition of interest, here abnormal pathology. Thus there are 258 positives and 86 negatives. The proportions of these two groups that have correct diagnoses based on the scan are thus $231/258 = 0.90$ and $54/86 = 0.63$ respectively. These two proportions have confusingly similar names which are formally defined as follows:

**Sensitivity** is the proportion of positives that are correctly identified by the test;

**Specificity** is the proportion of negatives that are correctly identified by the test.

We can thus say that, based on the sample studied, we would expect 90% of patients with abnormal pathology to have abnormal (positive) liver scans, while 63% of those with normal pathology would have normal (negative) liver scans.

At first sight these simple calculations appear to have answered the question posed, but there is more to these problems than meets the eye. We have answered the question from one direction only. In clinical practice the test result is all that is known, so we want to know how good the test is at predicting abnormality. In other words, what proportion of patients with abnormal test results are truly abnormal?

### 14.4.2 Positive and negative predictive values

The whole point of a diagnostic test is to use it to make a diagnosis, so we need to know what the probability is of the test giving the correct diagnosis, whether it is positive or negative. The sensitivity and specificity do not give us this information. Instead we must approach the data from the direction of the test results. Of the 263 patients with abnormal liver scans 231 had abnormal pathology, giving the proportion of correct diagnoses as 231/263 = 0.88. Similarly, among the 81 patients with normal liver scans the proportion of correct diagnoses was 54/81 = 0.67. These two proportions are given more sensible names, which are formally defined as follows:

**Positive predictive value** is the proportion of patients with positive test results who are correctly diagnosed;

**Negative predictive value** is the proportion of patients with negative test results who are correctly diagnosed.

The positive and negative predictive values give a direct assessment of the usefulness of the test in practice. Unfortunately, we still cannot stop the analysis because there is another essential aspect of the analysis to consider, which is invisible in the above calculations, and that is the **prevalence of abnormality**.

### 14.4.3 The effect of prevalence

The disadvantage of the sensitivity and specificity is that they do not assess the accuracy of the test in a clinically useful way. They do have the advantage, however, that they are not affected by the proportion of subjects with the abnormality, which we call the **prevalence**. It is assumed here that we know the patients' true status. See section 14.4.7 for further comment on this point.

The predictive values, in contrast, are clinically useful but depend very strongly on the prevalence. In the liver scan study the prevalence of abnormality was very high, being 258/344 = 0.75; that is, exactly three-quarters. In different clinical settings the prevalence of abnormality will vary greatly. Using the data in Table 14.6 I constructed Table 14.7 to show the results we would expect in a group of patients where the prevalence of abnormality is 0.25. Table 14.8 shows the analyses of the data for these

**Table 14.7** Predicted effect on liver scan results of a prevalence of abnormality of 0.25, based on data in Table 14.6

| | Pathology | | |
|---|---|---|---|
| Liver scan | Abnormal (+) | Normal (−) | Total |
| Abnormal (+) | 77 | 96 | 173 |
| Normal (−) | 9 | 162 | 171 |
| Total | 86 | 258 | 344 |

**Table 14.8** Analysis of liver scan data with prevalences of abnormality of 0.75 and 0.25

| | Prevalence | |
|---|---|---|
| | 0.75 | 0.25 |
| Sensitivity | 0.90 | 0.90 |
| Specificity | 0.63 | 0.63 |
| Positive predictive value | 0.88 | 0.45 |
| Negative predictive value | 0.67 | 0.95 |
| Total correct predictions | 0.83 | 0.69 |

two prevalences. As noted, the sensitivity and specificity are unchanged: these calculations are made on the columns of the table, and are not affected by the proportion of patients in each column. In contrast the predictive values of the test are based on the rows, and have changed a lot because they are affected by the prevalence of abnormality. The contrast between the data in Tables 14.6 and 14.7 is illustrated in Figure 14.4.

The effect of a lower prevalence is much as we would expect: the more uncommon is true abnormality the more sure we can be that a negative test indicates no abnormality, and the less sure that a positive result really

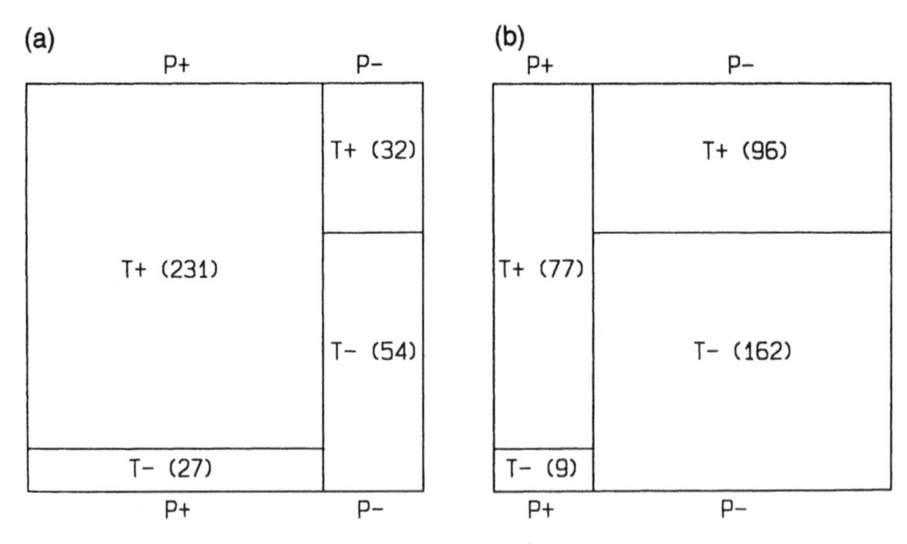


**Figure 14.4** Graphical illustration of (a) Table 14.6 and (b) Table 14.7. P indicates the pathology and T indicates the test. The sensitivity is depicted by the proportion of the area P+ that is labelled T+, and is the same in both figures. Likewise the specificity is the proportion of the area P– that is labelled T–, and this is the same in both figures. Conversely, the PPV is the proportion of the area labelled T+ that is P+, and is markedly different for the two figures. The same applies to the NPV.

indicates an abnormal patient. The predictive values of a test thus depend upon the prevalence of the abnormality in the patients being tested, which may not be known. **We should not take the predictive values observed in the sample as applying universally.**

### 14.4.4 Diagnosis based on a continuous measurement

So far I have considered the case where we wish to determine the presence or absence of some abnormality on the basis of the presence or absence of some symptom or test result. Another common situation arises when the diagnosis is to be made using a continuous measurement. I exclude here conditions such as hypertension, anaemia and perhaps obesity, which are *defined* by the value of a continuous measurement. We may have a single measurement or a score derived from combining two or more different measurements. Here the distinction between discriminant analysis based on logistic regression (section 12.5.2) and the methodology of diagnostic tests becomes decidedly blurred, as does that between diagnosis and prognosis.

Table 14.9 shows results of an HTLV-III (now HIV) antibody assay among patients with AIDS and healthy blood donors. If we wish to use the test to diagnose HIV seropositivity then we need to choose an appropriate cut-off. For each possible cut-off we can calculate the sensitivity and specificity of the test, and we can also calculate the positive and negative predictive values for any prevalence of seropositivity. The method for this last calculation is given in section 14.4.5.

Table 14.10 shows these calculations for the HTLV-III antibody assay results. Predictive values have been calculated assuming the prevalence of AIDS to be either 10% or 1% to illustrate the effect of the prevalence on

**Table 14.9** Results of enzyme-linked immunosorbent assay (ELISA) for HTLV-III among patients with AIDS and healthy blood donors (Weiss *et al.*, 1985). (Results expressed as the ratio of the mean absorbance of a pair of test samples divided by the mean absorbance of eight negative control wells)

| Ratio | Healthy blood donors | Patients with AIDS |
|---|---|---|
| < 2.0 | 202 (68%) | 0 (0%) |
| 2.0–2.99 | 73 (25%) | 2 (2%) |
| 3.0–3.99 | 15 (5%) | 7 (8%) |
| 4.0–4.99 | 3 (1%) | 7 (8%) |
| 5.0–5.99 | 2 (1%) | 15 (17%) |
| 6.0–11.99 | 2 (1%) | 36 (41%) |
| 12.0 + | 0 (0%) | 21 (24%) |
| Total | 297 (100%) | 88 (100%) |

**Table 14.10** Calculations of sensitivity, specificity, positive predictive value (PPV) and negative predictive value (NPV) for data in Table 14.9

| | | | Prevalence of HIV seropositivity | | | |
|---|---|---|---|---|---|---|
| | | | 10% | | 1% | |
| Cut-off for ratio | Sensitivity | Specificity | PPV | NPV | PPV | NPV |
| 2.0 | 1.00 | 0.68 | 0.26 | 1.00 | 0.03 | 1.00 |
| 3.0 | 0.98 | 0.93 | 0.59 | 0.997 | 0.12 | 0.9997 |
| 4.0 | 0.90 | 0.98 | 0.81 | 0.99 | 0.28 | 0.999 |
| 5.0 | 0.82 | 0.99 | 0.87 | 0.98 | 0.38 | 0.998 |
| 6.0 | 0.65 | 0.99 | 0.91 | 0.96 | 0.49 | 0.996 |
| 12.0 | 0.24 | 1.00 | 1.00 | 0.92 | 1.00 | 0.992 |

predictive values. There is no reason to use the prevalence in the study data (23%) which has no meaning because the two samples of subjects were selected independently. The appropriate figure to use will depend upon the characteristics of the population being studied.

The choice of a cut-off is not a statistical decision. Assuming that it is felt that the values in Table 14.10 show that the test is *clinically* useful, then the 'best' cut-off must be chosen according to the relative costs (not necessarily financial) associated with a false positive and false negative test results. This in turn will be related to the clinical action that will follow a positive test, in particular whether the test is a *screening* test or a *diagnostic* test (see section 14.4.7). It is not always necessary, however, to impose a cut-off, as we will see below. The need to do so depends on whether the aim is to make a diagnosis or a prognosis. Again, this is not a statistical issue.

We can arrive at a similar situation with the results of a multiple regression analysis. As we saw in section 12.4.8 a regression model can be used to derive a continuous score or prognostic index. When the outcome variable is binary and logistic regression is used, that prognostic index can be converted into a probability of the presence (or absence) of that outcome. In section 12.5.2 I described the application of logistic regression to the problem of discrimination. It is a small jump to the use of the same model for diagnosis; indeed, the two concepts are arguably the same.

In the next section the calculations are examined more closely.

### 14.4.5 Calculations

Table 14.11 shows a general representation of any diagnostic test based on a binary indicator, such as the presence or absence of a particular symptom

**Table 14.11** General representation of a diagnostic test

| | | Disease status Positive | Negative | Total |
|---|---|---|---|---|
| Test | Positive | $a$ | $b$ | $a + b$ |
| | Negative | $c$ | $d$ | $c + d$ |
| | Total | $a + c$ | $b + d$ | $n$ |

or test result. We can give names to the four cells:

| Test | Disease status | Name |
|---|---|---|
| + | + | True positive ($a$) |
| + | − | False positive ($b$) |
| − | + | False negative ($c$) |
| − | − | True negative ($d$) |

The quantities defined and discussed earlier are

$$\text{Sensitivity} = a/(a + c)$$
$$\text{Specificity} = d/(b + d)$$
$$\text{Positive predictive value} = a/(a + b)$$
$$\text{Negative predictive value} = d/(c + d)$$

The terms **false positive rate** and **false negative rate** are sometimes used, but these names are ambiguous. For example, the false negative rate might be $c/(c + d)$ or $c/(a + c)$, depending on your point of view.

The observed **prevalence** of disease in the study is $(a + c)/n$. If the study is carried out on a definable group of patients, such as those attending a particular clinic, then the prevalence may be useful, as may the calculation of positive and negative predictive values based on that prevalence. More generally, however, we may wish to consider the predictive ability of the test for groups with other prevalences of disease, such as different age groups or even the general population. These calculations depend upon **Bayes' theorem**, which is that

$$\text{Prob(disease}|\text{test positive)} = \frac{\text{Prob(test positive}|\text{disease)} \times \text{Prob(disease)}}{\text{Prob(test positive)}}$$

$$= \frac{\text{Prob(test positive}|\text{disease)} \times \text{Prob(disease)}}{\text{Prob(test positive}|\text{disease)} \times \text{Prob(disease)} + \text{Prob(test positive}|\text{no disease)} \times \text{Prob(no disease)}}$$

where Prob(disease|test positive) means the probability of disease when the test is positive, and so on. From the earlier definitions it is clear that

$$\text{Prob(disease)} = \text{prevalence of disease}$$

$$\text{Prob(disease}|\text{test positive)} = \text{positive predictive value (PPV)}$$

$$\text{Prob(test positive}|\text{disease)} = \text{sensitivity}$$

$$\text{Prob(test positive}|\text{ no disease)} = 1 - \text{specificity}$$

so that we can rewrite the above equation for the probability of disease when the test is positive as

$$\text{PPV} = \frac{\text{sensitivity} \times \text{prevalence}}{\text{sensitivity} \times \text{prevalence} + (1 - \text{specificity}) \times (1 - \text{prevalence})}.$$

By a similar argument we can show that the negative predictive value (NPV) is

$$\text{NPV} = \frac{\text{specificity} \times (1 - \text{prevalence})}{(1 - \text{sensitivity}) \times \text{prevalence} + \text{specificity} \times (1 - \text{prevalence})}.$$

Two consequences of these formulae are clear. Firstly, it is simple to estimate the predictive values for any prevalence of disease. The effect of varying the prevalence can be marked, as is seen in Table 14.10. Secondly, if we have no idea of the prevalence we cannot estimate the predictive value of the test. Another way of interpreting the prevalence is as the probability before the test is carried out that the subject has the disease, known as the **prior probability** of disease. The values of PPV and 1 − NPV are the revised estimates of the same probability for those subjects who are positive and negative to the test, and are known as **posterior probabilities**. The difference between the prior and posterior probabilities is one way of assessing the usefulness of the test.

We can extend these ideas to diagnosis based on a continuous measurement, by considering each possible cut-off in turn. Table 14.10 illustrated the procedure for the association between assay results and HIV seropositivity.

The sensitivity and specificity are proportions, and so we can calculate confidence intervals for them using the methods of section 10.2.1. When two diagnostic tests are compared on the same sample of individuals, the sensitivities and specificities are paired and so the appropriate confidence interval (section 10.4.1) and the McNemar test (section 10.7.5) should be used.

### 14.4.6 Two further ways of looking at diagnostic tests

*(This section can be omitted without loss of continuity.)*

The apparent simplicity of diagnostic test data, particularly when presented as a 2 by 2 table, is belied by the many ways of expressing the results.

Here I consider two further approaches that are more informative than simply looking at sensitivity and specificity.

*(a) The likelihood ratio*

For any test result we can compare the probability of getting that result if the patient truly had the condition of interest with the corresponding probability if they were healthy. The ratio of these probabilities is called the **likelihood ratio** (LR), and it is calculated as

$$\text{LR} = \frac{\text{Prob(positive test}|\text{disease)}}{\text{Prob(positive test}|\text{no disease)}} = \frac{\text{sensitivity}}{1 - \text{specificity}}.$$

We can consider the likelihood ratio as indicating the value of the test for increasing certainty about a positive diagnosis. The prevalence is the probability of disease before the test is performed. The *odds* of having the disease are thus given as prevalence/(1 − prevalence). Thus if the prevalence is 10%, the odds are 0.11, or 9 to 1 against the disease being present. We can call this figure the **pre-test odds**, and the odds corresponding to the positive predictive value as the **post-test odds**. It is not difficult mathematically to show that

$$\text{Post-test odds} = \text{pre-test odds} \times \text{likelihood ratio}$$

demonstrating how the likelihood ratio measures the change in certainty of diagnosis.

For the data in Table 14.6 the prevalence of abnormal pathology is 0.75, so the pre-test odds of disease are $0.75/(1 - 0.75) = 3.0$. The post-test odds of disease given a positive test are $0.878/(1 - 0.878) = 7.22$, and the likelihood ratio is $0.895/(1 - 0.628) = 2.406$, demonstrating the stated relation between these three quantities ($7.22 = 3.0 \times 2.406$). For the data in Table 14.7 the likelihood ratio is the same, but the pre-test odds of disease are $0.25/(1 - 0.25) = 0.33$. We can obtain the post-test odds as $2.406 \times 0.33 = 0.79$.

This approach may give further insight into the interpretation of diagnostic test data, but it does not add new information because the same quantities are used as before. As I have just shown, a high likelihood ratio may demonstrate that the test is useful but it does not necessarily indicate that a positive test is a good indicator of the presence of disease. For the data in Table 14.7, the low prevalence of 0.25 means that someone with a positive test is still more likely to be normal than abnormal – this is seen from both the post-test odds of 0.81 and the PPV of 0.45. Using odds rather than probabilities may be helpful, however, especially for seeing the usefulness of the test as assessed by the likelihood ratio (Ingelfinger *et al.*, 1987, p. 25).

*(b) ROC curve*

When a measurement is used to make a diagnosis the choice of the 'best' cut-off is not simple. A graphical approach is to plot the sensitivity versus 1 − specificity for each possible cut-off, and to join the points. The curve thus obtained is known as a 'receiver operating characteristic' curve or **ROC curve**, because the method originated in studies of signal detection by radar operators. For the data in Table 14.10 the curve would thus be based on the second and third columns. However, the ROC curve is not very helpful for these data because the specificities are so high that the 'curve' follows the *y* axis. If the 'cost' of a false negative result is the same as that of a false positive result, the best cut-off is that which maximizes the sum of the sensitivity and specificity, which is the point nearest the top left-hand corner. With different costs it is hard to note the best point from the graph.

The ROC method is perhaps most useful when comparing two or more competing methods. For a single test it does not add anything to a table but it is preferable when there are many possible cut-off values. Of course, the ROC curve, being based only on sensitivity and specificity, takes no account of the prevalence of the disease being tested for.

### 14.4.7 What is the patient's true condition?

In section 14.4.3 I observed that the sensitivity and specificity calculated from a sample of subjects are unrelated to the prevalence of abnormality. This may not always be the case. We can consider three ways of categorizing a patient – their true condition, the diagnosis, and the test results. When we calculate the sensitivity and specificity of the test we do this in relation to the diagnosis, but we do not necessarily know that the diagnosis is always correct. Unless the diagnosis is perfect, so that it always gives the patient's true status (positive or negative), we are evaluating the test's ability to predict the diagnosis rather than the patient's true disease status. In this case, the sensitivity and specificity of the test in relation to the true state *are* related to the prevalence of abnormality (Begg, 1987). This suggests that unless it is known that the diagnosis is almost always correct, it is wise to evaluate a diagnostic test on patients with the same prevalence of disease as those for whom the test will be used in future.

### 14.4.8 Discussion

The analysis of data from diagnostic tests requires no complicated mathematics. The main difficulty is not statistical, but rather the need to decide how good the test should be to be clinically valuable. The answer to this question is related to the prevalence of the disease in the subjects being tested. Two extremes are when we are testing high risk individuals, perhaps in a tertiary referral centre, and when we are screening an ostensibly healthy population for early signs of rare serious disease, such as cervical cancer. For screening tests it is very important to have high specificity and NPV. We do not want false negative results and are willing to accept a moderate number of false positive results. All those positive to the screening test will then be tested again, usually with a different test. Here the requirement will be a high sensitivity and PPV, because a positive result will probably lead to a diagnosis of disease and clinical intervention. A high specificity is also desirable, of course. The detection of HIV seropositivity is a good example of the case where the importance of a false positive diagnosis would have major consequences for the patient and so would a false negative diagnosis for someone receiving their blood in a transfusion. Another is the use of alpha-fetoprotein levels from amniocentesis to detect fetuses with Down's syndrome. These issues must be carefully weighed up when deciding where to put the cut-off between positive and negative diagnosis in the data in Table 14.9 or, indeed, whether it is wise to impose any cut-off.

One approach that could be adopted more frequently is to use the diagnostic test to divide subjects into three groups, with a central, 'uncertain' group who would be subjected to further testing. For the data shown in Table 14.9 Weiss *et al*., (1985) considered assay results between 3.0 and 5.0 as 'borderline'.

Finally, a link with the earlier sections of this chapter is that it is a requirement of a good diagnostic test that the result is repeatable and is subject to minimal inter-observer variation.

Further discussion of the methodology and interpretation of diagnostic tests can be found in the paper by Sheps and Schechter (1984), the series of articles from the Department of Clinical Epidemiology and Biostatistics at McMaster University (1983) and in the books by Galen and Gambino (1975) and Ingelfinger *et al*. (1987). The logic of clinical diagnosis and computer applications are reviewed by Macartney (1987).

## 14.5 REFERENCE INTERVALS

Diagnostic tests use patient data to classify individuals as either normal or abnormal. A related statistical problem is the description of variability in normal individuals, to provide a basis for assessing test results for other individuals. The most common form of presenting such data is as a range of values, or interval, which encompasses the values obtained from the majority of a sample of normal subjects. The **reference interval** is often referred to as a **normal range** or **reference range**. 'Reference interval' is a better term, both because it avoids confusion with Normal in the statistical sense, and also because the word 'range' suggests that values excluded are by definition abnormal.

Reference intervals are used most often in clinical chemistry, for example to provide a standard reference against which to assess cholesterol levels in blood samples from patients under investigation. As with diagnostic tests the calculations required are essentially simple and most of the problems are associated with interpretation. One point to note is that the procedure is equivalent to a diagnostic test where we know the specificity (usually 90% or 95%) but nothing else. Clearly such information should not be used *on its own* to make a diagnosis. Detailed discussion on the concepts of reference intervals are given in Solberg (1987) and the papers cited therein.

### 14.5.1 Selecting a sample

The concept of 'normality' is elusive, and any definition will be specific to the context. Reference intervals are often derived from samples taken in hospital from subjects subsequently found not to be seriously ill, but people in hospital are not normal in the sense of being representative of the healthy population. It is essential to describe how the reference subjects were selected and on what basis their health was determined.

Sample size is also an important consideration, and is discussed in section 14.5.3. Also there may be variation in the distribution of the measurement of interest between different groups of subjects. In particular it is frequently necessary to calculate separate intervals for males and females. There is often also variation by age, especially among children; this topic is considered in section 14.5.4.

### 14.5.2 Calculating the reference interval

The reference interval is simply the estimated range of values that includes a certain percentage of the values among the relevant population. As with other intervals discussed in earlier chapters, reference intervals usually encompass 90%, 95% or 99% of the values, with 95% the most frequently used. The same method is used whether both low and high values are considered suspicious or only those at one extreme.

There are two basic approaches to the calculation. We can either take the appropriate (per)centiles from the empirical distribution of the observations, or we can use the Normal distribution, perhaps after transforming the data. Many serum constituents, for example, have Lognormal distributions. The options are thus the same as for the general methods introduced in section 3.4 for summarizing the distribution of a set of observations. In that section the serum IgM values from 298 healthy children aged 0 to 6 years were analysed. In section 3.4.2 the $2\frac{1}{2}$th and $97\frac{1}{2}$th centiles were calculated as 0.2 and 2.0 g/l. The range of values from 0.2 and 2.0 thus defines a 95% reference interval using the percentile method. The distribution of IgM was skewed (Figure 3.3) but $\log_{10}$ IgM had a symmetrical distribution (Figure 3.13), with mean −0.158 and standard deviation 0.238.

If we can consider the distribution of $\log_{10}$ IgM as close to Normal we can use the standard Normal distribution to estimate the required centiles (see section 4.5.2). The 95% reference interval for $\log_{10}$ IgM is calculated as mean ±1.96SD, and the values are antilogged to give the 95% reference interval for IgM. We thus calculate first

$$-0.158 - (1.96 \times 0.238) \text{ and } -0.518 + (1.96 \times 0.238)$$

that is, −0.624 and 0.308, and back-transform these values (using $10^x$ as in section 3.4) to get a 95% reference interval for IgM as 0.24 to 2.03. The two approaches give very similar answers for these data.

As always there are advantages and disadvantages of the alternative approaches and each has strong advocates. The parametric approach depends on the data having a closely Normal distribution, perhaps after transformation. We can use a formal test of non-Normality, as described in section 7.5.3. The Normal plot for the log IgM data in Figure 14.5 shows that the data are indeed close to a Normal distribution. The alternative percentile approach makes no assumptions about the data, but is less reliable when the data are Normal.

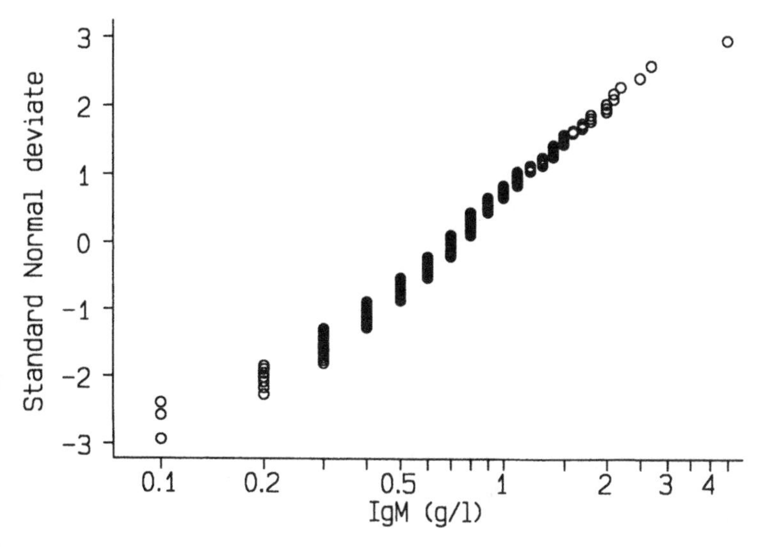


**Figure 14.5** Normal plot of log serum IgM data in children (Isaacs *et al.*, 1983).

### 14.5.3 Uncertainty and sample size

Whereas the parametric approach is based on estimates of the mean and standard deviation, the percentile approach is based on observations in the tails of the distribution. For both methods the reference interval is obtained as two values which are subject to sampling variability. Several samples from the same population of healthy individuals will give different reference intervals, with the variability depending on sample size. Samples from different populations would be even more variable, and the use of different types of machine to measure the quantity of interest would increase variability further. Table 14.12 shows mean fetal scalp blood pH and reference intervals from 14 different samples of women in 12 centres. Five different types of pH meter were used. There is marked variation in the reference intervals with two (numbers 3 and 14) hardly overlapping. Most noticeable, however, is the fact that most of the studies are very small, all but one being based on fewer than 50 subjects.

**Table 14.12** Reference intervals from 14 studies of fetal scalp blood pH (Lumley *et al.*, 1971)

| Study | Mean pH | 95% reference interval* | Sample size |
|---|---|---|---|
| 1 | 7.29 | 7.15 to 7.43 | 43 |
| 2 | 7.29 | 7.21 to 7.37 | 24 |
| 3 | 7.29 | 7.25 to 7.33 | 10 |
| 4 | 7.30 | 7.20 to 7.40 | 12 |
| 5 | 7.30 | 7.22 to 7.38 | 18 |
| 6 | 7.30 | 7.22 to 7.38 | 129 |
| 7 | 7.32 | 7.20 to 7.44 | 16 |
| 8 | 7.32 | 7.22 to 7.42 | 49 |
| 9 | 7.35 | 7.23 to 7.47 | 45 |
| 10 | 7.35 | 7.25 to 7.45 | 26 |
| 11 | 7.35 | 7.25 to 7.45 | 29 |
| 12 | 7.35 | 7.25 to 7.45 | 21 |
| 13 | 7.37 | 7.27 to 7.47 | 45 |
| 14 | 7.38 | 7.30 to 7.45 | 22 |

*mean ± 2SD

The standard error may be obtained for any estimated centile of the Normal distribution. For example, the values describing a 95% reference interval have a standard error of

$$\sqrt{\frac{s^2}{N} + \frac{1.96^2 s^2}{2N}}$$

where $s$ is the standard deviation of the observations. This is approximately equal to $s\sqrt{3/N}$. The widths of confidence intervals for the limits of 95% reference intervals for different sample sizes are shown in Figure 14.6. For sample sizes smaller than about 50 the values defining the reference interval themselves have a confidence interval wider than the standard

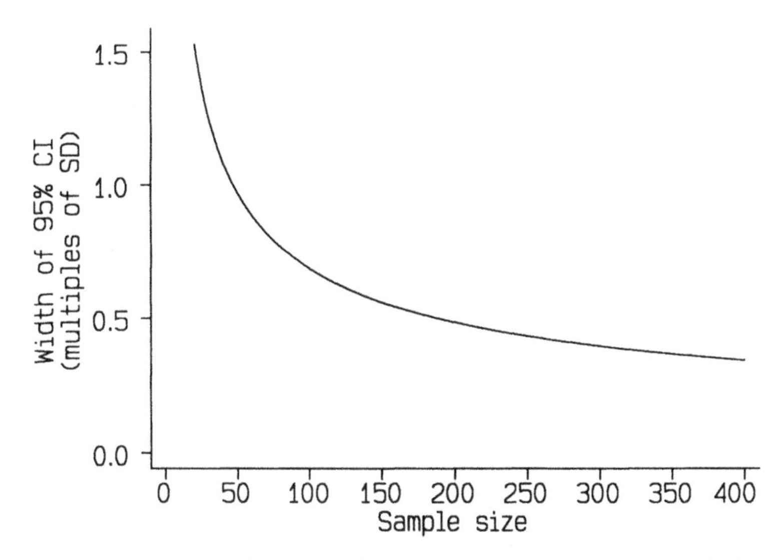


**Figure 14.6** Width of parametric 95% confidence interval for limits of reference interval as a multiple of the standard deviation if the data have a Normal distribution.

deviation of the observations. In order to reduce the uncertainty we need much larger samples, preferably of at least 200 observations. Reference intervals derived by the non-parametric percentile method have confidence intervals that are much wider than those shown in Figure 14.6 (Linnet, 1987). The parametric approach is therefore much better if we can make the data conform closely to a Normal distribution, unless we have a very large sample.

### 14.5.4 Relation to age

Many clinical and biochemical variables vary with age in healthy individuals. For example, as people get older their blood pressure tends to rise and they tend to put on weight. During childhood we are especially likely to find changes with age, and the same applies to both mother and fetus during pregnancy. It is important to investigate possible relations with age, especially for measurements on children or during pregnancy. Failure to do so may lead to the finding of a spurious change in prevalence of abnormality with age.

Not only the mean but also the standard deviation may vary with age. Further, the assessment of Normality needs to be made for small age groups. Regression can be used to fit a curve to the means and, if necessary, a separate curve to the standard deviations. The residuals from these analyses should show no relation to age. Careful analysis of the IgM data from children aged 6 months to 6 years showed that both the mean and standard deviation of log IgM increased slightly and then decreased in the $5\frac{1}{2}$ year period. Quadratic regression lines were fitted separately to the mean and SD of log IgM for 6 month age groups. These two curves were then combined to give mean ± 1.96SD at each age, and everything was antilogged to give the age-related reference interval shown in Figure 14.7.

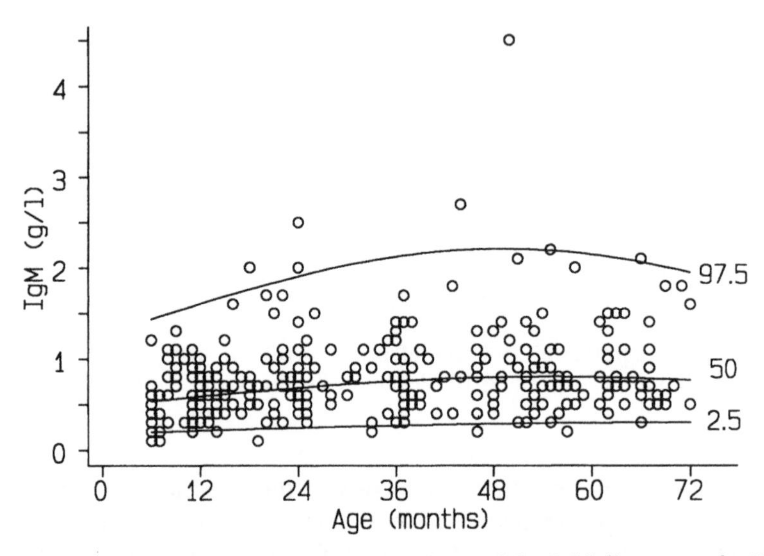


**Figure 14.7** 95% age-related reference interval for IgM (Isaacs *et al.*, 1983).

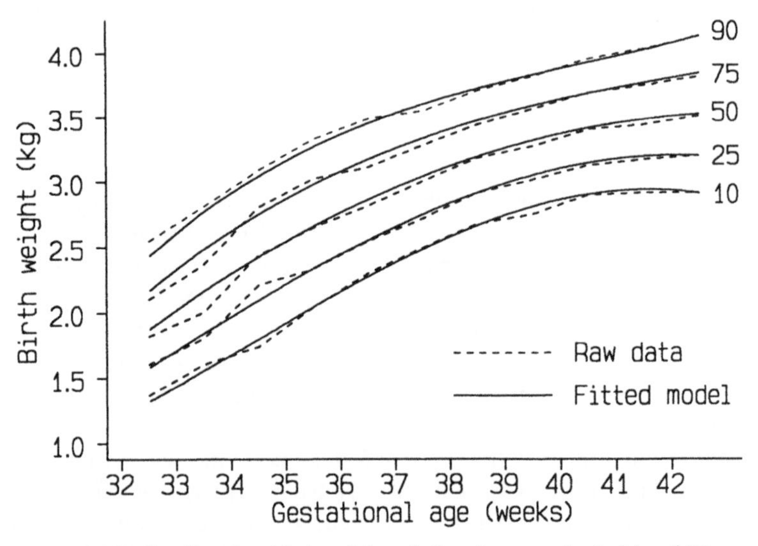


**Figure 14.8** Centiles for birthweight of first-born male babies (Altman and Coles, 1980), showing empirical (raw) centiles and curves derived from regression models.

Further details of the method are given in the original paper (Isaacs *et al.*, 1983).

Exactly the same statistical problem arises in constructing 'standards' of fetal or child growth. For example, as well as fitting quadratic curves to mean birthweight as shown in Figure 11.16, cubic curves were fitted to the standard deviations and several age-related centiles obtained, as shown in Figure 14.8 for first born male babies.

### 14.5.5 Discussion

It is common in clinical practice to classify subjects as normal or abnormal with regard to some clinical or biochemical measurement as an aid to decision-making and thus treatment. When data are available for normal (healthy) and abnormal (ill) subjects we have the type of data that form the basis of a diagnostic test, as discussed in section 14.4. If we wish to use the measurement itself to be a measure of abnormality, then we need to describe the variation among some defined group, usually of healthy subjects. The creation of a reference interval will, however, inevitably lead to the inference that subjects whose values fall outside the interval are abnormal. While this may be true, such an inference is not valid both because the interval by definition excludes a fixed small percentage of healthy subjects, and also because the values of the variable in ill subjects are not known. Where the measurement itself defines the condition, such as blood pressure above a certain level being termed 'hypertension', the logic becomes even more diffuse (Pickering, 1978).

From a statistical point of view, the most interesting question is whether to use the parametric method or the percentile method. While the percentile approach is attractive both in its simplicity and validity for all data sets, there are two important advantages of using the parametric method based on Normal distribution theory. Firstly, the confidence intervals for the values defining the reference interval are much narrower than for the equivalent percentile reference interval. Secondly, the use of the Normal distribution allows any subject's measurement to be expressed as a standard deviation score, and hence located at a particular percentile, which is much more informative than knowing whether they are inside or outside the reference interval. In other words, we can see *how* unusual a value is. (There is a strong analogy here to P values.) Where it is possible, therefore, to treat the data or some transformation of the data as Normal the parametric approach should be used.

The sample size should be large enough to restrict uncertainty about the limits of the reference interval, preferably with a bare minimum of 100 subjects for a parametric analysis and 200 for the percentile method. For age-related intervals it is important to smooth the data across ages. Apart from the fact that smoothly changing values are more plausible, there is much better statistical use of the data. In all cases, reports of new reference intervals should specify the criteria for inclusion of subjects and the statistical methods used.

## 14.6 SERIAL MEASUREMENTS

### 14.6.1 Introduction

Two types of study may yield a series of observations, or **serial measurements**, on each subject. Firstly, there are designed studies where repeated measurements are taken on each individual at specific times chosen in advance. Even when there are complete data for each individual, the appropriate analysis and interpretation of such data are not obvious. Secondly, data can arise from observational studies where multiple measurements are taken at unspecified times. With such data there may be doubts about the reason for the observations. For example, women with many measurements of blood pressure during pregnancy are likely to be a high risk group.

There are several approaches to analysing serial data, each with advantages and disadvantages. In particular some methods are complex both to perform and interpret, and some can be applied only to data at fixed time points. Here I shall consider a simple approach which gives useful results in most situations. It can be applied to experimental or observational data, and can thus be used for structured data sets with missing observations, which is a common phenomenon. A fuller discussion is given by Matthews *et al.* (1990). The method will be illustrated using the data in Table 14.13 and Figure 14.9, which show serum progesterone levels at several times up to two hours after nasal administration of progesterone for four groups of women.

### 14.6.2 The usual approach to analysis

The most common method of analysing data like these is to perform independent analyses at each time point, such as two-sample $t$ tests or one way analysis of variance. Frequently the data are displayed graphically by a plot joining the mean values at each time point, often with 'error bars' of $\pm 1$ standard error (or perhaps $\pm 1$ standard deviation). There are several important criticisms of this approach:

1. It ignores the design of the study, as no account is taken of the fact that the values at each time point are from the same individuals;
2. The curve joining the means may not be a good indicator of the typical curve for an individual, and will hide any variation in the shape of the curves for different individuals;

**Table 14.13** Serum levels of progesterone (nmol/l) after nasal administration in women (Dalton *et al.*, 1987)

| | Time after administration (min) | | | | | | | | | | Peak value (nmol/l) | Time to peak (min) |
|---|---|---|---|---|---|---|---|---|---|---|---|---|
| | 0 | 1 | 3 | 5 | 10 | 15 | 30 | 45 | 60 | 120 | | |
| Group 1 (0.2 ml of 100 mg/ml progesterone in one nostril) | | | | | | | | | | | | |
| 1 | 1.0 | — | 10.0 | 16.0 | 22.0 | 20.0 | 16.0 | — | 18.0 | 14.0 | 22.0 | 10 |
| 2 | 6.5 | 5.7 | 9.5 | 11.6 | 17.5 | 27.3 | 28.5 | 22.4 | 19.3 | 10.0 | 28.5 | 30 |
| 3 | 3.0 | 4.0 | 4.0 | 13.0 | 15.8 | 19.5 | 21.2 | 17.9 | 10.7 | 13.4 | 21.2 | 30 |
| 4 | 1.0 | 2.1 | 9.7 | — | 21.8 | — | 27.5 | — | 15.5 | 6.2 | 27.5 | 30 |
| 5 | 1.0 | 1.0 | 1.0 | 4.2 | 22.6 | 23.9 | 45.5 | 42.6 | 35.0 | 10.6 | 45.4 | 30 |
| 6 | 1.0 | 1.0 | 1.0 | 1.0 | 3.9 | 14.7 | 17.6 | 16.1 | 8.8 | 10.8 | 17.6 | 30 |
| Mean | 2.3 | 2.8 | 5.9 | 9.2 | 17.3 | 21.1 | 26.0 | 24.8 | 17.9 | 10.8 | 27.0 | 26.7 |
| (SE) | (0.9) | (0.9) | (1.8) | (2.8) | (2.9) | (3.5) | (4.4) | (6.1) | (3.8) | (1.1) | (4.0) | (3.3) |
| Group 2 (0.3 ml of 100 mg/ml progesterone in one nostril) | | | | | | | | | | | | |
| 7 | 1.0 | 1.5 | 5.0 | 11.0 | 16.0 | 23.0 | 15.0 | 9.0 | 6.0 | 5.0 | 23.0 | 15 |
| 8 | 1.0 | 1.0 | 6.5 | 20.0 | 22.5 | 27.8 | 19.0 | 9.0 | 8.2 | 8.0 | 27.8 | 15 |
| 9 | 1.0 | 1.0 | 7.3 | 7.5 | 18.0 | 20.0 | 18.9 | 12.8 | 6.3 | 4.8 | 20.0 | 15 |
| 10 | 3.0 | 2.5 | 2.0 | 2.7 | 3.4 | 3.6 | 14.0 | 7.3 | 7.7 | 4.7 | 14.0 | 30 |
| 11 | 8.3 | 7.5 | 9.6 | 11.0 | 11.5 | 15.7 | 15.2 | 15.8 | 14.0 | 11.5 | 15.8 | 45 |
| 12 | 6.2 | 5.9 | 6.8 | 7.7 | 9.0 | 9.3 | 12.1 | 12.2 | 11.0 | 9.0 | 12.2 | 45 |
| Mean | 3.2 | 3.2 | 6.2 | 10.0 | 13.4 | 16.6 | 15.7 | 11.0 | 8.1 | 7.1 | 18.8 | 27.5 |
| (SE) | (1.3) | (1.1) | (1.0) | (2.4) | (2.8) | (3.7) | (1.1) | (1.3) | (1.3) | (1.1) | (2.4) | (6.0) |

**Table 14.13** (*cont'd*) Serum levels of progesterone (nmol/l) after nasal administration in women

| | Time after administration (min) | | | | | | | | | | Peak value (nmol/l) | Time to peak (min) |
|---|---|---|---|---|---|---|---|---|---|---|---|---|
| | 0 | 1 | 3 | 5 | 10 | 15 | 30 | 45 | 60 | 120 | | |
| Group 3 (0.2 ml of 200 mg/ml progesterone in one nostril) | | | | | | | | | | | | |
| 13 | 8.4 | 10.8 | 8.1 | 7.8 | 8.5 | 12.0 | 19.8 | 22.2 | 25.2 | 40.5 | 40.5 | 120 |
| 14 | 3.5 | 3.2 | 3.4 | 3.3 | 8.5 | 9.4 | 14.5 | 12.7 | 11.5 | 10.2 | 14.5 | 30 |
| 15 | 3.5 | 4.0 | 4.8 | 3.5 | 3.7 | 13.0 | 12.5 | 15.0 | 22.0 | 10.5 | 22.0 | 60 |
| 16 | 3.7 | 3.2 | 4.3 | 4.5 | 5.5 | 8.5 | 10.3 | 11.1 | 8.0 | 6.0 | 11.1 | 45 |
| Mean | 4.8 | 5.3 | 5.2 | 4.8 | 6.7 | 10.7 | 14.3 | 15.3 | 16.7 | 16.8 | 22.0 | 63.8 |
| (SE) | (1.2) | (1.8) | (1.0) | (1.0) | (1.2) | (1.1) | (2.0) | (2.5) | (4.1) | (8.0) | (6.7) | (19.7) |
| Group 4 (0.2 ml of 100 mg/ml progesterone in each nostril) | | | | | | | | | | | | |
| 17 | 5.0 | 5.6 | 6.1 | 7.2 | 13.8 | 26.0 | 26.1 | 25.7 | 20.5 | 11.0 | 26.1 | 30 |
| 18 | 4.5 | 5.1 | 13.2 | 21.0 | 26.8 | 28.0 | 22.0 | 17.8 | 15.7 | 14.0 | 28.0 | 15 |
| 19 | 8.4 | 6.2 | 8.0 | 18.5 | 33.8 | 35.0 | 26.2 | 23.0 | 19.0 | 12.6 | 35.0 | 15 |
| 20 | 4.2 | 3.2 | 4.2 | 4.8 | 10.3 | 13.7 | 17.1 | 18.3 | 17.4 | 15.8 | 18.3 | 45 |
| Mean | 5.5 | 5.0 | 7.9 | 12.9 | 21.2 | 25.7 | 22.8 | 21.2 | 18.2 | 13.4 | 26.9 | 26.3 |
| (SE) | (1.0) | (0.7) | (1.9) | (4.0) | (5.5) | (4.4) | (2.2) | (1.9) | (1.0) | (1.0) | (3.4) | (7.2) |

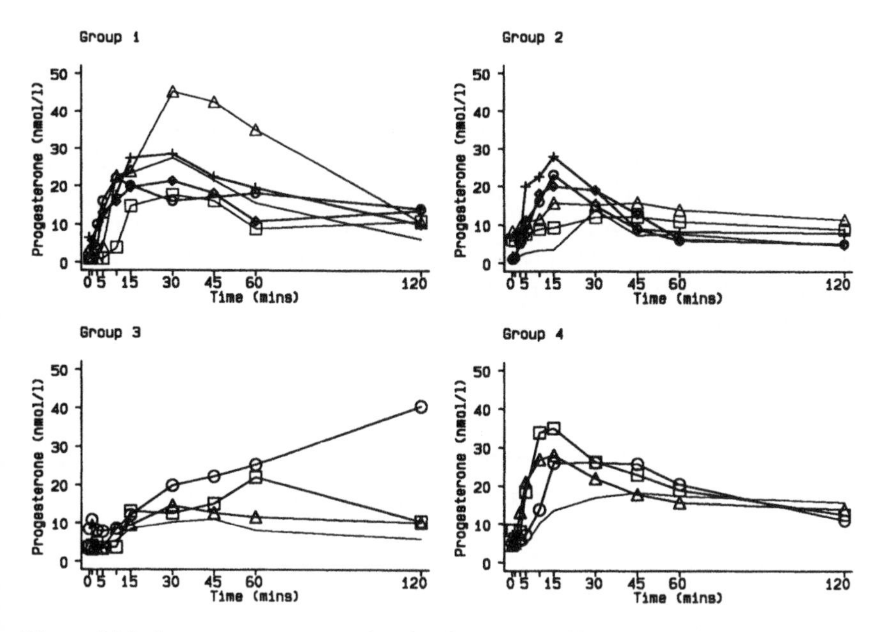


**Figure 14.9** Serum progesterone levels after nasal administration of progesterone in four groups of women. Data from Table 14.13.

3. It is difficult, if not impossible, to interpret the multiple non-independent P values that are obtained when different groups of subjects are compared;
4. No allowance can be made for any missing observations, so the data at different times may not relate to exactly the same group.

The first point above is the critical one, from which the others follow. It is not at all clear how we would interpret the analysis of the data in Figure 14.9 if, for example, the first two groups were significantly different only at 15 minutes. Further, should we take account of any differences in baseline (time zero) values in the two groups and, if so, how? The purpose of this type of study is usually to assess the response over time, so it is far better to tailor the analysis to the clinical objective.

### 14.6.3 Analysis using summary measures

Probably the most useful general approach to the analysis of serial measurements is to simplify the analysis by reducing each subject's data to certain features of particular interest. Either a statistical model may be fitted to each individual's data or the necessary quantities can be derived directly from the observed data. These **summary measures** are then analysed in the same way as if they were the original observations. Clearly this approach relies on the ability to choose summary measures of clinical relevance.

For clinical measurements the only commonly used model is to fit a linear regression of each subject's data on time. The slope of the line represents the rate of change of the measurement per unit of time (e.g. per hour). Clearly, linear regression is appropriate only for data which tend either to rise or fall systematically over time. Many data sets, such as that in Figure 14.9, have a general tendency to rise and then fall (or vice versa). It is unlikely that any simple statistical model would fit such data at all well.

A simpler and more common approach is to take summary statistics directly from the observed data, perhaps after some simple mathematical calculation. Some of the more frequent derived statistics are:

- mean of all the measurements (i.e. ignore the time response)
- height of peak
- time to reach peak
- time to reach a given level
- time to change by a given amount
- time above a given level
- time to achieve maximum change from original level (baseline)
- time to return (near) to baseline level
- change from first to last measurement
- final level (perhaps the average of the last few measurements)
- area under the curve (AUC)

Several of these suggestions incorporate some arbitrary definitions which should be chosen in advance of the analysis rather than after inspection of the data. Several are specifically aimed at data with peaks. Where initial values vary considerably the change from baseline may be used.

The AUC may be interpreted in some circumstances as the cumulative response to the intervention. The calculation is described in section 14.6.5. Note that for equally spaced observations the AUC, which is the hardest of these summary statistics to calculate, is virtually the same as the mean of all the measurements.

Dalton *et al.* (1987) used three measures to summarize the data in Figure 14.9: the time of the peak, the maximum increase from time zero and the AUC. In general it is reasonable to consider two or three derived statistics, but as in any study it is highly desirable to identify a single measure of primary interest. The choice of appropriate measures should relate to the study objectives. For example, if the study is one of treatment efficacy we may reasonably be most interested in the values at the end of the study, perhaps in relation to starting values. If the study is to evaluate the effectiveness of analgesics, then we would probably be interested in the rapid effectiveness of the drug, perhaps by looking at the timing of the peak and the level achieved, and perhaps also the time above some critical level.

Although the analysis of summary statistics is usually simple, there are some difficulties with this approach too:

1. it may be difficult to specify the feature(s) of major importance, because the study objective is too vague;
2. the choice of statistics to use may be influenced by inspecting the data;
3. it is difficult to study any possible variation between groups in the shape of the curves (but this is always difficult).

Against these disadvantages we must set some important further advantages; the ability to cope with missing observations (see Table 14.13) and variable timing of observations; the ability to handle the comparison of serial measurements for the same subjects under different conditions; and the ease of understanding and explaining the results (a notable problem with several alternative approaches). It may seem that when we analyse summary measures we discard a lot of data. In fact the large number of observations is more apparent than real, as consecutive readings in any patient will be very similar. The *patient* is the unit of investigation, so it is easier and more meaningful to handle such data when we have only one value per patient.

### 14.6.4 Graphical display

Because of the potentially misleading effect of plotting mean values at each time point it is important to examine graphs of individuals' data, and if possible to include these in the published paper. A graph will show very quickly if the curves are similar or dissimilar. Unfortunately, graphical display is effective only for small samples. Figure 14.9 showed the raw serum progesterone data in one form; an alternative is shown in Figure 14.10.

The summary measures can also be plotted. One interesting format for 'peaked' data is to plot the height of the peak against its time. Figure 14.11 shows such a plot for the progesterone data. This type of plot may reveal patterns that are not evident in other graphs. More generally, we can produce a scatter diagram of any two summary measures. The data in the example were collected at the same times for all subjects, but graphical display may be even more useful for data collected at varying times.

### 14.6.5 The area under the curve

The area under the curve (AUC) is a useful way of summarizing the information from a series of measurements on one individual. It is

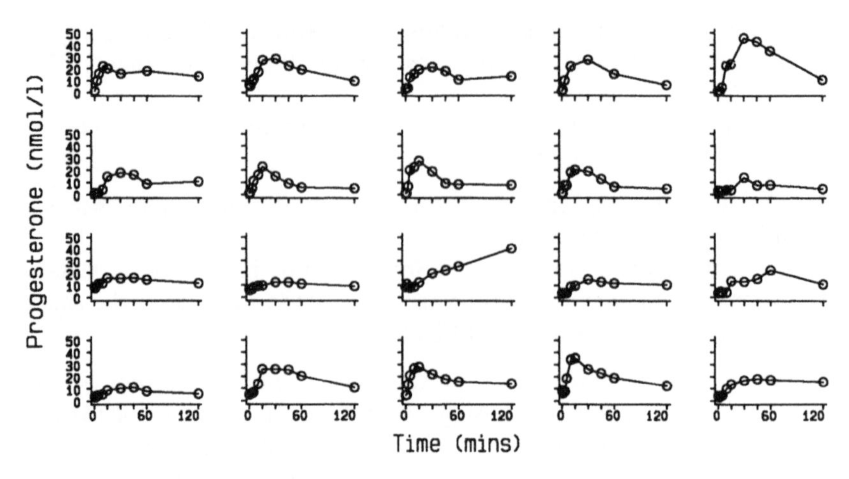


**Figure 14.10** Alternative display of serum progesterone data in Figure 14.9.

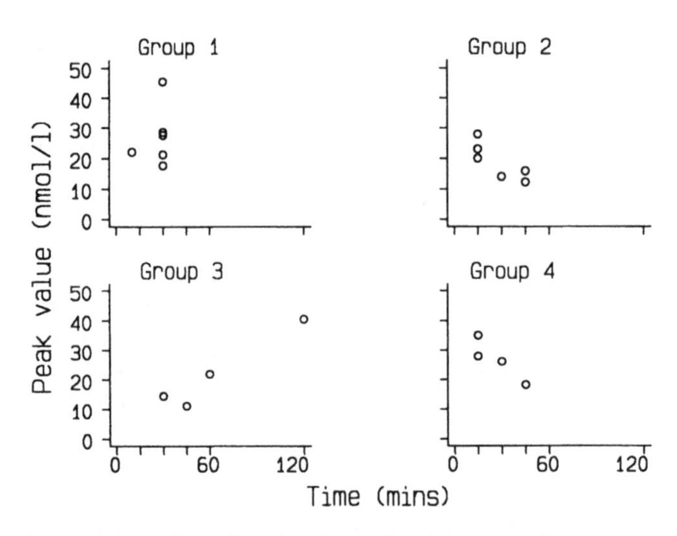


**Figure 14.11** Plot of peak values of progesterone by time.

frequently used in clinical pharmacology, where the AUC from serum levels can be interpreted as the total uptake or bioavailability of whatever had been administered.

The data are joined by straight lines to get a 'curve'. The AUC is usually calculated by adding the areas under the curve between each pair of consecutive observations. If we have measurements $y_1$ and $y_2$ at times $t_1$ and $t_2$, then the AUC between those two times is the product of the time difference and the average of the two measurements. Thus we get

$(t_2 - t_1)(y_1 + y_2)/2$. This is known as the **trapezium rule** because of the shape of each segment of the area under the curve.

If we have $n + 1$ measurements $y_i$ at times $t_i$ ($t = 0, \ldots, n$) then the AUC is calculated as

$$\frac{1}{2}\sum_{i=0}^{n-1}(t_{i+1} - t_i)(y_i + y_{i+1}).$$

The units of the AUC are the product of the units used for $y_i$ and $t_i$, for example nmol.min/l, and are not easy to understand. It may be useful to divide the AUC by the total time to get a sort of weighted average level over the time period.

The calculation for the first subject in Table 14.13 goes as follows. There were eight observations for this subject, so seven areas to calculate. We have

$$\begin{aligned}\text{AUC} &= 3 \times \left(\frac{1 + 10}{2}\right) + 2 \times \left(\frac{10 + 16}{2}\right) + 5 \times \left(\frac{16 + 22}{2}\right) + \ldots \\ &\quad + 60 \times \left(\frac{18 + 14}{2}\right) \\ &= 1930 \text{ nmol.min/l}.\end{aligned}$$

This value can also be expressed as an average level of $1930/120 = 16.1$ nmol/l.

We can calculate the AUC even when there are missing data, except when the final observation is missing.

### 14.6.6 Interpretation

Performing an analysis that does not relate to the questions of clinical interest often leads to incorrect inferences. When data are analysed separately at each of several time points it is common to see inferences based upon the time when groups become significantly different. Clearly the answer to this question will depend strongly on sample size, and has little if any scientific credibility. Presentation of all the raw data either in a table or figure is valuable, but neither may be feasible in a large study.

The use of summary statistics as the basis of statistical analysis avoids many difficulties by relating the analysis directly to one or more questions of specific interest. Interpretation is usually simplified by having one 'observation' per subject. Simple methods of estimation and hypothesis testing can be used.

## 14.7 CYCLIC VARIATION

Many measurements vary according to time of day. For example, most people's blood pressure is lowest at night and highest during the morning.

**Circadian variation** is also seen in many hormone levels and even our height tends to be slightly lower in the evening than in the morning.

Similarly, individual measurements and also population data may vary by month of the year. Table 14.14 shows the number of births with normal and abnormal cord blood IgE levels by month of birth in a study of over 5000 Belgian newborns. A high level of IgE is used to detect those predisposed to become allergic, and the study was carried out to confirm the results of a previous study that had found an association with month of birth.

**Table 14.14** Cord blood IgE by month of birth (Kimpen *et al.*, 1987)

| | Number of babies | | | |
|---|---|---|---|---|
| Month | Total | Normal IgE (≤ 1.0 IU/ml) | Abnormal IgE (> 1.0 IU/ml) | %Abnormal |
| January | 331 | 319 | 12 | 3.6 |
| February | 416 | 401 | 15 | 3.6 |
| March | 528 | 503 | 25 | 4.7 |
| April | 503 | 481 | 22 | 4.4 |
| May | 496 | 468 | 28 | 5.6 |
| June | 462 | 447 | 15 | 3.2 |
| July | 518 | 504 | 14 | 2.7 |
| August | 411 | 396 | 15 | 3.6 |
| September | 456 | 449 | 7 | 1.5 |
| October | 446 | 437 | 9 | 2.0 |
| November | 374 | 368 | 6 | 1.6 |
| December | 412 | 398 | 14 | 3.4 |

When data come from ordered groups we should examine directly the possibility of a *linear* trend. With data like the IgE values, which relate to months, the groups are ordered but are also cyclic. Clearly it makes no sense to look for a linear trend; rather, we should explore the possibility of a systematic *cyclic* trend. Data like these may arise from repeated measurement of the same individuals, or where the data at different times are from independent groups of subjects. When data at different times come from the same individuals this analysis is thus a special form of the analysis of serial measurements. Examples are the measurement of hormone levels throughout the menstrual cycle or blood pressure over 24 hours.

Several methods exist for analysing such data. Frequencies can be analysed using a non-parametric method given by Freedman (1979), for example to see if the incidence of new cases of disease varies seasonally. Continuous variables or proportions can be examined by fitting a **sinusoidal**

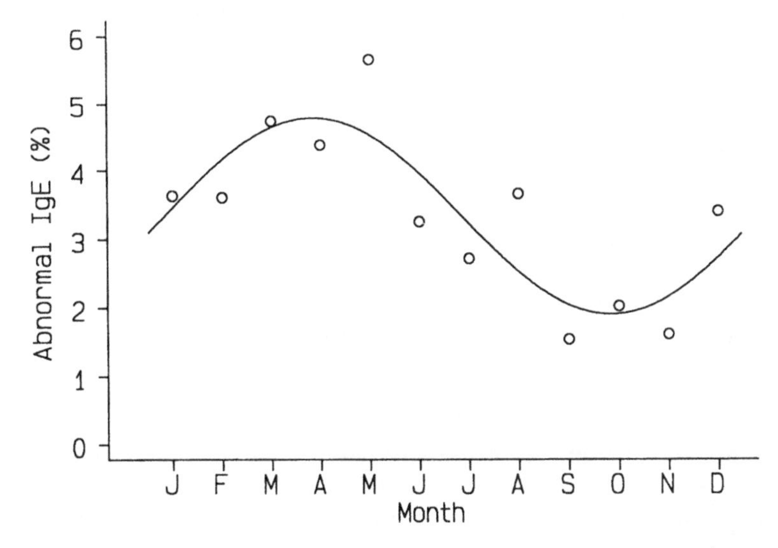


**Figure 14.12** Observed percentages of IgE values above 1.0 IU/ml and fitted sine curve.

(or **sine**) curve to the data. This analysis can be regarded as a complex form of regression. Figure 14.12 shows the observed proportions of abnormal IgE values together with the fitted curve. The analysis, which is not described here, shows a highly significant seasonal pattern.

Cyclic variation may require complicated statistical analysis. The purpose of introducing the topic here is to show again how the nature of the data needs to be considered explicitly when selecting the most appropriate analysis. I recommend expert statistical advice for data of this type.

## EXERCISES

14.1 The following table shows red cell volume measured simultaneously in 19 patients using radioactive ($^{51}Cr$) and non radioactive (biotin) cell labels (Cavill *et al.*, 1988):

| Patient | $^{51}Cr$ volume (ml) | Biotin volume (ml) |
|---|---|---|
| 1 | 1267 | 1954 |
| 2 | 1710 | 1651 |
| 3 | 1882 | 1887 |
| 4 | 1914 | 2043 |
| 5 | 1940 | 2054 |
| 6 | 1976 | 2075 |
| 7 | 2033 | 1976 |
| 8 | 2039 | 2120 |

| Patient | $^{51}Cr$ volume (ml) | Biotin volume (ml) |
|---|---|---|
| 9 | 2077 | 2061 |
| 10 | 2087 | 2152 |
| 11 | 2102 | 1894 |
| 12 | 2139 | 1982 |
| 13 | 2184 | 2153 |
| 14 | 2192 | 2288 |
| 15 | 2393 | 2628 |
| 16 | 2425 | 2495 |
| 17 | 2554 | 2463 |
| 18 | 2600 | 3186 |
| 19 | 3420 | 3488 |

The authors compared the two sets of data by the Wilcoxon matched pairs rank sum test, for which they got $P > 0.05$. They concluded that the comparison of methods 'showed no consistent clinically significant difference between the two'.

(a) Comment on their analysis and interpretation.
(b) Carry out a better analysis.
(c) What is the relevance of the fact that the patients had all been referred for the measurement of red cell volume.
(d) The largest differences between the methods are those for subjects 1 and 18. The biotin method is affected by prior consumption of eggs, and the authors note that 'at least one of these patients had had an egg for breakfast'. Should the analysis take account of this information?

14.2 Furst and Paulus (1975) reported a study to compare the metabolism of clonixin in 12 patients with rheumatoid arthritis and 12 normal controls. The drug was under investigation as an anti-inflammatory analgesic for treatment of rheumatoid arthritis. Serum clonixin levels were measured at 0, $\frac{1}{2}$, 1, 2, 4, 6 and 8 hours after administration of a single dose of three 250 mg tablets of clonixin. The authors did not report the initial (0 hour) values; the remaining data are shown below:

Patients with rheumatoid arthritis:

| | Clonixin levels ($\mu$g/ml) Time (hours) | | | | | |
|---|---|---|---|---|---|---|
| Patient | 0.5 | 1 | 2 | 4 | 6 | 8 |
| 1 | 12.70 | 32.20 | 42.00 | 19.80 | 7.09 | 2.10 |
| 2 | 18.48 | 40.24 | 45.87 | 15.61 | 5.58 | 3.25 |
| 3 | 6.70 | 20.60 | 27.70 | 11.49 | 2.48 | 0.56 |

| Patient | Clonixin levels (μg/ml) Time (hours) 0.5 | 1 | 2 | 4 | 6 | 8 |
|---|---|---|---|---|---|---|
| 4 | 24.20 | 16.20 | 7.84 | 5.30 | 0.38 | 0.00 |
| 5 | 14.70 | 28.30 | 31.90 | 16.08 | 9.20 | 3.60 |
| 6 | 6.55 | 29.17 | 33.30 | 15.17 | 3.17 | 0.00 |
| 7 | 41.70 | 29.40 | 16.90 | 7.04 | 3.48 | 2.56 |
| 8 | 1.49 | 47.26 | 32.78 | 15.89 | 4.72 | 2.61 |
| 9 | 13.04 | 19.08 | 39.47 | 12.42 | 4.91 | 2.86 |
| 10 | 29.28 | 44.94 | 45.72 | 12.71 | 4.43 | 1.67 |
| 11 | 8.61 | 20.34 | 44.33 | 6.74 | 2.15 | 1.11 |
| 12 | 28.10 | 56.10 | 36.68 | 19.10 | 5.62 | 1.82 |

Control subjects:

| Patient | Clonixin levels (μg/ml) Time (hours) 0.5 | 1 | 2 | 4 | 6 | 8 |
|---|---|---|---|---|---|---|
| 13 | 58.10 | 65.90 | 46.89 | 17.50 | 5.40 | 1.67 |
| 14 | 19.20 | 22.20 | 36.50 | 10.70 | 2.74 | 0.94 |
| 15 | 14.21 | 22.35 | 32.50 | 16.49 | 5.44 | 2.42 |
| 16 | 5.25 | 11.13 | 29.13 | 7.84 | 2.21 | 1.19 |
| 17 | 4.44 | 43.74 | 38.22 | 12.10 | 2.78 | 0.02 |
| 18 | 21.20 | 41.20 | 46.30 | 21.70 | 9.46 | 4.31 |
| 19 | 31.60 | 32.80 | 53.00 | 39.50 | 17.88 | 6.90 |
| 20 | 0.58 | 2.68 | 4.01 | 51.90 | 21.80 | 7.64 |
| 21 | 40.90 | 49.00 | 38.24 | 11.09 | 4.57 | 0.80 |
| 22 | 31.70 | 44.20 | 58.10 | 24.10 | 12.60 | 5.30 |
| 23 | 36.35 | 47.12 | 30.96 | 7.45 | 2.42 | 1.75 |
| 24 | 17.57 | 34.01 | 40.20 | 23.80 | 10.80 | 7.80 |

(a) Plot the mean levels in each group.
(b) Compare the peak levels and the area under the curve in the two groups using a suitable analysis assuming that the clonixin level is 0.0 at time zero. (The AUC is easy to calculate in a computer program, but is rather tedious to do by hand.)
(c) Are the plots from (a) a good representation of the data?

14.3 A search of the literature for studies concerning the polygraph (lie-detector) led to the assessment of the sensitivity and specificity of the machine as 0.76 and 0.63 respectively (Brett *et al.*, 1986). It is proposed that the polygraph be used in association with questioning potential blood donors about whether they are drug users. (Assuming that all non-drug users tell the truth.)

(a) If 5% of potential donors use drugs and a third of them lie about it, what proportion of blood donations will be from drug users?
(b) What proportion of people failing the polygraph test will be drug users?

14.4 Acute lower respiratory tract infection is one of the commonest causes of death among infants and under-5s in developing countries. A simple test is needed to identify those infants with acute respiratory infection who have lower respiratory tract infection (LRI) and should receive antibiotics from those with upper respiratory tract infection (URI). The following data come from a study of the usefulness of the respiratory rate for this purpose in infants (Cherian *et al.*, 1988):

| Respiratory rate (breaths/min) | Number of children (%) LRI | URI |
|---|---|---|
| 0–30 | 1 (1%) | 16 (11%) |
| 31–40 | 4 (3%) | 77 (51%) |
| 41–50 | 10 (7%) | 46 (30%) |
| 51–60 | 41 (29%) | 9 (6%) |
| 61+ | 86 (61%) | 3 (2%) |
| Total | 142 (100%) | 151 (100%) |

(a) Construct 2 × 2 tables for each of the four cut-offs 30, 40, 50 and 60 breaths/min relating low and high respiratory rate to the correct classification (LRI or URI). Which cut-off gives the best balance of sensitivity and specificity? (This is where their sum is a maximum.)
(b) The authors of the report estimated that the prevalence of LRI among all infants with acute respiratory infection in a developing country is 3%. Which cut-off gives the best balance of positive and negative predictive values when the prevalence is 3%?
(c) If a respiratory rate of >50 breaths/min is taken as an indication of LRI and all such children are treated with antibiotics, what proportion of treated infants will have been treated unnecessarily? What proportion of LRI infants would not get antibiotics?
(d) At present general practitioners cannot tell which infants have LRI and about 80% of infants with respiratory tract infection (LRI or URI) receive antibiotics. What would be the effect on the amount of antibiotics used of the policy suggested in (c)?

14.5 A study of observer variation was performed using radiographic diagnosis of caries on 3869 molars and premolars (Espeland and Handelman, 1989). The following table shows the results for three dentists. Teeth were diagnosed as sound (S) or carious (C).

| Dentist | | | |
|---|---|---|---|
| 1 | 2 | 3 | Frequency |
| S | S | S | 2128 |
| S | S | C | 1122 |
| S | C | S | 54 |
| S | C | C | 226 |
| C | S | S | 36 |
| C | S | C | 87 |
| C | C | S | 7 |
| C | C | C | 209 |

(a) Which pair of dentists agreed best?
(b) Is this a good level of agreement?

# 15
# Clinical trials

In a controlled trial, as in all experimental work, there is no need for the search for precision to throw sense out of the window.

Hill (1963)

## 15.1 INTRODUCTION

A clinical trial is a planned experiment on human beings which is designed to evaluate the effectiveness of one or more forms of treatment. Trials can be carried out to evaluate anything that may be considered a potential treatment in its widest sense, such as drugs, surgical procedures, physiotherapy, diet, acupuncture, health education, and so on. I shall use the term clinical trial to refer to any such study.

Clinical trials merit special attention because of their medical importance, some particular problems in design and analysis, and certain ethical problems. The methodology that is used was introduced into medical research about 50 years ago, with the most famous early example being a trial comparing streptomycin and bed rest with bed rest alone in the treatment of pulmonary tuberculosis (MRC, 1948). Comparative clinical trials were virtually unknown before the 1940s. Pocock (1983, p. 14) gives a summary of the historical development of clinical trials.

Within the pharmaceutical industry clinical trials are classified into one of four categories:

1. Phase I: Clinical pharmacology and toxicity;
2. Phase II: Initial clinical investigation;
3. Phase III: Full scale evaluation of treatment;
4. Phase IV: Postmarketing surveillance.

In this Chapter I shall consider only Phase III trials. They have the distinguishing feature that they involve direct comparison between two or more treatments. They are often referred to as **comparative trials** or **controlled trials**. Although some controlled trials are set up to compare more than two treatments I shall concentrate on the common two group case. I shall usually consider the two treatments to be an experimental treatment, perhaps a new drug, and a control treatment, which may be a standard treatment, a placebo, or even no treatment at all, depending on circumstances.

In practice the vast majority of comparative clinical trials have certain features in common which makes it possible to give general guidance on design, analysis and interpretation. Perhaps for this reason, clinical trials are probably the area of medical research where the integration of statistical ideas and methodology has been most successful.

The key idea of a clinical trial is that we wish to compare groups of patients who differ only with respect to their treatment. If the groups differ in some other way then the comparison of treatments is *biased*. If we can identify a bias then it may be possible to allow for its effect in the analysis, but unknown biases cannot be dealt with. The methods of design and analysis described in this chapter are aimed at the elimination of bias.

Deeper consideration of the issues covered in this chapter, as well as topics not covered here, can be found in several books devoted to clinical trials, of which that by Pocock (1983) is particularly recommended. In addition, the papers by Peto *et al*. (1976) and Pocock (1985) discuss some of the trickier issues. Lastly, much wisdom can be found in the chapter on clinical trials in the famous book by Bradford Hill (1984).

## 15.2 DESIGN OF CLINICAL TRIALS

### 15.2.1 The need for a comparison group

The introduction of a new treatment is a long and complex affair, and many apparently promising therapies fall by the wayside. It is natural to begin investigation by trying a new treatment on some patients to see what happens. This type of study is **uncontrolled**, so that any benefits or harmful effects seen in the patients will naturally be ascribed solely to the treatment. Such studies are usually **open**, where the clinician and the patients know what treatment each patient is getting. The investigator's natural enthusiasm for the new treatment may well influence his judgement of the patients' progress, and may also be transmitted to the patients and affect their well-being, especially for conditions where symptoms are subjective, such as degree of pain. Many early studies of this type have suggested that new treatments were highly effective, only for this apparent benefit to disappear on more careful examination. In some cases early results may lead to a treatment being adopted without what we would now consider to be adequate investigation. There are several instances of treatments being investigated after many years' clinical use and being found ineffective. One such was gastric freezing as a treatment for duodenal ulcer, which was discovered, adopted and abandoned within the space of seven years (Miao, 1977). A particularly marked example is the story of the epidemic in babies of retrolental fibroplasia leading to blindness. In the 1950s high doses of oxygen were given to very premature babies. However, the treatment of infants with early eye changes with adrenocorticotrophic hormone had a 75% success rate. Both the oxygen and hormone treatments had been adopted without the benefit of controlled trials. Only after several years of clinical use was it found, after clinical trials were belatedly carried out, that the hormone treatment was ineffective – 75% of such infants return to normal without treatment – and that the oxygen treatment was positively harmful; it caused the blindness in the first place (Silverman, 1985).

There is a place for uncontrolled experiments, designated above as Phase II trials, but they tend to give over-optimistic, and hence biased, results. Definitive assessment of a new treatment should be in relation to the effectiveness of an alternative treatment.

As we will see, there are major advantages if the two treatments are investigated concurrently, allocation of treatments to patients is by a random process, and neither the patient nor the clinician knows which treatment was received. The **randomized double-blind controlled** trial is usually taken as the 'gold standard' against which to judge the quality of the design of a trial.

### 15.2.2 Random allocation

A vital issue in design is to ensure that the allocation of treatments to patients is independent of the characteristics of the patients – in other words, it is carried out in an *unbiased* way. The most widely used method of unbiased treatment allocation is to use **random allocation** to determine which treatment each patient gets. As we saw in Chapter 5, random allocation gives all subjects the same chance of receiving either treatment, and is thus unbiased by definition. Another important reason for using random sampling is that statistical methods of analysis are based on what we expect to happen in random samples from populations with specified characteristics.

It is highly desirable that, as far as is possible, the groups of patients receiving the different treatments are very similar with regard to features that may affect how well they do, that is in their prognosis. For example, in most studies it is important that the age distribution of the groups is similar, because prognosis is very often related to age. There is no guarantee, however, that randomization will in fact lead to the groups being very similar. Any differences between the groups will have arisen by chance, but such differences can be at least inconvenient, and may lead to doubts being cast on the interpretation of the trial results. While it is possible to modify the analysis to take account of any differences between the groups at the start (see section 15.4), it is far better to try to control the problem at the design stage. Most obviously this can be done by using stratified randomization, as described in section 5.7.3. If we know in advance that there are a few key variables that are strongly prognostic then they can be incorporated into a stratified randomization scheme. As observed in section 5.7.3, it is essential that stratified randomization uses blocking, otherwise there is no benefit over simple randomization. There may well be other important variables that we cannot measure or have not identified, and we must rely on the randomization to balance them out. The benefits of having a stratified design are not widely accepted (Peto *et al.*, 1976; Meier, 1981), especially as the increased complexity gives more scope for errors in execution.

A different method of obtaining well-matched groups is to use the technique of **minimization** described in the next section.

### 15.2.3 Minimization

The desirability of random allocation in comparative studies was stressed in the previous section. The use of non-random controls in clinical trials severely lessens the credibility of the results.

Minimization is one non-random method, however, that can be used safely. Indeed, it has definite advantages over both simple or stratified random sampling, unless the sample size is large. The use of minimization will provide treatment groups very closely similar for several variables, even in small samples. It is especially suitable for smaller trials and for trials where small numbers of patients are recruited from each of several centres.

**Table 15.1** Some baseline characteristics of patients in a controlled trial of mustine versus talc in the control of pleural effusions in patients with breast cancer (Fentiman *et al.*, 1983)

| | Treatment | |
|---|---|---|
| | Mustine ($n$ = 23) | Talc ($n$ = 23) |
| Mean age (SE) | 50.3 (1.5) | 55.3 (2.2) |
| Stage of disease: | | |
| 1 or 2 | 52% | 74% |
| 3 or 4 | 48% | 26% |
| Mean interval in months between breast cancer diagnosis and effusion diagnosis (SE) | 33.1 (6.2) | 60.4 (13.1) |
| Postmenopausal | 43% | 74% |

Table 15.1 shows some characteristics of breast cancer patients randomized to receive either mustine or talc as a treatment for pleural effusions. Simple randomization was used in the small trial, and by chance the two treatment groups were noticeably different. Stratified randomization would have helped, but it is not feasible to stratify on several variables in such a small trial. With minimization the two groups would have been very similar with respect to all of these variables, and the results would have been more convincing.

Minimization is based on a completely different principle from randomization. If we regard the patients for the trial as arriving one at a time, then the first patient is given a treatment at random. For each subsequent patient we determine which treatment would lead to better balance between the groups with respect to the variables of interest. The patient is then randomized using a weighting (see section 5.7.1) in favour of the treatment which would minimize the imbalance. For example, we might use a weighting of 4 to 1, so that there is an 80% chance of each patient getting the treatment that minimizes the imbalance. The effect of this procedure is that the groups will be much more similar with regard to the chosen variables than they would be with simple randomization.

Suppose that the mustine vs talc trial had used minimization based on the four variables shown in Table 15.1. For each variable we can divide the possible values into two groups, as follows:

| | | | |
|---|---|---|---|
| Age (years) | $\leq 50$ | or | $> 50$ |
| Stage of disease | 1 or 2 | or | 3 or 4 |
| Time between diagnosis of cancer and diagnosis of effusions (months) | $\leq 30$ | or | $> 30$ |
| Menopausal status | Pre | or | Post |

Suppose that after 29 patients had entered this trial the numbers in each subgroup in each treatment group were as shown in Table 15.2. We now wish to enter into the trial a patient with the following characteristics: 57 years old; stage 3; time interval 22 months; postmenopausal. The numbers of women with this patient's characteristics already in the two treatment groups are shown in Table 15.3. As we wish to have the two groups as similar as possible, the preferable treatment for the new patient is that with the smaller total. Here we would use weighted randomization with a weighting in favour of talc.

After the patient is allocated to a treatment the numbers in each group are updated and the process is repeated for the next patient. If for any patient the totals for the two treatments are the same, then the choice should be made using simple (unweighted) randomization, as it is for the first patient. The method extends simply to variables with more than two categories and to trials of more than two treatments.

**Table 15.2** Characteristics of the first 29 patients in a clinical trial using minimization to allocate treatments

| | | Mustine ($n$ = 15) | Talc ($n$ = 14) |
|---|---|---|---|
| Age | ⩽ 50 | 7 | 6 |
| | > 50 | 8 | 8 |
| Stage | 1 or 2 | 11 | 11 |
| | 3 or 4 | 4 | 3 |
| Time interval | ⩽ 30 m | 6 | 4 |
| | > 30 m | 9 | 10 |
| Menopausal status | Pre | 7 | 5 |
| | Post | 8 | 9 |

**Table 15.3** Calculation of imbalance in patient characteristics for allocating treatment to the thirtieth patient

| | | Mustine ($n$ = 15) | Talc ($n$ = 14) |
|---|---|---|---|
| Age | > 50 | 8 | 8 |
| Stage | 3 or 4 | 4 | 3 |
| Time interval | ⩽ 30 m | 6 | 4 |
| Postmenopausal | | 8 | 9 |
| | Total | 26 | 24 |

The random component can be omitted from the allocation of treatments, so that each patient is automatically given the treatment which leads to less imbalance. Although the treatment that a particular patient receives depends in a complicated way upon the characteristics of the patients already entered into the trial, the absence of a random element introduces a small possibility of selection bias. It is preferable therefore to use weighted randomization.

Minimization is a valid alternative to ordinary randomization, and it has the important advantage, especially in small trials, that there will be only minor differences between the groups with respect to those variables used in the allocation process. It is particularly suitable to be performed with the aid of a computer program, but it is not difficult to perform 'by hand' if the record of the numbers of patients with each characteristic in each group is updated after each new patient has entered the trial.

### 15.2.4 Other methods of treatment allocation

Alternatives to random allocation may be divided into systematic (or **pseudo-random**) methods and non-random methods. Non-randomized trials can be further divided into those with concurrent or non-concurrent (or **historical**) controls.

*(a) Systematic allocation*

A common approach is to allocate treatments to patients according to the patient's date of birth or date of enrolment in the trial (such as giving treatment A to those with even dates, and treatment B to those with odd dates), by the terminal digit of the hospital number, or simply alternately into the different treatment groups. While all of these approaches are in principle unbiased, problems arise from the openness of the allocation system. Put crudely, it is a well-known phenomenon for the allocation to be altered by someone with access to the procedure. Further, knowledge of which treatment a patient is destined to receive can affect the decision about whether to enter that patient into the trial. While such actions are often taken for altruistic motives, the result is a biased allocation and quite possibly a worthless set of data.

Although systematic allocation appears unbiased, it is open to abuse and cannot be recommended unless there really is no alternative. The term 'pseudo-random' is misleading, as there is no random element and the method is definitely inferior to true random allocation.

*(b) Non-random concurrent controls*

The use of non-random controls leads to problems of interpretation, because it will usually be impossible to establish that the groups are comparable. Indeed, the groups may specifically differ in known ways but with unknown effect. For example, in the trial of vitamin supplementation versus placebo in relation to neural tube defects (Smithells *et al.*, 1980), discussed further below, the control group included women ineligible for the trial as well as women who refused to participate. Many studies have shown that there is a **volunteer bias**, with volunteers usually having a better prognosis than refusers. We should worry about bias whenever there is a systematic difference between the patients given different treatments, for example when the groups are taken from patients at different hospitals. Studies where the treatments are given as deemed appropriate by the clinician are especially unreliable.

*(c) Historical controls*

Probably the simplest approach to evaluating a new treatment is to compare a single group of patients all given the new treatment with a group previously treated with an alternative treatment. Often these will be two consecutive series of patients in the same hospital(s). Despite a few advocates, this approach is seriously flawed as we can never satisfactorily eliminate possible biases due to other factors that may have changed over time. Pocock (1977) showed that in 19 cases where the same therapy was used in two consecutive trials of cancer chemotherapy in the same institution there were large changes in the observed death rates, ranging from −46% to +24%. While some of the variation was probably due to small sample sizes, four of the differences were statistically significant at the 2% level. Sacks *et al.* (1983) compared trials of the same therapies in which randomized or historical controls were used, and found a consistent tendency for historically controlled trials to yield more optimistic results than randomized trials. The use of historical controls can only be justified in tightly controlled situations of relatively rare conditions, such as in evaluating therapies for advanced cancer.

The balance of opinion has now swung so far towards randomized trials that the results of non-randomized trials may cause major controversy. A recent example was the study of the possible benefit of vitamin supplementation at the time of conception in women at high risk of having a baby with a neural tube defect (NTD) (Smithells *et al.*, 1980). They found that the vitamin group subsequently had fewer NTD babies than the placebo control group, but because the study was not randomized the findings are not widely accepted, and the Medical Research Council is now running a large randomized trial to try to get a proper answer to the question.

### 15.2.5 Alternative designs

The simplest design for a clinical trial is called the **parallel group** design, in which two different groups of patients are studied concurrently. This is the design that has been implicit in this chapter so far. The most common alternative is the **crossover design**, which is described below together with some other less common designs that are worth knowing about.

*(a) Crossover design*

A crossover trial is one in which the same group of patients are given both (or all) treatments of interest in sequence. Here randomization is used to determine the order in which the treatments are received. The crossover design has some attractive features, in particular that the treatment comparison is 'within-subject' rather than 'between-subject', and that the sample size needed is smaller. There are some important disadvantages, however, which I shall describe in relation to a two-period crossover trial:

1. Patients may drop out after the first treatment, and so not receive the second treatment. Withdrawal may be related to side-effects. Treatment periods should be fairly short to minimize the risk of drop-out for other reasons.

2. There may be a **carry-over** of treatment effect from one period to the next, so that the results obtained during the second treatment are affected by what happened in the first period. In other words, the observed difference between the treatments will depend upon the order in which they were received. In the presence of such a **treatment-period interaction** the data for the second period may have to be discarded, severely weakening the power of the trial.
3. There may be some systematic difference between the two periods of the trial. For example, the observations in the second period may be somewhat lower than those in the first period, regardless of treatment. A small **period effect** is not too serious, as it applies equally to both treatments.
4. Crossover studies cannot be used for conditions which can be cured, and are most suitable when the effect of the treatment can be assessed quickly.

It is desirable to establish in advance that there will not be any carry-over treatment effect, but the information may be unavailable. A **wash-out** period is sometimes introduced between the treatment periods to try to eliminate carry-over effects. Because of the problems described, crossover studies are probably overused. Further discussion is given by Woods *et al*. (1989).

The analysis of crossover trials is explained and illustrated in section 15.4.10.

*(b) Within group (paired) comparisons*

Another type of within group design is when alternative treatments are investigated in the same subjects *at the same time*. It can be used for treatments that can be given independently to matching parts of the anatomy, such as limbs or eyes. The matched design has all the advantages of the crossover design, but none of the disadvantages, so is a very powerful design. Unfortunately, there are few circumstances in which it can be used.

The nearest equivalent to the paired within subject design is the matched pairs design, where pairs of subjects are matched for, say, age, sex and certain prognostic factors, and the two treatments are then allocated to the pair of subjects at random. This design can only be used easily when there is a pool of subjects that can be entered into the trial, in order to be able to find matched pairs. Where there are known important prognostic variables the design removes much of the between subject variation, and ensures that the subjects receiving each treatment have very similar characteristics.

*(c) Sequential designs*

Another type of design is the **sequential trial**, in which parallel groups are studied, but the trial continues until a clear benefit of one treatment is seen or it is unlikely that any difference will emerge. The main advantage of sequential trials is that they will be shorter than fixed length trials when there is a large difference in the effectiveness of the two treatments.

In sequential trials the data are analysed after each patient's results become available. Their use is therefore restricted to conditions where the outcome is known relatively quickly. There are problems with blinding (see section 15.2.6), and possibly also ethical difficulties.

A useful variation on this principle is the **group sequential trial**, in which the data are analysed after each block of patients has been seen, perhaps four or five times in all. This allows the trial to be planned more easily (regarding length) but also enables the trial to be stopped early if a clear treatment difference is seen.

In the right circumstances sequential trials are a good method, and they should be used more frequently.

*(d) Factorial designs*

One further type of design is called the **factorial design**, in which two treatments, say A and B, are simultaneously compared with each other and with a control. Patients are divided into four groups, who receive the control treatment, A only, B only, and both A and B. This design allows the investigation of the interaction (or 'synergy') between A and B. The factorial design is rarely used in clinical trials, but Pocock (1983, p. 139) describes some examples of its use.

*(e) Adaptive designs*

Ethical considerations have led some people to advocate **adaptive designs**, in which the proportion of subjects getting the inferior treatment diminishes as the trial proceeds. In other words, a patient's treatment depends to some extent on the outcome of treatment in previous patients in the trial. Apart from practical difficulties, such as needing to know quickly the results from each patient, it is questionable whether this design resolves any ethical problems. Adaptive designs have rarely been used.

*(f) Zelen's design*

Lastly, Zelen (1979) proposed a variation on the randomized trial that seems to avoid problems associated with getting informed consent. Half of the subjects are allocated at random to receive the standard treatment, and are treated as if they were not in a trial. The other half are offered the new experimental treatment, but they can choose to have the standard treatment if they wish. An essential feature of Zelen's proposal (Zelen, 1979) is that the two groups are analysed as originally randomized, regardless of which treatment those in the second group actually opted for. While this design has some useful features, it can only be of value when a high proportion of those offered the new treatment take it, which cannot be known in advance. This design has rarely been used, and many consider it unethical not to tell half the patients that they are in a trial. A variation is where both groups are told which treatment they have been allocated and are offered the chance to switch to the other. While resolving the ethical difficulty, there are possible difficulties associated with the necessary lack of blindness and loss of power if too many patients opt to change treatment. There does not seem to be much to recommend this design. Ellenberg (1984) gives further discussion.

### 15.2.6 Blindness

The key to a successful clinical trial is to avoid any biases in the comparison of the groups. Randomization deals with possible bias at the treatment allocation, but bias can also creep in while the study is being run. Both the patient and the doctor may be affected in the way they respectively respond and observe by knowledge of which treatment was given. For this reason, it is desirable that neither the patient nor the person evaluating the patient knows which treatment was given. Such a trial is called **double-blind**. If only the patient is unaware, as is sometimes the case, the trial is called **single-blind**. In several fields, such as surgery, it is often impossible for a study to be double-blind. Clinical trials should use the maximum degree of blindness that is possible.

In addition, the treatment allocation system should be set up so that the person entering patients does not know in advance which treatment the next person will get. A common way of doing this is to use a series of consecutively numbered sealed opaque envelopes, each containing a treatment specification. For stratified randomization, two or more sets of envelopes are needed. For drug trials the allocation may be carried out by the pharmacy, who will produce numbered bottles which do not indicate the treatment contained.

Double-blind trials clearly require that the different treatments should be indistinguishable to the patient and to whoever assesses the patient. For drug trials comparing two active treatments this may require the **double dummy** technique, in which each patient receives one of the active drugs and a dummy tablet that looks like the alternative active drug.

### 15.2.7 Placebos

When we wish to evaluate a new treatment for a condition there is the problem of what treatment to give to the control group. If (and only if) there is no existing standard beneficial treatment, then it is reasonable not to give the control group any active treatment. However, there are two reasons why it is desirable to give the control group patients an inert dummy or **placebo** treatment, rather than nothing. Firstly, the act of taking some treatment may itself have some benefit to the patient, so that if we give nothing at all to the control group then part of any benefit observed in the treated group could be due to the knowledge or belief that they had taken a treatment. This is known as the **placebo effect**. Secondly, in order for a study to be double-blind it is necessary for the two treatments to be indistinguishable. Placebo tablets should therefore be identical in appearance and taste to the active treatment, but pharmacologically inactive.

Many clinical trials do, in fact, find some apparent benefit of treatment in the placebo group, and there are often **side-effects** too. Without a comparison group, who may be given an alternative active treatment or a placebo, we cannot know how specific any benefit (or harm) is to the new treatment being investigated. For example, if there are as many reported headaches in the active and placebo treated groups, we would not consider headache as a side-effect of the active treatment.

Placebos can sometimes be used in non-drug trials too. In section 10.3 I described a trial that had used mock electrical stimulation as a control treatment. Likewise a control for acupuncture is easily set up by having needles inserted at the 'wrong' points. There may however be ethical problems associated with invasive placebos.

### 15.2.8 Selection of subjects

Clinical trials are a prime example of the principle that we collect data from a sample and use the results of the analysis to make inferences about the population of all such subjects. In order for this process to work it is clearly necessary to select a representative sample. In practice, however, many restrictions are usually placed on who is eligible to take part in a trial, and so extrapolation of the results to the population may be difficult. For example, a placebo-controlled trial was carried out in British doctors to see if daily aspirin would reduce the incidence of and mortality from stroke, myocardial infarction and other vascular conditions (Peto *et al.*, 1988). The investigators identified 20 000 doctors who were willing to participate but almost three-quarters of them were ineligible, either because they were already taking aspirin for some reason, because there were reasons why they could not take aspirin, or because they had a history of peptic ulcer, stroke or myocardial infarction. The doctors who took part in the study were therefore a selected group of more healthy individuals.

Figure 15.1 shows how patients with either low or high blood pressure would be excluded from a trial of a new hypertensive treatment, although for different reasons. Often the patients whom it is both ethical and reasonable to include in a trial are those most likely to benefit if the treatment is effective. In general, but not always, we do not expect treatment to do much for patients who already have an excellent prognosis, nor for those with a dreadful prognosis.

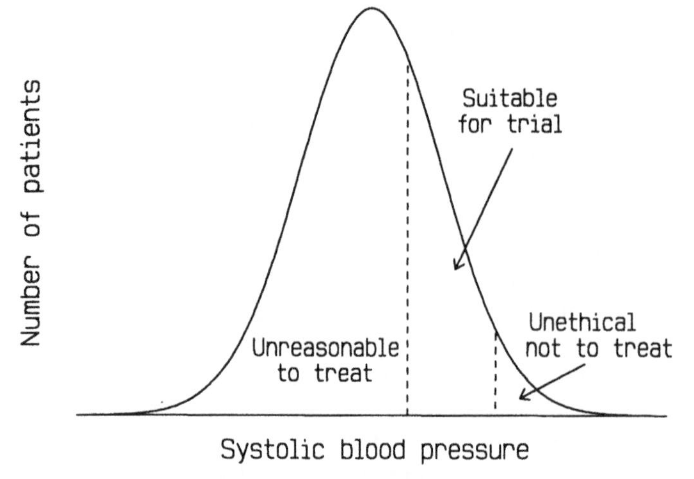


**Figure 15.1** Diagram showing the eligibility of patients for a trial of a new antihypertensive agent (based on Elwood, 1982).

Begg and Engstrom (1987) discussed the problem of over-restrictive eligibility criteria in cancer clinical trials, which can lead to most patients with a disease being ineligible for a trial. They suggest that many exclusion criteria are unnecessary. The more restrictive the exclusion criteria, the less generalizable will be the results of the trial. In large trials especially it is better not to be too restrictive, although in small trials there may be some advantage in keeping the study subjects more homogeneous, especially if simple randomization is used.

### 15.2.9 Ethical issues

A clinical trial is an experiment on human beings, so it is not surprising that there are several important ethical issues relating to clinical trials. One concerns the amount of information given to the patient. In general the patient should be invited to be in the trial, and should be told what the alternative treatments are (although they will usually not know which they will get). They can decline to be in the trial, in which case they will be treated normally. If they agree to participate they will often have to sign a form stating that they understand the trial. This **informed consent** is controversial, because it is likely that many patients do not really understand what they are told, and that they are not always told as much as they should be. There are some cases where it is not possible to get informed consent, for example when the patients are very young, very old, or unconscious. Also there are a few circumstances where it might be difficult to get people to agree to be randomized, such as in a trial comparing mastectomy with chemotherapy as a treatment for breast cancer.

From the clinical side, no doctor should participate in a clinical trial if he/she believes that one of the treatments being investigated is superior, and they should not enter any patient for which they think that a particular treatment is indicated. In other words, the ideal medical state to be in is one of ignorance: the trial is carried out because we do not know which treatment is better. It may be thought that an active treatment, which will have yielded promising results in uncontrolled observational studies, would be certain to be better than a placebo, but this is not always so. Further, even if the treatment is beneficial there may be unacceptable side-effects.

In many countries there are a large number of ethics committees set up to consider proposals to carry out clinical trials (and, indeed, any research involving human subjects). Interestingly, the problems relating to the design of the trial of vitamin supplementation around conception (Smithells *et al.*, 1980) stemmed largely from the refusal of ethics committees to sanction the randomized trial that was originally proposed. The study as performed *did*, of course, have the approval of the ethics committees. Ethics committees are usually concerned only with the welfare of the patient, and do not consider scientific, including statistical, issues.

Regarding design, it can be argued that non-randomized trials, especially those with non-concurrent (historical) controls, are unethical because, as shown earlier, the results of such trials are so unreliable. Similar comments can be levelled at any trial which uses suboptimal methodology, although it is not possible to draw a precise line between ethical and unethical studies.

More generally, any study (not necessarily a clinical trial) that uses substandard statistical methods, especially in design or analysis, may be deemed unethical for three reasons (Altman, 1982a):

1. the misuse of patients by exposing them to unjustified risk and inconvenience;
2. the misuse of resources, including the researchers' time, which could be better employed on more valuable activities; and
3. the consequences of publishing misleading results, which may include the carrying out of unnecessary further work.

Many of the ethical issues relating to clinical trials were dealt with by Bradford Hill (1963). Silverman (1985, p. 153) gives a more recent review of the main issues.

### 15.2.10 Outcome measures

In most clinical trials information about the effect of treatment is gathered in relation to many variables, sometimes on more than one occasion. There is the temptation to analyse each of the variables and look to see which differences between treatment groups are significant. This approach leads to misleading results, because multiple testing will invalidate the results of hypothesis tests. In particular, presenting only the most significant results, as if these were the only analyses performed, is fraudulent.

A preferable approach is to decide *in advance* of the analysis which outcome measure is of major interest, and focus attention on this variable when analysing the data. Other data can and should be analysed too, but these variables should be considered to be of secondary importance. Any interesting findings among the secondary variables should be interpreted rather cautiously, more as ideas for further research than as definitive results. Side-effects of treatment should be treated in this way.

Sometimes there really will be more than one major outcome measure. If there are two, then no great harm will come from analysing them both, perhaps taking a stricter cut-off for statistical significance. Sometimes it is possible to combine two variables into one, in particular when the variables of interest are alternative events, such as death or heart attack.

Finally, note that sample size calculations (see section 15.3) are based on a single variable.

### 15.2.11 Protocols

An important aspect of planning a clinical trial is to produce a **protocol**, which is a formal document outlining the proposed procedures for carrying out the trial.

Pocock (1983, pp. 28–31) suggests the following main features of a study protocol:

1. background and study objectives
2. specific objectives
3. patient selection criteria
4. treatment schedules
5. methods of patient evaluation
6. trial design
7. registration and randomization of patients
8. patient consent
9. required size of study
10. monitoring of trial progress
11. forms and data handling
12. protocol deviations
13. plans for statistical analysis
14. administrative responsibilities.

A protocol is necessary when applying for a grant to carry out a trial, and most of the above information will be required by the local ethics committee. Further, as well as aiding in the carrying out of a trial, a protocol makes the writing up of the results much easier as the introduction and methods section of the paper should be substantially the same as sections 1 to 9 above.

For multicentre studies a detailed protocol is essential, and it is strongly recommended for any clinical trial. Indeed, I recommend the drawing up of a proper protocol for *any* research project – most of the above categories are not specific to clinical trials.

## 15.3 SAMPLE SIZE

### 15.3.1 Introduction

In section 8.5.3 I introduced the concept of **power** in relation to hypothesis testing. The power of a test is the probability that a study of a given size would detect as statistically significant a real difference of a given magnitude. The medical literature contains many trials that were far too small to have a good chance of detecting clinically worthwhile differences between the treatments being investigated. It is clear from many reviews of published trials that the majority have been carried out with no statistical calculation of the appropriate sample size. Unless the true treatment effect is large, small trials can yield a statistically significant result only if, by chance, the observed difference in the sample is much larger than the real difference.

This section introduces statistical methods for calculating the appropriate sample size for comparing two independent groups of subjects (parallel group design), or for comparing paired observations (paired or crossover design). These methods are not specific to randomized trials, but apply to two group comparisons in general. While there is some artificiality in the approach, it is vastly preferable to the hit and miss approach that is so common. The calculations are based on the principles of hypothesis testing. Sample size calculations for more complicated trials, including sequential trials, will require statistical assistance, as will those where the main outcome of interest is survival time.

### 15.3.2 Sample size, hypothesis tests and power

We can use the power of a hypothesis test to calculate the appropriate sample size for a clinical trial if we can specify the smallest true difference between the treatments that would be clinically valuable. It is this requirement that is somewhat artificial and difficult to define. In practice, however, it is usually possible to specify the degree of benefit that the new treatment would need to have over the old one for it to be a worthwhile treatment.

The main idea behind the sample size calculations is to have a high chance of detecting, as statistically significant, a worthwhile effect *if it exists*, and thus to be reasonably sure that no such benefit exists if it is not found in the trial. The greater the power of the study, the more sure we can be, but greater power requires a larger sample, as we will see. It is common to require a power of between 80% and 90%. In effect, we try to make clinical importance and statistical significance agree, and thus reduce problems of interpretation.

The necessary sample size is usually obtained from complicated formulae or there are extensive tables available (Machin and Campbell, 1987), but it is much simpler to use a graphical method. Figure 15.2 shows a nomogram that can be used to calculate the appropriate sample size for all the situations considered in this chapter. It is simple to use and has the added

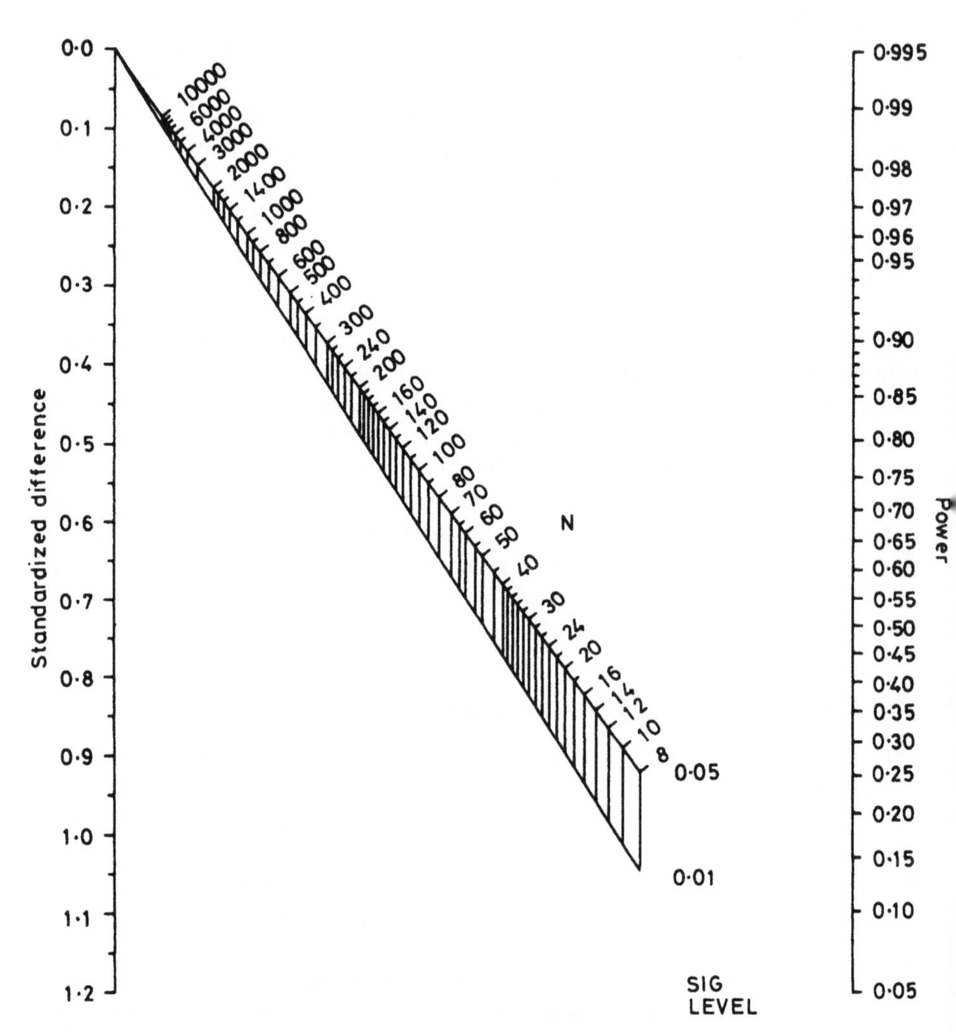


**Figure 15.2** Nomogram for calculating sample size or power (reproduced from Altman, 1982b, with permission).

advantage of being equally easy to use in reverse for determining the power of a study of given sample size.

I shall first consider the case where we intend to have two groups of equal size. The nomogram can be used, however, for unequal sample sizes, as I shall show later. All of the sample size calculations are based on the quantity known as the **standardized difference**. This is calculated in a different way for continuous or categorical outcome variables, but in principle it is based in each case on the ratio of the difference of interest to the standard deviation of the observations. In other words, we express the difference of interest as a multiple of the standard deviation. As we would expect, the smaller this ratio is the larger the required size of the trial.

*(a) Continuous data – two independent groups*

For studies of two independent groups of patients with a continuous outcome measure we need to specify the following quantities:

1. standard deviation of the variable (in each group) ($s$);
2. clinically relevant difference ($\delta$);
3. the significance level ($\alpha$ – two-sided);
4. the power ($1 - \beta$);

and it is assumed that the variable has a Normal distribution in the population. The total sample size is $N$.

The standardized difference is calculated simply as the ratio of the difference of interest to the standard deviation, that is $\delta/s$. We can use Figure 15.2 to calculate the necessary sample size from the standardized difference for any desired power, choosing either a 5% or 1% level of significance.

For example, suppose that we are planning a milk-feeding trial in five-year-old children, to see if a daily supplement of milk for a year will lead to an increased gain in height compared with a control group. (Such a study would in fact be difficult to carry out, for practical and ethical reasons.) We know from published data that at this age children grow on average about 6 cm in a year, with a standard deviation of 2 cm. Suppose that the effect of the milk on height gain will be considered important if it is at least 0.5 cm. We want a high probability of detecting such a difference, so we set the power to be 0.9 (90%) and choose a 1% significance level. The standardized difference is $0.5/2.0 = 0.25$. We can now use Figure 15.2 to calculate the necessary sample size. We 'draw' a straight line from the value 0.25 on the scale for the standardized difference to the value 0.90 on the scale for power and read off the value for $N$ on the line corresponding to $\alpha = 0.01$, which gives a total sample size of 900, i.e. 450 in each group.

There are several possible approaches if no estimate of the standard deviation is available. One way is to start the trial and use the data for the first patients to estimate the standard deviation and thus the sample size needed. Alternatively, the problem can be redefined in terms of the difference between the proportions above and below some chosen cut-off level, and then use the methods for proportions described below. For example, we may recast a trial of an antihypertensive agent in terms of the difference in the proportion of subjects whose systolic blood pressure is reduced to below 150 mm Hg, rather than a comparison of mean blood pressure. Another possibility is to specify the difference of interest directly in terms of the unknown standard deviation. For example, Guyatt *et al.* (1987) set up a trial to compare ambroxol and placebo in patients with chronic bronchitis, in which they used a questionnaire to derive a score for severity of symptoms. They did not know the standard deviation of these scores, so specified that they wished to be able to detect a difference between the groups of one standard deviation. The standardized difference was therefore 1.0, and the researchers had avoided the need to specify the standard deviation. All of these solutions involve some degree of subjectivity.

It is easy to calculate the sample size for any combination of input values $(s, \delta, \alpha, 1 - \beta)$, and we can always change the sample size by altering the input values. However, it is preferable to decide in advance what the requirements are. While some modest relaxation of these is acceptable, in general if the calculated sample size exceeds what seems practical, then the study can be extended either in time or by running the study at more centres. If it is not possible to get near to the required size of study, then the study may best be abandoned.

*(b) Continuous data – paired or within person studies*

The appropriate sample size for paired studies, or within person studies such as crossover trials, is obtained in a very similar way. The main difference is that the standard deviation we use is the standard deviation of the *changes* expected, which I shall call $s_d$. Unfortunately, an estimate of this standard deviation is often not available. If we do have a reasonable estimate of $s_d$, we can calculate the standardized difference as $2\delta/s_d$, and then use the nomogram as before. (Note the similarity to the formula for independent groups, apart from the multiplier of 2.)

*(c) Categorical data*

The nomogram in Figure 15.2 can also be used for studies which have a binary outcome variable. If the outcome variable has more than two categories it is necessary to create a binary variable of interest. For example, if patients are to be assessed as 'improved', 'no change' or 'worse', then the sample size calculation could be based on whether or not the patient has improved.

The calculation of sample size for comparing proportions makes use of the Normal approximation to the Binomial distribution, discussed in section 8.4.3. It is based on the following information:

1. the expected proportion with the specified outcome in each group ($p_1$ and $p_2$);
2. the significance level ($\alpha$ – two-sided);
3. the power ($1 - \beta$).

The usual way of thinking about specifying $p_1$ and $p_2$ is that previous knowledge should allow us to predict the proportion with the outcome in the control group (say $p_1$), and so we need to specify the proportion with the outcome in the experimental group that would represent an important improvement.

Given specified values of $p_1$ and $p_2$ we can calculate the standardized difference as

$$\frac{p_1 - p_2}{\sqrt{\bar{p}(1 - \bar{p})}}$$

where $\bar{p} = (p_1 + p_2)/2$.

For example, suppose we are planning a trial to compare two methods of helping smokers to give up smoking. One group is to be given a new kind of nicotine chewing gum and the other group will receive advice from their doctor and a booklet. On the basis of published evidence we expect that in the advice group 15% of smokers will remain non-smokers at 6 months. We would be interested in an improvement to 30% in the group given gum. The proportions to be compared are thus 0.30 and 0.15. Suppose that we want an 85% probability of detecting such a difference, if it really exists, as statistically significant at the 5% level. We can use the nomogram to work out the necessary sample size for the trial.

We have $p_1 = 0.30$ and $p_2 = 0.15$ so $\bar{p} = (0.30 + 0.15)/2 = 0.225$. Using the above formula the standardized difference is given as

$$\frac{0.30 - 0.15}{\sqrt{0.225(1 - 0.225)}}$$

or 0.36. We connect the standardized difference of 0.36 to the power of 0.85 in the nomogram in Figure 15.2 and read off the necessary sample size for the trial from the central axis corresponding to a significance level of 0.05, which gives $N = 280$. To meet the conditions specified for the trial we thus need to have 140 smokers in each group.

*(d) Unequal sample size*

The nomogram can be used for trials in which the sample size in the two groups will be different. Sometimes it is felt desirable or necessary to use unequal (weighted) randomization. As long as the imbalance is not great the loss in power is small.

To use the nomogram to plan a study with unequal groups, we must first calculate $N$ as if we were using equal groups and then calculate the modified sample size $N'$. If $k = n_1/n_2$ is the ratio of the sample sizes in the two groups, then the required total sample size is

$$N' = N(1 + k)^2/4k$$

and the two sample sizes are given by $N'/(1 + k)$ and $kN'/(1 + k)$. So, for example, if we wish to put twice as many subjects on the experimental treatment than on the control, we have $k = 2$, and so $N' = 9N/8$, a fairly small increase, but for $k = 3$ we have $N' = 16N/12$ which is an increase of a third over equal sample sizes.

*(e) Calculating power*

The nomogram can be used to calculate the power for a given sample size. We just connect by a straight line the relevant values for the sample size and standardized difference and read off the power of the study on the third scale.

To evaluate the power of a study with unequal sample sizes $n_1$ and $n_2$ we use the 'effective' sample size $N$, which is calculated as

$$N = 4N'k/(1 + k)^2$$

where $k = n_1/n_2$ and $N' = n_1 + n_2$.

*(f) Getting enough patients*

Often the sample size calculations reveal a required sample size that exceeds the recruiting capability of a single centre. Rather than carry out a trial that is low in power, it is often worth trying to get other centres to collaborate in a 'multicentre' trial, although there will be organizational difficulties to offset against the benefits of increased sample size.

A further problem is that the expected rate of accrual of patients to a trial can be much less than anticipated by the trial organizers. While this may be partly through over-optimism, it is often largely because of a failure to appreciate the effect of the trial's eligibility criteria. Restricting eligibility may lead to failure to achieve the planned sample size, and thus affect the usefulness of the trial as well as the generalizability of the results. Another factor here is the proportion of eligible patients who refuse to participate. If these rates cannot be reliably estimated, then it is prudent to make an allowance for them when planning the sample size for the trial.

Many of the difficulties can be avoided by having a pilot study, which is also valuable for assessing the quality of the data collection forms, and for checking the logistics of the trial, such as the expected time to examine each patient which affects the number that can be seen in a session. A pilot study may also provide more reliable estimates for use in sample size calculations.

## 15.4 ANALYSIS

The possibility of bias entering a trial at the treatment allocation or during the execution of a trial is well known, but there are also several less well known ways in which bias can arise during the analysis of clinical trial data.

In principle the analysis of clinical trial data should be straightforward, using relatively simple methods outlined in earlier chapters, such as *t* tests and $\chi^2$ tests. There are, however, several particular problems that arise in the analysis of clinical trials. I shall first consider the assessment of whether the treatment groups are comparable, then some possible causes of bias, and lastly analyses that are more complicated than simply comparing means or proportions in two groups. A fuller discussion of bias in analysis is given by May *et al.* (1981).

### 15.4.1 Comparison of entry characteristics

Randomization is a method of eliminating bias in the way that treatments are allocated to patients, but it does not guarantee that the characteristics of the different groups are similar. Methods for trying to keep the groups similar were discussed in section 15.2, but most trials use simple randomization with which it is possible to produce groups with quite different characteristics. For example, in a trial including 36 patients, even when we have 18 subjects in each group, any characteristic that is present in half of the subjects has a 6% chance of being at least twice as common in one treatment group as in the other. Such imbalance for a prognostic variable could have a marked effect on the results of the trial, and on their credibility.

The first analysis that should be carried out with data from a clinical trial is to summarize the entry or **baseline** characteristics of the patients in the two groups. It is important to show that the groups are similar with respect to variables that may affect the patient's response. For example, we would usually wish to be happy that the age distribution was similar in the different groups, as many outcomes are age-related. Smoking and stage of disease are other variables often looked at in this way.

The usual way of comparing the baseline characteristics of the groups is by performing hypothesis tests, but a moment's thought should suffice to see that this is unhelpful (Altman, 1985). If the randomization is performed fairly we *know* that any differences between the two treatment groups must be due to chance. A hypothesis test thus makes no sense. In any case the question at issue is whether the groups differ in a way that might affect their response to treatment, which is clearly a question of clinical importance rather than statistical significance. The only use of hypothesis testing is to judge whether the randomization was performed fairly, but this will only detect major failures. We expect 5% of tests to be significant at the 5% level.

While few trials will give results as close to expectation as that of Ueshima *et al.* (1987), in which 1 of 20 comparisons was statistically significant at the 5% level, we do not expect large discrepancies from chance. Collins *et al.* (1987) gave an example of extreme imbalance that is incompatible with proper randomization. Table 15.4 shows the nodal status of patients allocated to active treatment or control in two centres participating in a randomized trial in early breast cancer. The enormous imbalance in centre 2 can only be interpreted as indicating that the randomization at the centre was improper, and the results from that centre should be ignored.

**Table 15.4** Number of patients with different nodal status allocated to treatment or control in two centres participating in a randomized trial in early breast cancer (from Collins *et al.*, 1987)

| | Centre 1 | | Centre 2 | |
|---|---|---|---|---|
| | Treatment | Control | Treatment | Control |
| Nodal status | | | | |
| 0 | 62 (61%) | 65 (64%) | 27 (22%) | 63 (50%) |
| 1–3 | 29 (28%) | 28 (28%) | 39 (31%) | 44 (35%) |
| 4+ | 11 (11%) | 7 (7%) | 53 (42%) | 18 (14%) |
| Not known | 0 (0%) | 1 (1%) | 6 (5%) | 1 (1%) |
| Total | 102 (100%) | 101 (100%) | 125 (100%) | 126 (100%) |
| | $X^2 = 2.0$ on 2 df | | $X^2 = 35.4$ on 2 df | |
| | $P = 0.37$ | | $P < 0.00000001$ | |

(Excluding not knowns)

Imbalance in a baseline variable is only potentially important, in the sense of affecting the overall result of the trial, if that variable is related to the outcome variable. With proper randomization most variables will be distributed similarly in the different treatment groups. If there are one or more variables with known or suspected prognostic importance that are not very closely balanced we can see whether those variables really are related to the outcome variable, or we can simply adjust for them in the analysis, as discussed in section 15.4.6.

### 15.4.2 Main analysis

The main analysis of a clinical trial is the comparison of the pre-specified outcome measure(s) between the different treatment groups. As already noted, we can use the simple methods of analysis described in Chapters 9 and 10. For trials of independent groups we can use the two sample $t$ test, Mann-Whitney $U$ test, or $\chi^2$ test as appropriate and construct the associated confidence intervals. For paired or matched studies we can use the paired $t$ test, Wilcoxon paired test, or the McNemar test. Crossover trials require a particular form of analysis, which is described below.

There are, however, various possible complicating factors that may need to be considered, which are discussed in the next few sections.

### 15.4.3 Incomplete data

Data may be incomplete for several reasons. For example, occasional laboratory measurements will be missing because the samples taken were inadequate. It is important to use all the data available, and to specify if any observations are missing. Also, some information may simply not have been recorded. While it may seem reasonable to assume that a particular symptom was not present if it was not recorded, such inferences are in general unsafe and should be made only after careful consideration of the circumstances.

The most important problem with missing information relates to patients who drop out of the study before the end. Withdrawal may be by the clinician, perhaps because of side-effects. Alternatively, the patient may move to another area or just fail to return without reason. Efforts should be made to obtain at least some information regarding the status of these patients at the end of the trial, but some data are still likely to be missing. One possible approach is to assign the most optimistic outcome to all these patients and analyse the data, and then repeat the analysis with the most pessimistic outcome. If the two analyses yield similar results, and results also similar to those from an analysis in which these patients are simply excluded, then we can be fairly confident in the findings. The most common approach is simply to omit all such patients, which is reasonable if the number of withdrawals is not too great, and if the proportion withdrawing is similar in each treatment group. However, if there are many more withdrawals in one treatment group the results of the trial will be compromised, as it is likely that the withdrawals are treatment-related.

If the main outcome measure is the time to some event, such as death or recurrence of disease, then we can use some data for all patients, even those who withdraw (see Chapter 13).

### 15.4.4 Protocol violations

In many trials some patients will not have followed the protocol, either deliberately or accidentally. Included here are patients who actually receive the wrong treatment (i.e. not the one allocated) and patients who do not take their treatment, known as **non-compliers**. Also it is sometimes discovered after the trial has begun that a patient was not after all eligible for the trial.

The only safe way to deal with all of these situations is to **keep all randomized patients in the trial**. The analysis is thus based on the groups as randomized, and is known as an **intention to treat** analysis. Any other policy towards protocol violations will involve subjective decisions and will thus create an opportunity for bias. It is sometimes useful to perform an additional analysis of only those patients adhering to the protocol, but this cannot be taken as a completely fair comparison. For example, the exclusion of patients who did not comply with the protocol may bias the analysis. The analysis of the groups as randomized must be considered the main analysis.

### 15.4.5 Excluding some events

Sometimes the event of interest, such as myocardial infarction or death, occurs after randomization but before the treatment has commenced, or before it could have had an effect. The exclusion of such patients from the analysis is most unwise and may well lead to controversy. It is desirable to design a trial so that there is a minimal delay between randomization and the start of treatment. Sackett and Gent (1979) discuss this problem at some length.

A similar problem arises when the outcome of interest is death from a specific cause such as cancer. It is often unclear if a death is truly unrelated to the medical condition being treated and so it is generally unwise to exclude deaths from other causes.

### 15.4.6 Adjusting for other variables

If we suspect that the observed differences (imbalance) between the groups at the start of the trial may have affected the outcome we can take account of the imbalance in the analysis. Table 15.1 showed some of the baseline characteristics of patients in a trial where the groups look markedly different. The authors did not adjust for the large differences because none of them is statistically significant. We do not know what effect the imbalance may have had. With small trials it is quite common to have large imbalances that are not statistically significant but which could well be clinically important. (For small trials, therefore, simple randomization is not a good method of treatment allocation.)

Most clinical trials are based on the simple idea of comparing two groups with respect to a single variable of prime interest, for which the statistical analysis is straightforward. We may, however, wish to take one or more other variables into consideration in the analysis. One reason might be that the two groups were not similar with respect to baseline variables, as in Table 15.1. We can thus perform the analysis with and without adjustment. If the results are similar we can infer that the imbalance was not important, and can quote the simple comparison, but if the results are different we should use the adjusted analysis. Imbalance will only affect the results if the variable is related to the outcome measure. It will not matter if one group is on average much shorter than the other if height is unrelated to response to treatment. Table 15.1 shows imbalance for several variables which we might reasonably suppose would be related to outcome, so an adjusted analysis is strongly indicated. The use of some form of restricted randomization that is designed to give similar groups is thus desirable as it simplifies the subsequent analysis of the data.

Even if the groups had very similar characteristics it may still be desirable to adjust for another variable if we know in advance that the variable is strongly related to prognosis. Age is often such a variable. Adjustment for variables known to affect outcome can improve the power of the trial, although not greatly, by improving the precision with which we estimate the treatment effect. Again the effect of adjustment can be assessed by comparison with the unadjusted analysis. Further discussion is given in Altman (1985).

Adjusting for other variables requires the use of the analysis of co-variance or some form of multiple regression analysis, as described in Chapter 12.

### 15.4.7 Multiple outcome measures

I suggested in section 15.2.10 that where possible one outcome measure should be treated as the main focus of attention in the analysis. There may be other outcome measures, and these can be analysed using the same methods, but the findings given less emphasis. If there are genuinely several outcome measures of importance, then the P value considered statistically significant should be made smaller than the usual 5% to keep the risk of a Type I error small. One simple method is to use the Bonferroni correction, in which if there are $k$ variables being analysed then the P values are multiplied by $k$ (see section 9.8.4).

Smith *et al.* (1987) reviewed 66 clinical trials published in four major general journals: *Lancet, British Medical Journal, New England Journal of Medicine*, and the *Journal of the American Medical Association*. They found that the mean number of outcome measures analysed was 22. Appreciation of the dangers of multiple comparisons was rare. A review of 196 reports of trials of nonsteroidal anti-inflammatory drugs in rheumatoid arthritis (Gøtzsche, 1989) found that over 70 different outcome measures were used, with a median of eight per trial. In only 6% of trials was a main outcome variable chosen in advance.

Gøtzsche (1989) also highlighted the common error of multiple counting of measurements or side-effects. The 'sampling unit' (unit of investigation) of a clinical trial is the patient, so results should relate to patients rather than, for example, joints or teeth.

### 15.4.8 Changes from baseline

I observed in section 5.2 that a clinical trial is a longitudinal study. Although it is common to take the patients' status at the end of the study period as the outcome of interest, sometimes it is more appropriate to take the *change* from the pre-treatment, or baseline, measurement as the prime outcome measure. For example, in a trial comparing anti-asthma treatments, the improvements in each individual's lung function would be the focus of attention rather than their lung function at the end of the study. This analysis has the important advantage of removing any differences between the groups with respect to pre-treatment levels of the outcome variable. When changes from baseline are analysed it is misleading to perform separate analyses (either hypothesis tests or confidence intervals) within each treatment group. A better approach is to calculate each patient's change from baseline, and then compare directly the changes in the different groups.

### 15.4.9 Subgroup analyses

There is often interest in identifying which patients do well on a treatment and which do badly. We can answer a question like this by analysing the data separately for subsets of the data. We may, for example, re-do the analysis including only male patients, only patients less than 50, or those with a particular symptom. Subgroup analyses like these pose problems of interpretation similar to those resulting from multiple outcome measures. It is reasonable to carry out a small number of subgroup analyses *if these were specified in the protocol*, but on no account should the data be analysed in numerous different ways in the hope of discovering some significant comparison. An example of the dangers of searching through multiple subgroups is given by Collins *et al.* (1987), who showed that in a trial on patients with suspected acute myocardial infarction the benefit of treatment was four times as great for patients born under Scorpio than for patients born under all other signs put together.

In many cases the real question of interest is not whether the difference between the treatments is present in a subgroup of patients, but whether the treatment effect differs among two or more complementary subgroups. Thus, for example, in a placebo-controlled trial we may wish to know if the active treatment is more effective among younger patients than older patients. A common approach is to analyse separately the data for the younger and older patients and compare the two P values. This analysis makes comparisons *between* the two groups based on analyses carried out separately *within* each group, and is not a valid method. (A similar situation was described in the previous section.) The correct approach is to compare the difference between the treatments for the two age groups; in other words we look at the *interaction* between age and treatment. The possibility of an interaction can be examined within an appropriate multiple regression model, whether the outcome variable is continuous, binary or survival time. I recommend expert advice for this analysis. (See also Pocock, 1983, p. 213.) Note that this analysis is more like that from an observational study, and so we cannot infer causality from any association.

### 15.4.10 Crossover trials

Crossover trials were described in section 15.2.5. The analysis of a crossover trial will be illustrated using data from a trial comparing nicardipine, a calcium-channel blocker, and placebo in the treatment of Raynaud's phenomenon (Kahan *et al.*, 1987). The data, representing the number of attacks in two weeks, are shown in Table 15.5 separately for the groups having nicardipine followed by placebo and *vice versa*.

The analysis is simplified by calculating for each subject the difference ($d_i$) and average ($a_i$) of the observations in the two periods, and averaging these for each group as shown in Table 15.5. It is incorrect to ignore the design of the study and just perform a simple comparison of treatments. Before comparing the treatments there are two other tests that should be carried out. The correct analysis consists of three two sample $t$ tests or Mann-Whitney tests; $t$ tests are used here. (For categorical data we use $\chi^2$ tests.)

The possibility of a period effect is tested by a two sample $t$ test to compare the differences between the periods in the two groups of patients. If there was no general tendency for patients to do better in one of the periods we would expect the mean differences between the periods in the two groups to be of the same size but having opposite signs. The test for a period effect is thus a two sample $t$ test comparing $\bar{d}_1$ with $-\bar{d}_2$.

We investigate the possibility of a treatment–period interaction by noticing that in the absence of an interaction a patient's average response to the two treatments would be the same regardless of the order in which they were received. The test for interaction is thus a two sample $t$ test comparing $\bar{a}_1$ with $\bar{a}_2$.

If there is no period effect and no treatment-period interaction the analysis of a crossover trial is simple. However, it is important to investigate possible problems before carrying out the treatment comparison. Both a marked period effect and a treatment-period interaction are worrying because they mean that the observed magnitude of the treatment

**Table 15.5** Results from a randomized double-blind crossover trial comparing nicardipine (N) and placebo (P) in patients with Raynaud's phenomenon (Kahan *et al.*, 1987). The data are the number of attacks in two weeks. There was a one-week wash-out period between the two treatment periods

Group A: Nicardipine followed by placebo ($n$ = 10)

| | Period 1 Nicardipine | Period 2 Placebo | (1) − (2) | $\frac{(1) + (2)}{2}$ | P − N |
|---|---|---|---|---|---|
| | 16 | 12 | 4 | 14 | −4 |
| | 26 | 19 | 7 | 22.5 | −7 |
| | 8 | 20 | −12 | 14 | 12 |
| | 37 | 44 | −7 | 40.5 | 7 |
| | 9 | 25 | −16 | 17 | 16 |
| | 41 | 36 | 5 | 38.5 | −5 |
| | 52 | 36 | 16 | 44 | −16 |
| | 10 | 11 | −1 | 10.5 | 1 |
| | 11 | 20 | −9 | 15.5 | 9 |
| | 30 | 27 | 3 | 28.5 | −3 |
| Mean | 24.0 | 25.0 | −1.0 ($\bar{d}_1$) | 24.5 ($\bar{a}_1$) | 1.0 |
| SD | 15.61 | 10.84 | 9.87 | 12.50 | 9.87 |

Group B: Placebo followed by nicardipine ($n$ = 10)

| | Period 1 Placebo | Period 2 Nicardipine | (1) − (2) | $\frac{(1) + (2)}{2}$ | P − N |
|---|---|---|---|---|---|
| | 18 | 12 | 6 | 15 | 6 |
| | 12 | 4 | 8 | 8 | 8 |
| | 46 | 37 | 9 | 41.5 | 9 |
| | 51 | 58 | −7 | 54.5 | −7 |
| | 28 | 2 | 26 | 15 | 26 |
| | 29 | 18 | 11 | 23.5 | 11 |
| | 51 | 44 | 7 | 47.5 | 7 |
| | 46 | 14 | 32 | 30 | 32 |
| | 18 | 30 | −12 | 24 | −12 |
| | 44 | 4 | 40 | 24 | 40 |
| Mean | 34.3 | 22.3 | 12.0 ($\bar{d}_2$) | 28.3 ($\bar{a}_2$) | 12.0 |
| SD | 14.99 | 19.14 | 16.34 | 15.12 | 16.34 |

effect depends on the order in which the treatments were given. The latter is a more serious problem because it leads to a biased estimate of the treatment effect. (See also section 15.2.5.)

We can test the treatment effect by performing a one sample $t$ test on all 20 within subject differences between the two treatments. Because the two crossover groups may not be the same size it is preferable to consider the average effect in the two periods, which is equivalent to performing a two sample $t$ test to compare $\bar{d}_1$ and $\bar{d}_2$.

For this example the period effect and treatment–period interaction give $t = 1.82$ and $t = 0.613$ respectively, both on 18 degrees of freedom, giving $P = 0.09$ and $P = 0.55$. As neither is statistically significant we can go on to evaluate the treatment effect using a further two sample $t$ test, which gives $t = 2.154$ on 18 degrees of freedom ($P = 0.045$). The number of attacks in two weeks on nicardipine was on average 6.5 fewer than during two weeks on placebo, with a 95% confidence interval from 0.18 to 12.82. Although statistically significant at the 5% level, the magnitude of the effect of nicardipine is uncertain, reflecting the small sample size.

A problem with the analysis of crossover trials is that the important test for a possible treatment–period interaction is noted for its lack of statistical power. The above analysis is a good example, because Table 15.5 shows that patients in group 1 did nearly as well on placebo as they had on nicardipine, suggesting a long-lasting 'carry-over' effect of the active drug. Patients in group 2 showed a big improvement when they changed from placebo to nicardipine. This apparent interaction is not nearly statistically significant. The data from period 1 taken alone suggest that the true benefit of nicardipine might well be rather greater than indicated by the overall results of the trial.

In contrast Ueshima *et al.* (1987) found a marginally significant ($0.05 < P < 0.10$) treatment–period interaction in a crossover trial to investigate the possible effect on blood pressure of reducing alcohol intake. They discarded the data from the second period.

A graphical approach is to produce a scatter plot of the difference between the two periods against the average of the two periods, using different symbols to identify the two groups (Clayton and Hills, 1987). Vertical separation of the two groups is an indication of a difference between the treatments. If there is no treatment–period interaction there should be no horizontal difference between the groups, and the data for the two groups should lie symmetrically either side of the line $y = 0$, as in Figure 15.3(a). Figure 15.3(b) shows such a plot for the nicardipine trial, indicating both horizontal and vertical differences between the two groups, in line with the results already presented.

A comparison of baseline readings taken at the start of each period can show whether the washout period was successful. For example, Table 15.6

shows baseline data from a randomized crossover trial comparing rifampicin with phenobarbitone for treatment of pruritus in biliary cirrhosis. It is clear that patients in the first group had less severe pruritis at the beginning of the second period than at the start of the study. Thus either

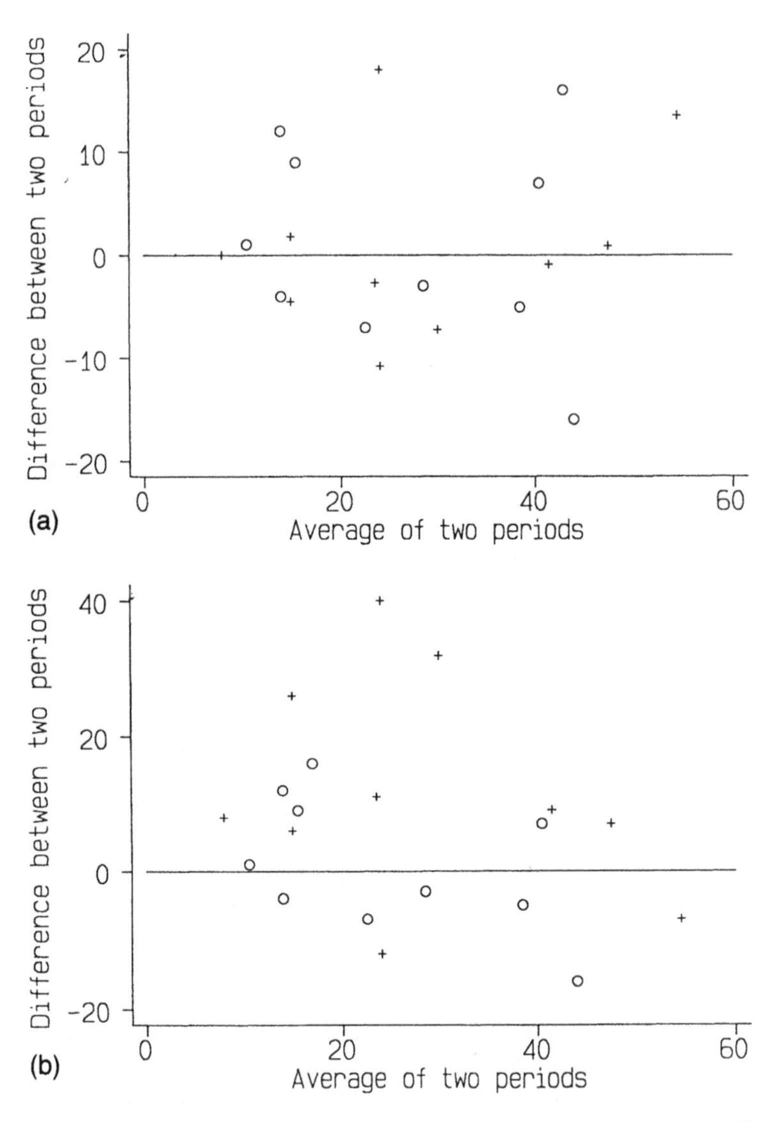


**Figure 15.3** (a) Ideal plot of the difference between the responses in the two periods against the average in the two periods showing the symmetry of the responses in the two groups (shown as ○ and +). (b) Plot of difference between periods against average of two periods for patients receiving nicardipine followed by placebo (○) or placebo followed by nicardipine (+) (data from Kahan *et al.*,1987).

**Table 15.6** Distribution of pruritus scores, from 0 (mild) to 3 (severe) before each period in a two-period crossover trial (Bachs *et al.*, 1989)

| | Pruritus score | | | |
|---|---|---|---|---|
| | 0 | 1 | 2 | 3 |
| Group 1 ($n$ = 12) | | | | |
| Before rifampicin | 0 | 2 | 5 | 5 |
| Before phenobarbitone* | 3 | 3 | 1 | 4 |
| Group 2 ($n$ = 10) | | | | |
| Before phenobarbitone | 0 | 2 | 2 | 6 |
| Before rifampicin | 0 | 2 | 2 | 6 |

*One patient dropped out after period 1.

the pruritus had been improved by the first treatment, so that a crossover trial was inappropriate, or the washout period was too short. In general, it is advantageous to incorporate baseline readings into the analysis, but this makes the analysis more complex.

Crossover trials are particularly vulnerable to the effects of patient withdrawal. If a patient withdraws after the first period they cannot be included in the analysis because they never received the other treatment. The randomized groups are thus compromised when there are withdrawals, especially when these are more common in one group. If there are many withdrawals it may be best to discard the data from the second period.

In a report of a crossover trial it is essential that any withdrawals from the trial are documented, with reasons. Also, the baseline characteristics of the two randomized groups should be described. Although this is routine in parallel group trials, most published reports of crossover trials do not give this information.

## 15.5 INTERPRETATION OF RESULTS

### 15.5.1 Single trials

In most cases the statistical analysis of a clinical trial will be simple, at least with respect to the main outcome measure, perhaps involving just a $t$ test or a Chi squared test. Interpretation seems straightforward, therefore, but for one difficulty. Inference from a sample to a population relies on the assumption that the trial participants are representative of all such patients. In most trials, however, participants are selected to conform to certain inclusion criteria, so extrapolation of results to other types of patient may not be warranted. For example, most trials of anti-hypertensive agents, such as beta-blocking drugs, are carried out on middle-aged men. Is it reasonable to assume that the results apply to women too, or to young or very old men? In the absence of any information to the contrary it is common to infer wider applicability of results, but the possibility that different groups would respond differently should be borne in mind. It is because of this possibility that subgroup analyses are carried out, as they may give clues about variation in the effectiveness of a treatment (or side-effects) for different groups of patients. Unfortunately, as indicated above, there is a risk of coming up with a misleading result as a consequence of carrying out several such analyses.

### 15.5.2 All published trials

In many fields there have been several similar clinical trials, and it is natural to want to assess all the evidence at once. The first thing that becomes apparent when looking at the results of a series of clinical trials of the same treatment is that the results vary, sometimes markedly. We would of course expect to see some variation in treatment effect, because of random variation, and should not necessarily be worried by it. The confidence interval for the treatment benefit observed in a single trial gives an idea of the range of treatment benefit likely to be observed in a series of trials of the same size.

A recent development has been a move towards the formal statistical analysis of data from all published trials to get an overall assessment of treatment effectiveness. The analysis is known either as an **overview** or a **meta-analysis** (Collins *et al.*, 1987). Overviews have often found a highly significant overall treatment benefit when most of the individual trials did not get a significant result. Again, this is not surprising, as many clinical trials are too small to detect anything other than an unrealistically huge treatment benefit. A common criticism of overviews is that they combine information from trials with different patient characteristics and designs. However, any trial may be considered as one of a series, representing just part of the spectrum of disease (Elwood, 1982), and so a clear picture emerging from an overview will indicate wider generalizability of results than is warranted from a single trial. It is important, though, to assess whether the results differ according to the nature of the trial.

A problem in performing overviews is that they usually are based on all the published trials. There is increasing evidence that medical journals exert **publication bias** (Begg and Berlin, 1988), perhaps unintentionally, by which it is easier to publish the results of a clinical trial in a journal if the treatment effect was significant than if it was not. Also authors make less effort to publish when the results are not significant. Such bias stems from the widespread but mistaken belief that non-significant results are uninteresting or uninformative or both. Here we see another possible benefit of expressing results as a confidence interval rather than an isolated P value.

Pooling all published trials will magnify any publication bias, and this is the major argument against overviews. However, it is better to use the available information in a systematic way than to rely on subjective assessment of the various trials. Although preferable, it is naturally exceedingly difficult to extract information about unpublished trials, but there have been a few cases where it has been done (for example, by Yusuf *et al.*, 1985).

## 15.6 WRITING UP AND ASSESSING CLINICAL TRIALS

For both writing up a clinical trial and assessing the quality of a published trial it is useful to have a check list of the important issues. Figure 16.2 in the next chapter shows the check list used by statisticians refereeing clinical trials for the *British Medical Journal*.

### 15.6.1 Writing a paper about a clinical trial

The check list in Figure 16.2 gives some idea of the information that should be included in a report about the design and execution of a trial. Further details can be found in Altman *et al.* (1989), Chalmers *et al.* (1981), Gardner *et al.* (1989), Grant (1989) and Simon and Wittes (1985). It is very important to account for all the patients that were originally randomized, indicating the numbers in each group that were withdrawn. It is better still, especially for large trials, to show what happened to all patients considered for entry to the trial – this can be done by a flow-chart (Hampton, 1981).

The results section should include information about the baseline characteristics of the different groups, especially with respect to known prognostic factors. Some comment on the comparability of the groups is needed – this should not be based on hypothesis testing.

Thereafter the results of between group comparisons should be presented, taking note of the problems of multiple outcome measures and subgroup analyses as discussed above.

### 15.6.2 Assessing published trials

Trials must be judged on the information that is included in the published report. We cannot *assume* a satisfactory answer to any of the questions on the check list if the information is not given. As Colton (1974, p. 269) noted: ‘It is the author’s onus to demonstrate that bias did not occur or was unlikely to have arisen’.

Many reviews have shown that the standard of published clinical trials leaves a lot to be desired. Most trials these days are randomized, but not all are as blind as they could be. Few trials seem to have been planned with regard to the sample size necessary to detect a clinically important treatment benefit. Common problems in reports of trials are the omission of the statistical method used to analyse the data, and failure to include or account for all the patients that were randomized. I discuss the quality of published papers in general more fully in the next chapter.

## EXERCISES

15.1 How would you assess the comparability of the treatment groups at baseline in the trial illustrated in Table 3.5?

15.2 In an open (unblinded) trial of the beta-blocker alprenolol given to patients after myocardial infarction, randomization to alprenolol or the standard treatment was at the time of admission to hospital (Ahlmark and Saetre, 1976). The start of medication was two weeks after admission, by which time 60% of the original 393 patients had been withdrawn from the trial. Reasons for withdrawal were mostly death, non-confirmation of myocardial infarction or contraindication for the beta-blocker. Of the 162 patients actually treated, 69 received alprenolol and 93 the control treatment.

(a) Why might the numbers of withdrawals have been different in the two groups?
(b) Is a hypothesis test to compare the proportions withdrawn in the two groups of any value?
(c) How could this problem have been avoided?

15.3 Thirteen patients with chronic skin disorders were studied in an open trial to assess the effect of aspirin on pruritus. No treatment was given on nights one or two, aspirin (900 mg) was given on the third and fourth nights, and no treatment was given on the fifth and sixth nights. On each night scratching was measured by a limb movement meter, and an assessment of itching was made by the patient the following morning using a 10 cm linear analogue scale. For each patient the data were averaged over each two day period. The results were presented in the paper (Daly and Shuster, 1986) as means (SE):

| | Before treatment | During treatment | After treatment |
|---|---|---|---|
| Linear analogue scale (cm) | 3.5 (0.5) | 3.3 (0.4) | 3.1 (0.5) |
| Nocturnal limb movements | 46.3 (10.0) | 38.8 (7.4) | 38.7 (5.5) |

The complete comment on this table was as follows: 'There was interindividual and intraindividual variation in itch and scratch throughout the study, but no consistent change in either measurement was recorded during aspirin treatment.'

(a) Comment on the design of this study.
(b) What can you say about the distribution across patients of the nocturnal limb movements score?
(c) How were the data analysed? How should the data have been analysed?
(d) How should the results have been presented?
(e) The authors stated: 'We found no effect of oral aspirin . . . We can therefore exclude the possibility that therapeutic doses of aspirin have a central effect on pruritus.' Why is this conclusion incorrect?

15.4 The table below shows the systolic blood pressures of 16 patients before and after one week's treatment with captopril or placebo. The data are from a randomized controlled trial carried out on insulin-dependent diabetic patients with nephropathy (Hommel *et al.*, 1986).

| | Captopril | | | Placebo | |
|---|---|---|---|---|---|
| | Baseline | After 1 week | | Baseline | After 1 week |
| 1 | 147 | 137 | 1 | 133 | 139 |
| 2 | 129 | 120 | 2 | 129 | 134 |
| 3 | 158 | 141 | 3 | 152 | 136 |
| 4 | 164 | 137 | 4 | 161 | 151 |
| 5 | 134 | 140 | 5 | 154 | 147 |
| 6 | 155 | 144 | 6 | 141 | 137 |
| 7 | 151 | 134 | 7 | 156 | 149 |
| 8 | 141 | 123 | | | |
| 9 | 153 | 142 | | | |

The authors performed paired $t$ tests on the data in each group. They found a significant drop in blood pressure in the captopril group, but the change in the placebo group was not significant. They concluded that 'captopril represents a valuable new drug for treating hypertension in diabetics dependent on insulin with nephropathy'.

(a) What is wrong with their analysis, and their interpretation of the results?
(b) Perform a correct analysis. What conclusions can be drawn about the effect of captopril on hypertension?

15.5 A randomized placebo-controlled trial was carried out to investigate the capacity of aspirin to prevent pregnancy-induced hypertension and preeclamptic toxaemia (Schiff *et al.*, 1989). The study was carried out on women at high risk of these conditions.

(a) How many patients would have been needed to have a 80% power of detecting as significant ($P < 0.05$) a reduction of one-third in the risk of hypertension from 30% to 20%?
(b) The actual sample size was 65. What was the power of the study to detect the difference considered in (a)?
(c) What reduction in risk of hypertension did the study have an 80% power to detect?
(d) The observed rates of hypertension were $\frac{11}{31}$ (36%) in the placebo group and $\frac{4}{34}$ (12%) in the aspirin group; the authors quoted $P = 0.024$ for this difference. They also quoted a relative risk (RR) of hypertension of 0.33 among the aspirin group. Calculate a 95% confidence interval for the RR, and comment on the authors' conclusion that large scale clinical trials are needed. (See also problem 10.7.)

# 16

# The medical literature

> One does feel that statistical techniques both of design and analysis are sometimes adopted rather as rituals designed to assuage the last holders of absolute power (editors of journals) and perhaps also regulatory agencies, and not because the techniques are appreciated to be scientifically important.
>
> Cox (1983)

## 16.1 INTRODUCTION

During this century clinical research has grown enormously as has its influence on clinical practice. Publication of research results, especially in a leading journal, will rapidly disseminate those findings all over the world. A paper in a peer-reviewed journal implies that the research is both scientifically sound and clinically worthwhile – it bestows both credibility and respectability on the work. This would be fine if all published papers were scientifically sound but, regrettably, the standard of research leaves much to be desired from the statistical point of view. Examples of substandard design and incorrect analysis can be seen in almost any issue of any medical journal.

The importance of sound design and analysis cannot be overemphasized. Clearly the conclusions from a study must rely on the methods having been correct. If the conclusions are unreliable because of faulty methodology, then the study cannot be clinically worthwhile. Worse, it may be clinically harmful by reason of the conclusions being misleading, and a clinically harmful study is surely unethical.

Thus, with some diffidence, in 1980 I suggested that the misuse of statistics was unethical (Altman, 1982a), a view which has subsequently been widely endorsed but never challenged. The ethical implications of substandard research (not just statistical errors) are:

1. the misuse of patients by exposing them to unjustified risk and inconvenience;
2. the misuse of resources, including the researchers' time, which could be better employed on more valuable activities; and

3. the consequences of publishing misleading results, which may include the carrying out of unnecessary further work.

In the extreme there may be a direct effect on patient care. In particular, there have been several examples of treatments that were widely used on the basis of promising results from uncontrolled studies, but were later shown by randomized trials to be ineffective (see section 15.2.1). Likewise, conflicting results from epidemiological studies may relate to methodological differences.

These remarks lead to three inevitable conclusions. First it behoves the researcher to take the greatest care in planning, executing, analysing and interpreting research. Second, care is needed too in reading and interpreting the research results from other investigators who may have disregarded the first point. As Albert (1981) has said: 'One of the most important skills a physician should have is the ability to critically analyse original contributions to the medical literature.' Third, the standard of statistics in published papers can be influenced by the editorial and refereeing policy of medical journals.

In this final chapter I shall briefly consider the growth of statistics within medical research, summarize the findings of reviews of the quality of statistics in published papers, consider the role of medical journals in improving the quality, and give guidance on reading and writing scientific papers.

## 16.2 THE GROWTH OF STATISTICS IN MEDICAL RESEARCH

It is not possible to pinpoint the introduction of statistical methods into medical research, but with a few notable exceptions we may look to the first quarter of this century. In 1929 a huge paper was published in a physiology journal expounding many of the main principles of statistical analysis and interpretation (Dunn, 1929). By 1937 the correct use of statistical methods in clinical research was considered important enough for the *Lancet* to publish a series of 15 articles on statistical methods by Austin Bradford Hill. These were quickly republished in book form; that this influential book remains in print 50 years later (Hill, 1984) pays tribute to its quality.

We might consider the modern rise of medical statistics to start either in 1937 or in 1948, when the report of the first well known randomized clinical trial was published. This was the Medical Research Council trial of streptomycin for pulmonary tuberculosis (Medical Research Council, 1948), in which Bradford Hill was a key influence. However, in general the introduction of statistics into medical research was slow. In 1954 the *British Medical Journal* reported a debate held by the Royal Statistical Society's

'Study Circle on Medical Statistics' (Anon, 1954). The motion was 'This house should welcome the growing influence of statistics in all branches of medicine'. The opposer of the motion made the remarkable observation that medicine was an art and statistics was a science, so statistics was out of place in medicine. More surprising, considering the forum, is that the motion was carried by only a narrow majority.

Much has happened since 1954, and statistical methods are now firmly entrenched in medicine. A good idea of the growth of statistics is given by a study of papers published by the journal *Pediatrics* in the years 1952, 1962, 1972 and 1982 (Hayden, 1983). As Table 16.1 shows, there was a large increase in the proportion of papers using statistical methods of analysis and a ten fold rise in the use of methods beyond simple $t$ and $\chi^2$ tests and correlation. The change in the latter was especially marked between 1972 and 1982. A similar study of the *New England Journal of Medicine* showed that 45% of papers published in 1978–79 used only simple methods of statistical analysis (Colditz and Emerson, 1985). Another study contrasted the statistical analyses in papers published in *Arthritis and Rheumatism* in 1967–68 and 1982 (Felson *et al.*, 1984). As Table 16.2 shows, they found some marked changes between the two periods. Papers published in 1982 contained many more statistical analyses, which may be at least partly due to the availability of computers. The proportion of papers containing statistical errors was much the same, but the nature of the errors had changed considerably.

**Table 16.1** Use of statistical procedures in *Pediatrics* (Hayden, 1983)

| | Year | | | |
|---|---|---|---|---|
| | 1952 | 1962 | 1972 | 1982 |
| Number of papers | 67 | 98 | 115 | 151 |
| No statistical procedures | 66% | 59% | 45% | 30% |
| Statistical procedures other than $t$, $\chi^2$ and $r$ | 3% | 5% | 12% | 35% |

Several authors have carried out a comprehensive study of journals to see which methods are in most frequent use. Table 16.3 shows the methods found in the review of the *New England Journal of Medicine* in 1978–79 in decreasing order of use, with the cumulative percentage of all papers that contained only methods that far down the table. We can see that the wide range of techniques listed covers most but not all published papers. The last ten years have seen a further increase in the use of more advanced statistical techniques, so that the proportion of papers which use methods not shown in Table 16.3 is likely to have increased.

**Table 16.2** Use of selected statistical methods in *Arthritis and Rheumatism* in 1967–68 and 1982, and numbers of errors found (Felson *et al.*, 1984)

| | 1967–68 ($n$ = 47) | 1982 ($n$ = 74) |
|---|---|---|
| Statistical method: | | |
| *t* test | 8 (17%) | 37 (50%) |
| Chi squared test | 9 (19%) | 22 (30%) |
| Linear regression | 1 (2%) | 18 (24%) |
| Multiple statistical tests | 4 (9%) | 30 (41%) |
| Error: | | |
| Undefined method | 14 (30%) | 7 (9%) |
| Inadequate description of measures of location or dispersion | 6 (13%) | 7 (9%) |
| Repeated observations treated as independent | 1 (2%) | 4 (5%) |
| Two groups compared on > 10 variables at 5% level | 3 (6%) | 28 (38%) |
| Multiple *t* tests instead of analysis of variance | 2 (4%) | 18 (24%) |
| Chi squared tests used when expected frequencies too small | 3 (6%) | 4 (5%) |
| At least one of above errors | 28 (60%) | 49 (66%) |

There is thus an enormous diversity of statistical methodology in the medical literature. Unfortunately, as shown in the next section, the reliability of the statistical information in published papers is worryingly low. Thus it is essential to be able to assess critically research papers, to which end it is necessary to be familiar with a large range of statistical concepts and methods. Apart from epidemiological methods, all of the topics listed in Table 16.3 are included in this book.

As well as changes in the methods of statistical analysis there has been a simultaneous change in the types of research design used. A review of the design of studies published in the *New England Journal of Medicine* over a similar period (1946–76) showed an increase in clinical trials, and in the proportion of trials that were controlled, but also a decrease in cohort studies in favour of cross-sectional studies (Fletcher and Fletcher, 1979). Much is written about clinical trials, but they still represent a small minority, perhaps only 5%, of all papers published in medical journals.

**Table 16.3** The most common statistical techniques in the *New England Journal of Medicine* in 1978–79 (Emerson and Colditz, 1983)

| Technique | Cumulative % of papers |
|---|---|
| 1 No statistical methods or descriptive methods only | 58 |
| 2 $t$ tests | 67 |
| 3 Contingency tables ($\chi^2$) | 73 |
| 4 Non-parametric tests | 75 |
| 5 Epidemiological methods | 77 |
| 6 Pearson correlation ($r$) | 79 |
| 7 Simple linear regression | 82 |
| 8 Analysis of variance | 84 |
| 9 Transformations | 86 |
| 10 Rank correlation | 87 |
| 11 Life table analysis | 89 |
| 12 Multiple regression | 90 |
| 13 Multiple comparisons | 92 |

## 16.3 STATISTICS IN PUBLISHED PAPERS

It is clear that the misuse of statistical methods has been a problem from the outset. As early as 1932, commenting on changes over the preceding 20 years, Greenwood wrote: 'Medical papers now frequently contain statistical analyses, and sometimes these analyses are correct, but the writers violate quite as often as before, the fundamental principles of statistical or of general logical reasoning' (Greenwood, 1932). In 1950 Hogben wrote 'Less than 1 per cent of research workers clearly apprehend the rationale of statistical techniques they commonly invoke' (Hogben, 1950). A much more recent comment contains the same message: 'It is nearly impossible to read an issue of leading cancer journals without giving rise to serious questions about study design, data collection, definitions of response, determination of results, and the reporting of results' (Hoogstraten, 1984). These assessments were not supported by systematic reviews of the content of published papers, but since the 1960s there have been many such reviews.

### 16.3.1 Reviews of the literature

The earliest comment I know of relating to the quality of statistics in medical journals is that by Dunn (1929), who observed that half of a series of published papers examined were not acceptable statistically. One of the first modern reviews was by Schor and Karten (1966) who examined 295 papers published in ten medical journals. They considered that 28% of the papers were statistically acceptable, 68% were deficient, and 5% were 'unsalvageable'. The many subsequent reviews of papers published in numerous different general and specialist journals have found a broadly similar picture. It is difficult to summarize these studies because of the wide range of criteria used by the reviewers, but they have typically found that about half of the papers examined included at least one statistical error. It is also hard to say how important these errors are. Certainly many minor errors will have no material bearing on the overall conclusions of a study, but some may lead to major errors of interpretation.

Most reviewers have looked at errors in statistical analysis, but some have looked at errors in design, especially for clinical trials. For example, Tyson *et al*. (1983) reviewed reports of 86 therapeutic trials in perinatal medicine published in four journals, using predetermined criteria. Their results are summarized in Table 16.4, and show major deficiencies in the papers examined. Some of the missing information may be due to poor reporting rather than bad design, but when reading a paper we cannot assume things that are not stated. For example, if a report of a clinical trial mentions that random allocation was used but offers no further information

**Table 16.4** Summary of review of 86 therapeutic trials in perinatal medicine (Tyson *et al.*, 1983)

| | % of studies fulfilling criteria | | |
|---|---|---|---|
| | Yes | Unclear | No |
| Statement of purpose | 94 | 6 | 0 |
| Clearly defined outcome variables | 74 | 1 | 25 |
| Planned prospective data collection | 48 | 30 | 22 |
| Predetermined sample size (or a sequential trial) | 3 | 16 | 71 |
| Sample size specified | 93 | 6 | 1 |
| Disease/health status of subjects specified ($n$ = 85) | 51 | 20 | 29 |
| Exclusion criteria specified ($n$ = 81) | 46 | 9 | 45 |
| Randomization (if feasible) appropriately performed and documented ($n$ = 69) | 9 | 12 | 79 |
| Blinding used, or lack of blinding unlikely to have biased results ($n$ = 83) | 49 | 47 | 4 |
| Adequate sample size | 15 | 44 | 41 |
| Statistical methods identified, appropriately used and interpreted | 26 | 0 | 74 |
| Recommendations/conclusions justified | 10 | 71 | 19 |

about the procedure used, we cannot assume that they really did randomize. Many researchers do not understand what 'random' means. Likewise, we cannot assume that the statistical methods were appropriate when, as is often the case, the methods are not identified. This is why the reviewers felt unable to judge whether the conclusions were justified in nearly three-quarters of the papers examined.

A comprehensive review of about 150 such studies has been carried out recently (Johnson and Altman, 1990; Altman and Johnson, 1990). It provides little evidence that the frequency of errors is diminishing over time, although it is likely that more recent reviewers have taken a harder line over what they considered to be errors.

Statistical errors can occur at any stage of a study: planning, design, execution, analysis, presentation and interpretation. When planning a study, it is possible to make incorrect judgements about the design or sample size if the findings of other published papers are accepted uncritically. However, the other stages of research, from design through to interpretation, are more obvious places where things can go wrong, and I shall consider each in turn. The examples given are by no means comprehensive.

### 16.3.2 Errors in design

Reviews of clinical trials have shown major deficiencies in the reporting of vital information relating to the design and execution of the trial. Perhaps more worryingly, they have also shown that a fair proportion of papers report studies that have used suboptimal design. For example, despite a huge literature urging the highest possible standards of design for clinical trials, studies are still commonly carried out without concurrent controls, or with concurrent but non-randomized controls, and blinding is not used when it could have been. A major worry is that studies with inferior designs are open to bias, and in particular may produce over-optimistic findings. Fletcher and Fletcher (1979) give several examples where conclusions based on weak research designs were later corrected by subsequent well designed studies. All reviews comparing the results of well designed and poorly designed clinical trials of the same treatments have found that the latter obtained larger treatment effects (Altman and Johnson, 1990). If, as is likely, the weaker studies are also smaller, then the effect of publication bias (see section 15.5.2) may be more severe.

The problems are not confined to clinical trials. Reviews of studies evaluating diagnostic tests have similarly been shown to have major deficiencies in design and reporting (Sheps and Schechter, 1984). However, outside the field of clinical trials it is harder to make general statements about the main errors that are made; Chapter 5 gave several examples of potential difficulties.

One reason for some of the problems is that many studies are not actually designed but rather 'happen'. They are based on an analysis of pre-existing data that were collected for some other purpose. While many reports of such studies admit that the study was retrospective, some pretend that the study was prospective, and thus planned, as it looks better to suggest that the idea came before the data. Symptoms of undesigned studies are variation in the treatments and methods of evaluation used, unequal numbers of observations for different subjects, many missing observations, and a general vagueness about what was done and why.

An example of the use of existing data is seen in many studies using fetal ultrasound measurements to develop reference standards. Virtually all published studies are based on the analysis of existing data, so that the number of observations per fetus varies and the measurements are not taken at pre-specified times. While a single routine ultrasound examination in early pregnancy is common, further ultrasound measurements are not usual unless there is some cause for clinical concern. Thus those fetuses that are represented several times in these data sets are likely to be atypical and quite possibly of a different size on average, so that the data are not what they purport to be. Green and Byar (1984) have discussed some of the problems that can arise from the analysis of data from registries rather than data collected for the purpose in hand.

Other design problems were referred to in Chapter 5. Examples are the choice of an inappropriate high risk sample to make inferences about the general population; choice of inappropriate controls in a case-control study; and the volunteer bias that arises when people can choose their treatment. Another example of a potential problem is the 'healthy worker effect', whereby people in employment are healthier than the general population; this needs to be considered in studies of possible adverse effects of industrial exposure to some hazard. Yet another is the use of different observers in a study to compare two alternative methods of measurement (see section 14.2). If each method is used by only one observer there is an inseparability (or 'confounding') of any systematic differences between the observers with any difference between the methods.

These few examples serve only to illustrate the wide variety of possible pitfalls. At the risk of repetition, I shall say again that the best time to seek expert statistical advice is when you are *planning* a study, so that any flaws of this sort can be spotted and rectified.

Lastly, there is the fundamental problem of having an inadequate sample size. As noted in section 8.5.4, a review by Freiman *et al.* (1978) showed that many published clinical trials that find a non-significant difference between treatments had little chance of detecting major treatment effects due to small sample sizes. Few published studies report that the sample size was chosen on the basis of power calculations. Indeed, the concept of sample size calculations seems almost unknown in medical research outside the field of clinical trials, although the same methods are equally applicable to all comparative studies and can be used in planning any investigation. For example, a recent paper has discussed sample size calculations for rheological studies (Stuart *et al.*, 1989).

Even when power calculations have been used to calculate sample size, the supply of subjects may not be as great as anticipated. It is common in clinical trials for the actual recruitment rate to fall far short of that anticipated, partly because of overestimation of the number of eligible subjects and partly because of their unwillingness to enter the trial.

Whereas P values can disguise the fact that a study was too small, a very wide confidence interval indicates the lack of useful information – this is one of the arguments in favour of the use of confidence intervals (see section 8.8).

### 16.3.3 Errors in execution

In prospective studies in particular, the collection of data may not go according to plan. Another way of expressing this idea is that the study plan or protocol is not strictly adhered to. Various problems that can occur in clinical trials were discussed in Chapter 15, notably with regard to the correct exclusion of ineligible subjects and ensuring that each patient received the treatment that was allocated to them. It might be thought that simple allocation schemes, such as those based on odd or even numbers, would be less prone to error, but this is not so. In the report of a study that used both odd and even date of operation and odd or even year of birth to allocate subjects to three different types of heart valve prothesis, the authors wrote: 'We found . . . that the randomisation procedure was not entirely consistent throughout the study period, partly because of supply difficulties and partly because the odd/even criteria were sometimes misunderstood' (Kuntze *et al.*, 1989). No further details were given. The mention of supply difficulties suggests that there may have been times when not all three devices were available, but we are not told how this was dealt with. The problems with odd and even dates suggest that this apparently simple scheme may indeed be harder to operate correctly than, for example, randomization using prepared envelopes, apart from this being an inferior design for other reasons. (Of course, the allocation system they used was not randomization, as they wrongly claimed.)

Missing data may be the consequence of a failure in the data collection system, for example arising from neglecting to consider what would happen during weekends or holidays. If the data are not examined until the end of the study, by the time that any problems are spotted it will be too late to rectify them.

### 16.3.4 Errors in analysis

Errors in analysis are regrettably common. In earlier chapters of this book I have warned against improper uses of the methods introduced. These warnings are based on knowledge that such misuses are common in medical journals. Thus the following basic errors are frequently made:

1. using methods of analysis when the assumptions are not met;
2. analysing paired data ignoring the pairing;
3. failing to take account of ordered categories;
4. treating multiple observations on one subject as independent;
5. using multiple paired comparisons instead of an analysis that considers all groups (e.g. analysis of variance);
6. performing within group analyses and then comparing groups by comparing P values or confidence intervals;
7. quoting confidence intervals that include impossible values.

I have described these errors as 'basic' because they demonstrate a lack of understanding of fundamental statistical concepts. They are not really excusable.

There are other errors, however, which may be equally or even more serious but where the error is more one of logic than technique. Some examples, all discussed in earlier chapters, are:

1. using correlation in method comparison studies;
2. using correlation to compare two sets of time-related observations;
3. assessing the comparability of two or more groups by means of hypothesis tests;
4. evaluating a diagnostic test solely by means of sensitivity and specificity.

There is perhaps rather more excuse for these errors being made as they are rather more subtle, although the errors have been written about many times in medical journals. There is little excuse for journals not detecting them when papers are submitted.

Another unacceptable practice is to base conclusions on a subset of the data. Apart from the fact that investigation of many subsets or subgroups will lead to a high probability that something will turn up (i.e. yield $P < 0.05$), presentation of a subset analysis as the main finding may distort the picture. An example is given in a clinical trial comparing two chemotherapy regimes in breast cancer patients (Lippman *et al.*, 1984). The overall comparison of time to progression of disease in the two groups was performed by the logrank test and gave $P = 0.26$. However, the authors also compared the time to progression among only those patients who responded to treatment, for whom there was a significant difference between the groups ($P = 0.009$). Only the latter analysis appears in the summary of the paper, with no mention that there was no overall significant difference. Either the proportion responding to treatment or time to progression (or survival time) might be considered a suitable end-point for this study, but the comparison must be based on all patients, not a selected subset.

### 16.3.5 Errors in presentation

With presentation of results too there are several common errors that abound in medical journals:

1. using standard errors (or confidence intervals) for descriptive information;
2. presenting means (or medians) of continuous data without any indication of variability;
3. presenting the results of a statistical analysis solely as a P value.

All but the last of these problems relate equally to numerical and graphical presentation.

*(a) Numerical precision*

One aspect of presentation that is often poor is the numerical precision used to present data and results. Spurious precision adds nothing to a paper and impairs its readability and credibility. It is hard to provide absolute rules, but the following guidelines may help. When presenting summary statistics or the results of analyses, such as means, standard deviations and regression equations, the precision of the original data should be borne in mind. Means should not usually be quoted to more than one further decimal place than the raw data, but standard errors and standard deviations may require one extra decimal place. Percentages do not need to be given to more than one decimal place at most, especially in small samples. If the numerator and denominator are given, as should usually be the case, then there is no reason not to quote percentages to the nearest integer. Test statistics such as $t$ and $X^2$ do not need to be given to more than two decimal places. Likewise P values do not need more than one or two significant digits, and it is not necessary to be specific below, say, 0.0001 (see section 8.10). Other specific advice is given in several earlier chapters.

Some examples of unnecessary (or spurious) precision, all from published papers, are:

$$P = 10^{-54}$$
$$P = 0.5254$$
$$r = 0.99299$$
$$\chi^2 = 0.7264$$

'86.95% of cases'

An example from a regression analysis is the following equation relating birth weight in kg (BWt) to chest circumference (CC) and mid-arm circumference (AC) (both in cm) (Bhargava *et al.*, 1985)

$$BWt = -3.0983527 + 0.142088CC + 0.158039AC$$

which purports to predict birthweight to the nearest $\frac{1}{10000}$ g! Many such examples may arise from exact transcription from computer output.

Lastly, a common problem found in many reviews of the literature is the use of the ± sign after a mean without specifying whether the number after the sign is the standard deviation or standard error. The ± usage has been around for many decades, but the ambiguity is so serious that several medical journals, including the *British Medical Journal* and *Lancet*, do not now allow its use, although most journals still do. Thus, for example, the phrase 'the mean blood pressure was 92.4 ± 7.1 mm Hg' would be changed to 'the mean blood pressure was 92.4 mm Hg (SD 7.1)' (or SE if that were the case). The preferred notation is unambiguous and also avoids the incorrect implications that the standard deviation (or standard error) can be positive or negative and that the range given by mean±SD (or mean±SE) is of especial interest.

*(b) Graphical presentation*

Although some results can be displayed only as a table or only as a graph, in cases where either is possible there is much uncertainty about which is preferable (journals will not allow the author to display the same data both ways). Again, I do not think it is possible to give simple general guidance. Results are given more accurately in tables, but many people find graphs preferable for seeing the message of the data. Graphs are most advantageous when they show data for individual subjects, for example as scatter diagrams or time trends, rather than summary information.

There is not room here for a comprehensive discussion of the dos and don'ts of graphical presentation. There are now several books devoted to the topic, of which that by Tufte (1983) is particularly worth reading. In the context of this section, however, it is worth considering some ways in which graphs can be misleading.

Scatter diagrams are a particularly valuable type of graph, and give meaning to a correlation or regression analysis. Likewise graphs that show all observations within several groups of subjects are far preferable to those showing just summary statistics. The contrast is illustrated by Figures 3.14 and 9.6, which show the same set of data in both styles. Graphs showing only summary statistics, such as means and standard errors (Figure 9.6), are rarely worth the space they occupy.

Common misleading features of graphs are:

1. the lack of a true zero on the vertical axis;
2. a change of scale in the middle of an axis (especially heinous in a

histogram);
3. three-dimensional effects;
4. failure to show coincident points in a scatter diagram;
5. showing a fitted regression line without a scatter diagram of the raw data;
6. superimposing two (or more) graphs with different vertical scales (especially when they do not start at zero);
7. plotting means without any indication of variability.

The last of these problems is common, and yet the addition of standard deviations or standard errors inevitably leads to a cluttered graph. As noted, this type of data may be better in a table. In the case of serial data, there are better approaches, as outlined in section 14.6.

Further discussion of these and many other issues can be found in Tufte (1983), Cleveland (1984) and Wainer (1984).

### 16.3.6 Errors in interpretation

It seems that the majority of errors in the interpretation of statistical analyses relate to hypothesis tests and P values. Many of these points have been covered in earlier chapters, but it is worth reiterating here that the P value is not, as is commonly wrongly stated, the probability that the observed effect is due to chance, but rather the probability of obtaining the observed effect (or a more unlikely one) when the null hypothesis is true. In other words, P assesses how likely it is to observe such an effect in a sample when there is no such difference in the population.

Another false interpretation is the belief that a P value of, say, 0.001 implies a stronger effect than $P = 0.01$. While this may be so, the P values do not demonstrate it.

Erroneous interpretations of 'significant' and 'not significant' P values abound. There is a common belief that the goal of research is a significant result, and consequently that a non-significant result implies that the research was unsuccessful. This attitude is seen in the frequent description of such study results as 'positive' and 'negative' respectively, and in the awful description of the latter as having 'failed to reach statistical significance'. An example of the contortion that this may lead to is the description of a result with $P = 0.05$ as 'probably significant'. Statistical significance is often used as the sole basis of the interpretation. Thus any significant effect, however small or implausible, is taken as real, and any non-significant effect is taken as indicating that there is 'no difference'. To use statistics in this way is to abdicate from any constructive thought about one's results.

The increasing use of confidence intervals may reduce the difficulties. Several leading medical journals have carried editorials or articles supporting the use of confidence intervals and some now expect authors to provide them for their main results (Gardner and Altman, 1989a). It is important in comparative studies that confidence intervals are calculated for the difference between groups, not for the results in each group separately.

The other frequent error in interpretation is to equate association and causation. As discussed in several chapters, an observed association does not necessarily imply that there is a causal relation. The only type of study where we can usually be safe in making such an inference is a well-conducted randomized controlled trial, where any difference in outcome may be taken as causally related to the difference in treatment. Otherwise great caution is needed in the interpretation of results, and causation cannot usually be inferred without other types of evidence. When the false inference is allied to a situation where the observed association itself may be spurious, as described in section 11.3, the scope for error is enormous.

Lastly, I must return to the basic idea of sample and population introduced in section 4.3. Most medical research is based on the principle of extrapolating findings from a sample to a population of interest. Clearly this exercise is crucially dependent upon the sample being representative of the population. In theory the sample should be a random one, but this is almost never the case. In practice, therefore, we need some way of assessing whether the sample may be considered representative, and this is usually done by means of describing the characteristics of the subjects in the sample, and sometimes comparing them with the known characteristics of the population. The whole process of statistical inference fails if the sample is not representative. This is why study results are heavily compromised by high dropout or refusal rates.

### 16.3.7 Errors of omission

Many reviews of the literature have included comments on how often important information was omitted. If the methods of analysis or key aspects of the design are not specified we should not assume that valid procedures were used.

Mosteller *et al*. (1980) examined 132 controlled trials in cancer and found that the method of statistical analysis was specified in only 46 (35%). The much better figure of 85% for clinical trials published in major journals (DerSimonian *et al*., 1982) still leaves scope for improvement (see also Table 16.2). If the data are paired or come from ordered categories it is important to know whether the methods used were appropriate. If the data are clearly not Normally distributed, we need to be assured that the method of analysis was appropriate. At a more basic level it is often unclear whether standard deviations or standard errors are presented. It is only occasionally possible to reanalyse the data from the information given in a paper and so verify which method was used, but this should not be necessary.

While the broad structure of the design of a study is usually clear from the report, crucial details may be missing. It is often unclear if all the observations were taken from different individuals. Methods of matching groups may be vague, and indeed we must doubt if matching was used when, as is not uncommon, the 'matched' groups are not of the same size. In randomized trials, the method of randomization is frequently omitted. DerSimonian *et al.* (1982) found that the method of randomization was reported in only 19% of the 67 trials that they examined. There are two aspects here: the method of generating the random number sequence, and the mechanism for allocating the treatments. Few papers give both of them, and the more important mechanism is rarely given (Altman and Doré, 1990). We cannot be sure that a trial really did use random allocation simply from the use of the word 'randomized' somewhere in the methods section, or even in the title (Kuntze *et al.*, 1989).

One way to see that a paper contains the necessary information is to use a checklist. Examples are discussed in section 16.4.

### 16.3.8 Consequences of statistical errors

Reviews of the literature typically report that about half of the papers examined contained a statistical error. However, the term 'error' encompasses an enormous variety of deviations from statistical purity and many errors will not be serious. At the trivial end we may not worry unduly about the presentation of some descriptive information as means with no indication of variability. Our reaction to an analysis where the method is not stated may depend on how 'obvious' it is what was done. For example, two by two tables of frequencies will almost certainly have been analysed by a Chi squared test, but there are many options for continuous data, not all of which will be reasonable in any particular case.

A further problem in assessing the typical 50% error rate is that there is no general agreement on what constitutes an error. On the other hand, there are other problems that are rarely considered in reviews, such as multiple comparisons or selective reporting of only those results that are significant.

In section 16.1 I gave three ethical implications of statistical errors: the misuse of patients, the misuse of resources and the consequences of publishing misleading results. The last of these can work in several ways, and will depend upon the nature of the results:

1. it may prove impossible to get ethics committee approval to carry out further research because a published study has found the experimental treatment beneficial, even though that study was flawed;
2. other scientists may be led to follow false lines of investigation;
3. future patients may receive an inferior treatment, either as a direct

consequence of the results of the study or possibly by the delay in the introduction of a truly effective treatment;
4. if the results go unchallenged the researchers may use the same inferior statistical methods in future research, and others may copy them.

The last of these applies whether or not the study reached inappropriate conclusions.

Some of these problems would, of course, be avoided if everyone was equally able to detect the errors, but it is much better if they can be detected by journals and the papers either not published or suitably amended. Unfortunately, almost any paper can get published somewhere, so however much journals continue to extend their statistical refereeing the problems will remain, as will the need for critical analysis.

### 16.3.9 Why are there so many statistical errors in published papers?

Mistakes in published papers can be ascribed to inadequate understanding of statistics by those using the methods, which in turn is due to inadequate statistical education. Undergraduate teaching of statistics can introduce some of the key statistical concepts, but provides inadequate preparation for the requirements of medical research. Several studies have shown that the statistical understanding by doctors of basic statistical methods and ideas is inadequate (Altman and Bland, 1991). If simple ideas are not well understood, we can hardly expect more complex methods to fare better.

Postgraduate courses are more appropriate for in-depth teaching of statistics, but few researchers have attended such a course. Other reasons for the widespread misuse of statistics have been considered by Altman and Bland (1991), and include misleading textbooks and easy access to computer programs. The recent tremendous increase in the availability of computers and statistical software has given wide access to complex methods of analysis, but there has not been an accompanying increase in understanding of those techniques.

Whatever the reasons, it is at best questionable whether ignorance is an adequate defence. Statistical methods of design and analysis are an essential component of sound medical research, and their use requires certain skills no less than the other components of the research. If those skills are not present within the research team they should be acquired by seeking expert advice. We can again find sound advice in this respect in the 1930s, in the editorial accompanying the first of Bradford Hill's *Lancet* articles: 'The time to allow for statistical factors is when an inquiry is being planned, not when it is completed' (Anon, 1937). Sadly many authors, editors, and even ethics committees remain unconvinced about the importance of correct statistics in medical research. Thus it is necessary to read published papers with some circumspection, even those published in the most illustrious journals. Section 16.4 gives advice on how to do this.

### 16.3.10 Role of the medical journals

It is self-evident that the standard of statistics in published papers could be greatly raised if journals ceased publishing papers containing major errors. Despite evidence that statistical refereeing can improve the standard of published papers, journals have in general been slow to take steps to judge the statistical component of submitted papers. It is still true that most journals' instructions to authors give far more attention to how the references are laid out than to what statistical information is required, and most do not even mention statistics. Like it or not, journals have a responsibility for publishing papers that are, as far as can be judged, scientifically sound. The quality of the medical literature is in their editorial hands.

As few members of the editorial staff of journals are likely to know much more statistics than the authors of papers, the statistical expertise must be obtained through expert refereeing. In a recent survey, 98 editors of medical journals were asked about their policy on statistical refereeing and replies were obtained from 83 (George, 1985). Only 16% had a policy that guaranteed a statistical review prior to publication, but 35% had either a statistical consultant or a statistician on the editorial board. There is clearly considerable scope for improvement in this respect (Altman, 1982c), although it must be acknowledged that there are probably not enough medical statisticians to look at all papers submitted to medical journals. Nevertheless, I believe that all journals should endeavour to obtain some statistical input. Further, they should publish their editorial policy regarding statistical refereeing, something which only 12% of the journals in the above-mentioned survey had done.

It is most unlikely that there will be a great improvement in the short term except perhaps in a few journals, so it is important to be a cautious reader of published papers. You should not accept research findings solely on the basis of the abstract of a paper, but rather should make a careful assessment of the authors' methods. Some guidance is given in the next section.

## 16.4 READING A SCIENTIFIC PAPER

It is enormously helpful when reading a paper to have a list of specific points to be looking out for. As noted by Colton (1974, p. 317), it is impossible to produce a set of questions that it would be appropriate to ask for every research paper. A partial solution is to have more than one; for example, Gardner *et al.* (1989) produced two checklists for statistical reviewers, one for general medical studies and one specifically for clinical trials. Other authors have proposed guidelines for reading reports on clinical trials (Simon and Wittes, 1985; Grant, 1989; Reisch *et al.*, 1989), epidemiological studies including case-control studies (Epidemiology Work Group, 1981; Lichtenstein *et al.*, 1987; Bracken, 1989), and evaluation of diagnostic and screening tests (Sheps and Schechter, 1984; Wald and Cuckle, 1989).

I shall follow the idea of having two different checklists for general studies and for clinical trials. Those shown in Figures 16.1 and 16.2 are heavily based on those in Gardner *et al.* (1989), but incorporate some extensions and clarifications. They were designed to aid the statistical refereeing of papers submitted to the *British Medical Journal*, but are equally applicable for assessing papers already published.

The questions in Figure 16.1 can be used to assess medical papers other than clinical trials. Most of the questions relate to important aspects of the design of the study and analysis of the data. Figure 16.2 shows a checklist for assessing reports of clinical trials. The questions relate to aspects of design and analysis that were discussed at length in the previous chapter. Aspects of design of particular importance relate to the description of efforts to eliminate the possibility of bias. As noted already, we cannot infer that a procedure was adopted if the relevant information is absent. For example, it is common to see papers describing trials as both randomized and double blind, but in the absence of any information beyond those three words we should not assume that the authors understand those terms. It is quite common to see methods of alternate allocation described as random; it is, of course, quite different and definitely inferior. A much more detailed assessment scheme for clinical trials was proposed by Chalmers *et al.* (1981).

It will be appreciated that for many of the questions in the checklists there is no unequivocal answer, and assessing a paper thus involves some subjectivity. Nevertheless, the use of these (or other) checklists makes it much easier to assess a paper, partly because it is always harder to detect omissions than errors in what is present.

The questions in the checklists are not equally important. Ideally we would like to see 'Yes' responses for all questions but few papers will achieve this. In practice we should be most concerned about possible bias in the design of the study. Indeed, if the design of the study is unacceptable for some reason, the paper is statistically unacceptable regardless of how the data were analysed. Next we would hope that the analysis was appropriate to the data, and that the conclusions were justified. Aspects of presentation, while not unimportant, are clearly less important than fundamental aspects of methodology.

STUDY DESIGN

| | | | |
|---|---|---|---|
| Is the objective of the study sufficiently described? | Yes | Unclear | No |
| Is the design of the study sufficiently described? | Yes | Unclear | No |
| Was the design of the study appropriate to the objective? | Yes | Unclear | No |
| Is the source of the subjects clearly described? | Yes | Unclear | No |
| Is the method of selection of the subjects clearly described (i.e. inclusion and exclusion criteria)? | Yes | Unclear | No |
| Was the sample of subjects appropriate with regard to the population to which the findings will be referred? | Yes | Unclear | No |
| Was the sample size based on pre-study considerations of statistical power? | Yes | Unclear | No |
| Is the design of the study acceptable? | Yes | | No |

CONDUCT OF STUDY

| | | | |
|---|---|---|---|
| Was a satisfactory (high) response rate achieved? | Yes | Unclear | No |

ANALYSIS AND PRESENTATION

| | | | |
|---|---|---|---|
| Is there a statement adequately describing or referencing all the statistical procedures used? | Yes | | No |
| Were the statistical methods used appropriate for the data? | Yes | Unclear | No |
| Were they used correctly? | Yes | Unclear | No |
| Is the presentation of statistical material (tables, graphical, numerical) satisfactory? | Yes | | No |
| Are sufficient analyses presented? | Yes | Unclear | No |
| Are confidence intervals given for the main results? | Yes | | No |

OVERALL ASSESSMENT

| | | | |
|---|---|---|---|
| Are the conclusions drawn from the statistical analyses justified? | Yes | Unclear | No |
| Is the paper statistically acceptable? | Yes | | No |

**Figure 16.1** Checklist for assessment of general medical papers.

STUDY DESIGN

| | | | |
|---|---|---|---|
| Is the objective of the trial sufficiently described? | Yes | Unclear | No |
| Is the design of the study sufficiently described? | Yes | Unclear | No |
| Is there a satisfactory statement of the diagnostic criteria for entry into the trial? | Yes | Unclear | No |
| Is the source of the subjects clearly described? | Yes | Unclear | No |
| Were the treatments well defined? | Yes | Unclear | No |
| Were the treatment groups studied concurrently? | Yes | Unclear | No |
| Was random allocation to treatment used? | Yes | Unclear | No |
| Is the method of creating the randomisation (e.g. tables of random numbers) described? | Yes | Unclear | No |
| Is the mechanism of treatment allocation (e.g. sealed envelopes) described? | Yes | Unclear | No |
| Was the mechanism of treatment allocation designed to eliminate bias? | Yes | Unclear | No |
| Was there an acceptably short delay from allocation to commencement of treatment? | Yes | Unclear | No |
| Was the potential degree of blindness used during the trial? | Yes | Unclear | No |
| Is there a satisfactory statement of criteria for outcome measures? | Yes | Unclear | No |
| Are the outcome measures appropriate? | Yes | Unclear | No |
| Is there a description of a pre-study calculation of sample size based on considerations of statistical power? | Yes | | No |
| Is the duration of post-treatment follow-up stated? | Yes | Unclear | No |
| Is the design of the study acceptable? | Yes | | No |

CONDUCT OF STUDY

| | | | |
|---|---|---|---|
| Were a high proportion of subjects followed up? | Yes | Unclear | No |
| Did a high proportion of subjects complete treatment? | Yes | Unclear | No |
| Are drop-outs described separately for each treatment group? | Yes | Unclear | No |
| Are side-effects of treatment described separately for each group? | Yes | Unclear | No |

ANALYSIS AND PRESENTATION

| | | | |
|---|---|---|---|
| Is there a statement adequately describing or referencing all the statistical procedures used? | Yes | | No |
| Are the baseline characteristics of each group presented adequately? | Yes | | No |
| Were the statistical methods used appropriate for the data? | Yes | Unclear | No |
| Were they used correctly? | Yes | Unclear | No |
| Have prognostic factors been adequately considered? | Yes | Unclear | No |
| Is the presentation of statistical material (tables, graphical, numerical) satisfactory? | Yes | | No |
| Are sufficient analyses presented? | Yes | Unclear | No |
| Are confidence intervals given for the main results? | Yes | | No |

OVERALL ASSESSMENT

| | | | |
|---|---|---|---|
| Are the conclusions drawn from the statistical analyses justified? | Yes | Unclear | No |
| Is the paper statistically acceptable? | Yes | | No |

**Figure 16.2** Checklist for assessment of reports of clinical trials.

## 16.5 WRITING A SCIENTIFIC PAPER

Medical journals give authors scant guidance regarding the statistical aspects of papers. Clearly there is much similarity between aspects of reading a paper and those of writing a paper, and the checklists in Figures 16.1 and 16.2 should give a good idea of the type of information that should be included in a paper. A much more comprehensive set of guidelines for authors is given by Altman *et al.* (1989), covering all aspects of statistics. The basic principle to be adhered to with respect to the statistical aspects of your research is that the methods should be described in sufficient detail to be fully understood, and so that anyone else with access to your raw data could, if desired, reproduce your results. Put more simply, you should describe clearly exactly what was done.

If your research had a useful objective, you have used a sensible design and adequate sample size, you have performed appropriate analyses and drawn reasonable inferences from your findings you should be able to get your paper published in a good journal. The most important aspect is unquestionably the design, because it is always possible to reanalyse your data. While I hope that after reading this book you will be able to carry out sensible analyses of your data, you may take comfort from the following comment:

> I cannot recall that during six years as editor of a major peer-reviewed journal I ever turned down a paper solely because statistical computations were in error, but a large proportion of disapprovals resulted from more fundamental problems of statistical design and concept, which can rarely be remedied after the fact.
>
> (Bailar, 1986)

Statistics is a relatively new field, and like medicine is subject to fashion. In recent years there has been a major shift in policy by many leading medical journals towards encouraging or even requiring authors to use confidence intervals when presenting their main results. The methods have been around for many decades, but have only belatedly become accepted in medicine. Perhaps a continuation of this process would be a decline in the use of hypothesis tests and the plethora of P values and asterisks that adorn most medical research papers (Evans *et al.*, 1988). I shall not predict such a development, but it seems likely that the next few years will see further changes in the use of statistics in medical journals. My hope is that we will begin to see a widespread reduction in the frequency of important statistical errors, whose presence compromises the integrity of the literature and may, ultimately, lead to adverse consequences for patients. Following the marked effect on the statistical quality of studies evaluating new drugs as a result of requirements of the regulatory authorities, there are signs of a more widespread increase in awareness of the importance of good design and correct analysis. To this end I hope that in this book I have succeeded in getting across the important concepts that underlie the statistical component of medical research. For example, it is not important to remember the formula for the confidence interval for a proportion (or any formula for that matter) – you can always look it up. It *is* important to understand what the confidence interval means. More generally it is essential to understand the key statistical concepts underlying study design and statistical inference.

I shall close with some comments of Mainland (1950), an anatomist who subsequently became a professor of statistics too. They are still as relevant as when he wrote them:

> Finally, it must be stressed again that, whatever sources of help are found and whatever techniques are employed, the investigator himself has to grasp the principles of statistical reasoning ... modern statistical principles are not something that we can take or leave as we wish, for they comprise the logic of the investigator in all fields, including the field of clinical research.

## EXERCISES

(*These problems are not specific to the material in this chapter*.)

16.1 If two studies' results yield $P < 0.001$ and $P = 0.02$, why is it not necessarily true, as noted in section 16.3.6, that the former has found a stronger effect than the latter?

16.2 If two identical studies yield $P < 0.001$ and $P = 0.2$, what are the possible explanations for the large difference?

16.3 The mean and standard deviation of the heights (in cm) of adult men and women in a population are as follows

| | Mean | SD |
|---|---|---|
| Men | 179.1 | 5.84 |
| Women | 171.7 | 5.75 |

Assuming that for both sexes height has a Normal distribution,

(a) What proportion of women are above the average height of men?
(b) If 60% of adults are female, what proportion of adults taller than 182.9 cm (six feet) are women?

16.4 The following table shows age-specific and total annual death rates per 1000 females in England and Wales in 1931–5 and 1983 (Office of

Population Censuses and Surveys *Mortality Statistics*).

| Age | Annual death rates/1000 1931–5 | 1983 |
|---|---|---|
| <1 | 54 | 9 |
| 1– 4 | 6.2 | 0.4 |
| 5– 9 | 2.1 | 0.2 |
| 10–14 | 1.4 | 0.2 |
| 15–19 | 2.2 | 0.3 |
| 20–24 | 2.8 | 0.3 |
| 25–34 | 3.1 | 0.5 |
| 35–44 | 4.3 | 1.2 |
| 45–54 | 8.0 | 3.6 |
| 55–64 | 17 | 10 |
| 65–74 | 43 | 24 |
| 75–84 | 109 | 64 |
| 85+ | 245 | 176 |
| All ages | 11.4 | 11.4 |

Over the fifty years there was a large decline in the death rate in every age group. What would explain the fact that the overall death rate per 1000 women of all ages was unchanged?

16.5 The following table shows the percentage of five year olds with five or more decayed, missing or filled teeth (% dmft) by social class, separately for children who had lived continuously in either an area with fluoridated water or in a nearby non-fluoridated area (Carmichael *et al*., 1989).

| Social class | % dmft Fluoridated | Non-fluoridated |
|---|---|---|
| I–II | 10 | 21 |
| III | 15 | 33 |
| IV–V | 21 | 45 |
| Unclassified | 20 | 47 |

(a) Is it reasonable to use a Chi squared test to compare % dmft by social class in the two areas?

(b) The actual numbers of children were as follows:

| Social class | dmft Fluoridated | Non-fluoridated |
|---|---|---|
| I–II | 12/117 | 12/ 56 |
| III | 26/170 | 48/146 |
| IV–V | 11/ 52 | 29/ 64 |
| Unclassified | 24/118 | 49/104 |
| Total | 73/457 | 138/370 |

Calculate a 95% confidence interval for the difference in % dmft in the total groups of children in the two areas.

(c) Is there a significant relation between % dmft and social class within each of the two areas?

(d) How might we assess whether the relation is stronger in the non-fluoridated than the fluoridated area?

(e) What is the name for such an effect?

16.6 The systolic blood pressure (SBP) of 50 pregnant women was measured simultaneously in the same arm using intra-arterial measurement (direct) and a sphygmomanometer (indirect) (Raftery and Ward, 1968). Arm circumference and weight were measured because there was some suggestion that they might affect the difference between the two measurements. The data are shown in the following table:

| | Age | Weight (kg) | Arm circumference (cm) | Systolic BP indirect (mm Hg) | Systolic BP direct (mm Hg) | Diff (I–D) |
|---|---|---|---|---|---|---|
| 1 | 32 | 78.2 | 29 | 115 | 127 | −12 |
| 2 | 25 | 67.8 | 25 | 122 | 147 | −25 |
| 3 | 35 | 71.7 | 26 | 118 | 144 | −26 |
| 4 | 41 | 60.8 | 24 | 127 | 158 | −31 |
| 5 | 30 | 78.7 | 33 | 110 | 125 | −15 |
| 6 | 29 | 87.8 | 31 | 146 | 131 | 15 |
| 7 | 20 | 68.9 | 26 | 127 | 127 | 0 |
| 8 | 38 | 70.5 | 25 | 126 | 126 | 0 |
| 9 | 31 | 68.0 | 29 | 81 | 97 | −16 |
| 10 | 39 | 72.6 | 28 | 127 | 140 | −13 |
| 11 | 36 | 53.3 | 31 | 127 | 132 | −5 |
| 12 | 23 | 53.3 | 23 | 80 | 85 | −5 |
| 13 | 25 | 46.0 | 22 | 89 | 116 | −27 |

| | Age | Weight (kg) | Arm circumference (cm) | Systolic BP indirect (mm Hg) | Systolic BP direct (mm Hg) | Diff (I–D) |
|---|---|---|---|---|---|---|
| 14 | 35 | 65.9 | 26 | 136 | 133 | 3 |
| 15 | 26 | 68.0 | 26 | 105 | 107 | −2 |
| 16 | 23 | 73.0 | 29 | 99 | 121 | −22 |
| 17 | 19 | 65.6 | 26 | 129 | 124 | 5 |
| 18 | 21 | 59.9 | 25 | 98 | 98 | 0 |
| 19 | 31 | 77.8 | 29 | 115 | 113 | 2 |
| 20 | 30 | 82.0 | 31 | 169 | 165 | 4 |
| 21 | 39 | 65.8 | 26 | 107 | 101 | 6 |
| 22 | 30 | 63.5 | 25 | 166 | 173 | −7 |
| 23 | 35 | 63.6 | 28 | 93 | 99 | −6 |
| 24 | 34 | 73.6 | 27 | 115 | 122 | −7 |
| 25 | 30 | 62.1 | 25 | 93 | 116 | −23 |
| 26 | 26 | 81.1 | 33 | 118 | 123 | −5 |
| 27 | 29 | 70.5 | 30 | 116 | 116 | 0 |
| 28 | 27 | 65.8 | 26 | 111 | 114 | −3 |
| 29 | 19 | 77.6 | 31 | 159 | 151 | 8 |
| 30 | 21 | 58.1 | 24 | 110 | 125 | −15 |
| 31 | 44 | 76.2 | 24 | 93 | 113 | −20 |
| 32 | 20 | 58.4 | 25 | 93 | 111 | −18 |
| 33 | 33 | 59.2 | 28 | 117 | 116 | 1 |
| 34 | 41 | 59.8 | 27 | 120 | 121 | −1 |
| 35 | 28 | 54.9 | 23 | 114 | 115 | −1 |
| 36 | 28 | 79.4 | 28 | 132 | 116 | 16 |
| 37 | 18 | 64.9 | 26 | 157 | 130 | 27 |
| 38 | 18 | 67.6 | 25 | 109 | 115 | −6 |
| 39 | 32 | 61.0 | 27 | 157 | 165 | −8 |
| 40 | 20 | 87.0 | 43 | 126 | 134 | −8 |
| 41 | 21 | 51.5 | 23 | 83 | 105 | −22 |
| 42 | 31 | 81.6 | 29 | 116 | 113 | 3 |
| 43 | 29 | 72.1 | 31 | 158 | 171 | −13 |
| 44 | 21 | 95.3 | 31 | 118 | 112 | 6 |
| 45 | 28 | 74.2 | 28 | 123 | 112 | 11 |
| 46 | 22 | 79.6 | 27 | 154 | 166 | −12 |
| 47 | 20 | 70.5 | 26 | 126 | 114 | 12 |
| 48 | 28 | 79.5 | 26 | 119 | 117 | 2 |
| 49 | 19 | 60.9 | 24 | 73 | 72 | 1 |
| 50 | 20 | 77.6 | 27 | 116 | 104 | 12 |

(a) Carry out an appropriate analysis to quantify the agreement between the directly and indirectly measured systolic blood pressures.

(b) Using the results from (a), for what proportion of women would the difference between the methods be expected to be within 10 mm Hg?

(c) Is there any relation between the differences and weight, arm circumference or age?

(d) The above table shows the data in the order in which the women were studied. The following table shows the mean and standard deviation of the indirect-direct differences in systolic blood pressure for the women taken in blocks of 10:

| Women | Difference in SBP (mm Hg) Mean | SD |
|---|---|---|
| 1–10 | −12.3 | 14.0 |
| 11–20 | −4.7 | 11.1 |
| 21–30 | −5.2 | 9.1 |
| 31–40 | −1.8 | 14.3 |
| 41–50 | 0.0 | 11.8 |
| Total | −4.8 | 12.5 |

What might explain the variation in the mean difference in SBP?

(e) Repeat (a) and (b) excluding the first ten women and contrast the answers with those obtained for all 50 women.

16.7 As part of a study of acute mountain sickness fifteen members of a climbing expedition to East Africa had plasma aldosterone measurements taken before and after a rapid ascent to 4300 m (Milledge *et al.*, 1989). The following table shows measurements taken at 09.00 at low and high altitudes over three days, together with a symptom score for acute mountain sickness (AMS) – high values mean worse symptoms.

| | | Plasma aldosterone (mmol/l) | | |
|---|---|---|---|---|
| Subject | AMS score | Low Day 1 | High Day 2 | High Day 3 |
| 1 | 1 | 68 | 151 | 188 |
| 2 | 1 | 153 | 49 | 77 |
| 3 | 7 | 110 | 141 | 95 |
| 4 | 9 | 238 | 286 | 143 |
| 5 | 11 | 204 | 242 | 84 |
| 6 | 11 | 141 | 263 | 63 |
| 7 | 11 | 183 | 233 | 121 |

| Subject | AMS score | Plasma aldosterone (mmol/l) Low Day 1 | High Day 2 | High Day 3 |
|---|---|---|---|---|
| 8 | 13 | 119 | 245 | 97 |
| 9 | 13 | 272 | 275 | 115 |
| 10 | 14 | 166 | 241 | 150 |
| 11 | 15 | 228 | 109 | 76 |
| 12 | 17 | 77 | 192 | 63 |
| 13 | 18 | 114 | 46 | 43 |
| 14 | 23 | 91 | 189 | 74 |
| 15 | 35 | 105 | 254 | 283 |

(a) Carry out an appropriate analysis of the plasma aldosterone levels on the three days. Which pairs of days are significantly different?
(b) Obtain a 95% confidence interval for the difference between plasma aldosterone levels on days 1 and 2.
(c) Examine the association between the AMS score and the change in plasma aldosterone between days 1 and 2.

16.8 In response to the criticism of the analysis of a crossover clinical trial of bran biscuits versus placebo biscuits in the diet of patients with irritable bowel syndrome, the first author wrote:

> 'In studies such as ours, however, given the relatively small numbers, a confidence interval . . . is likely to contain zero, be fairly wide and include both positive and negative values. Therefore this is not an appropriate setting for this form of analysis as the result always will be too diffuse to be meaningful' (Lucey, 1987).

Is this a reasonable argument?

# Appendix A
# Mathematical notation

## A1.1 INTRODUCTION

In this book repeated use is made of many mathematical expressions. These are explained in this appendix. Mathematical notation can be confusing, with the same letters used to denote different quantities in different situations, and with the same symbols used in different ways. Also, there may be several ways of depicting the same expression. A further problem is that while there is often a standard notation, in many cases there is not. Thus it can be confusing to look up the same item in two or more textbooks because they use different ways of expressing the same formula. To help a little, some entries below refer to common alternative forms of notation that may be encountered elsewhere, although they do not appear in this book.

The next three sections discuss basic ideas and the use of symbols and functions, after which there is a glossary of notation.

## A1.2 BASIC IDEAS

### A1.1.2 Variables

When we use a mathematical formula we need a simple way to refer to the values of a variable. For example, if we wish to express as a formula the idea that we calculate a person's age at death by subtracting their year of birth from the year in which they died, we replace each variable by a letter. Traditionally we often use $X$, $Y$ and $Z$ to indicate variables, so we could write the above calculation as

$$X = Y - Z$$

where $X$ represents age at death, $Y$ represents year of death, and $Z$ represents year of birth. It is common, but not universal, to use a capital letter to indicate a variable, and a small letter to indicate a value of that variable.

To denote a particular value of a variable we usually use a subscript. Thus to indicate the value of the variable $X$ for the fourth person in a sample, we write $x_4$. In the previous example $x_4$ represents the age at death of the fourth person.

Often we wish to denote the value for an unspecified individual, in which case we use $x_i$ to indicate the value of the variable $X$ for the '*i*th' subject in the sample. The letters $i$, $j$ and $k$ are often used in this way.

Unfortunately, a different use of subscripts can cause confusion. When we have many variables it is convenient to use subscripts to indicate the number of the variable, such as $X_1$, $X_2$, $X_3$, and so on. The exact meaning of the subscript ought to be clear from the context.

### A1.2.2 Statistics

Summary values derived from the raw data are called **statistics** – examples are means, standard deviations and proportions. We also use letters to denote these values in formulae. The mean of a variable called $X$ is denoted $\bar{x}$ (and pronounced 'x bar'), the standard deviation is denoted $s$, and a proportion is usually denoted as $p$. When we need to refer to more than one statistic of the same type in the same formula we use different subscripts. For example, we might use $p_1$ and $p_2$ to denote observed proportions in two samples. Again the meaning of the subscript should always be clear from the context.

### A1.2.3 Multiplication

Multiplication features in a high proportion of the formulae used in this book. There are several alternative methods of indicating that quantities are multiplied together. Apart from the usual multiplication sign, $\times$, we sometimes use a full stop, while in computer programming (but not in general use) we use an asterisk, $*$. Most confusingly, sometimes we use no symbol at all, relying on the idea that we multiply two adjacent separate quantities in a formula. This is because the multiplication sign looks very similar to the letter $x$ which is used a great deal in formulae, and a full stop could be confused with the decimal point.

Thus, for example, we have

$$2 \times (a + b) = 2 \cdot (a + b) = 2(a + b).$$

The last usage, without a symbol to indicate the multiplication, is the most common method. Thus when we multiply two quantities such $a$ and $b$ we write the product as $ab$. This is why we use a single letter to denote a variable.

### A1.2.4 Brackets

Brackets are used for grouping expressions, usually involving addition or subtraction, where the whole expression is part of a more complicated formula. A simple example was given in the preceding section; a more complicated example is

$$(a + b)(a + c)(b + d)(c + d)$$

a quantity calculated in Chapter 10 in which four sums of two frequencies are multiplied.

Quantities within brackets should be calculated before other parts of the calculation. Thus if we wish to evaluate

$$y = 2(a + b)$$

where $a = 13.5$ and $b = 7.1$, we have

$$y = 2(13.5 + 7.1) = 2(20.6) = 41.2.$$

For complicated formulae we often need to have one set of brackets within another. To make these easier to read we use different types of brackets, and usually have round brackets within square brackets within curly brackets. An example is

$$[p_1(1 - p_1) + p_2(1 - p_2)]/2.$$

### A1.2.5 Division

There are two ways of denoting division in formulae. To show, for example, the quantity $a + b$ divided by $c$ we can write either $(a + b)/c$ or $\frac{a+b}{c}$. The brackets in the first method are essential to distinguish $(a + b)/c$ from $a + \frac{b}{c}$. The upper quantity in a division is the **numerator** and the lower quantity is the **denominator**.

If the denominator involves multiple elements then brackets may be needed. For example, to denote $a + b$ divided by $c + d$ we use either $(a + b)/(c + d)$ or $\frac{a+b}{c+d}$. The symbol $\div$ is not usually used in mathematical notation.

### A1.2.6 Powers and square roots

When we multiply a quantity by itself we get the **square** of the original value, and if we multiply the result by the original value again we get its **cube**. Thus if we have a room that is 4.2 metres square, its area would be $4.2 \times 4.2 = 17.64$ square metres. If it is also 4.2 metres high, its volume is $4.2 \times 17.64 = 74.088$ cubic metres.

We denote the square of a number by a superscript of 2, and a cube with a superscript of 3. The floor area of the room is thus $4.2^2$ square metres and its volume is $4.2^3$ cubic metres. The superscript indicates the number of times we must multiply the value by itself, and is known as the **power**. More generally we write $x^k$ to indicate the value of $x$ to the power

$k$. Sometimes we need to evaluate $x^k$ when $k = 0$. The value of $x^0$ is 1, for any value of $x$.

The **square root** involves the reverse process. The square root of a number is the number that when squared gives the first number. For example, using the above example, 4.2 is the square root of 17.64. We write this as $\sqrt{17.64} = 4.2$. Alternative notation sometimes seen (but not used in this book) is $17.64^{1/2} = 4.2$. Similarly, the quantity $1/x$, which is known as the **reciprocal** of $x$, may be written as $x^{-1}$.

An example that combines the various features discussed so far is

$$\sqrt{\left[p(1-p)\left(\frac{1}{n_1}+\frac{1}{n_2}\right)\right]}.$$

### A1.2.7 Summation

A common feature of statistical formulae is the need to indicate the sum of a number of items. For example, the mean of a set of observations is calculated from the sum of all the observations divided by the number of observations. If we have $n$ observations denoted by $x_1, x_2, x_3, \ldots, x_n$ then, as described in Chapter 3, we can calculate the mean, $\bar{x}$, as

$$\bar{x} = (x_1 + x_2 + x_3 + \ldots + x_n)/n$$

but this is long-winded. We use the 'summation sign' $\Sigma$ (the Greek capital sigma) to indicate 'sum of', and can abbreviate the expression to

$$\bar{x} = \frac{1}{n}\sum_{i=1}^{n} x_i$$

where the symbols below and above the sigma indicate the range of values being added. In practice, it is usually obvious what these values are, so we use the shorthand $\Sigma x_i$ or $\Sigma x$. As with other examples already discussed, we use brackets to clarify what is being summed. Thus

$$\sum (y_i - a - bx_i)^2$$

indicates that we calculate $y_i - a - bx_i$ for each value of $i$, square them, and add them up for all values of $i$.

Note that $(\Sigma x)^2 = (\Sigma x) \times (\Sigma x)$ and is not the same as $\Sigma x^2$.

Sometimes we use two $\Sigma$ signs to indicate double summation. For example, the expression

$$\sum_{i=1}^{r}\sum_{j=1}^{c}\frac{(O_{ij} - E_{ij})^2}{E_{ij}}$$

means that the expression on the right is added for every combination of values of $i$ from 1 to $r$ and $j$ from 1 to $c$. Note the corresponding use of double subscripts. This formula appears in section 10.6.6.

### A1.2.8 Products

We sometimes need to indicate the product of a number of items; that is, we need to multiply them all together. If we have $n$ observations denoted as $x_1, x_2, x_3, \ldots, x_n$, then we can calculate their multiple product as

$$x_1 \times x_2 \times x_3 \times \ldots \times x_n$$

but this is long-winded. We use Π (the Greek capital pi) to indicate 'product of', and can abbreviate the expression to

$$\prod_{i=1}^{n} x_i$$

where the symbols below and above the letter pi indicate the range of values being multiplied. In practice, as with summation, it is usually obvious what these values are, so we use the shorthand $\Pi x_i$ or $\Pi x$.

### A1.2.9 Factorials

Another sort of product is the **factorial**. We write, for example, 5! (pronounced 'five factorial') to mean $5 \times 4 \times 3 \times 2 \times 1$. In general $x!$ means the product of all the integers from 1 up to $x$. We define $0! = 1$. Factorials are used in this book for Fisher's exact test, in section 10.7.3.

## A1.3 MATHEMATICAL SYMBOLS

$|\ldots|$ indicates the **absolute** value of the quantity between the vertical lines; that is, the sign is ignored. For example, $|-23.5| = |23.5| = 23.5$.

$\pm$ indicates 'plus or minus'. For example, the expression $a \pm b$ is shorthand for the *two* quantities $a + b$ and $a - b$.

**Bar** (e.g. $\bar{x}$) indicates the mean of the variable denoted by the letter, here $x$.

**Hat** (e.g. $\hat{p}$) indicates an **estimate** of the quantity denoted by the letter, here $p$.

$<$ and $>$ are used to indicate inequalities:

$a < b$: $a$ is **less than** $b$

$a > b$: $a$ is **greater than** $b$

$a \leq b$: $a$ is **less than or equal to** $b$

$a \geq b$: $a$ is **greater than or equal to** $b$

## A1.4 FUNCTIONS

Another common type of statistical notation is the mathematical function. This notation indicates a general relationship. For example, if we define a function $\mathrm{f}(x)$ so that $\mathrm{f}(x) = a + bx$, then we can write $y = \mathrm{f}(x)$ to mean $y = a + bx$. Here $\mathrm{f}(x)$ simply means a specified function or transformation of $x$. The most common function used in this book is $\log(x)$ indicating the logarithmic transformation. With this type of notation, it is understood that the name of the function, here 'log', describes what is done to the value in brackets. This use of brackets is thus different from that given above; in particular we do not interpret $\mathrm{f}(x)$ as f multiplied by $x$. To confuse matters further, in some cases we omit the brackets. Thus $\log(x)$ is often written simply as $\log x$.

### A1.4.1 Logarithms

Logarithms are mainly used in statistics to transform a set of observations to values with a more convenient distribution, in particular to make a skewed distribution closer to a Normal distribution. The logarithm (log) of a quantity $x$ is the value $y$ such that $x = \mathrm{e}^y$. Here e is the constant 2.718281. . . . The log of 1 is 0 and the log of 0 is minus infinity ($-\infty$). Log transformation can be used only for data where all values are positive. $\mathrm{Log}_\mathrm{e} x$ is known as the **natural** logarithm of $x$ to the base e, and is sometimes written $\ln x$. We sometimes use logarithms to the base 10, in which case $\log_{10} x$ is the value $y$ such that $x = 10^y$. The advantage of using logs to base 10 is that the numbers 10, 100, 1000, etc. become 1, 2, 3, etc. However, the use of logs to base e is much more common, and may be the only option in a computer package. There is no difference in the effect of taking logs to different bases; one gives values that are a constant multiple of the other. It is, however, important to clarify the base used if values are quoted in log units. We use brackets when necessary to make the meaning clear, as in $\log_\mathrm{e}(x - y)$.

The logarithm of the ratio of two quantities, say $f$ and $g$, is equal to the difference between their logarithms, i.e. $\log(f/g) = \log(f) - \log(g)$.

## A1.5 GLOSSARY OF NOTATION

The notation used in this book is briefly described below, along with a few items that do not appear but which may often be encountered.

$n_i$ or $N_i$ The sample size in the $i$th group of subjects.

$n$ or $N$ The total sample size.

$\bar{x}$ The mean of a sample of observations, where the individual observations are denoted by $x$ or $x_i$; it is pronounced 'x bar'. In some chapters observations are denoted by other letters such as $y$ or $d$, in which case the mean is $\bar{y}$ or $\bar{d}$.

$\mu$ The Greek letter mu, denoting the mean of a population.

*SD* or *sd* or *s* The standard deviation of a sample of observations. It is a measure of their variability around the mean.

$\sigma$ The Greek letter sigma, denoting the standard deviation of a population.

*SE* or *se* The standard error of a sample mean or some other estimated statistic. It is a measure of the uncertainty of such an estimate and is used to derive a confidence interval for the population value. The notation $SE(b)$ or $SE_b$ means 'the standard error of $b$'.

$p$ The proportion of a sample with a given characteristic. The proportion of the population with a given characteristic may also be called $p$, in which case the sample proportion is denoted $\hat{p}$.

$\Sigma$ The Greek capital letter sigma, denoting 'sum of'. See section A1.2.7.

$\Pi$ The Greek capital letter pi, denoting 'product of'. See section A1.2.8.

$\log_e x$ The natural logarithm of $x$ to the base e, also written $\ln x$. We sometimes use logarithms to the base 10, written $\log_{10} x$. Logarithms are explained in section A1.4.1. See also $e^x$.

$e^x$ The exponential function, denoting the inverse procedure to taking logarithms. It is sometimes called the antilogarithmic transformation. An alternative notation is $\exp(x)$.

$\alpha$ (a) The level of a hypothesis test; $1 - \alpha$ is the level of the confidence interval. To perform a test at a given level of $\alpha$, we compare the test statistic with the theoretical value of the appropriate sampling distribution which cuts off a proportion $\alpha$ of the distribution. Most commonly we use $\alpha$ equal to 0.05 or 0.01. Traditionally, the P value (see below) from a hypothesis test is compared with $\alpha$ and the test is 'significant' if $P < \alpha$. The modern attitude is to present the P value and not to consider the test as being a decision about whether or not the result is significant. $\alpha$ is also known as the Type I error rate. See section 8.5.
(b) The intercept of a regression line in the population. The sample intercept is denoted $a$.

$\beta$ (a) The Type II error rate associated with a hypothesis test. The power of a hypothesis test is $1 - \beta$, and is the probability that the P value will be lower than the prespecified significance level ($\alpha$) when the alternative hypothesis is true. See section 8.5.
(b) The slope of a regression line in the population. The sample slope is denoted $b$.

P The probability value, or significance level, from a hypothesis test. P is the probability of the data (or some more extreme data) arising by chance – that is, due to sampling variation only – when the null hypothesis is true. It is better to use P rather than p, which can be confused with an observed proportion.

$N_{1-\alpha/2}$ A value from the standard Normal distribution, which is the theoretical Normal distribution with mean 0 and standard deviation 1. The subscript represents the proportion of the distribution below the value $N_{1-\alpha/2}$. Thus $N_{0.975}$ is the value of the standard Normal distribution below which lies the bottom 0.975 or 97.5% of the distribution. Thus, for example, $N_{0.975} = 1.96$. The central $1 - \alpha$ or $100(1 - \alpha)\%$ of the distribution lies between $N_{\alpha/2}$ and $N_{1-\alpha/2}$. Because of the symmetry of the Normal distribution, $N_{\alpha/2} = -N_{1-\alpha/2}$ so that the central $100(1 - \alpha)\%$ of the distribution lies between $-N_{1-\alpha/2}$ and $N_{1-\alpha/2}$. For example, the central 95% of the Normal distribution lies between $-N_{0.975}$ and $N_{0.975}$, that is, between $-1.96$ and $+1.96$. A common alternative notation is $z$, used in this book for the value of the test statistic derived from a sample.

$t$ A value from 'Student's' $t$ distribution, the sampling distribution for means of small samples. We use $t$ for the value derived from a sample, and $t_{1-\alpha/2}(f)$ to indicate the appropriate value from the theoretical distribution, where $f$ denotes the number of degrees of freedom.

$\chi^2$ A value from the 'Chi squared' distribution, the sampling distribution for test statistics derived from tables of frequencies. We use $\chi^2$ or $X^2$ for the value derived from a sample, and $\chi^2_{1-\alpha}(f)$ to indicate the appropriate value from the theoretical distribution, where $f$ denotes the number of degrees of freedom.

$r$ The Pearson correlation coefficient calculated from a sample. The population correlation coefficient is denoted by the Greek letter rho ($\rho$). See Chapter 11.

$r_s$ The Spearman rank correlation coefficient calculated from a sample. See Chapter 11.

$F$ A value from the '$F$' distribution, the sampling distribution for the ratio of two variances. $F$ is also used for the sample value of the ratio of two variances.

$(x, y)$ The values corresponding to a point in a two-dimensional graph, such as a scatter diagram, sometimes called 'coordinates'. The mean of a set of values of the variables $X$ and $Y$ is denoted $(\bar{x}, \bar{y})$.

$\infty$ Infinity – the value larger than any imaginable number. Likewise $-\infty$ is the value less than any imaginable negative number. The values $\pm\infty$ are the extremities of a horizontal scale representing the values of a standard Normal distribution.

! Factorial, as in $5! = 5 \times 4 \times 3 \times 2 \times 1 = 120$. See section A1.2.9.

# Appendix B
# Statistical tables

This Appendix comprises twelve tables containing values to assist in the calculation of confidence intervals and P values for hypothesis tests. There is also a table of random numbers for use in random allocation or random sampling when designing studies.

More extensive tables can be found in Lentner (1982).

## INDEX OF TABLES



**Table B1 Normal distribution – areas in one tail ($z \rightarrow$ P)**

The tabulated values are the proportions of the standard Normal distribution below and above the value $z$, which is a standard Normal deviate. The tabulated values are also known as the lower and upper tail areas, or one-tailed P values, and are denoted $P_{lower}$ and $P_{upper}$. For negative values of $z$, the values of $P_{lower}$ and $P_{upper}$ should be interchanged. (Two-tailed P values are given in Table B2; $z$ values for specific P values are given in Table B3.)

Example: The lower and upper tail areas corresponding to $z = 1.24$ are 0.8925 and 0.1075.

| $z$ | $P_{lower}$ | $P_{upper}$ | $z$ | $P_{lower}$ | $P_{upper}$ | $z$ | $P_{lower}$ | $P_{upper}$ |
|---|---|---|---|---|---|---|---|---|
| 0.00 | 0.5000 | 0.5000 | | | | | | |
| 0.01 | 0.5040 | 0.4960 | 0.36 | 0.6406 | 0.3594 | 0.71 | 0.7611 | 0.2389 |
| 0.02 | 0.5080 | 0.4920 | 0.37 | 0.6443 | 0.3557 | 0.72 | 0.7642 | 0.2358 |
| 0.03 | 0.5120 | 0.4880 | 0.38 | 0.6480 | 0.3520 | 0.73 | 0.7673 | 0.2327 |
| 0.04 | 0.5160 | 0.4840 | 0.39 | 0.6517 | 0.3483 | 0.74 | 0.7704 | 0.2296 |
| 0.05 | 0.5199 | 0.4801 | 0.40 | 0.6554 | 0.3446 | 0.75 | 0.7734 | 0.2266 |
| 0.06 | 0.5239 | 0.4761 | 0.41 | 0.6591 | 0.3409 | 0.76 | 0.7764 | 0.2236 |
| 0.07 | 0.5279 | 0.4721 | 0.42 | 0.6628 | 0.3372 | 0.77 | 0.7794 | 0.2206 |
| 0.08 | 0.5319 | 0.4681 | 0.43 | 0.6664 | 0.3336 | 0.78 | 0.7823 | 0.2177 |
| 0.09 | 0.5359 | 0.4641 | 0.44 | 0.6700 | 0.3300 | 0.79 | 0.7852 | 0.2148 |
| 0.10 | 0.5398 | 0.4602 | 0.45 | 0.6736 | 0.3264 | 0.80 | 0.7881 | 0.2119 |
| 0.11 | 0.5438 | 0.4562 | 0.46 | 0.6772 | 0.3228 | 0.81 | 0.7910 | 0.2090 |
| 0.12 | 0.5478 | 0.4522 | 0.47 | 0.6808 | 0.3192 | 0.82 | 0.7939 | 0.2061 |
| 0.13 | 0.5517 | 0.4483 | 0.48 | 0.6844 | 0.3156 | 0.83 | 0.7967 | 0.2033 |
| 0.14 | 0.5557 | 0.4443 | 0.49 | 0.6879 | 0.3121 | 0.84 | 0.7995 | 0.2005 |
| 0.15 | 0.5596 | 0.4404 | 0.50 | 0.6915 | 0.3085 | 0.85 | 0.8023 | 0.1977 |
| 0.16 | 0.5636 | 0.4364 | 0.51 | 0.6950 | 0.3050 | 0.86 | 0.8051 | 0.1949 |
| 0.17 | 0.5675 | 0.4325 | 0.52 | 0.6985 | 0.3015 | 0.87 | 0.8078 | 0.1922 |
| 0.18 | 0.5714 | 0.4286 | 0.53 | 0.7019 | 0.2981 | 0.88 | 0.8106 | 0.1894 |
| 0.19 | 0.5753 | 0.4247 | 0.54 | 0.7054 | 0.2946 | 0.89 | 0.8133 | 0.1867 |
| 0.20 | 0.5793 | 0.4207 | 0.55 | 0.7088 | 0.2912 | 0.90 | 0.8159 | 0.1841 |
| 0.21 | 0.5832 | 0.4168 | 0.56 | 0.7123 | 0.2877 | 0.91 | 0.8186 | 0.1814 |
| 0.22 | 0.5871 | 0.4129 | 0.57 | 0.7157 | 0.2843 | 0.92 | 0.8212 | 0.1788 |
| 0.23 | 0.5910 | 0.4090 | 0.58 | 0.7190 | 0.2810 | 0.93 | 0.8238 | 0.1762 |
| 0.24 | 0.5948 | 0.4052 | 0.59 | 0.7224 | 0.2776 | 0.94 | 0.8264 | 0.1736 |
| 0.25 | 0.5987 | 0.4013 | 0.60 | 0.7257 | 0.2743 | 0.95 | 0.8289 | 0.1711 |
| 0.26 | 0.6026 | 0.3974 | 0.61 | 0.7291 | 0.2709 | 0.96 | 0.8315 | 0.1685 |
| 0.27 | 0.6064 | 0.3936 | 0.62 | 0.7324 | 0.2676 | 0.97 | 0.8340 | 0.1660 |
| 0.28 | 0.6103 | 0.3897 | 0.63 | 0.7357 | 0.2643 | 0.98 | 0.8365 | 0.1635 |
| 0.29 | 0.6141 | 0.3859 | 0.64 | 0.7389 | 0.2611 | 0.99 | 0.8389 | 0.1611 |
| 0.30 | 0.6179 | 0.3821 | 0.65 | 0.7422 | 0.2578 | 1.00 | 0.8413 | 0.1587 |
| 0.31 | 0.6217 | 0.3783 | 0.66 | 0.7454 | 0.2546 | 1.01 | 0.8438 | 0.1562 |
| 0.32 | 0.6255 | 0.3745 | 0.67 | 0.7486 | 0.2514 | 1.02 | 0.8461 | 0.1539 |
| 0.33 | 0.6293 | 0.3707 | 0.68 | 0.7517 | 0.2483 | 1.03 | 0.8485 | 0.1515 |
| 0.34 | 0.6331 | 0.3669 | 0.69 | 0.7549 | 0.2451 | 1.04 | 0.8508 | 0.1492 |
| 0.35 | 0.6368 | 0.3632 | 0.70 | 0.7580 | 0.2420 | 1.05 | 0.8531 | 0.1469 |

| $z$ | $P_{lower}$ | $P_{upper}$ | $z$ | $P_{lower}$ | $P_{upper}$ | $z$ | $P_{lower}$ | $P_{upper}$ |
|---|---|---|---|---|---|---|---|---|
| 1.06 | 0.8554 | 0.1446 | 1.46 | 0.9279 | 0.0721 | 1.86 | 0.9686 | 0.0314 |
| 1.07 | 0.8577 | 0.1423 | 1.47 | 0.9292 | 0.0708 | 1.87 | 0.9693 | 0.0307 |
| 1.08 | 0.8599 | 0.1401 | 1.48 | 0.9306 | 0.0694 | 1.88 | 0.9699 | 0.0301 |
| 1.09 | 0.8621 | 0.1379 | 1.49 | 0.9319 | 0.0681 | 1.89 | 0.9706 | 0.0294 |
| 1.10 | 0.8643 | 0.1357 | 1.50 | 0.9332 | 0.0668 | 1.90 | 0.9713 | 0.0287 |
| 1.11 | 0.8665 | 0.1335 | 1.51 | 0.9345 | 0.0655 | 1.91 | 0.9719 | 0.0281 |
| 1.12 | 0.8686 | 0.1314 | 1.52 | 0.9357 | 0.0643 | 1.92 | 0.9726 | 0.0274 |
| 1.13 | 0.8708 | 0.1292 | 1.53 | 0.9370 | 0.0630 | 1.93 | 0.9732 | 0.0268 |
| 1.14 | 0.8729 | 0.1271 | 1.54 | 0.9382 | 0.0618 | 1.94 | 0.9738 | 0.0262 |
| 1.15 | 0.8749 | 0.1251 | 1.55 | 0.9394 | 0.0606 | 1.95 | 0.9744 | 0.0256 |
| 1.16 | 0.8770 | 0.1230 | 1.56 | 0.9406 | 0.0594 | 1.96 | 0.9750 | 0.0250 |
| 1.17 | 0.8790 | 0.1210 | 1.57 | 0.9418 | 0.0582 | 1.97 | 0.9756 | 0.0244 |
| 1.18 | 0.8810 | 0.1190 | 1.58 | 0.9429 | 0.0571 | 1.98 | 0.9761 | 0.0239 |
| 1.19 | 0.8830 | 0.1170 | 1.59 | 0.9441 | 0.0559 | 1.99 | 0.9767 | 0.0233 |
| 1.20 | 0.8849 | 0.1151 | 1.60 | 0.9452 | 0.0548 | 2.00 | 0.9772 | 0.0228 |
| 1.21 | 0.8869 | 0.1131 | 1.61 | 0.9463 | 0.0537 | 2.01 | 0.9778 | 0.0222 |
| 1.22 | 0.8888 | 0.1112 | 1.62 | 0.9474 | 0.0526 | 2.02 | 0.9783 | 0.0217 |
| 1.23 | 0.8907 | 0.1093 | 1.63 | 0.9484 | 0.0516 | 2.03 | 0.9788 | 0.0212 |
| 1.24 | 0.8925 | 0.1075 | 1.64 | 0.9495 | 0.0505 | 2.04 | 0.9793 | 0.0207 |
| 1.25 | 0.8944 | 0.1056 | 1.65 | 0.9505 | 0.0495 | 2.05 | 0.9798 | 0.0202 |
| 1.26 | 0.8962 | 0.1038 | 1.66 | 0.9515 | 0.0485 | 2.06 | 0.9803 | 0.0197 |
| 1.27 | 0.8980 | 0.1020 | 1.67 | 0.9525 | 0.0475 | 2.07 | 0.9808 | 0.0192 |
| 1.28 | 0.8997 | 0.1003 | 1.68 | 0.9535 | 0.0465 | 2.08 | 0.9812 | 0.0188 |
| 1.29 | 0.9015 | 0.0985 | 1.69 | 0.9545 | 0.0455 | 2.09 | 0.9817 | 0.0183 |
| 1.30 | 0.9032 | 0.0968 | 1.70 | 0.9554 | 0.0446 | 2.10 | 0.9821 | 0.0179 |
| 1.31 | 0.9049 | 0.0951 | 1.71 | 0.9564 | 0.0436 | 2.11 | 0.9826 | 0.0174 |
| 1.32 | 0.9066 | 0.0934 | 1.72 | 0.9573 | 0.0427 | 2.12 | 0.9830 | 0.0170 |
| 1.33 | 0.9082 | 0.0918 | 1.73 | 0.9582 | 0.0418 | 2.13 | 0.9834 | 0.0166 |
| 1.34 | 0.9099 | 0.0901 | 1.74 | 0.9591 | 0.0409 | 2.14 | 0.9838 | 0.0162 |
| 1.35 | 0.9115 | 0.0885 | 1.75 | 0.9599 | 0.0401 | 2.15 | 0.9842 | 0.0158 |
| 1.36 | 0.9131 | 0.0869 | 1.76 | 0.9608 | 0.0392 | 2.16 | 0.9846 | 0.0154 |
| 1.37 | 0.9147 | 0.0853 | 1.77 | 0.9616 | 0.0384 | 2.17 | 0.9850 | 0.0150 |
| 1.38 | 0.9162 | 0.0838 | 1.78 | 0.9625 | 0.0375 | 2.18 | 0.9854 | 0.0146 |
| 1.39 | 0.9177 | 0.0823 | 1.79 | 0.9633 | 0.0367 | 2.19 | 0.9857 | 0.0143 |
| 1.40 | 0.9192 | 0.0808 | 1.80 | 0.9641 | 0.0359 | 2.20 | 0.9861 | 0.0139 |
| 1.41 | 0.9207 | 0.0793 | 1.81 | 0.9649 | 0.0351 | 2.21 | 0.9864 | 0.0136 |
| 1.42 | 0.9222 | 0.0778 | 1.82 | 0.9656 | 0.0344 | 2.22 | 0.9868 | 0.0132 |
| 1.43 | 0.9236 | 0.0764 | 1.83 | 0.9664 | 0.0336 | 2.23 | 0.9871 | 0.0129 |
| 1.44 | 0.9251 | 0.0749 | 1.84 | 0.9671 | 0.0329 | 2.24 | 0.9875 | 0.0125 |
| 1.45 | 0.9265 | 0.0735 | 1.85 | 0.9678 | 0.0322 | 2.25 | 0.9878 | 0.0122 |

| $z$ | $P_{lower}$ | $P_{upper}$ | $z$ | $P_{lower}$ | $P_{upper}$ | $z$ | $P_{lower}$ | $P_{upper}$ |
|---|---|---|---|---|---|---|---|---|
| 2.26 | 0.9881 | 0.0119 | 2.61 | 0.9955 | 0.0045 | 2.91 | 0.9982 | 0.0018 |
| 2.27 | 0.9884 | 0.0116 | 2.62 | 0.9956 | 0.0044 | 2.92 | 0.9982 | 0.0018 |
| 2.28 | 0.9887 | 0.0113 | 2.63 | 0.9957 | 0.0043 | 2.93 | 0.9983 | 0.0017 |
| 2.29 | 0.9890 | 0.0110 | 2.64 | 0.9959 | 0.0041 | 2.94 | 0.9984 | 0.0016 |
| 2.30 | 0.9893 | 0.0107 | 2.65 | 0.9960 | 0.0040 | 2.95 | 0.9984 | 0.0016 |
| 2.31 | 0.9896 | 0.0104 | 2.66 | 0.9961 | 0.0039 | 2.96 | 0.9985 | 0.0015 |
| 2.32 | 0.9898 | 0.0102 | 2.67 | 0.9962 | 0.0038 | 2.97 | 0.9985 | 0.0015 |
| 2.33 | 0.9901 | 0.0099 | 2.68 | 0.9963 | 0.0037 | 2.98 | 0.9986 | 0.0014 |
| 2.34 | 0.9904 | 0.0096 | 2.69 | 0.9964 | 0.0036 | 2.99 | 0.9986 | 0.0014 |
| 2.35 | 0.9906 | 0.0094 | 2.70 | 0.9965 | 0.0035 | 3.00 | 0.9987 | 0.0013 |
| 2.36 | 0.9909 | 0.0091 | 2.71 | 0.9966 | 0.0034 | 3.05 | 0.99886 | 0.00114 |
| 2.37 | 0.9911 | 0.0089 | 2.72 | 0.9967 | 0.0033 | 3.10 | 0.99903 | 0.00097 |
| 2.38 | 0.9913 | 0.0087 | 2.73 | 0.9968 | 0.0032 | 3.15 | 0.99918 | 0.00082 |
| 2.39 | 0.9916 | 0.0084 | 2.74 | 0.9969 | 0.0031 | 3.20 | 0.99931 | 0.00069 |
| 2.40 | 0.9918 | 0.0082 | 2.75 | 0.9970 | 0.0030 | 3.25 | 0.99942 | 0.00058 |
| 2.41 | 0.9920 | 0.0080 | 2.76 | 0.9971 | 0.0029 | 3.30 | 0.99952 | 0.00048 |
| 2.42 | 0.9922 | 0.0078 | 2.77 | 0.9972 | 0.0028 | 3.35 | 0.99960 | 0.00040 |
| 2.43 | 0.9925 | 0.0075 | 2.78 | 0.9973 | 0.0027 | 3.40 | 0.99966 | 0.00034 |
| 2.44 | 0.9927 | 0.0073 | 2.79 | 0.9974 | 0.0026 | 3.45 | 0.99972 | 0.00028 |
| 2.45 | 0.9929 | 0.0071 | 2.80 | 0.9974 | 0.0026 | 3.50 | 0.99977 | 0.00023 |
| 2.46 | 0.9931 | 0.0069 | 2.81 | 0.9975 | 0.0025 | 3.55 | 0.99981 | 0.00019 |
| 2.47 | 0.9932 | 0.0068 | 2.82 | 0.9976 | 0.0024 | 3.60 | 0.99984 | 0.00016 |
| 2.48 | 0.9934 | 0.0066 | 2.83 | 0.9977 | 0.0023 | 3.65 | 0.99987 | 0.00013 |
| 2.49 | 0.9936 | 0.0064 | 2.84 | 0.9977 | 0.0023 | 3.70 | 0.99989 | 0.00011 |
| 2.50 | 0.9938 | 0.0062 | 2.85 | 0.9978 | 0.0022 | 3.75 | 0.99991 | 0.00009 |
| 2.51 | 0.9940 | 0.0060 | 2.86 | 0.9979 | 0.0021 | 3.80 | 0.99993 | 0.00007 |
| 2.52 | 0.9941 | 0.0059 | 2.87 | 0.9979 | 0.0021 | 3.85 | 0.99994 | 0.00006 |
| 2.53 | 0.9943 | 0.0057 | 2.88 | 0.9980 | 0.0020 | 3.90 | 0.99995 | 0.00005 |
| 2.54 | 0.9945 | 0.0055 | 2.89 | 0.9981 | 0.0019 | 3.95 | 0.99996 | 0.00004 |
| 2.55 | 0.9946 | 0.0054 | 2.90 | 0.9981 | 0.0019 | 4.00 | 0.99997 | 0.00003 |
| 2.56 | 0.9948 | 0.0052 | | | | | | |
| 2.57 | 0.9949 | 0.0051 | | | | | | |
| 2.58 | 0.9951 | 0.0049 | | | | | | |
| 2.59 | 0.9952 | 0.0048 | | | | | | |
| 2.60 | 0.9953 | 0.0047 | | | | | | |

**Table B2 Normal distribution – two-tailed areas ($z \rightarrow$ P)**

The tabulated values are the proportions of the standard Normal distribution outside the range $\pm z$, where $z$ is a standard Normal deviate. The tabulated values are also known as two-tailed (or two-sided) P values. (One-tailed P values are given in Table Bl; $z$ values for specific P values are given in Table B3.)

Example: The two-tailed P value corresponding to $z$ = 1.24 is 0.2150.

| $z$ | P | $z$ | P | $z$ | P | $z$ | P |
|---|---|---|---|---|---|---|---|
| 0.00 | 1.0000 | | | | | | |
| 0.01 | 0.9920 | 0.31 | 0.7566 | 0.61 | 0.5419 | 0.91 | 0.3628 |
| 0.02 | 0.9840 | 0.32 | 0.7490 | 0.62 | 0.5353 | 0.92 | 0.3576 |
| 0.03 | 0.9761 | 0.33 | 0.7414 | 0.63 | 0.5287 | 0.93 | 0.3524 |
| 0.04 | 0.9681 | 0.34 | 0.7339 | 0.64 | 0.5222 | 0.94 | 0.3472 |
| 0.05 | 0.9601 | 0.35 | 0.7263 | 0.65 | 0.5157 | 0.95 | 0.3421 |
| 0.06 | 0.9522 | 0.36 | 0.7188 | 0.66 | 0.5093 | 0.96 | 0.3371 |
| 0.07 | 0.9442 | 0.37 | 0.7114 | 0.67 | 0.5029 | 0.97 | 0.3320 |
| 0.08 | 0.9362 | 0.38 | 0.7039 | 0.68 | 0.4965 | 0.98 | 0.3271 |
| 0.09 | 0.9283 | 0.39 | 0.6965 | 0.69 | 0.4902 | 0.99 | 0.3222 |
| 0.10 | 0.9203 | 0.40 | 0.6892 | 0.70 | 0.4839 | 1.00 | 0.3173 |
| 0.11 | 0.9124 | 0.41 | 0.6818 | 0.71 | 0.4777 | 1.01 | 0.3125 |
| 0.12 | 0.9045 | 0.42 | 0.6745 | 0.72 | 0.4715 | 1.02 | 0.3077 |
| 0.13 | 0.8966 | 0.43 | 0.6672 | 0.73 | 0.4654 | 1.03 | 0.3030 |
| 0.14 | 0.8887 | 0.44 | 0.6599 | 0.74 | 0.4593 | 1.04 | 0.2983 |
| 0.15 | 0.8808 | 0.45 | 0.6527 | 0.75 | 0.4533 | 1.05 | 0.2937 |
| 0.16 | 0.8729 | 0.46 | 0.6455 | 0.76 | 0.4473 | 1.06 | 0.2891 |
| 0.17 | 0.8650 | 0.47 | 0.6384 | 0.77 | 0.4413 | 1.07 | 0.2846 |
| 0.18 | 0.8572 | 0.48 | 0.6312 | 0.78 | 0.4354 | 1.08 | 0.2801 |
| 0.19 | 0.8493 | 0.49 | 0.6241 | 0.79 | 0.4295 | 1.09 | 0.2757 |
| 0.20 | 0.8415 | 0.50 | 0.6171 | 0.80 | 0.4237 | 1.10 | 0.2713 |
| 0.21 | 0.8337 | 0.51 | 0.6101 | 0.81 | 0.4179 | 1.11 | 0.2670 |
| 0.22 | 0.8259 | 0.52 | 0.6031 | 0.82 | 0.4122 | 1.12 | 0.2627 |
| 0.23 | 0.8181 | 0.53 | 0.5961 | 0.83 | 0.4065 | 1.13 | 0.2585 |
| 0.24 | 0.8103 | 0.54 | 0.5892 | 0.84 | 0.4009 | 1.14 | 0.2543 |
| 0.25 | 0.8026 | 0.55 | 0.5823 | 0.85 | 0.3953 | 1.15 | 0.2501 |
| 0.26 | 0.7949 | 0.56 | 0.5755 | 0.86 | 0.3898 | 1.16 | 0.2460 |
| 0.27 | 0.7872 | 0.57 | 0.5687 | 0.87 | 0.3843 | 1.17 | 0.2420 |
| 0.28 | 0.7795 | 0.58 | 0.5619 | 0.88 | 0.3789 | 1.18 | 0.2380 |
| 0.29 | 0.7718 | 0.59 | 0.5552 | 0.89 | 0.3735 | 1.19 | 0.2340 |
| 0.30 | 0.7642 | 0.60 | 0.5485 | 0.90 | 0.3681 | 1.20 | 0.2301 |

| z | P | z | P | z | P | z | P |
|---|---|---|---|---|---|---|---|
| 1.21 | 0.2263 | 1.61 | 0.1074 | 2.01 | 0.0444 | 2.41 | 0.0160 |
| 1.22 | 0.2225 | 1.62 | 0.1052 | 2.02 | 0.0434 | 2.42 | 0.0155 |
| 1.23 | 0.2187 | 1.63 | 0.1031 | 2.03 | 0.0424 | 2.43 | 0.0151 |
| 1.24 | 0.2150 | 1.64 | 0.1010 | 2.04 | 0.0414 | 2.44 | 0.0147 |
| 1.25 | 0.2113 | 1.65 | 0.0989 | 2.05 | 0.0404 | 2.45 | 0.0143 |
| 1.26 | 0.2077 | 1.66 | 0.0969 | 2.06 | 0.0394 | 2.46 | 0.0139 |
| 1.27 | 0.2041 | 1.67 | 0.0949 | 2.07 | 0.0385 | 2.47 | 0.0135 |
| 1.28 | 0.2005 | 1.68 | 0.0930 | 2.08 | 0.0375 | 2.48 | 0.0131 |
| 1.29 | 0.1971 | 1.69 | 0.0910 | 2.09 | 0.0366 | 2.49 | 0.0128 |
| 1.30 | 0.1936 | 1.70 | 0.0891 | 2.10 | 0.0357 | 2.50 | 0.0124 |
| 1.31 | 0.1902 | 1.71 | 0.0873 | 2.11 | 0.0349 | 2.51 | 0.0121 |
| 1.32 | 0.1868 | 1.72 | 0.0854 | 2.12 | 0.0340 | 2.52 | 0.0117 |
| 1.33 | 0.1835 | 1.73 | 0.0836 | 2.13 | 0.0332 | 2.53 | 0.0114 |
| 1.34 | 0.1802 | 1.74 | 0.0819 | 2.14 | 0.0324 | 2.54 | 0.0111 |
| 1.35 | 0.1770 | 1.75 | 0.0801 | 2.15 | 0.0316 | 2.55 | 0.0108 |
| 1.36 | 0.1738 | 1.76 | 0.0784 | 2.16 | 0.0308 | 2.56 | 0.0105 |
| 1.37 | 0.1707 | 1.77 | 0.0767 | 2.17 | 0.0300 | 2.57 | 0.0102 |
| 1.38 | 0.1676 | 1.78 | 0.0751 | 2.18 | 0.0293 | 2.58 | 0.0099 |
| 1.39 | 0.1645 | 1.79 | 0.0735 | 2.19 | 0.0285 | 2.59 | 0.0096 |
| 1.40 | 0.1615 | 1.80 | 0.0719 | 2.20 | 0.0278 | 2.60 | 0.0093 |
| 1.41 | 0.1585 | 1.81 | 0.0703 | 2.21 | 0.0271 | 2.61 | 0.0091 |
| 1.42 | 0.1556 | 1.82 | 0.0688 | 2.22 | 0.0264 | 2.62 | 0.0088 |
| 1.43 | 0.1527 | 1.83 | 0.0672 | 2.23 | 0.0257 | 2.63 | 0.0085 |
| 1.44 | 0.1499 | 1.84 | 0.0658 | 2.24 | 0.0251 | 2.64 | 0.0083 |
| 1.45 | 0.1471 | 1.85 | 0.0643 | 2.25 | 0.0244 | 2.65 | 0.0080 |
| 1.46 | 0.1443 | 1.86 | 0.0629 | 2.26 | 0.0238 | 2.66 | 0.0078 |
| 1.47 | 0.1416 | 1.87 | 0.0615 | 2.27 | 0.0232 | 2.67 | 0.0076 |
| 1.48 | 0.1389 | 1.88 | 0.0601 | 2.28 | 0.0226 | 2.68 | 0.0074 |
| 1.49 | 0.1362 | 1.89 | 0.0588 | 2.29 | 0.0220 | 2.69 | 0.0071 |
| 1.50 | 0.1336 | 1.90 | 0.0574 | 2.30 | 0.0214 | 2.70 | 0.0069 |
| 1.51 | 0.1310 | 1.91 | 0.0561 | 2.31 | 0.0209 | 2.71 | 0.0067 |
| 1.52 | 0.1285 | 1.92 | 0.0549 | 2.32 | 0.0203 | 2.72 | 0.0065 |
| 1.53 | 0.1260 | 1.93 | 0.0536 | 2.33 | 0.0198 | 2.73 | 0.0063 |
| 1.54 | 0.1236 | 1.94 | 0.0524 | 2.34 | 0.0193 | 2.74 | 0.0061 |
| 1.55 | 0.1211 | 1.95 | 0.0512 | 2.35 | 0.0188 | 2.75 | 0.0060 |
| 1.56 | 0.1188 | 1.96 | 0.0500 | 2.36 | 0.0183 | 2.76 | 0.0058 |
| 1.57 | 0.1164 | 1.97 | 0.0488 | 2.37 | 0.0178 | 2.77 | 0.0056 |
| 1.58 | 0.1141 | 1.98 | 0.0477 | 2.38 | 0.0173 | 2.78 | 0.0054 |
| 1.59 | 0.1118 | 1.99 | 0.0466 | 2.39 | 0.0168 | 2.79 | 0.0053 |
| 1.60 | 0.1096 | 2.00 | 0.0455 | 2.40 | 0.0164 | 2.80 | 0.0051 |

| $z$ | P | $z$ | P | $z$ | P |
|---|---|---|---|---|---|
| 2.81 | 0.0050 | 2.91 | 0.0036 | 3.10 | 0.00194 |
| 2.82 | 0.0048 | 2.92 | 0.0035 | 3.20 | 0.00137 |
| 2.83 | 0.0047 | 2.93 | 0.0034 | 3.30 | 0.00097 |
| 2.84 | 0.0045 | 2.94 | 0.0033 | 3.40 | 0.00067 |
| 2.85 | 0.0044 | 2.95 | 0.0032 | 3.50 | 0.00047 |
| 2.86 | 0.0042 | 2.96 | 0.0031 | 3.60 | 0.00032 |
| 2.87 | 0.0041 | 2.97 | 0.0030 | 3.70 | 0.00022 |
| 2.88 | 0.0040 | 2.98 | 0.0029 | 3.80 | 0.00014 |
| 2.89 | 0.0039 | 2.99 | 0.0028 | 3.90 | 0.00010 |
| 2.90 | 0.0037 | 3.00 | 0.0027 | 4.00 | 0.00006 |

**Table B3 The Normal distribution – standard Normal deviates corresponding to specific two-tailed areas (P → $z$)**

The tabulated values of $z$ are the standard Normal deviates corresponding to given two-tailed P values. For the two-sided hypothesis test where the test statistic has a standard Normal distribution, the P value is less than a tabulated value of P if the test statistic is greater than the corresponding value of $z$. In the notation of Appendix A, $z = N_{1-\alpha/2}$ where $P = \alpha$. The values of $z$ are also used to construct confidence intervals for statistics with a Normal sampling distribution.

Example: For an observed test statistic $z = 2.91$ we have $P < 0.01$

| P | $z$ |
|---|---|
| 1.0 | 0.000 |
| 0.9 | 0.126 |
| 0.8 | 0.253 |
| 0.7 | 0.385 |
| 0.6 | 0.524 |
| 0.5 | 0.674 |
| 0.4 | 0.842 |
| 0.3 | 1.036 |
| 0.2 | 1.282 |
| 0.1 | 1.645 |
| 0.05 | 1.960 |
| 0.02 | 2.326 |
| 0.01 | 2.576 |
| 0.001 | 3.291 |
| 0.0001 | 3.891 |

**Table B4 The *t* distribution**

The tabulated values of the $t$ distribution correspond to given two-tailed P values for different degrees of freedom. For the two-sided hypothesis test where the test statistic has a $t$ distribution, the P value is less than a tabulated value of P if the test statistic is greater than the tabulated $t$ value. In the notation of Appendix A, the tabulated values are $t_{1-\alpha/2}$ where $P = \alpha$.

Example: For an observed test statistic $t = 3.21$ on 20 degrees of freedom we have $P < 0.01$.

| Degrees of | Two-tailed probability (P) | | | | | |
|---|---|---|---|---|---|---|
| freedom | 0.2 | 0.1 | 0.05 | 0.02 | 0.01 | 0.001 |
| 1 | 3.078 | 6.314 | 12.706 | 31.821 | 63.657 | 636.619 |
| 2 | 1.886 | 2.920 | 4.303 | 6.965 | 9.925 | 31.599 |
| 3 | 1.638 | 2.353 | 3.182 | 4.541 | 5.841 | 12.924 |
| 4 | 1.533 | 2.132 | 2.776 | 3.747 | 4.604 | 8.610 |
| 5 | 1.476 | 2.015 | 2.571 | 3.365 | 4.032 | 6.869 |
| 6 | 1.440 | 1.943 | 2.447 | 3.143 | 3.707 | 5.959 |
| 7 | 1.415 | 1.895 | 2.365 | 2.998 | 3.499 | 5.408 |
| 8 | 1.397 | 1.860 | 2.306 | 2.896 | 3.355 | 5.041 |
| 9 | 1.383 | 1.833 | 2.262 | 2.821 | 3.250 | 4.781 |
| 10 | 1.372 | 1.812 | 2.228 | 2.764 | 3.169 | 4.587 |
| 11 | 1.363 | 1.796 | 2.201 | 2.718 | 3.106 | 4.437 |
| 12 | 1.356 | 1.782 | 2.179 | 2.681 | 3.055 | 4.318 |
| 13 | 1.350 | 1.771 | 2.160 | 2.650 | 3.012 | 4.221 |
| 14 | 1.345 | 1.761 | 2.145 | 2.624 | 2.977 | 4.140 |
| 15 | 1.341 | 1.753 | 2.131 | 2.602 | 2.947 | 4.073 |
| 16 | 1.337 | 1.746 | 2.120 | 2.583 | 2.921 | 4.015 |
| 17 | 1.333 | 1.740 | 2.110 | 2.567 | 2.898 | 3.965 |
| 18 | 1.330 | 1.734 | 2.101 | 2.552 | 2.878 | 3.922 |
| 19 | 1.328 | 1.729 | 2.093 | 2.539 | 2.861 | 3.883 |
| 20 | 1.325 | 1.725 | 2.086 | 2.528 | 2.845 | 3.850 |
| 21 | 1.323 | 1.721 | 2.080 | 2.518 | 2.831 | 3.819 |
| 22 | 1.321 | 1.717 | 2.074 | 2.508 | 2.819 | 3.792 |
| 23 | 1.319 | 1.714 | 2.069 | 2.500 | 2.807 | 3.768 |
| 24 | 1.318 | 1.711 | 2.064 | 2.492 | 2.797 | 3.745 |
| 25 | 1.316 | 1.708 | 2.060 | 2.485 | 2.787 | 3.725 |
| 26 | 1.315 | 1.706 | 2.056 | 2.479 | 2.779 | 3.707 |
| 27 | 1.314 | 1.703 | 2.052 | 2.473 | 2.771 | 3.690 |
| 28 | 1.313 | 1.701 | 2.048 | 2.467 | 2.763 | 3.674 |
| 29 | 1.311 | 1.699 | 2.045 | 2.462 | 2.756 | 3.659 |
| 30 | 1.310 | 1.697 | 2.042 | 2.457 | 2.750 | 3.646 |

| Degrees of freedom | Two-tailed probability (P) | | | | | |
|---|---|---|---|---|---|---|
| | 0.2 | 0.1 | 0.05 | 0.02 | 0.01 | 0.001 |
| 31 | 1.309 | 1.696 | 2.040 | 2.453 | 2.744 | 3.633 |
| 32 | 1.309 | 1.694 | 2.037 | 2.449 | 2.738 | 3.622 |
| 33 | 1.308 | 1.692 | 2.035 | 2.445 | 2.733 | 3.611 |
| 34 | 1.307 | 1.691 | 2.032 | 2.441 | 2.728 | 3.601 |
| 35 | 1.306 | 1.690 | 2.030 | 2.438 | 2.724 | 3.591 |
| 36 | 1.306 | 1.688 | 2.028 | 2.434 | 2.719 | 3.582 |
| 37 | 1.305 | 1.687 | 2.026 | 2.431 | 2.715 | 3.574 |
| 38 | 1.304 | 1.686 | 2.024 | 2.429 | 2.712 | 3.566 |
| 39 | 1.304 | 1.685 | 2.023 | 2.426 | 2.708 | 3.558 |
| 40 | 1.303 | 1.684 | 2.021 | 2.423 | 2.704 | 3.551 |
| 41 | 1.303 | 1.683 | 2.020 | 2.421 | 2.701 | 3.544 |
| 42 | 1.302 | 1.682 | 2.018 | 2.418 | 2.698 | 3.538 |
| 43 | 1.302 | 1.681 | 2.017 | 2.416 | 2.695 | 3.532 |
| 44 | 1.301 | 1.680 | 2.015 | 2.414 | 2.692 | 3.526 |
| 45 | 1.301 | 1.679 | 2.014 | 2.412 | 2.690 | 3.520 |
| 46 | 1.300 | 1.679 | 2.013 | 2.410 | 2.687 | 3.515 |
| 47 | 1.300 | 1.678 | 2.012 | 2.408 | 2.685 | 3.510 |
| 48 | 1.299 | 1.677 | 2.011 | 2.407 | 2.682 | 3.505 |
| 49 | 1.299 | 1.677 | 2.010 | 2.405 | 2.680 | 3.500 |
| 50 | 1.299 | 1.676 | 2.009 | 2.403 | 2.678 | 3.496 |
| 51 | 1.298 | 1.675 | 2.008 | 2.402 | 2.676 | 3.492 |
| 52 | 1.298 | 1.675 | 2.007 | 2.400 | 2.674 | 3.488 |
| 53 | 1.298 | 1.674 | 2.006 | 2.399 | 2.672 | 3.484 |
| 54 | 1.297 | 1.674 | 2.005 | 2.397 | 2.670 | 3.480 |
| 55 | 1.297 | 1.673 | 2.004 | 2.396 | 2.668 | 3.476 |
| 56 | 1.297 | 1.673 | 2.003 | 2.395 | 2.667 | 3.473 |
| 57 | 1.297 | 1.672 | 2.002 | 2.394 | 2.665 | 3.470 |
| 58 | 1.296 | 1.672 | 2.002 | 2.392 | 2.663 | 3.466 |
| 59 | 1.296 | 1.671 | 2.001 | 2.391 | 2.662 | 3.463 |
| 60 | 1.296 | 1.671 | 2.000 | 2.390 | 2.660 | 3.460 |
| 70 | 1.294 | 1.667 | 1.994 | 2.381 | 2.648 | 3.435 |
| 80 | 1.292 | 1.664 | 1.990 | 2.374 | 2.639 | 3.416 |
| 90 | 1.291 | 1.662 | 1.987 | 2.368 | 2.632 | 3.402 |
| 100 | 1.290 | 1.660 | 1.984 | 2.364 | 2.626 | 3.390 |
| 110 | 1.289 | 1.659 | 1.982 | 2.361 | 2.621 | 3.381 |
| 120 | 1.289 | 1.658 | 1.980 | 2.358 | 2.617 | 3.373 |
| 130 | 1.288 | 1.657 | 1.978 | 2.355 | 2.614 | 3.367 |
| 140 | 1.288 | 1.656 | 1.977 | 2.353 | 2.611 | 3.361 |
| 150 | 1.287 | 1.655 | 1.976 | 2.351 | 2.609 | 3.357 |

**Table B5 The Chi squared ($\chi^2$) distribution**

The tabulated values of $\chi^2$ are values of the Chi squared distribution corresponding to given two-tailed P values for different degrees of freedom. For the two-sided hypothesis test where the test statistic has a Chi squared distribution, the P value is less than a tabulated value of P if the test statistic $X^2$ is greater than the corresponding value of $\chi^2$.

Example: For an observed test statistic $X^2 = 5.91$ on 2 degrees of freedom we have $0.1 > P > 0.05$.

| Degrees of freedom | Two-tailed probability (P) | | | | | |
|---|---|---|---|---|---|---|
| | 0.2 | 0.1 | 0.05 | 0.02 | 0.01 | 0.001 |
| 1 | 1.642 | 2.706 | 3.841 | 5.412 | 6.635 | 10.827 |
| 2 | 3.219 | 4.605 | 5.991 | 7.824 | 9.210 | 13.815 |
| 3 | 4.642 | 6.251 | 7.815 | 9.837 | 11.345 | 16.268 |
| 4 | 5.989 | 7.779 | 9.488 | 11.668 | 13.277 | 18.465 |
| 5 | 7.289 | 9.236 | 11.070 | 13.388 | 15.086 | 20.517 |
| 6 | 8.558 | 10.645 | 12.592 | 15.033 | 16.812 | 22.457 |
| 7 | 9.803 | 12.017 | 14.067 | 16.622 | 18.475 | 24.322 |
| 8 | 11.030 | 13.362 | 15.507 | 18.168 | 20.090 | 26.125 |
| 9 | 12.242 | 14.684 | 16.919 | 19.679 | 21.666 | 27.877 |
| 10 | 13.442 | 15.987 | 18.307 | 21.161 | 23.209 | 29.588 |
| 11 | 14.631 | 17.275 | 19.675 | 22.618 | 24.725 | 31.264 |
| 12 | 15.812 | 18.549 | 21.026 | 24.054 | 26.217 | 32.909 |
| 13 | 16.985 | 19.812 | 22.362 | 25.472 | 27.688 | 34.528 |
| 14 | 18.151 | 21.064 | 23.685 | 26.873 | 29.141 | 36.123 |
| 15 | 19.311 | 22.307 | 24.996 | 28.259 | 30.578 | 37.697 |
| 16 | 20.465 | 23.542 | 26.296 | 29.633 | 32.000 | 39.252 |
| 17 | 21.615 | 24.769 | 27.587 | 30.995 | 33.409 | 40.790 |
| 18 | 22.760 | 25.989 | 28.869 | 32.346 | 34.805 | 42.312 |
| 19 | 23.900 | 27.204 | 30.144 | 33.687 | 36.191 | 43.820 |
| 20 | 25.038 | 28.412 | 31.410 | 35.020 | 37.566 | 45.315 |
| 21 | 26.171 | 29.615 | 32.671 | 36.343 | 38.932 | 46.797 |
| 22 | 27.301 | 30.813 | 33.924 | 37.659 | 40.289 | 48.268 |
| 23 | 28.429 | 32.007 | 35.172 | 38.968 | 41.638 | 49.728 |
| 24 | 29.553 | 33.196 | 36.415 | 40.270 | 42.980 | 51.179 |
| 25 | 30.675 | 34.382 | 37.652 | 41.566 | 44.314 | 52.620 |

**Table B6 The *F* distribution**

The tabulated values of the *F* distribution correspond to given one-tailed P values for different degrees of freedom for the numerator ($n_1$) and denominator ($n_2$). For the one-sided hypothesis test where the test statistic has an *F* distribution, the P value is less than a tabulated value of P if the test statistic is greater than the tabulated value of *F*.

Example: For an observed test statistic $F = 3.21$ on 2 and 20 degrees of freedom we have $0.1 > P > 0.05$.

**Table B6**

| | | $n_1$ | | | | | | | | | | | | | |
|---|---|---|---|---|---|---|---|---|---|---|---|---|---|---|---|
| $n_2$ | P | 1 | 2 | 3 | 4 | 5 | 6 | 7 | 8 | 9 | 10 | 12 | 15 | 20 | ∞ |
| 1 | 0.1 | 39.9 | 49.5 | 53.6 | 55.8 | 57.2 | 58.2 | 59.1 | 59.7 | 60.1 | 60.5 | 61.0 | 61.5 | 62.0 | 63.3 |
| | 0.05 | 161.4 | 199.5 | 215.8 | 224.7 | 230.4 | 234.2 | 237.0 | 239.1 | 240.8 | 242.1 | 244.2 | 246.2 | 248.3 | 254.3 |
| | 0.01 | 4051.8 | 4999.5 | 5403.5 | 5624.8 | 5763.8 | 5859.2 | 5928.6 | 5981.3 | 6022.7 | 6056.1 | 6106.6 | 6157.6 | 6209.0 | 6365.9 |
| 2 | 0.1 | 8.53 | 9.00 | 9.16 | 9.24 | 9.29 | 9.33 | 9.35 | 9.37 | 9.38 | 9.39 | 9.41 | 9.43 | 9.44 | 9.49 |
| | 0.05 | 18.51 | 19.00 | 19.16 | 19.25 | 19.30 | 19.33 | 19.35 | 19.37 | 19.38 | 19.40 | 19.41 | 19.43 | 19.45 | 19.50 |
| | 0.01 | 98.50 | 99.00 | 99.17 | 99.25 | 99.30 | 99.33 | 99.36 | 99.75 | 99.78 | 99.80 | 99.83 | 99.87 | 99.90 | 99.50 |
| 3 | 0.1 | 5.54 | 5.46 | 5.39 | 5.34 | 5.31 | 5.28 | 5.27 | 5.25 | 5.24 | 5.23 | 5.22 | 5.20 | 5.18 | 5.13 |
| | 0.05 | 10.13 | 9.55 | 9.28 | 9.12 | 9.01 | 8.94 | 8.89 | 8.85 | 8.81 | 8.79 | 8.74 | 8.70 | 8.66 | 8.53 |
| | 0.01 | 34.11 | 30.82 | 29.46 | 28.71 | 28.24 | 27.91 | 27.67 | 27.49 | 27.34 | 27.23 | 27.05 | 26.87 | 26.69 | 26.13 |
| 4 | 0.1 | 4.54 | 4.32 | 4.19 | 4.11 | 4.05 | 4.01 | 3.98 | 3.95 | 3.94 | 3.92 | 3.90 | 3.87 | 3.84 | 3.76 |
| | 0.05 | 7.71 | 6.94 | 6.59 | 6.39 | 6.26 | 6.16 | 6.09 | 6.04 | 6.00 | 5.96 | 5.91 | 5.86 | 5.80 | 5.63 |
| | 0.01 | 21.20 | 18.00 | 16.69 | 15.98 | 15.52 | 15.21 | 14.98 | 14.80 | 14.66 | 14.55 | 14.37 | 14.20 | 14.02 | 13.46 |
| 5 | 0.1 | 4.06 | 3.78 | 3.62 | 3.52 | 3.45 | 3.40 | 3.37 | 3.34 | 3.32 | 3.30 | 3.27 | 3.24 | 3.21 | 3.10 |
| | 0.05 | 6.61 | 5.79 | 5.41 | 5.19 | 5.05 | 4.95 | 4.88 | 4.82 | 4.77 | 4.74 | 4.68 | 4.62 | 4.56 | 4.36 |
| | 0.01 | 16.26 | 13.27 | 12.06 | 11.39 | 10.97 | 10.67 | 10.46 | 10.29 | 10.16 | 10.05 | 9.89 | 9.72 | 9.55 | 9.02 |
| 6 | 0.1 | 3.78 | 3.46 | 3.29 | 3.18 | 3.11 | 3.05 | 3.01 | 2.98 | 2.96 | 2.94 | 2.90 | 2.87 | 2.84 | 2.72 |
| | 0.05 | 5.99 | 5.14 | 4.76 | 4.53 | 4.39 | 4.28 | 4.21 | 4.15 | 4.10 | 4.06 | 4.00 | 3.94 | 3.87 | 3.67 |
| | 0.01 | 13.74 | 10.92 | 9.78 | 9.15 | 8.75 | 8.47 | 8.26 | 8.10 | 7.98 | 7.87 | 7.72 | 7.56 | 7.40 | 6.88 |

**Table B6** (*cont.*)

| $n_2$ | P | $n_1$: 1 | 2 | 3 | 4 | 5 | 6 | 7 | 8 | 9 | 10 | 12 | 15 | 20 | ∞ |
|---|---|---|---|---|---|---|---|---|---|---|---|---|---|---|---|
| 7 | 0.1 | 3.59 | 3.26 | 3.07 | 2.96 | 2.88 | 2.83 | 2.78 | 2.75 | 2.72 | 2.70 | 2.67 | 2.63 | 2.59 | 2.47 |
| | 0.05 | 5.59 | 4.74 | 4.35 | 4.12 | 3.97 | 3.87 | 3.79 | 3.73 | 3.68 | 3.64 | 3.57 | 3.51 | 3.44 | 3.23 |
| | 0.01 | 12.25 | 9.55 | 8.45 | 7.85 | 7.46 | 7.19 | 6.99 | 6.84 | 6.72 | 6.62 | 6.47 | 6.31 | 6.16 | 5.65 |
| 8 | 0.1 | 3.46 | 3.11 | 2.92 | 2.81 | 2.73 | 2.67 | 2.62 | 2.59 | 2.56 | 2.54 | 2.50 | 2.46 | 2.42 | 2.29 |
| | 0.05 | 5.32 | 4.46 | 4.07 | 3.84 | 3.69 | 3.58 | 3.50 | 3.44 | 3.39 | 3.35 | 3.28 | 3.22 | 3.15 | 2.93 |
| | 0.01 | 11.26 | 8.65 | 7.59 | 7.01 | 6.63 | 6.37 | 6.18 | 6.03 | 5.91 | 5.81 | 5.67 | 5.52 | 5.36 | 4.86 |
| 9 | 0.1 | 3.36 | 3.01 | 2.81 | 2.69 | 2.61 | 2.55 | 2.51 | 2.47 | 2.44 | 2.42 | 2.38 | 2.34 | 2.30 | 2.16 |
| | 0.05 | 5.12 | 4.26 | 3.86 | 3.63 | 3.48 | 3.37 | 3.29 | 3.23 | 3.18 | 3.14 | 3.07 | 3.01 | 2.94 | 2.71 |
| | 0.01 | 10.56 | 8.02 | 6.99 | 6.42 | 6.06 | 5.80 | 5.61 | 5.47 | 5.35 | 5.26 | 5.11 | 4.96 | 4.81 | 4.31 |
| 10 | 0.1 | 3.29 | 2.92 | 2.73 | 2.61 | 2.52 | 2.46 | 2.41 | 2.38 | 2.35 | 2.32 | 2.28 | 2.24 | 2.20 | 2.06 |
| | 0.05 | 4.96 | 4.10 | 3.71 | 3.48 | 3.33 | 3.22 | 3.14 | 3.07 | 3.02 | 2.98 | 2.91 | 2.84 | 2.77 | 2.54 |
| | 0.01 | 10.04 | 7.56 | 6.55 | 5.99 | 5.64 | 5.39 | 5.20 | 5.06 | 4.94 | 4.85 | 4.71 | 4.56 | 4.41 | 3.91 |
| 12 | 0.1 | 3.18 | 2.81 | 2.61 | 2.48 | 2.39 | 2.33 | 2.28 | 2.24 | 2.21 | 2.19 | 2.15 | 2.10 | 2.06 | 1.90 |
| | 0.05 | 4.75 | 3.89 | 3.49 | 3.26 | 3.11 | 3.00 | 2.91 | 2.85 | 2.80 | 2.75 | 2.69 | 2.62 | 2.54 | 2.30 |
| | 0.01 | 9.33 | 6.93 | 5.95 | 5.41 | 5.06 | 4.82 | 4.64 | 4.50 | 4.39 | 4.30 | 4.16 | 4.01 | 3.86 | 3.36 |
| 15 | 0.1 | 3.07 | 2.70 | 2.49 | 2.36 | 2.27 | 2.21 | 2.16 | 2.12 | 2.09 | 2.06 | 2.02 | 1.97 | 1.92 | 1.76 |
| | 0.05 | 4.54 | 3.68 | 3.29 | 3.06 | 2.90 | 2.79 | 2.71 | 2.64 | 2.59 | 2.54 | 2.48 | 2.40 | 2.33 | 2.07 |
| | 0.01 | 8.68 | 6.36 | 5.42 | 4.89 | 4.56 | 4.32 | 4.14 | 4.00 | 3.89 | 3.80 | 3.67 | 3.52 | 3.37 | 2.87 |

**Table B6** (*cont.*)

| $n_2$ | P | $n_1$ 1 | 2 | 3 | 4 | 5 | 6 | 7 | 8 | 9 | 10 | 12 | 15 | 20 | $\infty$ |
|---|---|---|---|---|---|---|---|---|---|---|---|---|---|---|---|
| 20 | 0.1 | 2.97 | 2.59 | 2.38 | 2.25 | 2.16 | 2.09 | 2.04 | 2.00 | 1.96 | 1.94 | 1.89 | 1.84 | 1.79 | 1.61 |
| | 0.05 | 4.35 | 3.49 | 3.10 | 2.87 | 2.71 | 2.60 | 2.51 | 2.45 | 2.39 | 2.35 | 2.28 | 2.20 | 2.12 | 1.84 |
| | 0.01 | 8.10 | 5.85 | 4.94 | 4.43 | 4.10 | 3.87 | 3.70 | 3.56 | 3.46 | 3.37 | 3.23 | 3.09 | 2.94 | 2.42 |
| 30 | 0.1 | 2.88 | 2.49 | 2.28 | 2.14 | 2.05 | 1.98 | 1.93 | 1.88 | 1.85 | 1.82 | 1.77 | 1.72 | 1.67 | 1.46 |
| | 0.05 | 4.17 | 3.32 | 2.92 | 2.69 | 2.53 | 2.42 | 2.33 | 2.27 | 2.21 | 2.16 | 2.09 | 2.01 | 1.93 | 1.62 |
| | 0.01 | 7.56 | 5.39 | 4.51 | 4.02 | 3.70 | 3.47 | 3.30 | 3.17 | 3.07 | 2.98 | 2.84 | 2.70 | 2.55 | 2.01 |
| 40 | 0.1 | 2.84 | 2.44 | 2.23 | 2.09 | 2.00 | 1.93 | 1.87 | 1.83 | 1.79 | 1.76 | 1.71 | 1.66 | 1.61 | 1.38 |
| | 0.05 | 4.08 | 3.23 | 2.84 | 2.61 | 2.45 | 2.34 | 2.25 | 2.18 | 2.12 | 2.08 | 2.00 | 1.92 | 1.84 | 1.51 |
| | 0.01 | 7.31 | 5.18 | 4.31 | 3.83 | 3.51 | 3.29 | 3.12 | 2.99 | 2.89 | 2.80 | 2.66 | 2.52 | 2.37 | 1.80 |
| 60 | 0.1 | 2.79 | 2.39 | 2.18 | 2.04 | 1.95 | 1.87 | 1.82 | 1.77 | 1.74 | 1.71 | 1.66 | 1.60 | 1.54 | 1.29 |
| | 0.05 | 4.00 | 3.15 | 2.76 | 2.53 | 2.37 | 2.25 | 2.17 | 2.10 | 2.04 | 1.99 | 1.92 | 1.84 | 1.75 | 1.39 |
| | 0.01 | 7.08 | 4.98 | 4.13 | 3.65 | 3.34 | 3.12 | 2.95 | 2.82 | 2.72 | 2.63 | 2.50 | 2.35 | 2.20 | 1.60 |
| 120 | 0.1 | 2.75 | 2.35 | 2.13 | 1.99 | 1.90 | 1.82 | 1.77 | 1.72 | 1.68 | 1.65 | 1.60 | 1.54 | 1.48 | 1.19 |
| | 0.05 | 3.92 | 3.07 | 2.68 | 2.45 | 2.29 | 2.18 | 2.09 | 2.02 | 1.96 | 1.91 | 1.83 | 1.75 | 1.66 | 1.25 |
| | 0.01 | 6.85 | 4.79 | 3.95 | 3.48 | 3.17 | 2.96 | 2.79 | 2.66 | 2.56 | 2.47 | 2.34 | 2.19 | 2.03 | 1.38 |
| $\infty$ | 0.1 | 2.71 | 2.30 | 2.08 | 1.94 | 1.85 | 1.77 | 1.72 | 1.67 | 1.63 | 1.60 | 1.55 | 1.49 | 1.42 | 1.13 |
| | 0.05 | 3.84 | 3.00 | 2.60 | 2.37 | 2.21 | 2.10 | 2.01 | 1.94 | 1.88 | 1.83 | 1.75 | 1.67 | 1.57 | 1.17 |
| | 0.01 | 6.63 | 4.61 | 3.78 | 3.32 | 3.02 | 2.80 | 2.64 | 2.51 | 2.41 | 2.32 | 2.18 | 2.04 | 1.88 | 1.24 |

**Table B7 Pearson's correlation coefficient (*r*)**

If the observed correlation coefficient, $r$, exceeds the tabulated value, the associated two-tailed P value is less than the value at the top of the column. For negative values of $r$ ignore the sign. For partial correlation coefficients reduce the sample size by 1.

Example: For an observed value of $r = 0.43$ from a sample of 39, the two-tailed P value is $P < 0.01$.

| Sample | Two-tailed probability (P) | | | | | |
|---|---|---|---|---|---|---|
| size | 0.2 | 0.1 | 0.05 | 0.02 | 0.01 | 0.001 |
| 3 | 0.9511 | 0.9877 | 0.9969 | 0.9995 | 0.9999 | 1.0000 |
| 4 | 0.8000 | 0.9000 | 0.9500 | 0.9800 | 0.9900 | 0.9990 |
| 5 | 0.6870 | 0.8054 | 0.8783 | 0.9343 | 0.9587 | 0.9911 |
| 6 | 0.6084 | 0.7293 | 0.8114 | 0.8822 | 0.9172 | 0.9741 |
| 7 | 0.5509 | 0.6694 | 0.7545 | 0.8329 | 0.8745 | 0.9509 |
| 8 | 0.5067 | 0.6215 | 0.7067 | 0.7887 | 0.8343 | 0.9249 |
| 9 | 0.4716 | 0.5822 | 0.6664 | 0.7498 | 0.7977 | 0.8983 |
| 10 | 0.4428 | 0.5494 | 0.6319 | 0.7155 | 0.7646 | 0.8721 |
| 11 | 0.4187 | 0.5214 | 0.6021 | 0.6851 | 0.7348 | 0.8470 |
| 12 | 0.3981 | 0.4973 | 0.5760 | 0.6581 | 0.7079 | 0.8233 |
| 13 | 0.3802 | 0.4762 | 0.5529 | 0.6339 | 0.6835 | 0.8010 |
| 14 | 0.3646 | 0.4575 | 0.5324 | 0.6120 | 0.6614 | 0.7800 |
| 15 | 0.3507 | 0.4409 | 0.5140 | 0.5923 | 0.6411 | 0.7604 |
| 16 | 0.3383 | 0.4259 | 0.4973 | 0.5742 | 0.6226 | 0.7419 |
| 17 | 0.3271 | 0.4124 | 0.4821 | 0.5577 | 0.6055 | 0.7247 |
| 18 | 0.3170 | 0.4000 | 0.4683 | 0.5425 | 0.5897 | 0.7084 |
| 19 | 0.3077 | 0.3887 | 0.4555 | 0.5285 | 0.5751 | 0.6932 |
| 20 | 0.2992 | 0.3783 | 0.4438 | 0.5155 | 0.5614 | 0.6788 |
| 21 | 0.2914 | 0.3687 | 0.4329 | 0.5034 | 0.5487 | 0.6652 |
| 22 | 0.2841 | 0.3598 | 0.4227 | 0.4921 | 0.5368 | 0.6524 |
| 23 | 0.2774 | 0.3515 | 0.4132 | 0.4815 | 0.5256 | 0.6402 |
| 24 | 0.2711 | 0.3438 | 0.4044 | 0.4716 | 0.5151 | 0.6287 |
| 25 | 0.2653 | 0.3365 | 0.3961 | 0.4622 | 0.5052 | 0.6178 |
| 26 | 0.2598 | 0.3297 | 0.3882 | 0.4534 | 0.4958 | 0.6074 |
| 27 | 0.2546 | 0.3233 | 0.3809 | 0.4451 | 0.4869 | 0.5974 |
| 28 | 0.2497 | 0.3172 | 0.3739 | 0.4372 | 0.4785 | 0.5880 |
| 29 | 0.2451 | 0.3115 | 0.3673 | 0.4297 | 0.4705 | 0.5790 |
| 30 | 0.2407 | 0.3061 | 0.3610 | 0.4226 | 0.4629 | 0.5703 |

| Sample size | Two-tailed probability (P) 0.2 | 0.1 | 0.05 | 0.02 | 0.01 | 0.001 |
|---|---|---|---|---|---|---|
| 31 | 0.2366 | 0.3009 | 0.3550 | 0.4158 | 0.4556 | 0.5620 |
| 32 | 0.2327 | 0.2960 | 0.3494 | 0.4093 | 0.4487 | 0.5541 |
| 33 | 0.2289 | 0.2913 | 0.3440 | 0.4032 | 0.4421 | 0.5465 |
| 34 | 0.2254 | 0.2869 | 0.3388 | 0.3972 | 0.4357 | 0.5392 |
| 35 | 0.2220 | 0.2826 | 0.3338 | 0.3916 | 0.4296 | 0.5322 |
| 36 | 0.2187 | 0.2785 | 0.3291 | 0.3862 | 0.4238 | 0.5254 |
| 37 | 0.2156 | 0.2746 | 0.3246 | 0.3810 | 0.4182 | 0.5189 |
| 38 | 0.2126 | 0.2709 | 0.3202 | 0.3760 | 0.4128 | 0.5126 |
| 39 | 0.2097 | 0.2673 | 0.3160 | 0.3712 | 0.4076 | 0.5066 |
| 40 | 0.2070 | 0.2638 | 0.3120 | 0.3665 | 0.4026 | 0.5007 |
| 41 | 0.2043 | 0.2605 | 0.3081 | 0.3621 | 0.3978 | 0.4950 |
| 42 | 0.2018 | 0.2573 | 0.3044 | 0.3578 | 0.3932 | 0.4896 |
| 43 | 0.1993 | 0.2542 | 0.3008 | 0.3536 | 0.3887 | 0.4843 |
| 44 | 0.1970 | 0.2512 | 0.2973 | 0.3496 | 0.3843 | 0.4791 |
| 45 | 0.1947 | 0.2483 | 0.2940 | 0.3457 | 0.3801 | 0.4742 |
| 46 | 0.1925 | 0.2455 | 0.2907 | 0.3420 | 0.3761 | 0.4694 |
| 47 | 0.1903 | 0.2429 | 0.2876 | 0.3384 | 0.3721 | 0.4647 |
| 48 | 0.1883 | 0.2403 | 0.2845 | 0.3348 | 0.3683 | 0.4601 |
| 49 | 0.1863 | 0.2377 | 0.2816 | 0.3314 | 0.3646 | 0.4557 |
| 50 | 0.1843 | 0.2353 | 0.2787 | 0.3281 | 0.3610 | 0.4514 |
| 51 | 0.1825 | 0.2329 | 0.2759 | 0.3249 | 0.3575 | 0.4473 |
| 52 | 0.1806 | 0.2306 | 0.2732 | 0.3218 | 0.3542 | 0.4432 |
| 53 | 0.1789 | 0.2284 | 0.2706 | 0.3188 | 0.3509 | 0.4393 |
| 54 | 0.1772 | 0.2262 | 0.2681 | 0.3158 | 0.3477 | 0.4354 |
| 55 | 0.1755 | 0.2241 | 0.2656 | 0.3129 | 0.3445 | 0.4317 |
| 56 | 0.1739 | 0.2221 | 0.2632 | 0.3102 | 0.3415 | 0.4280 |
| 57 | 0.1723 | 0.2201 | 0.2609 | 0.3074 | 0.3385 | 0.4244 |
| 58 | 0.1708 | 0.2181 | 0.2586 | 0.3048 | 0.3357 | 0.4210 |
| 59 | 0.1693 | 0.2162 | 0.2564 | 0.3022 | 0.3328 | 0.4176 |
| 60 | 0.1678 | 0.2144 | 0.2542 | 0.2997 | 0.3301 | 0.4143 |
| 70 | 0.1550 | 0.1982 | 0.2352 | 0.2776 | 0.3060 | 0.3850 |
| 80 | 0.1448 | 0.1852 | 0.2199 | 0.2597 | 0.2864 | 0.3611 |
| 90 | 0.1364 | 0.1745 | 0.2072 | 0.2449 | 0.2702 | 0.3412 |
| 100 | 0.1292 | 0.1654 | 0.1966 | 0.2324 | 0.2565 | 0.3242 |
| 110 | 0.1231 | 0.1576 | 0.1874 | 0.2216 | 0.2446 | 0.3095 |
| 120 | 0.1178 | 0.1509 | 0.1793 | 0.2122 | 0.2343 | 0.2967 |
| 130 | 0.1131 | 0.1449 | 0.1723 | 0.2039 | 0.2252 | 0.2853 |
| 140 | 0.1090 | 0.1396 | 0.1660 | 0.1965 | 0.2170 | 0.2752 |
| 150 | 0.1052 | 0.1348 | 0.1603 | 0.1898 | 0.2097 | 0.2660 |

For $n > 60$, $r\sqrt{\frac{n-2}{1-r^2}}$ has a $t$ distribution with $n - 2$ degrees of freedom.

**Table B8 Spearman's rank correlation coefficient ($r_s$)**

If the observed rank correlation coefficient, $r_s$, exceeds the tabulated value, the associated two-tailed P value is less than the value at the top of the column. For negative values of $r_s$ ignore the sign. For partial correlation coefficients reduce the sample size by 1.

Example: For an observed value of $r_s = 0.43$ from a sample of 19, the two-tailed P value is $0.1 > P > 0.05$.

| Sample | | | Two-tailed probability (P) | | | |
|---|---|---|---|---|---|---|
| size | 0.2 | 0.1 | 0.05 | 0.02 | 0.01 | 0.002 |
| 4 | 0.8000 | 0.8000 | | | | |
| 5 | 0.7000 | 0.8000 | 0.9000 | 0.9000 | | |
| 6 | 0.6000 | 0.7714 | 0.8286 | 0.8857 | 0.9429 | |
| 7 | 0.5357 | 0.6786 | 0.7450 | 0.8571 | 0.8929 | 0.9643 |
| 8 | 0.5000 | 0.6190 | 0.7143 | 0.8095 | 0.8571 | 0.9286 |
| 9 | 0.4667 | 0.5833 | 0.6833 | 0.7667 | 0.8167 | 0.9000 |
| 10 | 0.4424 | 0.5515 | 0.6364 | 0.7333 | 0.7818 | 0.8667 |
| 11 | 0.4182 | 0.5273 | 0.6091 | 0.7000 | 0.7455 | 0.8364 |
| 12 | 0.3986 | 0.4965 | 0.5804 | 0.6713 | 0.7273 | 0.8182 |
| 13 | 0.3791 | 0.4780 | 0.5549 | 0.6429 | 0.6978 | 0.7912 |
| 14 | 0.3626 | 0.4593 | 0.5341 | 0.6220 | 0.6747 | 0.7670 |
| 15 | 0.3500 | 0.4429 | 0.5179 | 0.6000 | 0.6536 | 0.7464 |
| 16 | 0.3382 | 0.4265 | 0.5000 | 0.5824 | 0.6324 | 0.7265 |
| 17 | 0.3260 | 0.4118 | 0.4853 | 0.5637 | 0.6152 | 0.7083 |
| 18 | 0.3148 | 0.3994 | 0.4716 | 0.5480 | 0.5975 | 0.6904 |
| 19 | 0.3070 | 0.3895 | 0.4579 | 0.5333 | 0.5825 | 0.6737 |
| 20 | 0.2977 | 0.3789 | 0.4451 | 0.5203 | 0.5684 | 0.6586 |
| 21 | 0.2909 | 0.3688 | 0.4351 | 0.5078 | 0.5545 | 0.6455 |
| 22 | 0.2829 | 0.3597 | 0.4241 | 0.4963 | 0.5426 | 0.6318 |
| 23 | 0.2767 | 0.3518 | 0.4150 | 0.4852 | 0.5306 | 0.6186 |
| 24 | 0.2704 | 0.3435 | 0.4061 | 0.4748 | 0.5200 | 0.6070 |
| 25 | 0.2646 | 0.3362 | 0.3977 | 0.4654 | 0.5100 | 0.5962 |
| 26 | 0.2588 | 0.3299 | 0.3894 | 0.4564 | 0.5002 | 0.5856 |
| 27 | 0.2540 | 0.3236 | 0.3822 | 0.4481 | 0.4915 | 0.5757 |
| 28 | 0.2490 | 0.3175 | 0.3749 | 0.4401 | 0.4828 | 0.5660 |
| 29 | 0.2443 | 0.3113 | 0.3685 | 0.4320 | 0.4744 | 0.5567 |
| 30 | 0.2400 | 0.3059 | 0.3620 | 0.4251 | 0.4665 | 0.5479 |

For $n > 30$, $r\sqrt{\dfrac{n-2}{1-r_s^2}}$ has a $t$ distribution with $n - 2$ degrees of freedom.

**Table B9 Wilcoxon one sample (or matched pairs) test**

If the sum of positive (or negative) ranks is equal to the tabulated values or is outside the range shown (i.e is not between the tabulated values), the P value of the test is less than the value at the top of the column. The sample size shown, $n$, is the number of non-zero differences.

Example: For a rank sum of 8 from a sample of 11 we look along the row for $n = 11$ from the left until we find the last column where the value 8 is not between the tabulated values, which gives $P < 0.05$. A rank sum of 7 would give $P < 0.02$.

| | Two-tailed probability (P) | | | | | |
|---|---|---|---|---|---|---|
| $n$ | 0.2 | 0.1 | 0.05 | 0.02 | 0.01 | 0.001 |
| 4 | 0–10 | – | – | – | – | – |
| 5 | 2–13 | 0–15 | – | – | – | – |
| 6 | 3–18 | 2–19 | 0–21 | – | – | – |
| 7 | 5–23 | 3–25 | 2–26 | 0–28 | – | – |
| 8 | 8–28 | 5–31 | 3–33 | 1–35 | 0–36 | – |
| 9 | 10–35 | 8–37 | 5–40 | 3–42 | 1–44 | – |
| 10 | 14–41 | 10–45 | 8–47 | 5–50 | 3–52 | – |
| 11 | 17–49 | 13–53 | 10–56 | 7–59 | 5–61 | 0–66 |
| 12 | 21–57 | 17–61 | 13–65 | 9–69 | 7–71 | 1–77 |
| 13 | 26–65 | 21–70 | 17–74 | 12–79 | 9–82 | 2–89 |
| 14 | 31–74 | 25–80 | 21–84 | 15–90 | 12–93 | 4–101 |
| 15 | 36–84 | 30–90 | 25–95 | 19–101 | 15–105 | 6–114 |
| 16 | 42–94 | 35–101 | 29–107 | 23–113 | 19–117 | 9–127 |
| 17 | 48–105 | 41–112 | 34–119 | 28–125 | 23–130 | 11–142 |
| 18 | 55–116 | 47–124 | 40–131 | 32–139 | 27–144 | 14–157 |
| 19 | 62–128 | 53–137 | 46–144 | 37–153 | 32–158 | 18–172 |
| 20 | 69–141 | 60–150 | 52–158 | 43–167 | 37–173 | 21–189 |
| 21 | 77–154 | 67–164 | 58–173 | 49–182 | 42–189 | 26–205 |
| 22 | 86–167 | 75–178 | 66–187 | 55–198 | 48–105 | 30–223 |
| 23 | 95–181 | 83–193 | 73–203 | 62–214 | 54–222 | 35–241 |
| 24 | 104–196 | 91–209 | 81–219 | 69–231 | 61–239 | 40–260 |
| 25 | 114–211 | 100–225 | 89–236 | 76–249 | 68–257 | 45–280 |

For $n > 25$ the rank sum ($R$) has an approximately Normal distribution with mean $M = n(n+1)/4$ and standard deviation

$$S = \sqrt{n(n+1)(2n+1)/24}.$$

The test statistic $(R - M)/S$ is evaluated using Table B2.

**Table B10 The Mann-Whitney test (Wilcoxon two sample test)**

For a comparison of two groups of size $n_1$ and $n_2$, where $n_1 \leq n_2$, if the sum of the ranks in the smaller group is equal to the tabulated values or is outside the range shown (i.e. is not between the tabulated values), the P value of the test is less than the value at the top of the column.

Example: For a rank sum of 29 from a sample of 6 compared with a sample of 11 we look along the row for $n_1 = 6$ and $n_2 = 11$ from the left until we find the last column where the value 29 is not between the tabulated values, which gives $P < 0.02$. A rank sum of 28 would give $P < 0.01$.

| | | Two-tailed probability (P) | | | | |
|---|---|---|---|---|---|---|
| $n_1$ | $n_2$ | 0.1 | 0.05 | 0.02 | 0.01 | 0.001 |
| 3 | 3 | 6–15 | – | – | – | – |
| 3 | 4 | 6–18 | – | – | – | – |
| 4 | 4 | 11–25 | 10–26 | – | – | – |
| 2 | 5 | 3–13 | – | – | – | – |
| 3 | 5 | 7–20 | 6–21 | – | – | – |
| 4 | 5 | 12–28 | 11–29 | 10–30 | – | – |
| 5 | 5 | 19–36 | 17–38 | 16–39 | 15–40 | – |
| 2 | 6 | 3–15 | – | – | – | – |
| 3 | 6 | 8–22 | 7–23 | – | – | – |
| 4 | 6 | 13–31 | 12–32 | 11–33 | 10–34 | – |
| 5 | 6 | 20–40 | 18–42 | 17–43 | 16–44 | – |
| 6 | 6 | 28–50 | 26–52 | 24–54 | 23–55 | – |
| 2 | 7 | 3–17 | – | – | – | – |
| 3 | 7 | 8–25 | 7–26 | 6–27 | – | |
| 4 | 7 | 14–34 | 13–35 | 11–37 | 10–38 | – |
| 5 | 7 | 21–44 | 20–45 | 18–47 | 16–49 | – |
| 6 | 7 | 29–55 | 27–57 | 25–59 | 24–60 | – |
| 7 | 7 | 39–66 | 36–69 | 34–71 | 32–73 | 28–77 |
| 2 | 8 | 4–18 | 3–19 | – | – | – |
| 3 | 8 | 9–27 | 8–28 | 6–30 | – | – |
| 4 | 8 | 15–37 | 14–38 | 12–40 | 11–41 | – |
| 5 | 8 | 23–47 | 21–49 | 19–51 | 17–53 | – |
| 6 | 8 | 31–59 | 29–61 | 27–63 | 25–65 | 21–69 |
| 7 | 8 | 41–71 | 38–74 | 35–77 | 34–78 | 29–83 |
| 8 | 8 | 51–85 | 49–87 | 45–91 | 43–93 | 38–98 |

| $n_1$ | $n_2$ | Two-tailed probability (P) 0.1 | 0.05 | 0.02 | 0.01 | 0.001 |
|---|---|---|---|---|---|---|
| 2 | 9 | 4–20 | 3–21 | – | – | – |
| 3 | 9 | 10–29 | 8–31 | 7–32 | 6–33 | – |
| 4 | 9 | 16–40 | 14–42 | 13–43 | 11–45 | – |
| 5 | 9 | 24–51 | 22–53 | 20–55 | 18–57 | 15–60 |
| 6 | 9 | 33–63 | 31–65 | 28–68 | 26–70 | 22–74 |
| 7 | 9 | 43–76 | 40–79 | 37–82 | 35–84 | 30–89 |
| 8 | 9 | 54–90 | 51–93 | 47–97 | 45–99 | 40–104 |
| 9 | 9 | 66–105 | 62–109 | 59–112 | 56–115 | 50–121 |
| 2 | 10 | 4–22 | 3–23 | – | – | – |
| 3 | 10 | 10–32 | 9–33 | 7–35 | 6–36 | – |
| 4 | 10 | 17–43 | 15–45 | 13–47 | 12–48 | – |
| 5 | 10 | 26–54 | 23–57 | 21–59 | 19–61 | 15–65 |
| 6 | 10 | 35–67 | 32–70 | 29–73 | 27–75 | 23–79 |
| 7 | 10 | 45–81 | 42–84 | 39–87 | 37–89 | 31–95 |
| 8 | 10 | 56–96 | 53–99 | 49–103 | 47–105 | 41–111 |
| 9 | 10 | 69–111 | 65–115 | 61–119 | 58–122 | 52–128 |
| 10 | 10 | 82–128 | 78–132 | 74–136 | 71–139 | 63–147 |
| 2 | 11 | 4–24 | 3–25 | – | – | – |
| 3 | 11 | 11–34 | 9–36 | 7–38 | 6–39 | – |
| 4 | 11 | 18–46 | 16–48 | 14–50 | 12–52 | – |
| 5 | 11 | 27–58 | 24–61 | 22–63 | 20–65 | 16–69 |
| 6 | 11 | 37–71 | 34–74 | 30–78 | 28–80 | 23–85 |
| 7 | 11 | 47–86 | 44–89 | 40–93 | 38–95 | 32–101 |
| 8 | 11 | 59–101 | 55–105 | 51–109 | 49–111 | 42–118 |
| 9 | 11 | 72–117 | 68–121 | 63–126 | 61–128 | 53–136 |
| 10 | 11 | 86–134 | 81–139 | 77–143 | 73–147 | 65–155 |
| 11 | 11 | 100–153 | 96–157 | 91–162 | 87–166 | 78–175 |
| 2 | 12 | 5–25 | 4–26 | – | – | – |
| 3 | 12 | 11–37 | 10–38 | 8–40 | 7–41 | – |
| 4 | 12 | 19–49 | 17–51 | 15–53 | 13–55 | – |
| 5 | 12 | 28–62 | 26–64 | 23–67 | 21–69 | 16–74 |
| 6 | 12 | 38–76 | 35–79 | 32–82 | 30–84 | 24–90 |
| 7 | 12 | 49–91 | 46–94 | 42–98 | 40–100 | 33–107 |
| 8 | 12 | 62–106 | 58–110 | 53–115 | 51–117 | 43–125 |
| 9 | 12 | 75–123 | 71–127 | 66–132 | 63–135 | 55–143 |
| 10 | 12 | 89–141 | 84–146 | 79–151 | 76–154 | 67–163 |
| 11 | 12 | 104–160 | 99–165 | 94–170 | 90–174 | 81–183 |
| 12 | 12 | 120–180 | 115–185 | 109–191 | 105–195 | 95–205 |

| $n_1$ | $n_2$ | Two-tailed probability (P) 0.1 | 0.05 | 0.02 | 0.01 | 0.001 |
|---|---|---|---|---|---|---|
| 2 | 13 | 5–27 | 4–28 | 3–29 | – | – |
| 3 | 13 | 12–39 | 10–41 | 8–43 | 7–44 | – |
| 4 | 13 | 20–52 | 18–54 | 15–57 | 13–59 | 10–62 |
| 5 | 13 | 30–65 | 27–68 | 24–71 | 22–73 | 17–78 |
| 6 | 13 | 40–80 | 37–83 | 33–87 | 31–89 | 25–95 |
| 7 | 13 | 52–95 | 48–99 | 44–103 | 41–106 | 34–113 |
| 8 | 13 | 64–112 | 60–116 | 56–120 | 53–123 | 45–131 |
| 9 | 13 | 78–129 | 73–134 | 68–139 | 65–142 | 56–151 |
| 10 | 13 | 92–148 | 88–152 | 82–158 | 79–161 | 69–171 |
| 11 | 13 | 108–167 | 103–172 | 97–178 | 93–182 | 83–192 |
| 12 | 13 | 125–187 | 119–193 | 113–199 | 109–203 | 98–214 |
| 13 | 13 | 142–209 | 136–215 | 130–221 | 125–226 | 114–237 |
| 2 | 14 | 6–28 | 4–30 | 3–31 | – | – |
| 3 | 14 | 13–41 | 11–43 | 8–46 | 7–47 | – |
| 4 | 14 | 21–55 | 19–57 | 16–60 | 14–62 | 10–66 |
| 5 | 14 | 31–69 | 28–72 | 25–75 | 22–78 | 17–83 |
| 6 | 14 | 42–84 | 38–88 | 34–92 | 32–94 | 26–100 |
| 7 | 14 | 54–100 | 50–104 | 45–109 | 43–111 | 35–119 |
| 8 | 14 | 67–117 | 62–122 | 58–126 | 54–130 | 46–138 |
| 9 | 14 | 81–135 | 76–140 | 71–145 | 67–149 | 58–158 |
| 10 | 14 | 96–154 | 91–159 | 85–165 | 81–169 | 71–179 |
| 11 | 14 | 112–174 | 106–180 | 100–186 | 96–190 | 85–201 |
| 12 | 14 | 129–195 | 123–201 | 116–208 | 112–212 | 100–224 |
| 13 | 14 | 147–217 | 141–223 | 134–230 | 129–235 | 116–248 |
| 14 | 14 | 166–240 | 160–246 | 152–254 | 147–259 | 134–272 |
| 2 | 15 | 6–30 | 4–32 | 3–33 | – | – |
| 3 | 15 | 13–44 | 11–46 | 9–48 | 8–49 | – |
| 4 | 15 | 22–58 | 20–60 | 17–63 | 15–65 | 10–70 |
| 5 | 15 | 33–72 | 29–76 | 26–79 | 23–82 | 18–87 |
| 6 | 15 | 44–88 | 40–92 | 36–96 | 33–99 | 26–106 |
| 7 | 15 | 56–105 | 52–109 | 47–114 | 44–117 | 36–125 |
| 8 | 15 | 69–123 | 65–127 | 60–132 | 56–136 | 47–145 |
| 9 | 15 | 84–141 | 79–146 | 73–152 | 69–156 | 60–165 |
| 10 | 15 | 99–161 | 94–166 | 88–172 | 84–176 | 73–187 |
| 11 | 15 | 116–181 | 110–187 | 103–194 | 99–198 | 87–210 |
| 12 | 15 | 133–203 | 127–209 | 120–216 | 115–221 | 103–233 |
| 13 | 15 | 152–225 | 145–232 | 138–239 | 133–244 | 119–258 |
| 14 | 15 | 171–249 | 164–256 | 156–264 | 151–269 | 137–283 |
| 15 | 15 | 192–273 | 184–281 | 176–289 | 171–294 | 156–309 |

For larger samples, the sum of the ranks in the smaller group, $T$, has an approximately Normal distribution with mean $M = n_1(n_1 + n_2 + 1)/2$ and standard deviation

$$S = \sqrt{n_2 M/6}.$$

The test statistic $(T - M)/S$ is evaluated using Table B2.

**Table B11 Ranks for obtaining a confidence interval for the median**

The tabulated values are ranks of the observations that provide approximate 90%, 95% or 99% confidence intervals for the population median based on a single sample of data.

Example: The 99% confidence interval for the population median calculated from a sample of size 56 is given by the observations with ranks 18 and 39.

| Sample | Level of confidence | | |
|---|---|---|---|
| size | 90% | 95% | 99% |
| 6 | 1, 6 | 1, 6 | – |
| 7 | 1, 7 | 1, 7 | – |
| 8 | 2, 7 | 1, 8 | 1, 8 |
| 9 | 2, 8 | 2, 8 | 1, 9 |
| 10 | 2, 9 | 2, 9 | 1, 10 |
| 11 | 3, 9 | 2, 10 | 1, 11 |
| 12 | 3, 10 | 3, 10 | 2, 11 |
| 13 | 4, 10 | 3, 11 | 2, 12 |
| 14 | 4, 11 | 3, 12 | 2, 13 |
| 15 | 4, 12 | 4, 12 | 3, 13 |
| 16 | 5, 12 | 4, 13 | 3, 14 |
| 17 | 5, 13 | 5, 13 | 3, 15 |
| 18 | 6, 13 | 5, 14 | 4, 15 |
| 19 | 6, 14 | 5, 15 | 4, 16 |
| 20 | 6, 15 | 6, 15 | 4, 17 |
| 21 | 7, 15 | 6, 16 | 5, 17 |
| 22 | 7, 16 | 6, 17 | 5, 18 |
| 23 | 8, 16 | 7, 17 | 5, 19 |
| 24 | 8, 17 | 7, 18 | 6, 19 |
| 25 | 8, 18 | 8, 18 | 6, 20 |
| 26 | 9, 18 | 8, 19 | 7, 20 |
| 27 | 9, 19 | 8, 20 | 7, 21 |
| 28 | 10, 19 | 9, 20 | 7, 22 |
| 29 | 10, 20 | 9, 21 | 8, 22 |
| 30 | 11, 20 | 10, 21 | 8, 23 |
| 31 | 11, 21 | 10, 22 | 8, 24 |
| 32 | 11, 22 | 10, 23 | 9, 24 |
| 33 | 12, 22 | 11, 23 | 9, 25 |
| 34 | 12, 23 | 11, 24 | 10, 25 |
| 35 | 13, 23 | 12, 24 | 10, 26 |

| Sample size | Level of confidence 90% | 95% | 99% |
|---|---|---|---|
| 36 | 13, 24 | 12, 25 | 10, 27 |
| 37 | 14, 24 | 13, 25 | 11, 27 |
| 38 | 14, 25 | 13, 26 | 11, 28 |
| 39 | 14, 26 | 13, 27 | 12, 28 |
| 40 | 15, 26 | 14, 27 | 12, 29 |
| 41 | 15, 27 | 14, 28 | 12, 30 |
| 42 | 16, 27 | 15, 28 | 13, 30 |
| 43 | 16, 28 | 15, 29 | 13, 31 |
| 44 | 17, 28 | 16, 29 | 14, 31 |
| 45 | 17, 29 | 16, 30 | 14, 32 |
| 46 | 17, 30 | 16, 31 | 14, 33 |
| 47 | 18, 30 | 17, 31 | 15, 33 |
| 48 | 18, 31 | 17, 32 | 15, 34 |
| 49 | 19, 31 | 18, 32 | 16, 34 |
| 50 | 19, 32 | 18, 33 | 16, 35 |
| 51 | 20, 32 | 19, 33 | 16, 36 |
| 52 | 20, 33 | 19, 34 | 17, 36 |
| 53 | 21, 33 | 19, 35 | 17, 37 |
| 54 | 21, 34 | 20, 35 | 18, 37 |
| 55 | 21, 35 | 20, 36 | 18, 38 |
| 56 | 22, 35 | 21, 36 | 18, 39 |
| 57 | 22, 36 | 21, 37 | 19, 39 |
| 58 | 23, 36 | 22, 37 | 19, 40 |
| 59 | 23, 37 | 22, 38 | 20, 40 |
| 60 | 24, 37 | 22, 39 | 20, 41 |
| 61 | 24, 38 | 23, 39 | 21, 41 |
| 62 | 25, 38 | 23, 40 | 21, 42 |
| 63 | 25, 39 | 24, 40 | 21, 43 |
| 64 | 25, 40 | 24, 41 | 22, 43 |
| 65 | 26, 40 | 25, 41 | 22, 44 |
| 66 | 26, 41 | 25, 42 | 23, 44 |
| 67 | 27, 41 | 26, 42 | 23, 45 |
| 68 | 27, 42 | 26, 43 | 23, 46 |
| 69 | 28, 42 | 26, 44 | 24, 46 |
| 70 | 28, 43 | 27, 44 | 24, 47 |

| Sample size | Level of confidence 90% | 95% | 99% |
|---|---|---|---|
| 71 | 29, 43 | 27, 45 | 25, 47 |
| 72 | 29, 44 | 28, 45 | 25, 48 |
| 73 | 29, 45 | 28, 46 | 26, 48 |
| 74 | 30, 45 | 29, 46 | 26, 49 |
| 75 | 30, 46 | 29, 47 | 26, 50 |
| 76 | 31, 46 | 29, 48 | 27, 50 |
| 77 | 31, 47 | 30, 48 | 27, 51 |
| 78 | 32, 47 | 30, 49 | 28, 51 |
| 79 | 32, 48 | 31, 49 | 28, 52 |
| 80 | 33, 48 | 31, 50 | 29, 52 |
| 81 | 33, 49 | 32, 50 | 29, 53 |
| 82 | 34, 49 | 32, 51 | 29, 54 |
| 83 | 34, 50 | 33, 51 | 30, 54 |
| 84 | 34, 51 | 33, 52 | 30, 55 |
| 85 | 35, 51 | 33, 53 | 31, 55 |
| 86 | 35, 52 | 34, 53 | 31, 56 |
| 87 | 36, 52 | 34, 54 | 32, 56 |
| 88 | 36, 53 | 35, 54 | 32, 57 |
| 89 | 37, 53 | 35, 55 | 32, 58 |
| 90 | 37, 54 | 36, 55 | 33, 58 |
| 91 | 38, 54 | 36, 56 | 33, 59 |
| 92 | 38, 55 | 37, 56 | 34, 59 |
| 93 | 39, 55 | 37, 57 | 34, 60 |
| 94 | 39, 56 | 38, 57 | 35, 60 |
| 95 | 39, 57 | 38, 58 | 35, 61 |
| 96 | 40, 57 | 38, 59 | 35, 62 |
| 97 | 40, 58 | 39, 59 | 36, 62 |
| 98 | 41, 58 | 39, 60 | 36, 63 |
| 99 | 41, 59 | 40, 60 | 37, 63 |
| 100 | 42, 59 | 40, 61 | 37, 64 |

For sample larger than 100, the required ranks are the nearest integers to

$$\frac{n}{2} - \left(N_{1-\alpha/2} \times \frac{\sqrt{n}}{2}\right) \text{ and } 1 + \frac{n}{2} + \left(N_{1-\alpha/2} \times \frac{\sqrt{n}}{2}\right),$$

where $\alpha = 0.1$, 0.05 or 0.01. Values of $N_{1-\alpha/2}$ are given in Table B3.

**Table B12 The Shapiro-Francia $W'$ test of non-Normality**

The P value is the smallest for which the tabulated value exceeds the observed value of $W'$, i.e. small values of $W'$ indicate non-Normality.

Example: An observed value of $W' = 0.851$ from a sample of 18 gives $P < 0.02$.

| Sample | Probability (P) | | | | | |
|---|---|---|---|---|---|---|
| size | 0.2 | 0.1 | 0.05 | 0.02 | 0.01 | 0.001 |
| 10 | 0.9010 | 0.8728 | 0.8445 | 0.8063 | 0.7765 | 0.6710 |
| 11 | 0.9068 | 0.8804 | 0.8537 | 0.8174 | 0.7890 | 0.6872 |
| 12 | 0.9120 | 0.8871 | 0.8618 | 0.8273 | 0.8001 | 0.7021 |
| 13 | 0.9166 | 0.8930 | 0.8690 | 0.8361 | 0.8101 | 0.7156 |
| 14 | 0.9208 | 0.8984 | 0.8755 | 0.8441 | 0.8192 | 0.7281 |
| 15 | 0.9245 | 0.9032 | 0.8814 | 0.8514 | 0.8275 | 0.7395 |
| 16 | 0.9279 | 0.9076 | 0.8868 | 0.8580 | 0.8350 | 0.7501 |
| 17 | 0.9309 | 0.9115 | 0.8916 | 0.8640 | 0.8419 | 0.7599 |
| 18 | 0.9337 | 0.9152 | 0.8961 | 0.8695 | 0.8483 | 0.7690 |
| 19 | 0.9363 | 0.9185 | 0.9001 | 0.8746 | 0.8541 | 0.7774 |
| 20 | 0.9387 | 0.9216 | 0.9039 | 0.8793 | 0.8595 | 0.7853 |
| 21 | 0.9409 | 0.9244 | 0.9074 | 0.8837 | 0.8646 | 0.7927 |
| 22 | 0.9429 | 0.9270 | 0.9106 | 0.8877 | 0.8692 | 0.7997 |
| 23 | 0.9448 | 0.9295 | 0.9136 | 0.8915 | 0.8736 | 0.8061 |
| 24 | 0.9465 | 0.9317 | 0.9164 | 0.8950 | 0.8777 | 0.8123 |
| 25 | 0.9482 | 0.9339 | 0.9190 | 0.8983 | 0.8815 | 0.8180 |
| 30 | 0.9550 | 0.9427 | 0.9299 | 0.9121 | 0.8976 | 0.8424 |
| 35 | 0.9601 | 0.9494 | 0.9382 | 0.9225 | 0.9098 | 0.8612 |
| 40 | 0.9642 | 0.9546 | 0.9446 | 0.9307 | 0.9194 | 0.8761 |
| 45 | 0.9674 | 0.9588 | 0.9498 | 0.9373 | 0.9271 | 0.8882 |
| 50 | 0.9701 | 0.9622 | 0.9541 | 0.9427 | 0.9335 | 0.8982 |
| 55 | 0.9723 | 0.9651 | 0.9577 | 0.9472 | 0.9388 | 0.9066 |
| 60 | 0.9742 | 0.9676 | 0.9607 | 0.9511 | 0.9433 | 0.9137 |
| 65 | 0.9759 | 0.9697 | 0.9633 | 0.9544 | 0.9472 | 0.9199 |
| 70 | 0.9773 | 0.9716 | 0.9656 | 0.9573 | 0.9506 | 0.9252 |
| 75 | 0.9786 | 0.9732 | 0.9676 | 0.9598 | 0.9536 | 0.9299 |
| 80 | 0.9797 | 0.9746 | 0.9694 | 0.9621 | 0.9562 | 0.9340 |
| 85 | 0.9807 | 0.9759 | 0.9710 | 0.9641 | 0.9585 | 0.9376 |
| 90 | 0.9816 | 0.9771 | 0.9724 | 0.9659 | 0.9606 | 0.9409 |
| 95 | 0.9825 | 0.9781 | 0.9737 | 0.9675 | 0.9625 | 0.9439 |
| 100 | 0.9832 | 0.9791 | 0.9748 | 0.9689 | 0.9642 | 0.9465 |

| Sample size | Probability (P) 0.2 | 0.1 | 0.05 | 0.02 | 0.01 | 0.001 |
|---|---|---|---|---|---|---|
| 110 | 0.9845 | 0.9807 | 0.9768 | 0.9715 | 0.9672 | 0.9511 |
| 120 | 0.9856 | 0.9821 | 0.9786 | 0.9736 | 0.9697 | 0.9550 |
| 130 | 0.9866 | 0.9833 | 0.9800 | 0.9755 | 0.9718 | 0.9583 |
| 140 | 0.9874 | 0.9844 | 0.9813 | 0.9771 | 0.9737 | 0.9612 |
| 150 | 0.9881 | 0.9853 | 0.9824 | 0.9785 | 0.9753 | 0.9637 |
| 160 | 0.9888 | 0.9861 | 0.9834 | 0.9797 | 0.9767 | 0.9658 |
| 170 | 0.9893 | 0.9868 | 0.9843 | 0.9808 | 0.9780 | 0.9677 |
| 180 | 0.9899 | 0.9875 | 0.9851 | 0.9817 | 0.9791 | 0.9695 |
| 190 | 0.9903 | 0.9881 | 0.9858 | 0.9826 | 0.9801 | 0.9710 |
| 200 | 0.9907 | 0.9886 | 0.9864 | 0.9834 | 0.9811 | 0.9724 |

**Table B13 Random digits**

These numbers are used for random allocation, as described in section 5.7.

| | | | | | | | | | | | | | | | | | | | |
|---|---|---|---|---|---|---|---|---|---|---|---|---|---|---|---|---|---|---|---|
| 47 | 44 | 76 | 60 | 72 | 56 | 99 | 20 | 20 | 52 | 49 | 05 | 78 | 58 | 50 | 62 | 86 | 52 | 11 | 88 |
| 31 | 60 | 26 | 13 | 69 | 74 | 80 | 71 | 48 | 73 | 72 | 18 | 60 | 58 | 20 | 55 | 59 | 06 | 67 | 02 |
| 72 | 89 | 83 | 91 | 86 | 62 | 78 | 86 | 95 | 07 | 16 | 11 | 59 | 55 | 14 | 98 | 62 | 04 | 11 | 23 |
| 31 | 40 | 99 | 54 | 61 | 99 | 32 | 30 | 43 | 80 | 92 | 42 | 19 | 28 | 69 | 90 | 04 | 88 | 30 | 98 |
| 03 | 49 | 79 | 75 | 46 | 76 | 56 | 99 | 54 | 46 | 67 | 32 | 57 | 03 | 75 | 44 | 10 | 82 | 77 | 73 |
| | | | | | | | | | | | | | | | | | | | |
| 36 | 61 | 26 | 31 | 49 | 40 | 74 | 86 | 32 | 36 | 15 | 39 | 15 | 12 | 89 | 68 | 52 | 51 | 10 | 08 |
| 91 | 72 | 12 | 92 | 31 | 66 | 91 | 99 | 48 | 42 | 67 | 16 | 14 | 69 | 67 | 23 | 42 | 74 | 51 | 43 |
| 42 | 73 | 76 | 68 | 86 | 75 | 21 | 91 | 72 | 38 | 44 | 79 | 58 | 48 | 95 | 63 | 53 | 86 | 56 | 77 |
| 32 | 95 | 21 | 17 | 27 | 63 | 06 | 14 | 24 | 05 | 81 | 30 | 23 | 30 | 82 | 53 | 62 | 76 | 36 | 99 |
| 57 | 24 | 32 | 29 | 46 | 60 | 82 | 90 | 81 | 31 | 03 | 67 | 43 | 07 | 91 | 93 | 45 | 73 | 20 | 57 |
| | | | | | | | | | | | | | | | | | | | |
| 89 | 11 | 77 | 99 | 94 | 29 | 35 | 71 | 10 | 56 | 46 | 70 | 29 | 10 | 20 | 90 | 28 | 39 | 43 | 73 |
| 35 | 83 | 73 | 68 | 20 | 40 | 89 | 24 | 06 | 32 | 08 | 38 | 06 | 73 | 59 | 38 | 78 | 13 | 04 | 60 |
| 84 | 85 | 95 | 45 | 52 | 26 | 42 | 34 | 22 | 49 | 81 | 11 | 90 | 19 | 37 | 46 | 17 | 07 | 96 | 13 |
| 56 | 80 | 93 | 52 | 82 | 71 | 55 | 76 | 17 | 20 | 69 | 37 | 87 | 54 | 29 | 56 | 72 | 83 | 18 | 15 |
| 97 | 62 | 98 | 71 | 39 | 03 | 75 | 35 | 84 | 20 | 86 | 17 | 26 | 63 | 75 | 61 | 61 | 98 | 57 | 82 |
| | | | | | | | | | | | | | | | | | | | |
| 79 | 36 | 13 | 72 | 99 | 09 | 78 | 61 | 77 | 71 | 13 | 91 | 49 | 07 | 46 | 21 | 49 | 96 | 90 | 79 |
| 34 | 96 | 98 | 54 | 89 | 85 | 76 | 99 | 11 | 27 | 36 | 33 | 93 | 88 | 53 | 10 | 68 | 12 | 34 | 49 |
| 69 | 56 | 88 | 97 | 43 | 29 | 63 | 67 | 99 | 32 | 78 | 26 | 87 | 02 | 31 | 37 | 95 | 44 | 79 | 57 |
| 09 | 17 | 78 | 78 | 02 | 13 | 13 | 34 | 96 | 42 | 55 | 09 | 11 | 69 | 26 | 95 | 95 | 50 | 23 | 93 |
| 83 | 17 | 39 | 84 | 16 | 70 | 25 | 40 | 20 | 94 | 68 | 10 | 90 | 91 | 90 | 16 | 83 | 18 | 25 | 03 |

| | | | | | | | | | | | | | | | | | | | |
|---|---|---|---|---|---|---|---|---|---|---|---|---|---|---|---|---|---|---|---|
| 24 | 23 | 36 | 44 | 14 | 10 | 15 | 02 | 70 | 78 | 27 | 07 | 91 | 84 | 89 | 26 | 03 | 75 | 66 | 39 |
| 39 | 87 | 30 | 20 | 41 | 78 | 19 | 39 | 76 | 16 | 99 | 68 | 54 | 58 | 91 | 69 | 32 | 72 | 02 | 41 |
| 75 | 18 | 53 | 77 | 83 | 85 | 46 | 03 | 68 | 87 | 92 | 23 | 98 | 70 | 88 | 12 | 55 | 80 | 66 | 63 |
| 33 | 93 | 39 | 24 | 81 | 41 | 60 | 48 | 13 | 08 | 67 | 68 | 05 | 27 | 38 | 55 | 86 | 19 | 56 | 28 |
| 22 | 52 | 01 | 86 | 71 | 74 | 89 | 71 | 27 | 01 | 52 | 15 | 89 | 69 | 79 | 97 | 61 | 55 | 36 | 46 |
| 19 | 77 | 57 | 91 | 08 | 91 | 51 | 18 | 84 | 66 | 24 | 89 | 92 | 19 | 27 | 00 | 83 | 43 | 12 | 13 |
| 79 | 82 | 45 | 59 | 28 | 38 | 40 | 73 | 47 | 29 | 07 | 45 | 12 | 32 | 69 | 09 | 43 | 64 | 62 | 14 |
| 93 | 69 | 09 | 97 | 30 | 86 | 70 | 58 | 24 | 98 | 73 | 25 | 90 | 23 | 90 | 30 | 01 | 90 | 51 | 77 |
| 17 | 59 | 81 | 59 | 51 | 21 | 47 | 75 | 72 | 12 | 05 | 74 | 72 | 65 | 56 | 33 | 50 | 22 | 13 | 03 |
| 01 | 04 | 85 | 55 | 83 | 85 | 55 | 26 | 03 | 66 | 02 | 71 | 34 | 07 | 75 | 46 | 16 | 24 | 48 | 27 |
| 68 | 46 | 94 | 08 | 31 | 14 | 42 | 38 | 87 | 20 | 40 | 14 | 32 | 65 | 22 | 48 | 74 | 66 | 23 | 52 |
| 45 | 49 | 01 | 21 | 29 | 68 | 50 | 14 | 66 | 64 | 95 | 95 | 71 | 32 | 03 | 75 | 22 | 76 | 53 | 43 |
| 92 | 65 | 74 | 48 | 88 | 79 | 36 | 17 | 18 | 30 | 15 | 26 | 05 | 54 | 61 | 18 | 96 | 73 | 99 | 63 |
| 55 | 20 | 00 | 95 | 21 | 15 | 41 | 30 | 52 | 22 | 32 | 10 | 09 | 63 | 64 | 51 | 59 | 06 | 78 | 53 |
| 15 | 08 | 01 | 56 | 89 | 99 | 15 | 17 | 60 | 07 | 02 | 65 | 83 | 40 | 90 | 05 | 97 | 65 | 40 | 71 |
| 55 | 81 | 61 | 65 | 62 | 26 | 05 | 37 | 73 | 53 | 95 | 94 | 53 | 26 | 31 | 56 | 74 | 00 | 10 | 28 |
| 03 | 21 | 36 | 98 | 89 | 58 | 02 | 91 | 97 | 74 | 51 | 73 | 33 | 25 | 60 | 78 | 38 | 35 | 75 | 82 |
| 02 | 91 | 31 | 26 | 57 | 07 | 57 | 75 | 61 | 38 | 38 | 22 | 23 | 48 | 64 | 53 | 93 | 21 | 99 | 00 |
| 06 | 09 | 83 | 81 | 53 | 81 | 60 | 65 | 13 | 21 | 93 | 55 | 95 | 27 | 02 | 20 | 87 | 18 | 44 | 63 |
| 71 | 69 | 84 | 48 | 28 | 76 | 73 | 86 | 19 | 48 | 34 | 08 | 50 | 72 | 84 | 00 | 68 | 80 | 12 | 79 |

**Table B13** (*cont*)

| | | | | | | | | | | | | | | | | | | | |
|---|---|---|---|---|---|---|---|---|---|---|---|---|---|---|---|---|---|---|---|
| 27 | 30 | 09 | 49 | 12 | 64 | 43 | 56 | 79 | 75 | 00 | 76 | 06 | 79 | 40 | 67 | 91 | 47 | 13 | 53 |
| 91 | 71 | 11 | 65 | 87 | 95 | 58 | 68 | 40 | 08 | 03 | 70 | 03 | 58 | 87 | 71 | 24 | 54 | 38 | 28 |
| 92 | 90 | 76 | 09 | 48 | 95 | 92 | 16 | 79 | 24 | 27 | 22 | 28 | 17 | 18 | 15 | 26 | 77 | 44 | 71 |
| 05 | 87 | 71 | 16 | 87 | 80 | 11 | 42 | 74 | 59 | 44 | 69 | 24 | 53 | 95 | 19 | 67 | 43 | 63 | 22 |
| 34 | 84 | 28 | 25 | 87 | 15 | 58 | 15 | 70 | 38 | 27 | 70 | 95 | 40 | 75 | 08 | 70 | 69 | 93 | 51 |
| 67 | 91 | 71 | 45 | 69 | 30 | 14 | 45 | 33 | 49 | 68 | 50 | 04 | 92 | 57 | 14 | 91 | 97 | 23 | 60 |
| 73 | 33 | 45 | 55 | 88 | 48 | 64 | 06 | 43 | 92 | 18 | 58 | 39 | 84 | 29 | 98 | 58 | 91 | 42 | 42 |
| 58 | 67 | 08 | 35 | 62 | 90 | 74 | 47 | 58 | 16 | 19 | 25 | 62 | 35 | 74 | 50 | 11 | 97 | 17 | 18 |
| 06 | 57 | 93 | 89 | 35 | 35 | 91 | 80 | 59 | 87 | 09 | 96 | 30 | 17 | 64 | 82 | 83 | 88 | 76 | 31 |
| 68 | 94 | 16 | 54 | 82 | 15 | 58 | 06 | 40 | 27 | 19 | 61 | 50 | 50 | 58 | 11 | 96 | 66 | 34 | 20 |
| 65 | 37 | 23 | 24 | 16 | 86 | 00 | 72 | 16 | 22 | 42 | 61 | 71 | 54 | 11 | 39 | 84 | 88 | 97 | 79 |
| 94 | 72 | 49 | 22 | 91 | 48 | 61 | 69 | 97 | 72 | 45 | 29 | 71 | 70 | 83 | 25 | 37 | 12 | 40 | 88 |
| 25 | 55 | 80 | 41 | 97 | 86 | 34 | 73 | 65 | 13 | 10 | 64 | 97 | 16 | 12 | 17 | 03 | 45 | 33 | 16 |
| 57 | 91 | 28 | 59 | 37 | 90 | 86 | 84 | 33 | 89 | 58 | 78 | 01 | 08 | 27 | 93 | 05 | 50 | 29 | 43 |
| 61 | 54 | 50 | 45 | 02 | 01 | 49 | 86 | 88 | 76 | 85 | 24 | 75 | 20 | 36 | 28 | 50 | 01 | 19 | 67 |
| 44 | 86 | 92 | 60 | 09 | 75 | 09 | 25 | 03 | 63 | 97 | 30 | 44 | 19 | 63 | 71 | 69 | 77 | 07 | 15 |
| 07 | 49 | 94 | 38 | 94 | 03 | 62 | 14 | 22 | 21 | 16 | 37 | 26 | 19 | 10 | 23 | 09 | 84 | 28 | 87 |
| 35 | 13 | 11 | 93 | 80 | 12 | 54 | 95 | 10 | 65 | 63 | 51 | 99 | 36 | 73 | 69 | 41 | 89 | 14 | 20 |
| 33 | 27 | 80 | 92 | 30 | 55 | 33 | 26 | 55 | 70 | 50 | 05 | 19 | 88 | 27 | 72 | 39 | 37 | 52 | 85 |
| 40 | 64 | 39 | 62 | 67 | 36 | 34 | 22 | 71 | 23 | 96 | 71 | 91 | 35 | 02 | 16 | 08 | 58 | 02 | 69 |

| | | | | | | | | | | | | | | | | | | | |
|---|---|---|---|---|---|---|---|---|---|---|---|---|---|---|---|---|---|---|---|
| 97 | 95 | 27 | 05 | 71 | 96 | 46 | 04 | 60 | 32 | 56 | 33 | 17 | 08 | 24 | 29 | 73 | 34 | 93 | 49 |
| 03 | 41 | 36 | 64 | 62 | 56 | 49 | 46 | 79 | 96 | 31 | 38 | 48 | 84 | 27 | 54 | 79 | 14 | 61 | 93 |
| 30 | 51 | 05 | 71 | 61 | 98 | 84 | 49 | 08 | 85 | 08 | 60 | 93 | 67 | 69 | 79 | 63 | 62 | 89 | 74 |
| 65 | 06 | 72 | 60 | 50 | 63 | 39 | 97 | 07 | 89 | 85 | 34 | 75 | 39 | 02 | 72 | 13 | 54 | 30 | 94 |
| 96 | 77 | 85 | 16 | 97 | 53 | 17 | 52 | 99 | 01 | 90 | 22 | 66 | 53 | 52 | 67 | 20 | 06 | 60 | 78 |
| 30 | 38 | 05 | 49 | 03 | 20 | 34 | 74 | 71 | 66 | 06 | 01 | 25 | 16 | 76 | 29 | 05 | 48 | 61 | 47 |
| 27 | 66 | 31 | 41 | 41 | 42 | 27 | 31 | 55 | 95 | 17 | 32 | 65 | 54 | 77 | 08 | 33 | 31 | 35 | 17 |
| 35 | 76 | 27 | 08 | 71 | 42 | 53 | 51 | 84 | 46 | 50 | 80 | 46 | 33 | 27 | 56 | 10 | 17 | 87 | 30 |
| 59 | 85 | 30 | 79 | 54 | 83 | 94 | 60 | 03 | 28 | 44 | 49 | 81 | 96 | 14 | 84 | 73 | 65 | 87 | 35 |
| 57 | 68 | 50 | 11 | 67 | 92 | 19 | 74 | 93 | 45 | 64 | 70 | 49 | 04 | 43 | 87 | 14 | 33 | 20 | 44 |
| 28 | 58 | 77 | 49 | 61 | 39 | 33 | 84 | 54 | 82 | 80 | 67 | 45 | 67 | 07 | 99 | 81 | 06 | 95 | 59 |
| 45 | 83 | 16 | 23 | 64 | 02 | 14 | 28 | 66 | 89 | 06 | 81 | 50 | 56 | 50 | 32 | 48 | 11 | 97 | 07 |
| 11 | 11 | 92 | 70 | 62 | 07 | 75 | 02 | 86 | 87 | 72 | 10 | 43 | 50 | 51 | 99 | 00 | 86 | 85 | 57 |
| 99 | 37 | 54 | 21 | 76 | 95 | 71 | 29 | 34 | 92 | 79 | 01 | 35 | 83 | 48 | 80 | 29 | 63 | 46 | 53 |
| 37 | 17 | 17 | 58 | 68 | 89 | 89 | 64 | 76 | 15 | 13 | 08 | 47 | 05 | 86 | 22 | 23 | 76 | 25 | 31 |
| 90 | 93 | 08 | 00 | 09 | 39 | 83 | 54 | 06 | 47 | 28 | 93 | 13 | 11 | 37 | 50 | 26 | 64 | 34 | 58 |
| 81 | 76 | 66 | 75 | 93 | 77 | 72 | 95 | 39 | 89 | 92 | 72 | 15 | 40 | 48 | 96 | 52 | 83 | 21 | 58 |
| 15 | 31 | 15 | 47 | 93 | 55 | 48 | 48 | 78 | 96 | 36 | 77 | 00 | 98 | 21 | 34 | 69 | 30 | 47 | 31 |
| 05 | 96 | 48 | 09 | 40 | 50 | 78 | 72 | 30 | 11 | 39 | 45 | 98 | 45 | 31 | 17 | 80 | 00 | 43 | 93 |
| 84 | 14 | 44 | 28 | 42 | 71 | 19 | 16 | 22 | 19 | 25 | 74 | 58 | 47 | 66 | 62 | 79 | 39 | 70 | 51 |

**Table B13** (*cont*)

| | | | | | | | | | | | | | | | | | | | |
|---|---|---|---|---|---|---|---|---|---|---|---|---|---|---|---|---|---|---|---|
| 70 | 73 | 73 | 30 | 22 | 14 | 59 | 65 | 46 | 11 | 16 | 68 | 25 | 46 | 96 | 89 | 32 | 98 | 96 | 45 |
| 80 | 12 | 00 | 19 | 09 | 11 | 41 | 75 | 97 | 78 | 22 | 55 | 64 | 61 | 47 | 39 | 00 | 79 | 88 | 06 |
| 77 | 34 | 44 | 42 | 80 | 55 | 29 | 25 | 55 | 83 | 88 | 57 | 08 | 65 | 36 | 63 | 68 | 67 | 71 | 22 |
| 69 | 17 | 52 | 89 | 32 | 16 | 07 | 33 | 25 | 54 | 70 | 76 | 09 | 82 | 40 | 54 | 53 | 78 | 88 | 66 |
| 86 | 54 | 95 | 80 | 49 | 45 | 47 | 59 | 31 | 57 | 58 | 56 | 66 | 29 | 34 | 57 | 98 | 95 | 61 | 88 |
| 95 | 50 | 38 | 03 | 92 | 65 | 41 | 66 | 59 | 75 | 25 | 70 | 58 | 63 | 99 | 70 | 86 | 44 | 69 | 39 |
| 89 | 86 | 81 | 70 | 80 | 34 | 95 | 72 | 28 | 01 | 15 | 99 | 58 | 55 | 52 | 62 | 88 | 48 | 10 | 80 |
| 09 | 25 | 43 | 50 | 45 | 40 | 66 | 62 | 86 | 21 | 69 | 66 | 58 | 30 | 71 | 39 | 05 | 36 | 58 | 09 |
| 46 | 00 | 41 | 44 | 69 | 81 | 30 | 34 | 33 | 56 | 73 | 25 | 98 | 82 | 19 | 97 | 61 | 56 | 09 | 47 |
| 31 | 74 | 00 | 85 | 48 | 49 | 91 | 34 | 83 | 76 | 07 | 01 | 22 | 14 | 71 | 65 | 24 | 63 | 56 | 85 |
| 42 | 82 | 02 | 00 | 26 | 65 | 19 | 92 | 09 | 12 | 57 | 53 | 00 | 39 | 80 | 59 | 82 | 03 | 19 | 14 |
| 44 | 23 | 29 | 76 | 67 | 04 | 88 | 78 | 22 | 02 | 17 | 94 | 51 | 26 | 50 | 84 | 84 | 90 | 66 | 23 |
| 76 | 81 | 90 | 15 | 75 | 85 | 18 | 79 | 65 | 43 | 91 | 15 | 93 | 25 | 54 | 07 | 91 | 40 | 06 | 19 |
| 68 | 81 | 53 | 17 | 20 | 14 | 41 | 15 | 50 | 18 | 42 | 52 | 99 | 16 | 28 | 08 | 47 | 12 | 46 | 02 |
| 92 | 92 | 95 | 78 | 09 | 56 | 10 | 89 | 02 | 81 | 96 | 97 | 46 | 94 | 16 | 19 | 97 | 19 | 81 | 29 |
| 49 | 06 | 01 | 66 | 76 | 62 | 60 | 97 | 48 | 41 | 93 | 12 | 95 | 23 | 90 | 12 | 46 | 28 | 38 | 69 |
| 77 | 62 | 07 | 45 | 07 | 11 | 25 | 40 | 46 | 58 | 58 | 49 | 20 | 20 | 65 | 52 | 35 | 60 | 47 | 61 |
| 93 | 66 | 53 | 25 | 24 | 63 | 61 | 73 | 51 | 34 | 06 | 75 | 88 | 47 | 86 | 46 | 82 | 05 | 91 | 24 |
| 15 | 44 | 16 | 15 | 14 | 85 | 65 | 81 | 67 | 55 | 70 | 16 | 92 | 89 | 37 | 99 | 14 | 10 | 97 | 76 |
| 01 | 56 | 26 | 85 | 58 | 64 | 48 | 85 | 01 | 17 | 01 | 11 | 87 | 06 | 77 | 26 | 87 | 98 | 06 | 72 |

**Sources of Tables in Appendix B**

B1 derived using NAG* routine.
B2 derived using NAG* routine.
B3 adapted from Lentner (1982) with permission.
B4 derived using NAG* routine.
B5 adapted from Fisher and Yates (1963) with permission.
B6 derived using NAG* routine.
B7 derived using NAG* routine.
B8 from Glasser and Winter (1961) with corrections, with permission of *Biometrika* trustees.
B9 adapted from Lentner (1982) with permission.
B10 adapted from Lentner (1982) with permission.
B11 from Gardner and Altman (1989c, p. 119) with permission.
B12 directly from formulae in Royston (1983).
B13 obtained using random number generator in STATA.

---

*NAG Fortran Library (Numerical Algorithms Group, 1987).

# Answers to exercises

These solutions do not in general include the graphs that would usually be produced routinely as part of the analysis.
Common abbreviations are:

| | |
|---|---|
| SD | standard deviation |
| SE | standard error |
| CI | confidence interval |
| df | degrees of freedom |

## CHAPTER 3

3.1 (a) Censored.
(b) We do not know the upper limit of SI. The uncensored data show that the distributions are positively skewed (skewed to the right).
(c) The data are skewed and some values are censored.
(d) 3.8 and 22.3 respectively.
(e) 1135 mg.
(f) Without adverse reactions / With adverse reactions

| Without adverse reactions | | With adverse reactions | |
|---|---|---|---|
| 2 | | 2 | 99 |
| 3 | 135799 | 3 | 89 |
| 4 | 1234489 | 4 | 1244669999 |
| 5 | 1337899 | 5 | 01113333347799 |
| 6 | 11457 | 6 | 12237788 |
| 7 | 122 | 7 | 4 |

(g) The median ages of the two groups are easily obtained from the stem-and-leaf diagrams as 52 and 53, suggesting that adverse reactions are not age-related.

3.2 (a) The answer depends upon the interpretation of 'more likely'. The Figure shows that more accidents involve professional pilots than any other group, but gives no information of the risk per individual.
(b) When the figures are adjusted for the amount of flying in each group it is clear that professional pilots had much the lowest risk. The highest risks were among housewives and students. The different answers are explained by the strong negative relation between the amount of flying and the risk of an accident.

3.3 Figure 3.12 shows the $2\frac{1}{2}$, 25, 50, 75 and $97\frac{1}{2}$ centiles. The ranks of the required observations are thus the sample size plus 1 (299) multiplied by 0.025, 0.25, 0.5, 0.75 and 0.975. These values are 7.475, 74.75, 149.5, 224.25 and 291.525. The observations with ranks either side of these values can be found from Table 3.4 (it helps to calculate a column of cumulative frequencies), and interpolation used to get the required centiles. However, in each case the observations with ranks either side of the required rank are the same, so the centiles of the distribution of IgM are obtained simply as 0.2, 0.5, 0.7, 1.0 and 2.0 g/l.

## CHAPTER 4

4.1 0.023 or 2.3% (from Table B1).

4.2 Following the method given in section 4.9.1, we need to calculate the probabilities of obtaining 0, 1, or 2 pints of group B blood. We thus need to calculate the number of ways of choosing these numbers from a sample of 100, which are:

$$\binom{100}{0} = 1$$

$$\binom{100}{1} = \binom{100}{0} \times 100/1 = 100$$

$$\binom{100}{2} = \binom{100}{1} \times 99/2 = 4950$$

Using the formula in section 4.9.1, the required probability is

$$(0.08)^0(0.92)^{100} + 100(0.08)^1(0.92)^{99} + 4950(0.08)^2(0.92)^{98}$$

$$= 0.00024 + 0.00208 + 0.00895 = 0.0113.$$

The probability of getting fewer than three pints of group B blood is about 1 in 100, or 0.01.

4.3 As the probability of a boy is slightly greater than the probability of a girl, the sequence with the most boys is most likely, which is the last sequence. The other two sequences are equally likely.

4.4 (a) 0.0013.
(b) $20\,000 \times 0.0013 = 26$.

4.5 (a) The question can be reversed, so that we wish to evaluate the necessary sample size so that the probability of all the children being negative to the test is $< 0.05$. In mathematics, we require the sample size $m$, such that $0.9^m < 0.05$. It is simple to show, by trial and error, that we need $m = 29$. (If your maths is good, you might have evaluated $m$ as the smallest integer greater than $\log(0.05)/\log(0.9)$.)
(b) It has no effect.

4.6 At the start the minimum height was $(172 - 175.8)/5.84 = -0.65$

standard deviations from the mean. From Table B1, the proportion of men taller than this would be 0.7422 (about 74%). At the end of the 25 year period the minimum height was $(172 - 179.1)/5.84 = -1.22$ standard deviations from the mean. From Table B1, the proportion of men above the minimum is now 0.8888, or about 89%. The proportion of ineligible men has more than halved.

4.7 If there is no change in the true blood pressure, each of a sequence of three measurements is equally likely to be in between the other two. The probability that the third measurement will *not* fall between the first two is thus two thirds (0.67), discounting the possibility of equal measurements. There is no reason to expect the third measurement to be between the first two and no reason to discard measurements as unreliable if they do not. If the intention is to use the average of the three readings in an analysis, the averages would be less well estimated for those with only two values.

4.8 (a) The probability of each child being unaffected is 0.75. The probability of two children being unaffected is $0.75^2 = 0.56$, as these are independent events.
(b) The probability is 0.75. Each child has the same probability, regardless of the outcome for previous children.
(c) The probability of both parents being heterozygous for the abnormal gene is $\frac{1}{22} \times \frac{1}{22} = 0.0021$. The expected number of babies with cystic fibrosis per year is thus $0.25 \times 3500 \times 0.0021$, which is about 2.

## CHAPTER 5

5.1 (a) No, it is definitely wrong. If we want to see if a group of subjects has shifted its behaviour in some way we should re-examine the whole group. To study only a selected subset is to bias the sample being re-examined and thus to bias the results.
(b) The response rate in the second study was 69% which is rather poor. The non-responders, nearly a third of the sample, might well be atypical (this is what is usually found), and could well include heavier drinkers. For example, some may have been too ill to respond through a drink-related illness. Thus the high rate of non-response could have biased the results. The authors should have compared the characteristics of responders and non-responders with respect to their responses to the first survey. The paper does not give the response rate to the first study. If it was also around 70%, which is quite likely, then the final sample interviewed at the second survey would be even more highly selected.
(c) It is not a good idea, because drinking habits are not consistent throughout the year.
(d) No. First, we cannot necessarily interpret two simultaneous

changes over time as being causally related. Second, we would expect them to have found a reduction in the reported alcohol consumption, because the sample was biased to include only those drinking in the first study. If they had re-interviewed only those not drinking in the first study, we would expect them to have found an increase. This is one form of the phenomenon known as 'regression to the mean', and occurs when we remeasure a quantity on a sample selected by a restricted range of the same quantity on a previous occasion. Thus even when there has been no change over time, this study would be expected to have shown a decrease in alcohol consumption.

(e) No. For reasons given above, they are by no means representative. Further, they are a *sample*, not a *population*.

(f) The interpretation is not valid for the reasons noted above.

(g) No.

5.2 (a) It was a cross-sectional study.

(b) If the population of interest is taken as all menopausal British women, then the representativeness of this general practice is relevant. We have no information about this, although it does not seem unreasonable to carry out this type of study in a single practice. All 132 women born in 1930 were investigated, so there was no selection bias. However, we are assuming that the register of patients is accurate and complete, and the fact that 21/132 were not contactable casts some doubt on this. Of these 132 women, only 31 were actually studied, for the various reasons stated. Most of the exclusions are reasonable, although it is not clear why the unmarried women were excluded. The sample appears reasonably representative.

(c) The major problem with this study is that if the use of the pill delays the menopause then at the time of the study some women who will have had their menopause delayed will still have been premenopausal and so excluded from the study. The design does not allow the research objective to be investigated.

(d) This is a question that could be answered by a cohort study. If the researcher had taken, for example, all the women born in 1930 and waited until they had all reached the menopause, then he could make a valid comparison. However, it should be noted that it is not really good practice to lump together all pill users regardless of the length of pill use or the age at which it was taken. The cohort design would allow these factors to be investigated in relation to the age of menopause.

5.3 (a) Baseball players are clearly not truly representative of the population, but it is impossible to assess whether it matters in this particular case. However, it appears that there might have been a higher proportion of left-handers (14%) than we would expect in the population.

(b) If the prevalence of left-handedness had increased during the twentieth century, or if the prevalence within different social groups (with different mortality rates) had changed. Both of these are likely.
(c) The analysis would be biased towards including those born a long time ago as most recent players would still be alive. It is likely that left-handedness was less common earlier in the century than it is now. These two facts mean that the analysis would be biased towards earlier death among left-handers. Further, it is misleading to analyse mean age at death excluding those still alive. The correct analysis of survival data, which takes account of data for survivors too, is described in Chapter 13.
(d) It would be desirable to take a cohort of people born at about the same time, for example all those in the same year at school. In order to get a reasonable proportion of deaths, the survivors would need to be at least 70. It is most unlikely that such data are available and a prospective study would take a very long time! The baseball data would yield a more valid answer if analysed using an appropriate method, and if year of birth was considered in the analysis.

## CHAPTER 7

7.1 Figure A7.1 shows a scatter diagram of the data. The point that is most distant from the general trend is in the bottom left-hand corner, corresponding to patient 19. This patient's wedge pressure was actually 28 mm Hg.

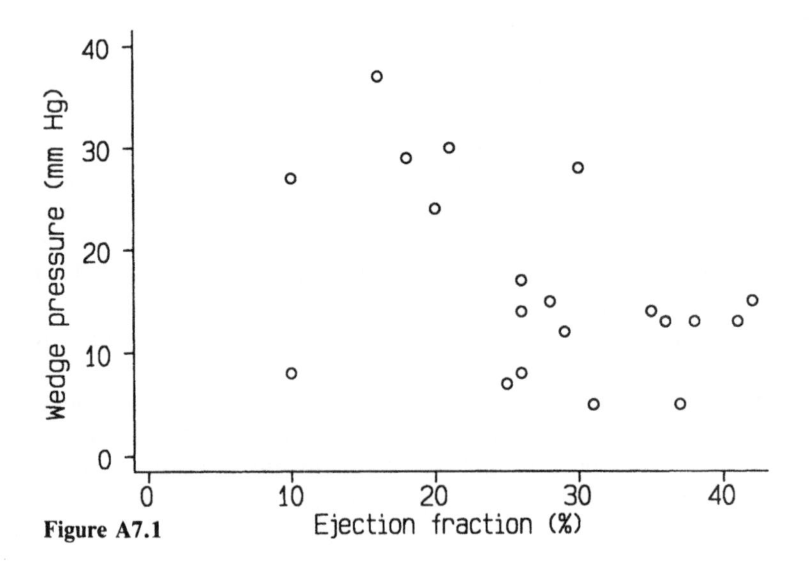


**Figure A7.1**

7.2 The following table shows the calculations:

| $T_4$ | $\log_e T_4$ | P | Normal score |
|---|---|---|---|
| 171 | 5.14 | 0.0309 | −1.868 |
| 257 | 5.55 | 0.0802 | −1.403 |
| 288 | 5.66 | 0.1296 | −1.128 |
| 295 | 5.69 | 0.1790 | −0.919 |
| 396 | 5.98 | 0.2284 | −0.744 |
| 397 | 5.98 | 0.2778 | −0.589 |
| 431 | 6.07 | 0.3272 | −0.448 |
| 435 | 6.08 | 0.3765 | −0.315 |
| 554 | 6.32 | 0.4259 | −0.187 |
| 568 | 6.34 | 0.4753 | −0.062 |
| 795 | 6.68 | 0.5247 | 0.062 |
| 902 | 6.80 | 0.5741 | 0.187 |
| 958 | 6.86 | 0.6235 | 0.315 |
| 1004 | 6.91 | 0.6728 | 0.448 |
| 1104 | 7.01 | 0.7222 | 0.589 |
| 1212 | 7.10 | 0.7716 | 0.744 |
| 1283 | 7.16 | 0.8210 | 0.919 |
| 1378 | 7.23 | 0.8704 | 1.128 |
| 1621 | 7.39 | 0.9198 | 1.403 |
| 2415 | 7.79 | 0.9691 | 1.868 |

The Normal scores can be obtained in many statistics packages. Otherwise they can be obtained by using Table B1 'in reverse'. The Normal plot of these data is very straight, as is shown in Figure A7.2.

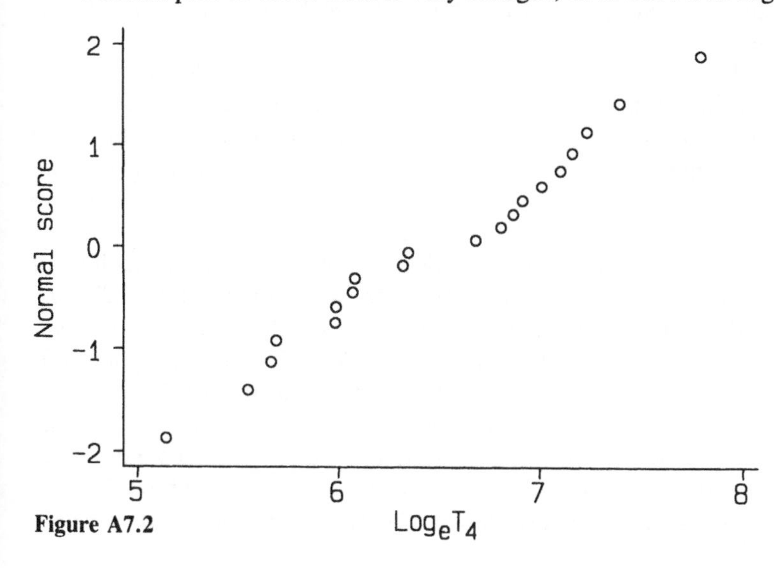


**Figure A7.2**

7.3 The terminal digits (or penultimate digits in the case of dose of SA) are distributed as follows:

| | Digit | | | | | | | | | | |
|---|---|---|---|---|---|---|---|---|---|---|---|
| | 0 | 1 | 2 | 3 | 4 | 5 | 6 | 7 | 8 | 9 | Total |
| Age | 1 | 11 | 6 | 10 | 7 | 2 | 2 | 7 | 5 | 14 | 65 |
| SA | 2 | 24 | 0 | 6 | 0 | 10 | 20 | 0 | 0 | 3 | 65 |
| SI | 16 | 0 | 5 | 3 | 4 | 2 | 3 | 4 | 7 | 4 | 48 |

Digit preference is a likely phenomenon for measurements, but would not be expected for information such as age. Nevertheless, the large number of ages ending in 9 is rather odd.

Both SA and SI show dramatic digit preference which is hard to explain. That for the total dose of SA is peculiar, especially as it represents the sum of doses given over at least six months. The SI is the ratio of two percentages, so the surfeit of zeros suggests imprecise recording.

7.4 Almost half (27/60) of the values end in zero. The other terminating digits are fairly evenly spread. This effect may be due to different observers reporting data to different precision.

## CHAPTER 8

8.1 (a) The larger hospital, simply because there are more births.
(b) The day to day variation in the proportion of boys will be greater in the smaller hospital, so it is more likely to have more than 60% of babies being boys on any day.

8.2 (a) The SE of the mean is $SD/\sqrt{n}$, which is $2.3629/\sqrt{8} = 0.8354$.
(b) The 95% CI for the mean is the range from mean $-1.96$ SE to mean $+1.96$ SE, so the width of the CI is $2 \times 1.96 \times$ SE. For this to be equal to 0.5 mmol/l we need $SE = \frac{0.5}{2 \times 1.96} = 0.1276$. Assuming that we still have $SD = 2.3629$, then we would have $2.3629/\sqrt{N} = 0.1276$ which gives $N = (2.3629/0.1276)^2 = 343$.

8.3 Another way of phrasing the question is, 'What is the probability of the number in one group being less than 40 or more than 60?'. The sampling distribution for the proportion of patients allocated a particular treatment is the Binomial distribution. The SD of the distribution is $\sqrt{np(1-p)}$. Here $p = 0.5$, so the SD is $\sqrt{100 \times 0.5 \times 0.5} = 5$. Using the Normal approximation, which is excellent for $p = 0.5$, the required probability is the two-tailed area corresponding to $z = (60 - 50)/5 = 2.0$, which from Table B2 is 0.0455, or about 5%.

8.4 The use of a one-tailed test should always be specified and justified.

The justification, which I believe is rarely appropriate, is that the experimenters are only interested in a difference in a particular direction. Results of previous analyses are not an adequate justification for performing a one-tailed test.

## CHAPTER 9

9.1 (a) If the changes have a reasonably Normal distribution, then a CI could be obtained using the $t$ distribution as described in sections 9.4.1 and 9.5.1, and a paired $t$ test could be used (or, equivalently, a one sample $t$ test of the differences). A Wilcoxon test for matched data could be used if the differences had a reasonably symmetric but non-Normal distribution.

A Normal plot of the changes is quite straight, and the $W'$ test gives $W' = 0.98$, $P = 0.96$, so either of the above methods is appropriate. Because the changes have a nearly Normal distribution they will give very similar results. Using the parametric approach, the 95% confidence interval for the mean change in supine heart rate in the countermeasure group is 1.38 to 12.38 beats/min. The paired $t$ test gives $t = 2.65$ $(P = 0.017)$. The data thus appear to show that the countermeasure has reduced heart rate, but the correct approach is to compare this group with a group who did not adopt the countermeasure, as discussed below.

(b) The changes in heart rate in the group not adopting the countermeasure were not significantly non-Normal $(W' = 0.865, P = 0.10)$, and the SDs in the two groups were very similar, so we can use a two sample $t$ test to compare the changes in heart rate in the two groups. The difference between the mean changes is 10.56 and the 95% CI is 1.62 to 19.50, giving some evidence in support of the effectiveness of the countermeasure. The two sample $t$ test gives $t = 2.44$ $(P = 0.023)$.

(c) It is incorrect to analyse multiple observations on the same individuals as if they were from different people. Here the effect is likely to be minimal as only two astronauts were included twice. The duplicate data were not identified in the paper.

(d) In clinical research it is highly undesirable to let subjects choose their own treatments. No clinical trial conducted in this way would have credibility. Ideally (from the research point of view) the astronauts should have been randomized to receive the dietary countermeasure, but this was not set up as a prospective study. The likely homogeneity of the astronauts, for example with respect to fitness, would probably lessen the volunteer effect. Clearly the pre-flight heart rates in the two groups were very similar, which strengthens the findings. In the end the validity of the results is a matter of judgement.

9.2 (a) The paired $t$ test gives $t = 1.85$, $P = 0.08$. However, the test assumes that the differences have a reasonably Normal distribution, which is clearly not the case here.

(b) Even after log transformation of the original data the differences between the log values have a skewed distribution. Although the paired $t$ test gives $t = 2.77$, $P = 0.01$, it is better to use the Wilcoxon matched pairs signed ranks test, which gives $z = 2.91$, $P = 0.004$.

9.3 As was shown in Figures 9.2 and 9.3, log transformation makes these data much nearer to Normal. The mean $\log_e T_4$ counts for the Hodgkin's and non-Hodgkin's disease patients were 6.487 and 6.089 respectively, giving a difference of 0.398 (SE = 0.212). The 90% CI is 0.041 to 0.756. The antilogs of these values are 1.04 and 2.13, which give a 90% CI for the ratio of the $T_4$ counts in the two groups. The best estimate of the ratio is $\exp(0.398) = 1.49$.

9.4 The linear analogue scale data do not meet the distributional assumptions for parametric methods based on the $t$ distribution. The groups can be compared using the non-parametric Mann-Whitney test, which gives $z = 3.29$, $P = 0.001$. There is thus strong evidence that nausea was less severe in patients receiving the active treatment.

A 95% confidence interval for the difference in median scores can be obtained using the method described by Campbell and Gardner (1989), and is 15 to 49 mm. In general estimates and confidence intervals are of limited value for data like these as the measurements have no straightforward interpretation.

9.5 (a) The SDs can be calculated by multiplying the SEs by $\sqrt{n}$ to give

| Cigarettes | $n$ | Mean | SD |
|---|---|---|---|
| 1-9 | 25 | 0.31 | 0.40 |
| 10-19 | 57 | 0.42 | 0.75 |
| 20-29 | 99 | 0.87 | 1.89 |
| 30-39 | 38 | 1.03 | 1.54 |
| > 40 | 28 | 1.56 | 3.02 |
| Unspecified | 25 | 0.56 | 0.80 |

As in all cases the SD is greater than the mean (and negative values are impossible), the urinary cotinine excretion values are highly skewed to the right.

(b) Some form of analysis of trend, such as within a one way analysis of variance.

(c) If the data are to be analysed by analysis of variance then we require *standard deviations* to be similar (in theory the groups are samples from populations with the same standard deviation). There is no such requirement for standard errors, which are partly dependent on sample size. As shown above, the data do not meet this requirement. If log transformation would yield similar SDs and reasonably Normal distributions, then a linear trend could be applied in a one way analysis of variance. The 'unspecified' group would have to be excluded. The simplest approach would be to calculate the rank correlation between number of cigarettes smoked and urinary cotinine level.

(d) There are three reasons why this analysis is not valid:

(i) the data are highly skewed within each group;

(ii) the SDs vary enormously;

(iii) the use of multiple comparisons of pairs of groups is an inferior method of assessing whether there is a relation between smoking and urinary cotinine levels as it takes no account of the ordering of the groups.

9.6 The P values associated with paired Wilcoxon tests of the data for Groups 1 and 2 are 0.01 and 0.09, which are not so far apart. More revealing are the means and standard deviations of the changes:

| | Mean | SD |
|---|---|---|
| Group 1 | −0.078 | 0.073 |
| Group 2 | −0.071 | 0.129 |

The mean changes in the two groups are almost the same.

The correct way to compare the groups is by testing directly the difference between the changes in the two groups. A two sample $t$ test gives $t = 0.16$ on 22 degrees of freedom ($P = 0.88$). The SDs are rather different, so that the assumptions of the $t$ test may not be considered reasonable. A similar result is, however, obtained from a Mann-Whitney test ($z = 0.89$, $P = 0.37$). There is thus no evidence to support the idea that the groups differ.

9.7 (a) The post-treatment scores should be compared by the Mann-Whitney test because the data are not suitable for the $t$ test. This analysis gives $z = 3.22$ ($P = 0.001$), strong evidence that gestrinone is more effective than placebo in improving the scores of these patients.

(b) The same method can be applied to the changes in scores. This analysis gives $z = 2.71$ ($P = 0.007$), a result which is only slightly weaker. Alternatively the sign test could be used to compare the groups with respect to positive or negative changes.

9.8 The Mann-Whitney test could be used. As it is a test based on ranks, the censored values recorded as >80.0 would all have the same rank. As there are so many ties at this value the adjustment for ties would be desirable. Also, the SI values clearly have a skewed distribution, indicating that a non-parametric method would be suitable. An alternative, but less satisfactory, approach would be to compare the proportions above a given cut-off using methods described in the next chapter.

## CHAPTER 10

10.1 (a) It is essential to use an analysis appropriate for *paired* data. The proportions negative to croton oil and DNCB were 44/173 = 25.4% and 69/173 = 39.9% respectively. A 95% CI for the difference between these proportions, using the method given in section 10.4, is from 5% to 24%. The hypothesis test that the proportions of patients negative to the two skin tests are the same is evaluated by calculating

$$z = \frac{48 - 23}{\sqrt{48 + 23}} = 2.97$$

which, from Table B2, corresponds to P = 0.003. There is thus strong evidence that fewer of these patients show negative reactions to croton oil than DNCB.

(b) The proportions of patients with a positive reaction to DNCB are 75%, 67% and 41% for stages I, II and III respectively. The Chi squared test for trend gives $X^2_{trend} = 14.04$ on 1 degree of freedom (P = 0.0002). There is strong evidence therefore that DNCB reactivity is related to stage of cancer.

10.2 (a) The author seems to have concluded that $P > 0.05$ means that there is no effect present. However, the P value is 0.08 and so only slightly greater than 0.05.

(b) The test considered in (a) is not appropriate because it ignored the fact that the groups were ordered. The aim of the study was explicitly to study the relation between testosterone level (examined by the proxy measure of the sex ratio of siblings) and level of singing voice, so the Chi squared test for trend should be used. The test gives $X^2 = 8.92$ on 1 degree of freedom, which is highly significant (P = 0.003). We can therefore infer that there is a relation between level of singing voice and sex ratio of siblings, assuming that the test is a valid one (but see below). This does not, of course, directly answer the question about testosterone levels as they were not measured on this sample.

(c) It was chosen after inspecting the data, so the P value is not valid. In any case, it is not sensible to ignore the ordering – the trend test is far preferable.

(d) The value of $X^2$ for part of the table cannot exceed the value for the whole table. The correct value for this comparison is $X^2 = 9.44$ on 2 degrees of freedom.

(e) The observations are not independent, as the 422 siblings related to only 195 singers. Large families will carry more influence than small ones.

(f) It is not easy to say how important the non-independence is. If this is considered to be a preliminary study, leading to a study with direct analysis of testosterone levels if the results look suggestive (as they do), then it is probably not too important. In any case, there is no simple statistical way round the problem. We could study only singers with one sibling; choose one sibling at random for each singer; take each singer's oldest sibling, none of which would be very satisfactory. A completely valid statistical analysis would be highly complex.

10.3 (a) Yes, but it was not necessary. The observed frequencies were 2 and 20, but the expected frequencies (under the null hypothesis) were about 10 so the Chi squared test could have been used.

(b) The confidence intervals are based on the Normal approximation. This is not valid for the very small proportion in the placebo group, and has led to an impossible negative lower limit. More fundamentally, it is not helpful to give confidence intervals for each group separately. The 95% confidence interval for the *difference* in proportions is much more useful; it is 16% to 39%.

10.4 (a) The Mann-Whitney test or the Chi squared test for trend could be used. Each would require scores to be given to each column. These could reasonably be equally spaced; most obviously the values 1 to 8 could be used.

(b) The Mann-Whitney test is hard to apply when the samples are so large (most computer programs cannot perform the test on a table, but would require data for the 3469 children). The Chi squared test can be applied equally easily regardless of sample size. The overall comparison of the eight groups gives $X^2 = 7.83$ on 7 degrees of freedom ($P = 0.35$), and the trend test gives $X^2_{trend} = 0.04$ on 1 degree of freedom ($P = 0.84$). These figures indicate that the variation seen is likely to be due to chance and not to a tendency for boys to sleep longer than girls or *vice versa*.

10.5 (a) There is only one Chi squared test for a $2 \times 2$ table, which can be interpreted as either a comparison of the proportions in each row or in each column. The two tests described should have given the same answer.

(b) The correct test statistic is either $X^2 = 15.90$ ($P = 0.0001$) or $X^2_c = 13.93$ ($P = 0.0002$) depending on whether Yates' correction is used. Thus both of the quoted results were incorrect.

10.6 It is clear from the table that some patients had more than one of the three habits, as would be expected. It is incorrect, therefore, to calculate $X^2$ for the full $4 \times 3$ table. If we knew each patient's habits, then a complex regression analysis could be performed, using methods described in Chapter 12. From the available data we could construct 3 × 2 tables for each habit and calculate the test statistic $X^2$ on 2 degrees of freedom.

10.7 The proportions of women developing hypertension were 0.1176 (4/34) in the aspirin group and 0.3548 (11/31) in the placebo group. The difference is 0.24 with a wide 95% CI from 0.04 to 0.44. The Chi squared test with Yates' correction gives $X^2 = 3.89$ (P = 0.049). There is thus a suggestion that aspirin may reduce the risk of hypertension among pregnant women, but the wide CI points to considerable uncertainty about the magnitude of the effect.

10.8 From the information given a 2 × 2 table can be constructed as follows:

| | | Cases | | |
|---|---|---|---|---|
| | | + | − | Total |
| Controls | + | 38 | 8 | 46 |
| | − | 20 | 20 | 40 |
| Total | | 58 | 28 | 86 |

where + and − refer to presence or absence of exposure to loud noise at work.

(a) The proportions of cases and controls reporting exposure to loud noise were 0.674 (58/86) and 0.535 (46/86). The difference in proportions is 0.14, with the 95% CI of 0.02 to 0.26. The proportions can be compared using McNemar's test, which gives

$$z_c = 11/\sqrt{28} = 2.08 \text{ (P = 0.04)}.$$

(b) The odds ratio is estimated as 20/8 = 2.5. The 95% CI (method not given in Chapter 10) is 1.05 to 6.56.

## CHAPTER 11

11.1 (a) Yes. The censored survival time was also the longest and thus gets the highest rank. The method cannot generally be used for survival data because the censored data mean that the order of survival times cannot be determined.

(b) The Pearson correlation coefficient could be calculated but it would be severely inflated by the very long survival time (even ignoring the censoring). The distribution of survival times is highly skewed, so rank correlation is far preferable here.

(c) The changes in lactate, bicarbonate and pH have Spearman rank correlation coefficients with survival time of 0.63, −0.67 and −0.42 respectively, so the strongest relation is with changes in bicarbonate. Note that bicarbonate and pH have negative associations with survival while for lactate the correlation is positive.

11.2 (a) The linear regression equation is

$$\text{RMR} = 811.23 + 7.0595 \times \text{weight}$$

and the residual SD is 157.91 kcal/24hr.

(b) A scatter diagram shows no obvious relation between the residuals and weight. The test of Normality of the residuals gives $W' = 0.955$, $P > 0.05$. The distribution is reasonably Normal – the largest residual relates to the woman with the highest RMR. Overall, there is no reason to reject the validity of the analysis.

(c) The SE of the slope of the regression line is 0.9776 kcal/24 hr, so the 95% CI is

$$7.0595 - 2.018 \times 0.9776 \text{ to } 7.0595 + 2.018 \times 0.9776$$

or 5.09 to 9.03 kcal/24 hr.

(d) The SD of the residuals is 157.91 kcal/24 hr, so the narrowest prediction interval (at the mean value of body weight) is about twice this amount either side of the predicted value. Thus it is not possible to predict RMR from body weight to within 250 kcal/24 hr.

11.3 (a) The regression of $\log_e$Vcf on blood glucose gives the equation

$$\log_e \text{Vcf} = 0.115 + 0.0148 \times \text{blood glucose}.$$

The residual SD is 0.2167.

(b) The test of Normality of the residuals from this regression line gives $W' = 0.936$, $P > 0.1$. The residuals after log transformation are thus more nearly Normal than those from the analysis of the raw data.

(c) From the regression equation using the raw values of Vcf (Table 11.6) the predicted Vcf is $1.10 + 0.0220 \times 16 = 1.45$%/sec. The 95% prediction interval is $1.45 \pm 2.080 \times 0.229$ or 0.97 to 1.93%/sec. From the above regression equation using log transformed Vcf, the predicted Vcf is $\exp(0.115 + 0.0148 \times 16) = e^{0.352} = 1.42$%/sec. The 95% prediction interval is $\exp(0.352 \pm 2.080 \times 0.164)$ or 1.01 to 2.00%/sec. The two equations thus give similar answers for someone with a blood glucose of 16 mmol/l.

11.4 The values for the last two subjects are identical, suggesting a transcription error or the inadvertent inclusion of the same patient twice.

11.5 The correlations between log creatinine clearance (CC), log digoxin clearance (DC) and urine flow are:

| | $r$ | P |
|---|---|---|
| DC CC | 0.838 | < 0.0001 |
| DC flow | 0.515 | 0.002 |
| CC flow | 0.322 | 0.06 |

These figures support the first statement but do not appear to support the second. A better answer is obtained by considering all three variables at once, by calculating the partial correlation coefficients. The partial correlation coefficient between DC and CC adjusting for urine flow is 0.83 ($P < 0.0001$), and that between DC and flow adjusting for CC is 0.47 (0.005), hardly different from the simple correlation coefficients. The data thus support the first but not the second of the statements about digoxin clearance.

## CHAPTER 12

12.1 (a) (i) A paired $t$ test or, equivalently, a two way analysis of variance.

(ii) Same as (i).

(b) The data of interest can be rewritten as

| | Diet | |
|---|---|---|
| Subject | N | O |
| 1 | 0.31 | 0.77 |
| 2 | 0.26 | 0.43 |
| 3 | 0.16 | 0.25 |
| 4 | 0.27 | 0.39 |
| 5 | 0.18 | 0.25 |

The mean and SD of the differences between the diets (O–N) are 0.182 and 0.160, so the paired $t$ test gives $t = 2.545$. The appropriate value of the $t$ distribution ($t_{0.975}$) on 4 degrees of freedom is 2.776, so the difference is not quite statistically significant at the 5% level ($P = 0.06$). The 95% CI for the mean difference is $0.182 \pm 2.776 \times 0.160/\sqrt{5}$ or −0.02 to 0.38. The two way analysis of variance, with factors diet and subject, gives $F = 6.48$ for the comparison between the diets – this is the square of the $t$ value as expected.

12.2 Backwards stepwise multiple regression yields the following model

$$\text{FRC} = 286.94 - 4.1965 \times \text{age} - 2.0386 \times \text{FEV}_1.$$

The residual SD is 26.7, compared with the SD of the raw FRC values which was 43.7, indicating that the model explains a good proportion of the variability in FRC. The value of $R^2$ is 66%.

A test of Normality of the residuals gives $W' = 0.966$, $P > 0.2$, indicating that the residuals have a closely Normal distribution.

12.3 (a) Recipient and donor ages can be compared by two sample $t$ tests, as can the log index values (the raw index values are skewed). The results of these are

| | No GvHD | | GvHD | | | |
|---|---|---|---|---|---|---|
| | Mean | SD | Mean | SD | $t$ | P |
| Recip age | 22.4 | 5.18 | 28.4 | 8.10 | 2.73 | 0.01 |
| Donor age | 23.1 | 6.69 | 29.0 | 8.07 | 2.43 | 0.02 |
| Log index | 0.111 | 0.860 | 1.115 | 0.662 | 3.92 | 0.0006 |

The type of leukaemia and whether the donor had been pregnant can be related to GvHD by Chi squared tests:

| | Type of leukaemia | | | | Donor pregnancy | |
|---|---|---|---|---|---|---|
| | AML | ALL | CML | | No | Yes |
| No GvHD | 6 | 12 | 2 | No GvHD | 18 | 2 |
| GvHD | 5 | 4 | 8 | GvHD | 9 | 8 |

$X^2 = 7.497$ on 2 df (P = 0.02) $X^2 = 4.66$ on 1 df (P = 0.03)

Thus all five variables are significantly different between the groups of patients who did and did not develop GvHD. This suggests that it might be possible to find a logistic regression model that discriminates usefully between the groups.

(b) The results given here relate to backward stepwise multiple logistic regression with the following potential explanatory variables: recipient's age, donor's age, donor pregnancy, log index, and two dummy variables indicating whether the patient did (1) or did not (0) have ALL and CML. Using the 5% level of statistical significance to decide whether to retain a variable in the analysis, the following model is obtained:

| Variable | Coefficient | SE | $z$ | P |
|---|---|---|---|---|
| Constant | −2.546 | | | |
| CML | 2.251 | 1.106 | 2.035 | 0.04 |
| Pregnancy | 2.496 | 1.101 | 2.266 | 0.02 |
| Log index | 1.488 | 0.720 | 2.067 | 0.04 |

All three variables in this model are only moderately significant.

For each patient we can calculate the probability of GvHD on the basis of this model, and relate these to what actually happened. The probability $p$ is obtained from the logistic regression model:

$$l = \text{logit}(p)$$
$$= -2.546 + 2.251 \times \text{CML} + 2.496 \times \text{pregnancy} + 1.488 \times \text{log index}$$

or

$$p = \exp(l)/[1 + \exp(l)].$$

It should be remembered that the assessment of a model using the same data that were used to derive the model will give a slightly optimistic picture. It is best to use new data to test a model.

(c) For a binary variable in a logistic regression model, the odds ratio is given by $e^b$ where $b$ is the estimated regression coefficient. This corresponds to the increased odds associated with being in the group coded 1 compared to the group coded 0.

For CML we have $OR = e^{2.251} = 9.5$ and for pregnancy we have $OR = e^{2.496} = 12.1$. 90% CIs are obtained as $e^{b \pm 1.645 SE(b)}$. For CML these values are 1.54 and 58.6; for pregnancy they are 1.98 and 74.2. Both CIs are extremely wide, showing that precise estimates cannot be obtained from a sample this small.

12.4 (a) $e^{1.167} = 3.21$

(b) $1000 \times 1.167/0.0106 = 110\,094$. Smoking 20 cigarettes per day is equal to $20 \times 365 = 7300$ per year, so a total of about 110 000 cigarettes is equivalent to smoking 20 per day for about 15 years.

(c) The total number of cigarettes smoked is $20 \times 365 \times 30 = 219\,000$, so the odds ratio is $\exp(1.167 + 219 \times 0.0106) = 32.7$. This is ten times the odds ratio for family history in a non-smoker.

12.5 (a) The multiple regression model is

| Variable | Coefficient | SE | $t$ | P |
|---|---|---|---|---|
| Constant | −6.7459 | 4.3923 | −1.536 | 0.14 |
| Age | −0.0260 | 0.0241 | −1.080 | 0.29 |
| Sex | −0.8029 | 0.5120 | −1.568 | 0.13 |
| Height | 0.0880 | 0.0252 | 3.497 | 0.002 |

Only height is statistically significant in this model. The residual SD is 1.185 and $R^2 = 0.54$. The residual SD is the SD of the differences between the observed values and those predicted by the regression model. This represents a considerable reduction in comparison with the SD of 1.657 for the raw lung capacity values, but still indicates a large prediction error in some cases. For 5% of cases we would expect the model to err by more than about 2.37 l (twice the residual SD), which is more than a third of the mean lung volume (which is 6.05 l).

(b) The linear regression equation of lung volume on height is

$$\text{lung volume} = -9.869 + 0.0951 \times \text{height}.$$

The SE of the slope is 0.0184 and the residual SD is 1.227, and $R^2 = 0.47$. These values suggest that the multiple regression model fits the data only marginally better than the linear regression on height, as was indicated by the non-significant coefficients for age and sex in the first model.

(c) Using the above results of linear regression of lung volume on height, the 95% prediction interval for someone with average lung capacity is

$$6.047 \pm 2.042 \times 1.227\sqrt{1 + 1/32}$$

or 3.50 to 8.59 l.

(d) The simple way is to carry out separate regressions for males and females, which give slopes of 0.0736 and 0.0745.

However, the correct way to test the hypothesis that the slopes are the same is by fitting a multiple regression model including an interaction term. As we would expect from the similar slopes just given, the interaction is nowhere near to being statistically significant. As we have also seen that there was no significant effect of sex in the multiple regression model, we can reasonably conclude that the relation between lung volume and height is the same for males and females.

## CHAPTER 13

13.1 If we take the three values censored before the end of the experiment as events, we get

$$O_1 = 7; \quad E_1 = 10.2339; \quad O_2 = 15; \quad E_2 = 11.7661$$

giving $X^2 = 1.91$, $P = 0.17$. The evidence for a difference is now much weaker.

13.2 (a) Because the longest survival time is so much greater than the next longest, the meaningful early part of the curve will be severely compressed at the left hand side. The graph is much more useful if this patient is excluded. As noted in section 13.8.2, stopping the curve when there are only five patients still alive will usually give a more reliable visual impression.

(b) The logrank test is used to compare survival in different groups of patients. Where the variable of interest is continuous, as here, we can create groups of patients corresponding to broad ranges of values and perform the logrank test for trend.

A common approach is to divide the patients into three equal sized groups. Groups of size 10, 10 and 9 give the following results:

| Variable | Logrank $X^2$ Overall (2 df) | Trend (1 df) | P |
|---|---|---|---|
| Lactate | 10.19 | 9.47 | 0.002 |
| Bicarbonate | 17.26 | 15.01 | 0.0001 |
| pH | 6.10 | 4.62 | 0.03 |

For each variable the trend is statistically significant, and most of the variation between groups is due to the trend. Thus the changes in all of the three variables are related to survival time.

(c) Cox regression models of each of the three variables treated either as continuous or split into three groups as in the previous analysis are summarized in the following table:

| | Continuous | | | Grouped | | |
|---|---|---|---|---|---|---|
| | $b$ | SE($b$) | P | $b$ | SE($b$) | P |
| Lactate | −0.071 | 0.019 | 0.001 | −0.061 | 0.022 | 0.01 |
| Bicarbonate | 0.186 | 0.051 | 0.001 | 0.087 | 0.022 | 0.0001 |
| pH | 3.921 | 1.704 | 0.03 | 0.965 | 0.395 | 0.02 |

The regression coefficients, $b$, should not be directly compared for the two types of analysis. All three variables are significantly associated with survival by either method, but the level of significance differs. In general, the grouped analysis will give a very similar answer to the logrank test for trend.

If the three variables are all entered into a Cox model together only bicarbonate is statistically significant.

13.3 (a) The opposite signs mean that high values of one variable and low values of the other variable are associated with an increased risk of dying. A positive regression coefficient means that high values of that variable are associated with worse survival, and conversely for a negative coefficient. Thus the model predicts that survival is worse for non-CML patients and those with GvHD.

(b) We need to calculate the prognostic index for each group of patients. These are as follows:

| | | PI |
|---|---|---|
| non-GvHD | non-CML | 0.000 |
| non-GvHD | CML | −2.508 |
| GvHD | non-CML | 2.306 |
| GvHD | CML | −0.202 (= −2.508 + 2.306) |

The relative risk of dying relative to the non-GvHD non-CML group is simply $e^{PI}$ as the PI for that group is zero. Thus the risks of dying in the other groups relative to non-GvHD non-CML patients are

| | | |
|---|---|---|
| non-GvHD | CML | 0.08 |
| GvHD | non-CML | 10.03 |
| GvHD | CML | 0.82 |

(c) The 95% CI is given by the range $e^{2.306-1.96\times0.5898}$ to $e^{2.306+1.96\times0.5898}$, or 3.16 to 31.9.
(d) A Cox model based on such a small sample would be extremely unreliable, as is indicated by the wide CI given above. It is the number of 'events', here deaths, that determines the power of a Cox analysis, not the number of subjects.

## CHAPTER 14

14.1 (a) The Wilcoxon test (or the *t* test) assesses whether the values obtained by the two methods differ *on average*. It is essential also to consider how well they agree for individual patients, which cannot be done by a hypothesis test.
(b) A simple analysis is based on calculating the 95% limits of agreement from the mean and SD of the differences between the two methods, and by plotting the differences against the average of the two values.

The mean and SD of the differences ($^{51}$Cr−biotin) are −85.0 and 221.9 ml respectively, so the 95% limits of agreement are −529 to +359 ml. This very wide range is completely disguised by the non-significant Wilcoxon test. Figure A14.1 shows the differences plotted against the average of the two values. There is no evidence that the magnitude of the differences varies with red cell volume. The 95% limits of agreement are shown as solid lines.
(c) The red cell volumes of these patients may be systematically different from those in the healthy population. It does not necessarily follow that the methods would agree equally badly (or equally well) in a different population with a different range of red cell volumes.
(d) If one method is affected by consumption of eggs then it would be advisable to exclude patients who had eaten eggs. In contrast, it would be completely invalid to omit some patients simply because

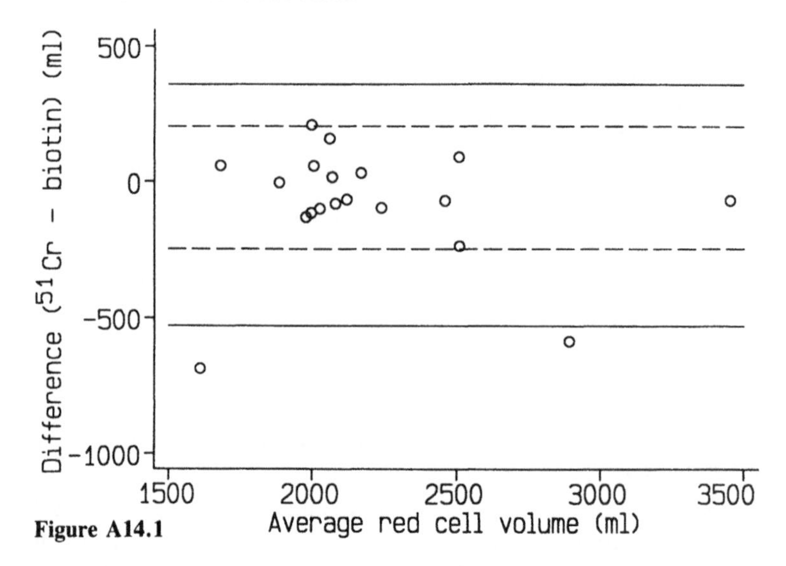

**Figure A14.1**

their data were discrepant. The authors' comment is curious, as they do not say which of the patients had eaten an egg. If the two patients with suspect values are excluded, the mean and SD of the between method differences become −20.2 and 112.2 ml, a considerable improvement. The revised limits of agreement are shown in Figure A14.1 as dashed lines.

14.2 (a) The means are plotted in Figure A14.2. The means for the two groups show a very similar pattern.

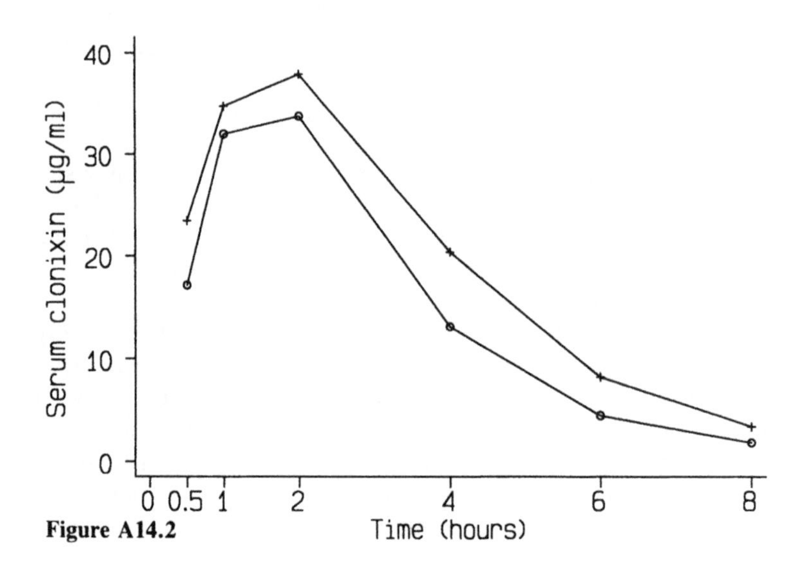

**Figure A14.2**

(b) The mean and SD of the peak values and areas under the curves for the two groups are

| | Rheumatoid arthritis patients | | Controls | |
|---|---|---|---|---|
| | Mean | SD | Mean | SD |
| Peak | 39.96 | 9.13 | 46.12 | 10.58 |
| AUC | 120.05 | 33.61 | 154.93 | 48.23 |

The two groups can be compared by two sample $t$ tests, which give $t = 1.53$ (P = 0.14) and $t = 2.06$ (P = 0.052) respectively. (Mann-Whitney tests give very similar results.) There is thus some evidence that the area under the curve is lower among patients with rheumatoid arthritis.

(c) The individual curves shown in Figure A14.3 show considerable variation – many look very different from the mean curves. It is a matter of judgement whether the means are a good representation of the overall pattern.

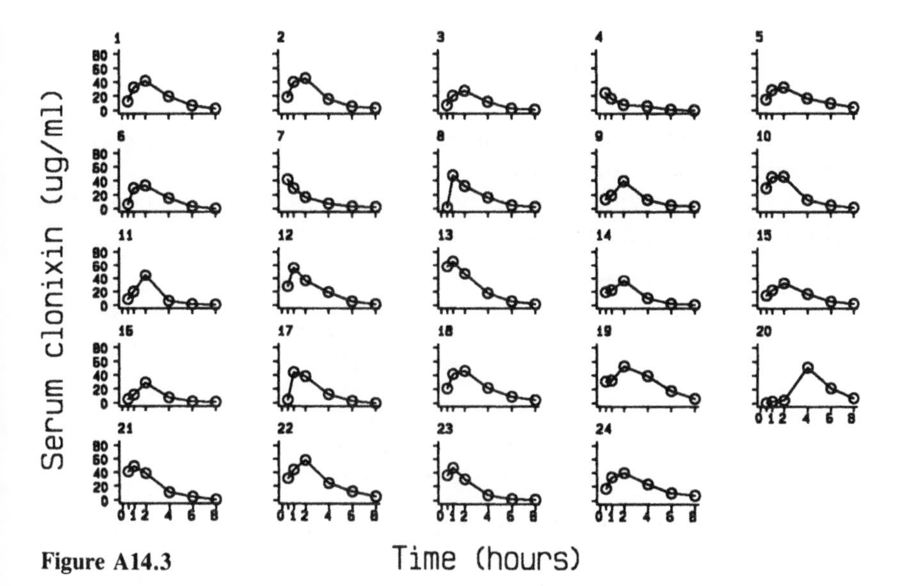


**Figure A14.3**

14.3 (a) The two thirds of drug users who admitted the fact would not be allowed to give blood. Among the other third we would expect 0.24 (24%) to pass the test, and thus give blood. Among the non-drug users we would expect 0.63 (63%) to pass the test and give blood.

Thus the proportion of blood donors who would be drug users is

$$\frac{0.24 \times 0.33 \times 0.05}{0.24 \times 0.33 \times 0.05 + 0.63 \times 0.95} = 0.007.$$

(b) Among the two thirds of drug users who lied, we would expect 0.76 (76%) to fail the polygraph test. Among non-drug users we would expect 0.37 (37%) to fail the test too. Thus the expected proportion of drug users among those failing the test is

$$\frac{0.76 \times 0.33 \times 0.05}{0.76 \times 0.33 \times 0.05 + 0.37 \times 0.95} = 0.035.$$

In other words, almost all of those rejected by the test (about 96%) would be non-drug users. To pick up one drug user it would be necessary to reject falsely about 27 genuine donors.

14.4 (a) Taking the cut-off as respiratory rates less than or equal to 30, 40, 50 or 60 breaths/min gives

| Cut-off | Sensitivity | Specificity |
|---|---|---|
| 30 | 141/142 = 99% | 16/151 = 11% |
| 40 | 137/142 = 96% | 93/151 = 62% |
| 50 | 127/142 = 89% | 139/151 = 92% |
| 60 | 86/142 = 61% | 148/151 = 98% |

The best cut-off is 50 breaths/min, with an overall correct assessment for 266/293 = 91% of infants.

(b) Using the formulae for the positive and negative predictive values (PPV and NPV) given in section 14.4.5, the required values are

| Cut-off | PPV | NPV |
|---|---|---|
| 30 | 3.3% | 99.8% |
| 40 | 7% | 99.8% |
| 50 | 26% | 99.6% |
| 60 | 49% | 98.8% |

With low prevalence, as here, the NPV is usually not helpful. The PPV increases as the cut off level rises, so the 'best' choice to maximize correct predictions is a cut-off of 60 breaths/min. However, as we have seen, with this cut-off nearly half of the infants with LRI would be missed. A cut-off of 50 breaths/min would mean that nearly all infants with LRI would be identified, but that more of the infants identified by the test would not have LRI (false positives) compared with a cut-off of 60 breaths/min. Note that about half of the study sample had LRI – they were inpatients and thus unrepresentative of the general population of infants with acute respiratory infection where the prevalence of LRI is much lower.

(c) The PPV is the proportion of those infants with respiratory rate $>50$ who have LRI, which is 26%. Thus if all infants with a respiratory rate above the cut-off are treated with antibiotics, 74% of them will have been treated 'unnecessarily'. The sensitivity is 89% at this cut-off, which means that 89% of LRI infants would receive antibiotics. Thus 11% would not get antibiotics. At the lower cut-off of 40 breaths/min the proportion with LRI treated with antibiotics would be rather higher (96%) but only 7% of those treated would have LRI. It should be clear that the choice of cut-off must be made on non-statistical considerations.

(d) If all infants above the cut-off are treated then 89% of LRI infants and 8% of URI infants would be treated. Taking the proportion with LRI as 3%, the proportion treated would be $0.89 \times 0.03 + 0.08 \times 0.97 = 0.10$. Thus only 10% of infants would be treated with antibiotics, representing an enormous saving in cost. Even using a cutoff of 40 breaths/min the proportion treated would be $0.96 \times 0.03 + 0.38 \times 0.97 = 0.40$, which would cost half as much as the existing policy.

14.5 (a) For each pair of dentists each tooth can be categorized SS, SC, CS or CC by aggregating the relevant rows of the table. The resulting $2 \times 2$ tables can be assessed by calculating kappa, as follows:

| | SS | SC | CS | CC | kappa | %agree |
|---|---|---|---|---|---|---|
| 1 v 2 | 3520 | 280 | 123 | 216 | 0.46 | 97% |
| 1 v 3 | 2182 | 1348 | 43 | 296 | 0.18 | 64% |
| 2 v 3 | 2164 | 1209 | 61 | 435 | 0.26 | 67% |

Also shown is the percentage agreement. Thus the best agreement is between dentists 1 and 2. Dentist 3 considered that there were many more carious teeth (1644) than the other two observers (339 and 496).

(b) A kappa value of 0.46 is not usually considered to be especially good agreement, but dentists 1 and 2 agreed about 97% of the teeth examined. This discrepancy is because they both considered the large majority of teeth to be sound. Among the 619 teeth which at least one of dentists 1 and 2 considered carious, they agreed on only 216 (35%). Good agreement depends upon circumstances, not upon the kappa value (and certainly not upon the P value – because of the huge sample size, all the above kappa values are highly statistically significant).

## CHAPTER 15

15.1 Differences in baseline values in the treatment groups for variables which might affect patient prognosis could affect the result of the trial. It is the magnitude of the imbalance that is important – statistical significance is irrelevant. In Table 3.5, the differences are trivial except perhaps for pain at presentation. As pain score was also the outcome measure for the trial this imbalance could be important. It may therefore be reasonable to analyse the change in pain from baseline rather than the value at the end of the study. (In fact, in this study the authors noted that the baseline pain score was not prognostic.) When there is imbalance in a variable for which the prognostic value is unknown, the outcome can be examined in relation to the values of that variable for each treatment group. Imbalance in a prognostic variable is handled by adjusting the comparison of treatment groups using regression analysis, see section 15.4.

15.2 (a) Only those allocated alprenolol would have been withdrawn because of contraindication for the beta-blocker. The two groups, apart from being of unequal size, would thus have been non-comparable, and the trial results would be unsound.
(b) No.
(c) By not allocating treatments (randomizing) until immediately before starting treatment.

15.3 (a) This was an uncontrolled trial, which is not a proper way to evaluate a treatment. Another very poor feature of this study was that the study was 'open', so that the patients knew when they were taking aspirin. Further, the study was extremely small, especially bearing in mind that the measurements were highly variable.
(b) The standard deviations are obtained as SE × $\sqrt{13}$, or 36.1, 26.7 and 19.8 for the three sets of observations. The data are thus skewed, especially before treatment, because the SD is more than half the mean.
(c) The paper gives no indication about how the data were analysed (if at all). An appropriate analysis would be a paired Wilcoxon test to compare any two sets of data, or a paired $t$ test if the differences were reasonably Normal. Two way analysis of variance could be used to compare all three groups simultaneously. As noted, however, these analyses would be of limited value because there was no comparison group.
(d) The mean and SD (or SE) of the within-subject changes would be valuable, as would a CI for the changes.
(e) For the reasons already given, the design of this study was inappropriate to answer the question. The data do in fact show some improvement, although it is implied that this was not statistically

significant. Confidence intervals would be very wide. It is totally wrong to suggest that on the basis of this small study the possibility of an effect of aspirin can be excluded.

15.4 (a) Paired $t$ tests for the two groups give $t = 4.23$ (on 8 df; $P = 0.003$) and $t = 1.58$ (on 6 df; $P = 0.17$). The highly significant changes in one group only may suggest that there is indeed a difference between the groups. However, these are within group analyses whereas the whole point of a clinical trial is to compare the groups directly. We should do this using a two sample $t$ test on the values after one week of treatment or on the changes in systolic blood pressure, not via an indirect comparison of P values from independent analyses. The authors' interpretation is not valid.
(b) The means (SD) of the changes for the two groups are 12.67 (8.99) and 4.71 (7.91) respectively, and the $t$ test gives $t = 1.85$ (14 df; $P = 0.09$). (Likewise, a comparison of the one week blood pressures gives $t = 1.65$ (14 df; $P = 0.12$).) There is thus some weak evidence that the groups may differ – the conclusion drawn by the authors is not supported by a correct analysis.

15.5 (a) As described in section 15.3, the standardized difference here is

$$\frac{0.3 - 0.2}{\sqrt{0.25 \times 0.75}} = 0.23.$$

Using the nomogram in Figure 15.2, the required sample size is 600 (300 per group).
(b) About 15%.
(c) A standardized difference of 0.7 gives 80% power with a sample of size 65. Taking the risk of hypertension in the placebo group as 0.3, we have

$$\frac{0.3 - p_a}{\sqrt{\bar{p}(1 - \bar{p})}} = 0.7$$

where $p_a$ is the proportion developing hypertension in the aspirin group and $\bar{p}$ is the average of 0.3 and $p_a$. This equation can be solved mathematically or by trial and error; the answer is $p_a = 0.04$. The trial was clearly too small to have a good chance of detecting all but a very large benefit of treatment.
(d) The Chi squared test with Yates' correction gives $X^2 = 3.89$ ($P = 0.049$). The P value quoted is one-sided, although there is no comment to that effect in the paper. The result is thus only marginally significant. The RR of 0.33 has a very wide 95% CI from 0.12 to 0.93. The authors are right to interpret their findings cautiously, and to suggest that a larger trial would be needed to confirm (or not) the benefit of aspirin in this setting.

## CHAPTER 16

16.1 The P value is a measure of the strength of evidence against the null hypothesis. It does not indicate the magnitude of the observed effect. Two clinical trials of different sizes may yield the same treatment effect but different P values. For continuous variables the P value also depends upon the variability (see exercise 9.6).

16.2 If we do not consider 'identical' to refer to sample size, then one reason could be variation in the numbers of patients studied. Two identical studies of the same size would not be expected to yield exactly the same results. The observed effects (and P values) would tend to be closer if the studies were large than if they were small. Dramatically different results for large studies may mean that the studies were not as 'identical' as claimed. For example, there may be differences between patients in different countries or between laboratories.

16.3 (a) Assuming a Normal distribution, the average height of men can be expressed as $(179.1 - 171.7)/5.75$ standard deviations above the mean height of women. This value is 1.287. From Table B1 the upper tail areas corresponding to standard Normal deviates of 1.25 and 1.30 are 0.1056 and 0.0968, so the required value is 0.10 or 10%.

(b) The probability of a man being taller than 182.9 cm is the upper tail area of the Normal distribution corresponding to $z = (182.9 - 179.1)/5.84 = 0.65$, which from Table B1 is 0.2578. For women we require the tail area corresponding to $z = (182.9 - 171.7)/5.75 = 1.95$, which is 0.0256. If 60% of adults are women the proportion of adults taller than 182.9 cm who are women is given by

$$\frac{0.6 \times 0.0256}{0.4 \times 0.2578 + 0.6 \times 0.0256}$$

$$= 0.1296 \text{ or } 13\%.$$

16.4 The age-structure of the population has changed markedly, with the proportion of older people being much higher than it was. The total death rate, which is calculated by multiplying the age-specific rates and the numbers at risk, is unchanged because the age-specific reductions in rates are counterbalanced by the greater numbers of elderly people.

16.5 (a) No, because the figures are percentages. Although it is a method of comparing proportions (or percentages) the Chi squared test must be performed on frequencies.

(b) The percentages are $73/457 = 16.0\%$ and $138/370 = 37.3\%$, so the difference is 21%. The 95% confidence interval is 15% to 27%. Because the sample is large the interval is quite narrow.

(c) The simplest way to assess a trend is to use the Chi squared test for trend. It is reasonable to give equally spaced scores to the three social class groups (such as −1, 0 and 1). Those children whose social class was unclassified must be excluded. The proportions being compared were shown at the beginning of the problem. The Chi squared tests give $X^2_{trend} = 3.64$ (P = 0.06) and $X^2_{trend} = 7.69$ (P = 0.006).

(d) Although the trend is significant (at the 5% level) in one group but not the other, we should not infer that the relation is present only within the non-fluoridated area. The simplest way to compare the trends is to use the regression approach to estimate the change in %dmft for each change in social class category (section 11.15.2) and compare the slopes (section 11.12.1). Alternatively, all the data could be analysed at once in a complicated logistic regression analysis.

(e) The technical term for such a heterogeneity of effect is 'interaction'.

16.6 (a) A graph of the differences between the indirect and direct measurements against their average shows no tendency for the differences to be related to the level of blood pressure. The mean and SD of differences were −4.80 and 12.46 respectively, so 95% limits of agreement are −29.72 to 20.12 mm Hg.

(b) The values −10 and +10 are respectively −0.42 and 1.18 SDs from the mean. Assuming that the differences come from a Normal population, the probability of a difference larger than 10 in either direction is the probability of being less than −10 plus the probability of being greater than 10, which (from Table B1) is 0.3372 + 0.1190 = 0.4562, or about 46%. Alternatively, we can take the observed proportion as an estimate, which is 22/50 = 0.44 or 44%. (This method is less reliable when the differences are Normal.)

(c) Pearson correlation coefficients are 0.32 ($P < 0.01$) with weight, 0.18 ($P > 0.10$) with arm circumference and −0.24 ($P > 0.05$) with age. There is thus some evidence that the discrepancy between the direct and indirect measurements increases with body weight. The slope of the regression line is 0.394 (SE = 0.167), indicating an estimated increase in the difference between the methods of 4 mm Hg per 10 kg additional body weight.

(d) It could be due to a 'learning effect' with the new direct method of measurement. The rank correlation between the differences and the order of measurement is 0.37 ($P < 0.01$).

(e) The Mean and SD of the differences between the measurements from the last 40 women are −2.93 and 11.47 mm Hg, so that the 95% limits of agreement are −25.87 and 20.01. These limits are not much narrower than those derived using the data from all 50 women.

16.7 (a) The data for the three days can be examined by a two way analysis of variance. The means and SDs for the three days are:

| | Mean | SD |
|---|---|---|
| Day 1 | 151.27 | 62.37 |
| Day 2 | 194.40 | 78.77 |
| Day 3 | 111.47 | 61.14 |

As the SDs are similar it is likely that the assumptions for a parametric analysis will be met, but the residuals should be checked after fitting the model. The comparison of the three times within the analysis of variance gives $F = 7.24$ on 2 and 28 degrees of freedom (P = 0.003). The Shapiro-Francia $W'$ test of the residuals from this model gives $W' = 0.992$ (P = 0.97), showing that the residuals have a distribution very close to Normal.

As there is highly significant variation among the days it is reasonable to examine each pair of days using $t$ tests with the SE based on the residual SD from the analysis of variance (which is 59.7175 mmol/l). These tests give:

| | Difference | $t$ | P | P* |
|---|---|---|---|---|
| Day 1 v Day 2 | 43.13 | 1.98 | 0.06 | 0.17 |
| Day 1 v Day 3 | −39.80 | −1.82 | 0.08 | 0.24 |
| Day 2 v Day 3 | −82.93 | −3.80 | 0.0007 | 0.002 |

where P* is P multiplied by 3 (the Bonferroni adjustment). Days 2 and 3 are highly significantly different, even after the Bonferroni correction. The other differences are not significant, but the mean changes in plasma aldosterone are quite large.

(b) The residual SD should also be used to construct a CI for the difference between any pair of means. The 95% CI for the difference between the means on days 1 and 2 is given by $43.13 \pm 2.048 \times 59.7175 \times \sqrt{\frac{1}{15} + \frac{1}{15}}$, or −1.53 to 87.79 mmol/l. This wide CI suggests that there may well be a real change in plasma aldosterone associated with a rapid change from low to high altitude, but a larger study would be needed to investigate this possibility.

(c) The correlation coefficient between the mountain sickness score (AMS) and the change in plasma aldosterone is −0.36 (P = 0.19). There is little evidence that the two variables are related.

16.8 No, this is not a reasonable argument. It is true that the confidence interval will be wide. This is not meaningless, but rather indicates that the study was too small to enable precise conclusions to be drawn.

# REFERENCES

Ahlmark, G. and Saetre, H. (1976) Long-term treatment with beta-blockers after myocardial infarction. *Eur. J. Clin. Pharmacol.*, **10**, 77–83. [Ex 15.2]

Albert, D. A. (1981) Deciding whether the conclusions of studies are justified: a review. *Med. Decision Making*, **1**, 265–75. [16.1]

Altman, D. G. (1982a) Misuse of statistics is unethical. In *Statistics in Practice* (eds S. M. Gore and D. G. Altman), London, British Medical Association, 1–2. [15.2.9, 16.1]

Altman, D. G. (1982b) How large a sample? In *Statistics in Practice* (eds S. M. Gore and D. G. Altman), London, British Medical Association, 6–8. [15.3.2]

Altman, D. G. (1982c) Improving the quality of statistics in medical journals. In *Statistics in Practice* (eds S. M. Gore and D. G. Altman), London, British Medical Association, 21–4. [16.3.10]

Altman, D. G. (1985) Comparability of randomised groups. *Statistician*, **34**, 125–36. [15.4.1, 15.4.6]

Altman, D. G. and Bland, J. M. (1991) Improving doctors' understanding of statistics. *J. Roy. Statist. Soc.*, A. (in press). [16.3.9]

Altman, D. G. and Coles, E. C. (1980) Assessing birth weight-for-dates on a continuous scale. *Ann. Hum. Biol.*, **7**, 35–44. [11.12.2, 14.5.4]

Altman, D. G. and Doré, C. J. (1990) Randomisation and baseline comparisons in clinical trials. *Lancet*, **335**, 149–53. [16.3.7]

Altman, D. G. and Gardner, M. J. (1989) Confidence intervals for regression and correlation. In *Statistics with Confidence* (eds M. J. Gardner and D. G. Altman), London, British Medical Journal, 34–49. [11.12.1]

Altman, D. G., Gore, S. M., Gardner, M. J. and Pocock, S. J. (1989) Statistical guidelines for contributors to medical journals. In *Statistics with Confidence* (eds M. J. Gardner and D. G. Altman), London, British Medical Journal, 83–100. [15.6.1, 16.5]

Altman, D. G. and Johnson, A. L. (1990) A survey of reviews of the quality of statistics in the medical literature. III. Findings (in preparation) [16.3.1, 16.3.2]

Altman, D. G. and Royston, J. P. (1988) The hidden effect of time. *Stat. Med.*, **7**, 629–37. [7.7.2]

Amess, J. A. L., Burman, J. F., Rees, G. M., *et al.* (1978) Megaloblastic haemopoiesis in patients receiving nitrous oxide. *Lancet*, **ii**, 339–42. [9.8.2]

Andréasson, S., Allebeck, P., Engström, A. and Rydberg, U. (1987) Cannabis and schizophrenia. A longitudinal study of Swedish conscripts. *Lancet*, **ii**, 1483–6. [5.11.2, 5.14]

Anon (1937) Mathematics and medicine. *Lancet*, **i**, 31. [16.3.9]

Anon (1954) Numbering off. *Br. Med. J.*, **1**, 1314. [16.2]

Anon (1978) The anomaly that wouldn't go away. *Lancet*, **ii**, 978. [11.17]

Apgar, V. (1953) Proposal for new method of evaluation of newborn infants, *Anesth. Analg.*, **32**, 260–7. [2.4.4]

Apgar, V., Holaday, D. A., James, L. S., *et al.* (1958) Evaluation of the newborn infant – second report. *J. Am. Med. Ass.*, **168**, 1985–8. [2.4.4]

Armitage, P. and Berry, G. (1987) *Statistical Methods in Medical Research*, 2nd

edn, Oxford: Blackwell. [6.7, 7.6.1, 9.6.5, 9.8.2, 12.3.4, 13.2.2]
Ayesh, R., Mitchell, S. C., Waring, R. H., *et al.* (1987) Sodium aurothiomalate toxicity and sulphoxidation capacity in rheumatoid arthritic patients. *Br. J. Rheumatol.*, **26**, 197–201. [Ex 3.1, Ex 10.5]
Bachs, L., Parés, A., Elena, M., *et al.* (1989) Comparison of rifampicin with phenobarbitone for treatment of pruritis in biliary cirrhosis. *Lancet*, **i**, 574–6. [15.4.10]
Bagot, M., Mary, J.-Y., Heslan, M., *et al.* (1988) The mixed epidermal cell lymphocyte-reaction is the most predictive factor of acute graft-versus-host disease in bone marrow graft recipients. *Br. J. Haematol.*, **70**, 403–9. [Ex 12.3]
Bailar, J. C. (1986) Communicating with a scientific audience. In *Medical Uses of Statistics* (eds J. C. Bailar and F. Mosteller), Waltham, Mass.: NEJM Books, 325–37. [16.5]
Bailar, J. C., Louis, T. A., Lavori, P. W. and Polansky, M. (1984) A classification for biomedical research reports. *N. Engl. J. Med.*, **311**, 1482–7. [5.2.4, 5.14]
Baker, C. J., Kasper, D. L., Edwards, M. S. and Schiffman, G. (1980) Influence of preimmunization antibody levels on the specificity of the immune response to related polysaccharide antigens. *N. Engl. J. Med.*, **303**, 173–8. [Ex 9.2]
Barnes, D. M., Lammie, G. A., Millis, R. R., *et al.* (1988) An immunohistochemical evaluation of c-erbB-2 expression in human breast carcinoma. *Br. J. Cancer*, **58**, 448–52. [13.3.1]
Begg, C. B. (1987) Biases in the assessment of diagnostic tests. *Stat. Med.*, **6**, 411–23. [14.4.7]
Begg, C. B. and Berlin, J. A. (1988) Publication bias: a problem in interpreting medical data (with discussion). *J. Roy. Statist. Soc. A.*, **151**, 419–63. [15.5.2]
Begg, C. B. and Engstrom, P. F. (1987) Eligibility and extrapolation in cancer clinical trials. *J. Clin. Oncol.*, **5**, 962–8. [15.2.8]
Begg, T. B. and Hearns, J. B. (1966) Components in blood viscosity. The relative contributions of haematocrit, plasma fibrinogen and other proteins. *Clin. Sci.*, **31**, 87–93. [11.5]
Bhargava, S. K., Ramji, S., Kumar, A., *et al.* (1985) Mid-arm and chest circumferences at birth as predictors of low birth weight and neonatal mortality in the community. *Br. Med. J.*, **291**, 1617–19. [16.3.5]
Blackwell, R. and Chang, A. (1988) Video display terminals and pregnancy. A review. *Br. J. Obstet. Gynaecol.*, **95**, 446–53. [Ex 4.4]
Bland, J. M. and Altman, D. G. (1986) Statistical methods for assessing agreement between two methods of clinical measurement. *Lancet*, **i**, 307–10. [11.3.4, 14.2, 14.2.2, 14.2.3, 14.2.6]
Bland, J. M. and Altman, D. G. (1988) Misleading statistics: errors in textbooks, software and manuals. *Int. J. Epidemiol.*, **17**, 245–7. [6.3, 6.5]
Bland, M. (1987) *An Introduction to Medical Statistics*, Oxford: University Press. [9.6.4, 13.2.2]
Blomqvist, N. (1986) On the bias caused by regression toward the mean in studying the relation between change and initial value. *J. Clin. Periodontol.*, **13**, 34–7. [11.3.5]
Booze, C. F. (1977) Epidemiologic investigation of occupation, age, and exposure in general aviation accidents. *Aviat. Space Environ. Med.*, **48**, 1081–91. [3.1, Ex 3.2]
Boyd, N. F., Wolfson, C., Moskowitz, M., *et al.* (1982) Observer variation in the interpretation of xeromammograms. *J. Nat. Cancer Inst.*, **68**, 357–63. [14.3]
Bracken, M. B. (1989) Reporting observational studies. *Br. J. Obstet. Gynaecol.*, **96**, 383–8. [16.4]

Breslow, N. E. and Day, N. E. (1980) *Statistical Methods in Cancer Research. Volume 1 – The analysis of case-control studies*, Lyon: IARC. [5.10.6, 5.14, 10.11.2]
Breslow, N. E. and Day, N. E. (1987) *Statistical Methods in Cancer Research. Volume II – The design and analysis of cohort studies*, Oxford: University Press/IARC. [5.10.4, 5.11, 5.14]
Brett, A. S., Phillips, M. and Beary, J. F. (1986) Predictive power of the polygraph: can the 'lie detector' really detect liars? *Lancet*, **i**, 544–7. [Ex 14.3]
Brostoff, J., Pack, S. and Merrett, T. (1984) A new multiple specific IgE assay – MAST. *Lancet*, **i**, 748–9. [14.3.1, 14.3.5]
Brown, G. W. (1984) Discriminant analysis. *Am. J. Dis. Child*, **138**, 395–400. [12.6]
Bungo, M. W., Charles, J. B. and Johnson, P. C. (1985) Cardiovascular deconditioning during space flight and the use of saline as a countermeasure to orthostatic intolerance. *Aviat. Space Environ. Med.*, **56**, 985–90. [Ex 9.1]
Burns, K. C. (1984) Motion sickness incidence: distribution of time to first emesis and comparison of some complex motion conditions. *Aviat. Space Environ. Med.*, **50**, 521–7. [13.2.1, 13.3.1]
Buyse, M. (1984) Quality control in multi-centre cancer clinical trials. In *Cancer Clinical Trials. Methods and Practice* (eds M. E. Buyse, M. J. Staquet and R. J. Sylvester), Oxford: University Press, 102–23. [7.7.8]
Campbell, M. J. and Gardner, M. J. (1989) Calculating confidence intervals for some non-parametric analyses. In *Statistics with Confidence* (eds M. J. Gardner and D. G. Altman), London: British Medical Journal, 71–9. [9.6.3, Ans 9.4]
Campogrande, M., Todros, T. and Brizzolara, M. (1977) Prediction of birthweight by ultrasound measurements of the fetus. *Br. J. Obstet. Gynaecol.*, **84**, 175–8. [11.16]
Carmichael, C. L., Rugg-Gunn, A. J. and Ferrell, R. S. (1989) The relationship between fluoridation, social class and caries experience in 5-year-old children in Newcastle and Northumberland in 1987. *Br. Dent. J.*, **167**, 57–61. [Ex 16.5]
Caruana, M. P., Lahiri, A., Cashman, P. M. M., *et al.* (1988) Effects of chronic congestive heart failure secondary to coronary artery disease on the circadian rhythm of blood pressure and heart rate. *Am. J. Cardiol.*, **62**, 755–9. [Ex 7.1]
Cavill, I., Trevett, D., Fisher, J. and Hoy, T. (1988) The measurement of the total volume of red cells in man: a non-radioactive approach using biotin. *Br. J. Haematol.*, **70**, 491–3. [Ex 14.1]
Centerwall, B. S., Armstrong, C. W., Funkhouser, L. S. and Elzay, R. P. (1986) Erosion of dental enamel among competitive swimmers at a gas-chlorinated swimming pool. *Am. J. Epidemiol.*, **123**, 641–7. [10.7]
Chalmers, T. C., Smith, H., Blackburn, B., *et al.* (1981) A method for assessing the quality of a randomized control trial. *Controlled Clin. Trials.*, **2**, 31–49. [15.6.1, 16.4]
Cherian, T., John, T. J., Simoes, E., *et al.* (1988) Evaluation of simple clinical signs for the diagnosis of acute lower respiratory tract infection. *Lancet*, **ii**, 125–8. [Ex 14.4]
Christensen, E. (1987) Multivariate survival analysis using Cox's regression model. *Hepatology*, **7**, 1346–58. [13.6.3]
Christensen, E., Neuberger, J., Crowe, J., *et al.* (1985) Beneficial effect of azathioprine and prediction of prognosis in primary biliary cirrhosis: final results of an international trial. *Gastroenterology* **89**, 1084–91. [4.5, 4.6, 7.5.3, 7.7.2, 13.6.1]
Clayton, D. and Hills, M. (1987) A two-period crossover trial. In: *The Statistical*

*Consultant in Action* (eds D. J. Hand and B. S. Everitt), Cambridge: University Press, 42–57. [15.4.10]

Cleveland, W. S. (1984) Graphs in scientific publications. *Am. Stat.*, **38**, 261–9. [16.3.5]

Colditz, G. A. and Emerson, J. D. (1985) The statistical content of published medical research: some implications for biomedical education. *Med. Educ.*, **19**, 248–55. [16.2]

Collins, R., Gray, R., Godwin, J. and Peto, R. (1987) Avoidance of large biases and large random errors in the assessment of moderate treatment effects: the need for systematic overviews. *Stat. Med.*, **6**, 245–50. [15.4.1, 15.4.9, 15.5.2]

Colton, T. (1974) *Statistics in Medicine,* Boston: Little, Brown. [1.3, 15.6.2, 16.4]

Cooper, G. S. and Zangwill, L. (1989) An analysis of the quality of research reports in the *Journal of General Internal Medicine*. *J. Gen. Intern. Med.*, **4**, 232–6. [14.]

Cox, D. R. (1972) Regression models and life tables. *J. Roy. Statist. Soc. B.*, **34**, 187–220. [13.6]

Cox, D. R. (1982) Statistical significance tests. *Br. J. Clin. Pharmacol.,* **14**, 325–31. [8.8.1]

Cox, D. R. (1983) Discussion of paper by P. Armitage. *J. Roy. Statist. Soc. A,* **146**, 332–3. [16.]

Cuckle, H. S., Wald, N. J. and Lindenbaum, R. H. (1986) Cord serum alpha-fetoprotein and Down's syndrome. *Br. J. Obstet. Gynaecol.*, **93**, 408–10. [5.10.1]

Cuzick, J. (1985) A Wilcoxon-type test for trend. *Stat. Med.,* **4**, 87–90. [9.8.7]

Dallal, G. E. (1988) Statistical microcomputing – like it is. *Am. Stat.*, **42**, 212–16. [6.3, 6.4, 6.5]

Dalton, M. E., Bromham, D. R., Ambrose, C. L., *et al*. (1987) Nasal absorption of progesterone in women. *Br. J. Obstet. Gynaecol.*, **94**, 84–8. [14.6.1, 14.6.3]

Daly, B. M. and Shuster, S. (1986) Effect of aspirin on pruritis. *Br. Med. J.*, **293**, 907. [Ex 15.3]

Davis, P. J. M. (1985) The oral contraceptive pill and the menopause. *Update*, 15 April, 799–802. [Ex 5.2]

Department of Clinical Epidemiology and Biostatistics, McMaster University (1983) Interpretation of diagnostic data. *Can. Med. Assoc. J.*, **129**, 429–32, 559–64, 586, 705–10, 832–5, 947–54, 1093–9. [14.4.8]

De Pauw, M. and Buyse, M. (1984) Design of forms for cancer clinical trials. In: *Cancer Clinical Trials. Methods and Practice* (eds M. E. Buyse, M. J. Staquet and R. J. Sylvester). Oxford: University Press, 64–82. [6.7]

DerSimonian, R., Charette, L. J., McPeek, B. and Mosteller, F. (1982) Reporting on methods in clinical trials. *N. Engl. J. Med.*, **306**, 1332–7. [16.3.7]

Dittrich, H., Gilpin, E., Nicod, P., *et al*. (1988) Acute myocardial infarction in women: influence of gender on mortality and prognostic variables. *Am. J. Cardiol.*, **62**, 1-7. [8.4.2]

Doll, R. and Hill, A. B. (1950) Smoking and carcinoma of the lung. Preliminary report. *Br. Med. J.*, **ii**, 739–48. [4.1]

Drum, D. E. and Christacapoulos, J. S. (1972) Hepatic scintigraphy in clinical decision making. *J. Nucl. Med.*, **13**, 908–15. [14.4]

Dunn, H. L. (1929) Application of statistical methods in physiology. *Physiol. Rev.*, **9**, 275–398. [16.2, 16.3.1]

Elashoff, J. D. (1983) Surviving proportional hazards. *Hepatology*, **3**, 1031–5. [13.6.3]

Ellenberg, J. H. and Nelson, K. B. (1980) Sample selection and the natural history of disease. Studies of febrile seizures. *J. Am. Med. Ass.,* **243**, 1337–40. [5.11.1]

Ellenberg, S. S. (1984) Randomization designs in comparative clinical trials. *N. Engl. J. Med.*, **310**, 1404–8. [15.2.5]
Elwood, P. C. (1982) Randomised controlled trials: sampling. *Br. J. Clin. Pharmacol.* **13**, 631–6. [15.2.8, 15.5.2]
Emerson, J. D. and Colditz, G. A. (1983) Use of statistical analysis in the *New England Journal of Medicine. N. Engl. J. Med.*, **309**, 709–13. [16.2]
Epidemiology Work Group of the Interagency Regulatory Liaison Group (1981) Guidelines for the documentation of epidemiological studies. *Am. J. Epidemiol.*, **114**, 609–13. [16.4]
Espeland, M. A. and Handelman, S. L. (1989) Using latent class models to characterize and assess relative error in discrete measurements. *Biometrics*, **45**, 587–99. [Ex 14.5]
Evans, S. J. W., Mills, P. and Dawson, J. (1988) The end of the p value? *Br. Heart J.*, **60**, 177–80. [16.5]
Feingold, K. R., Browner, W. S. and Siperstein, W. D. (1989) Prospective studies of muscle capillary basement membrane width in prediabetics. *J. Clin. Endocrinol. Metab.*, **69**, 784–9. [Ex 8.2]
Feinstein, A. R. (1985) Tempest in a P-pot? *Hypertension*, **7**, 313–18. [11.8]
Feinstein, A. R. (1988) Scientific standards in epidemiologic studies of the menace of daily life. *Science*, **242**, 1257–63. [1.1, 5.14]
Felson, D. T., Cupples, L. A. and Meenan, R. F. (1984) Misuse of statistical methods in *Arthritis and Rheumatism.* 1982 versus 1967–68. *Arthritis Rheumatism*, **27**, 1018–22. [16.2]
Fentiman, L. S., Rubens, R. D. and Hayward, J. L. (1983) Control of pleural effusions in patients with breast cancer. A randomized trial. *Cancer*, **52**, 737–9. [15.2.3]
Fentress, D. W., Masek, B. J., Mehegan, J. E. and Benson, H. (1986) Biofeedback and relaxation–response in the treatment of pediatric migraine. *Dev. Med. Child Neurol.* **28**, 139–46. [9.8.6]
Festing, M. F. W. (1981) The 'defined' animal and the reduction of animal use. In: *New Perspectives in Animal Experimentation* (ed. D. Sperlinger). Chichester: Wiley, 285–306. [5.7.4]
Fisher, R. A. and Yates, F. (1963) *Statistical Tables for Biological, Agricultural and Medical Research*, 6th edn. Edinburgh: Oliver and Boyd. [App. B]
Fleiss, J. L. (1981) *Statistical Methods for Rates and Proportions,* 2nd edn. New York: Wiley. [10.5, 10.8.2, 10.10, 10.11.2, 10.11.3, 14.3.4]
Fleming, D. M. and Crombie, D. L. (1987) Prevalence of asthma and hay fever in England and Wales. *Br. Med. J.*, **294**, 279–83. [8.3]
Fletcher, R. H. and Fletcher, S. W. (1979) Clinical research in general medical journals. A 30-year perspective. *N. Engl. J. Med.*, **301**, 180–3. [16.2, 16.3.2]
Frame, S., Moore, J., Peters, A. and Hall, D. (1985) Maternal height and shoe size as predictors of pelvic disproportion: an assessment. *Br. J. Obstet. Gynaecol.*, **92**, 1239–45. [10.8.2]
Freedman, L. S. (1979) The use of a Kolmogorov-Smirnov type statistic in testing hypotheses about seasonal variation. *J. Epidemiol. Comm. Health.*, **33**, 223–8. [14.7]
Freiman, J. A., Chalmers, T. C., Smith, H. and Kuebler, R. R. (1978) The importance of beta, the type II error and sample size in the design and interpretation of the randomized control trial. Survey of 71 'negative' trials. *N. Engl. J. Med.*, **299**, 690–4. [8.5.4, 16.3.2]
Furst, D. E. and Paulus, H. E. (1975) Lack of effect of rheumatoid arthritis on clonixin metabolism. *Clin. Pharmacol. Ther.*, **17**, 622–6. [Ex 14.2]

Galen, R. S. and Gambino, S. R. (1975) *Beyond Normality: the predictive value and efficiency of medical diagnosis*, New York: Wiley. [14.4.8]
Gardner, M. J. and Altman, D. G. (1989a) Estimating with confidence. In: *Statistics with Confidence* (eds M. J. Gardner and D. G. Altman), London: British Medical Journal, 3–5. [8.8, 16.3.6]
Gardner, M. J. and Altman, D. G. (1989b) Estimation rather than hypothesis testing: confidence intervals rather than P values. In: *Statistics with Confidence* (eds M. J. Gardner and D. G. Altman), London: British Medical Journal, 6–19. [8.8.1]
Gardner, M. J. and Altman, D. G. (eds) (1989c) *Statistics with Confidence*, London: British Medical Journal. [App B]
Gardner, M. J., Machin, D. and Campbell, M. J. (1989) Use of check lists in assessing the statistical content of medical studies. In: *Statistics with Confidence*. (eds M. J. Gardner, D. G. Altman) London: *British Medical Journal*, 101–8. [15.6.1, 16.4]
Gart, J. J., Krewski, D., Lee, P. N., *et al*. (1986) *Statistical Methods in Cancer Research. Volume III – The design and analysis of long-term animal experiments*, Lyon: IARC, 29–32. [5.7.4]
Gehlbach, S. H. (1982) *Interpreting the Medical Literature. A clinician's guide*, Lexington Mass.: D. C. Heath and Co. [5.14]
George, S. L. (1985) Statistics in medical journals: a survey of current policies and proposals for editors. *Med. Pediatr. Oncol.*, **13**, 109–12. [16.3.10]
Gibbons, R. D. and Davis, J. M. (1984) The price of beer and the salaries of priests: analysis and display of longitudinal psychiatric data. *Arch. Gen. Psychiatry*, **41**, 1183–4. [5.13]
Gibson, T., Grahame, R., Harkness, J., *et al*. (1985) Controlled comparison of short-wave diathermy treatment with osteopathic treatment in non-specific low back pain. *Lancet*, **i**, 1258–61. [3.5.1]
Glasser, G. J. and Winter R. F. (1961) Critical values of the coefficient of rank correlation for testing the hypothesis of independence. *Biometrika*, **48**, 444–8. [App B]
Gore, S. M. (1982) Assessing methods – transforming the data. In: *Statistics in Practice* (eds S. M. Gore and D. G. Altman), London: British Medical Association, 67–9. [7.6.1]
Gøtzsche, P. C. (1989) Methodology and overt and hidden bias in reports of 196 double-blind trials of non-steroidal antiinflammatory drugs in rheumatoid arthritis. *Controlled Clin. Trials*, **10**, 31–56. [15.4.7]
Gould, B. A., Hornung, R. S., Kieso, H. A., *et al*. (1985) Is the blood pressure the same in both arms? *Clin. Cardiol.*, **8**, 423–6. [5.4, 8.5.1]
Grant, A. (1989) Reporting controlled trials. *Br. J. Obstet. Gynaecol.*, **96**, 397–400. [15.6.1, 16.4]
Gray-Donald, K. and Kramer, M. S. (1988) Causality inference in observational vs. experimental studies. An empirical comparison. *Am. J. Epidemiol.*, **127**, 885–92. [5.9]
Green, S. B. and Byar, D. P. (1984) Using observational data from registries to compare treatments: the fallacy of omnimetrics. *Stat. Med.*, **3**, 361–70. [16.3.2]
Greenwood, M. (1932) What is wrong with the medical curriculum? *Lancet*, **i**, 1269–70. [16.3]
Greenwood, M. (1948) The statistician and medical research. *Br. Med. J.*, **2**, 467–8. [Preface]
Guyatt, G. H., Townsend, M., Kazim, F. and Newhouse, M. T. (1987) A controlled trial of ambroxol in chronic bronchitis. *Chest*, **92**, 618–20. [15.3.2]

Halkin, H., Sheiner, L. B., Peck, C. C. and Melmon, K. L. (1975) Determinants of the renal clearance of digoxin. *Clin. Pharmocol. Ther.*, **17**, 385–94. [Ex 11.4]

Halpern, D. F. and Coren, S. (1988) Do right-handers live longer? *Nature*, **333**, 213. [1.1, 5.14, Ex 5.3]

Hampton, J. R. (1981) Presentation and analysis of the results of clinical trials in cardiovascular disease. *Br. Med. J.*, **282**, 1371–3. [15.6.1]

Hayden, G. F. (1983) Biostatistical trends in *Pediatrics*: implications for the future. *Pediatrics*, **72**, 84–7. [16.2]

Hayes, R. J. (1988) Methods for assessing whether change depends on initial value. *Stat. Med.*, **7**, 915–27. [11.3.5]

Hill, A. B. (1963) Medical ethics and controlled trials. *Br. Med. J.*, **i**, 1043–9. [15., 15.2.9]

Hill, A. B. (1984) *A Short Textbook of Medical Statistics*, 11th edn, London: Hodder and Stoughton. [15.1, 16.2]

Hofacker, C. F. (1983) Abuse of statistical packages: the case of the general linear model. *Am. J. Physiol.*, **245**, R299–R302. [6]

Hogben, L. (1950) *Chance and Choice by Cardpack and Chessboard*, Volume 1, New York: Chanticleer Press Unnumbered page. [16.3]

Hommel, E., Parving, H.-H., Mathiesen, E., *et al.* (1986) Effect of captopril on kidney function in insulin-dependent diabetic patients with nephropathy. *Br. Med. J.*, **293**, 467–70. [Ex 15.4]

Hoogstraten, B. (1984) Reporting treatment results in solid tumours. In: *Cancer Clinical Trials. Methods and Practice.* (eds M. E. Buyse, M. J. Staquet, and R. J. Sylvester), Oxford: University Press, 139–56. [16.3]

Hughes, R. E. and Jones, E. (1985) Intake of dietary fibre and the age of menarche. *Ann. Hum. Biol.*, **12**, 325–32. [11.4]

Hulse, J. A., Jackson, D., Grant, D. B., *et al.* (1979) Different measurements of thyroid function in hypothyroid infants diagnosed by screening, *Acta Paediatr. Scand. Suppl.*, **277**, 21–5. [9.6.5]

Ingelfinger, J. A., Mosteller, F., Thibodeau, L. A. and Ware, J. H. (1987) *Biostatistics in Clinical Medicine,* 2nd edn, New York: Macmillan. [14.4.6, 14.4.8]

Isaacs, D., Altman, D. G., Tidmarsh, C. E., *et al.* (1983) Serum immunoglobulin concentrations in preschool children measured by laser nephelometry: reference ranges for IgG, IgA, IgM. *J. Clin. Pathol.* **36**, 1193–6. [3.3.1, 14.5.2, 14.5.4]

James, W. H. (1985) Dizygotic twinning, birth weight and latitude. *Ann. Hum. Biol.*, **12**, 441–7. [11.5]

Johnson, A. L. and Altman, D.G. (1990) A survey of reviews of the quality of statistics in the medical literature. I. Methods and bibliography (pre-1987). In preparation [16.3.1]

Kahan, A., Amor, B., Menkès, C. J., *et al.* (1987) Nicardipine in the treatment of Raynaud's phenomenon: a randomized double-blind trial. *Angiology*, **38**, 333–7 [15.4.10]

Kahneman, D. and Tversky, A. (1982) Subjective probability: a judgement of representativeness. In *Judgement under Uncertainty: Heuristics and Biases* (eds D. Kahneman, P. Slovic and A. Tversky), Cambridge: University Press, 32–47 [Ex 8.1]

Karacan, I., Fernández-Salas, A., Coggins, W. S., *et al.* (1976) Sleep electrocephalographic–electrooculographic characteristics of chronic marijuana users: part 1. *Ann. NY Acad. Sci.*, **282**, 348–74. [10.4, 10.4.1]

Kendell, R. E., de Roumanie, M. and Ritson, E. B. (1983) Influence of an increase in excise duty on alcohol consumption and its adverse effects. *Br. Med.*

*J.*, **287**, 809–11 [Ex 5.1]
Kimpen, J., Callaert, H., Embrechts, P. and Bosmans, E. (1987) Cord blood IgE and month of birth. *Arch. Dis. Child.*, **62**, 478–82. [14.7]
Kirwan, J. R., Byron, M. A., Winfield, J., *et al*. (1979) Circumferential measurements in the assessment of synovitis of the knee. *Rheumatol. Rehab.*, **18**, 78–84. [14.2.4]
Kitson, T. (1984) The ultimate mile. *New Scientist*, **103** (1415), 34. [11.14]
Koehn, H. D. and Mostbeck, A. (1981) Age-dependence of immunoreactive trypsin concentrations in serum. *Clin. Chem.*, **27**, 502. [9.8.5]
Kuntze, C. E. E., Ebels, T., Eijgelaar, A. and Homan van der Heide, J. N. (1989) Rates of thromboembolism with three different mechanical heart valve prostheses: randomised study. *Lancet*, **i**, 514–17. [16.3.3, 16.3.7]
Kurjak, A., Latin, V. and Polak, J. (1978) Ultrasonic recognition of two types of growth retardation by measurement of four fetal dimensions. *J. Perinat. Med.*, **6**, 102–8. [10.11.1]
Lachenbruch, P. A. (1977) Some misuses of discriminant analysis. *Meth. Inform. Med.*, **16**, 255–8. [12., 12.6]
Lam, K. C., Lai, C. L., Ng, R. P., *et al*. (1981) Deleterious effect of prednisolone in HBsAg-positive chronic active hepatitis. *N. Engl. J. Med.*, **304**, 380–6. [Ex 8.4]
Landis, J. R. and Koch, G. G. (1977) The measurement of observer agreement for categorical data. *Biometrics*, **33**, 159–74. [14.3.1]
Langhoff-Roos, J., Lindmark, G., Gustavson, K-H., *et al*. (1987) Relative effect of parental birth weight on infant birth weight at term. *Clin. Genet.*, **32**, 240–8. [12.4]
Leitch, I., Hytten, F. E. and Billewicz, W. Z. (1959) The maternal and neonatal weights of some mammalia. *Proc. Zool. Soc. Lond.*, **133**, 11–28. [11.2, 11.2.1]
Lentner, C. (Ed.) (1982) *Geigy Scientific Tables*, Volume 2, 8th edn, Basle: Ciba-Geigy. [4.9.1, App. B]
Lewith, G. T. and Machin, D. (1981) A randomised trial to evaluate the effect of infra-red stimulation of local trigger points, versus placebo, on the pain caused by cervical osteoarthrosis. *Int. J. Acupuncture Electro-Therapeut. Res.*, **6**, 277–84. [10.3, 10.7.1]
Lichtenstein, M. J., Mulrow, C. D. and Elwood, P. C. (1987) Guidelines for reading case-control studies. *J. Chron. Dis.*, **40**, 893–903. [5.14, 16.4]
Light, I. M., Avery, A. and Grieve, A. M. (1987) Immersion suit insulation: the effect of dampening on survival estimates. *Aviat. Space Environ. Med.*, **58**, 964–9. [12.3.5]
Lind, T., Godfrey, K. A., Otun, H. and Philips, P. R. (1984) Changes in serum uric acid concentrations during normal pregnancy. *Br. J. Obstet. Gynaecol.*, **91**, 128–32. [3.5.1, 9.10]
Linnet, K. (1987) Two-stage transformation systems for normalisation of reference distributions evaluated. *Clin. Chem.*, **33**, 381–6. [14.5.3]
Lippman, M. E., Cassidy, J., Wesley, M. and Young, R. C. (1984) A randomized attempt to increase the efficacy of cytotoxic chemotherapy in metastatic breast cancer by hormonal synchronization. *J. Clin. Oncol.*, **2**, 28–36. [16.3.4]
Lucey, M. R. (1987) The need for confidence intervals in reporting clinical trials. *Gut*, **28**, 916–17. [Ex 16.8]
Lumley, J., McKinnon, L. and Wood, C. (1971) Lack of agreement on normal values for fetal scalp blood. *J. Obstet. Gynaecol. Br. Commwlth.*, **78**, 13–21. [14.5.3]
Lyster, W. R. (1984) Bass singers have a more masculine sex ratio in their siblings

than tenors. *IRCS Med. Sci.*, **12**, 234. [Ex 10.2]

Macartney, F. J. (1987) Diagnostic logic. *Br. Med. J.*, **295**, 1325–31. [14.4.8]

Macfarlane, A. and Mugford, M. (1984) *Birth Counts. Statistics of pregnancy and childbirth*, London: HMSO, 49. [3.1]

Macgregor, I. D. M. and Balding, J. W. (1988) Bedtimes and family size in English schoolchildren. *Ann. Hum. Biol.*, **15**, 435–41. [Ex 10.4]

Machin, D. and Campbell, M. J. (1987) *Statistical Tables for the Design of Clinical Trials*, Oxford: Blackwell. [13.7, 15.3.2]

Mackenzie, S. G. and Lippman, A. (1989) An investigation of report bias in a case-control study of pregnancy outcome. *Am. J. Epidemiol.*, **129**, 65–75. [5.10.3]

Mainland, D. (1950) Statistics in clinical research: some general principles. *Ann. NY Acad. Sci.*, **52**(6), 922–30 [16.5]

Manocha, S., Choudhuri, G. and Tandon, B.N. (1986) A study of dietary intake in pre- and post-menstrual period. *Hum. Nut.: Appl. Nut.*, **40A**, 213–16. [9.4, 9.5]

Maron, D. J., Telch, M. J., Killen, J. D. *et al.* (1986) Correlates of seat-belt use by adolescents: implications for health promotion. *Prev. Med.*, **15**, 614–23. [8.8.4]

Martin, T. R. and Bracken, M. B. (1987) The association between low birth weight and caffeine consumption during pregnancy. *Am. J. Epidemiol.*, **126**, 813–21. [5.11.2, 10.6.1]

Maskin, C. S., Ocken, S., Chadwick, B. and Le Jemtel, T. H. (1985) Comparative systemic and renal effects of dopamine and angiotensin-converting enzyme inhibition with enalaprilat in patients with heart failure. *Circulation*, **72**, 846–52. [12.3.1]

Matsukura, S., Taminato, T., Kitano, N., *et al.* (1984) Effects of environmental tobacco smoke on urinary cotinine excretion in nonsmokers. *N. Engl. J. Med.*, **311**, 828–32. [Ex 9.5]

Matthews, J. N. S., Altman, D. G., Campbell, M. J. and Royston, J. P. (1990) Analysis of serial measurements in medical research. *Br. Med. J.*, **300**, 230–5. [14.6.1]

Mattila, K. J., Nieminen, M. S., Valtonen, V. V., *et al.* (1989) Association between dental health and acute myocardial infarction. *Br. Med. J.*, **298**, 779–82. [5.10.6]

May, G. S., DeMets, D. L., Friedman, L., *et al.* (1981) The randomized clinical trial: bias in analysis. *Circulation*, **64**, 669–73. [15.4]

Mayes, L. C., Horwitz, R. I. and Feinstein, A. R. (1988) A collection of 56 topics with contradictory results in case-control research. *Int. J. Epidemiol.*, **17**, 680–5. [5.10.6]

Mazess, R. B., Peppler, W. W. and Gibbons, M. (1984) Total body composition by dual-photon ($^{153}$Gd) absorptiometry. *Am. J. Clin. Nut.*, **40**, 834–9. [11.2, 11.4, 11.8]

Medical Research Council (MRC) (1948) Streptomycin treatment of pulmonary tuberculosis. *Br. Med. J.*, **ii**, 769–82. [15.1, 16.2]

Meier, P. (1981) Stratification in the design of a clinical trial. *Controlled Clin. Trials*, **1**, 355–61. [15.2.2]

Miao, L. L. (1977) Gastric freezing: an example of the evaluation of medical therapy by randomized clinical trials. In *Costs, Risks, and Benefits of Surgery* (eds J. P. Bunker, B.A. Barnes and F. Mosteller), New York: Oxford University Press, 198–211. [15.2.1]

Milledge, J. S., Beeley, J. M., McArthur, S. and Morice, A. M. (1989) Atrial natriuretic peptide, altitude and acute mountain sickness. *Clin. Sci.*, **77**, 509–14. [Ex 16.7]

Morris, J. A. and Gardner, M. J. (1989) Calculating confidence intervals for relative risks, odds ratios, and standardized ratios and rates. In *Statistics with Confidence* (eds M. J. Gardner and D. G. Altman), London: British Medical Journal, 50–63. [10.11.2]

Moses, L. E. (1987) Graphical methods in statistical analysis. *Ann. Rev. Publ. Health*, **8**, 309–53. [3.7.3]

Moses, L. E., Emerson, J. D. and Hosseini, H. (1984) Analyzing data from ordered categories. *N. Engl. J. Med.*, **311**, 442–8. [10.8.2, 10.13]

Mosteller, F., Gilbert, J. P. and McPeek, B. (1980) Reporting standards and research strategies for controlled trials. Agenda for the editor. *Controlled Clin. Trials*, **1**, 37–58. [16.3.7]

Nanji, A. A. and French, S. W. (1985) Relationship between pork consumption and cirrhosis. *Lancet*, **i**, 681–3. [11.8]

Ng, R. P., Lam, K. C., Lai, C. L. and Wu, P. C. (1981) Prednisolone in HBsAg-positive chronic active hepatitis. *N. Engl. J. Med.*, **305**, 283. [Ex 8.4]

Noller, K. L. and Melton, L. J. (1985) Study design in perinatal medicine. *Am. J. Perinatol.*, **2**, 250–5. [5.]

Norton, P. G. and Dunn, E. V. (1985) Snoring as a risk factor for disease: an epidemiological survey. *Br. Med. J.*, **291**, 630–2. [10.8.2, 12.5]

Numerical Algorithms Group (1987) *The NAG Fortran Library – Mark 12*. Oxford: Numerical Algorithms Group. [App B]

Oldham, P. D. (1979) Per cent of predicted as the limit of normal in pulmonary function testing: a statistically valid approach. *Thorax*, **34**, 569. [14.]

Oldham, P. D. (1985) The fluoridation of the Strathclyde Regional Council's water supply: opinion of Lord Jauncey *in causa* Mrs Catherine McColl against Strathclyde Regional Council: a review. *J. Roy. Statist. Soc. A.*, **148**, 37–44. [1.1]

O'Neill, S., Leahy, F., Pasterkamp, H. and Tal, A. (1983) The effects of chronic hyperinflation, nutritional status, and posture on respiratory muscle strength in cystic fibrosis. *Am. Rev. Respir. Dis.*, **128**, 1051–4. [3.2, 12.4]

Otulana, B., Mist, B. A., Scott, J. P., *et al*. (1989) The effect of recipient lung size on lung physiology after heart–lung transplantation. *Transplantation*, **48**, 625–9. [Ex 12.5]

Owen, O. E., Kavle, E., Owen, R. S., *et al*. (1986) A reappraisal of caloric requirements in healthy women. *Am. J. Clin. Nutr.*, **44**, 1–19. [Ex 11.2]

Oye, R. K. and Shapiro, M. K. (1984) Reporting from chemotherapy trials. Does response make a difference in patient survival? *J. Am. Med. Ass.*, **252**, 2722–5. [13.5.3]

Peeters, P. H. M., Verbeek, A. L. M., Hendriks, J. H. C. L., *et al*. (1987) The predictive value of positive test results in screening for breast cancer by mammography in the Nijmegen programme. *Br. J. Cancer*, **56**, 667–71. [12.5.2]

Peto, R., Gray, R., Collins, R., *et al*. (1988) Randomised trial of prophylactic daily aspirin in British male doctors. *Br. Med. J.*, **296**, 313–16. [15.2.8]

Peto, R., Pike, M. C., Armitage, P., *et al*. (1976) Design and analysis of randomized clinical trials requiring prolonged observation of each patient. I. Introduction and design. *Br. J. Cancer*, **34**, 585–612. [13.1, 13.7, 15.1, 15.2.2]

Peto, R., Pike, M. C., Armitage, P., *et al*. (1977) Design and analysis of randomized clinical trials requiring prolonged observation of each patient. II. Analysis and examples. *Br. J. Cancer*, **35**, 1–39. [13.1, 13.3.1, 13.5, 13.7]

Pickering, G. (1978) Normotension and hypertension: the mysterious viability of the false. *Am. J. Med.*, **65**, 561–3. [14.5.5]

Pisani, P., Berrino, F., Macaluso, M., *et al*. (1986) Carrots, green vegetables and

lung cancer: a case-control study. *Int. J. Epidemiol.*, **15**, 463–8. [5.10.1]
Pocock, S. J. (1977) Randomised clinical trials. *Br. Med. J.*, **i**, 1661. [15.2.4]
Pocock, S. J. (1983) *Clinical Trials: A Practical Approach*, Chichester, Wiley. [5.14, 6.7, 15.1, 15.2.5, 15.2.11, 15.4.9]
Pocock, S.J. (1985) Current issues in the design and interpretation of clinical trials. *Br. Med. J.*, **290**, 39–42. [15.1]
Prentice, A. M., Black, A. E., Coward, W. A., *et al.* (1986) High levels of energy expenditure in obese women. *Br. Med. J.*, **292**, 983–7. [9.6.1]
Preston-Martin, S., Thomas, D. C., Wright, W. E. and Henderson, B. E. (1989) Noise trauma in the aetiology of acoustic neuromas in men in Los Angeles County, 1978–1985. *Br. J. Cancer*, **59**, 783–6. [Ex 10.8]
Raftery, E. B. and Ward, A. P. (1968) The indirect method of recording blood pressure. *Cardiovasc. Res.*, **2**, 210–18. [Ex 16.6]
Ramirez, A., Craig, T. K. J., Watson, J. P., *et al.* (1989) Stress and relapse of breast cancer. *Br. Med. J.*, **298**, 291–3. [10.11.2]
Ramsdale, D. R., Faragher, E. B., Bennett, D. H., *et al.* (1982) Preoperative prediction of significant coronary artery disease in patients with valvular heart disease. *Br. Med. J.*, **284**, 223–6. [Ex 12.4]
Rantakallio, P. and Mäkinen, H. (1984) Number of teeth at the age of one year in relation to maternal smoking. *Ann. Hum. Biol.*, **11**, 45–52. [3.3.3, 12.4.10]
Reading, V. M. and Weale, R. A. (1986) Eye strain and visual display units. *Lancet*, **i**, 905–6. [10.8.1]
Reisch, J. S., Tyson, J. E. and Mize, S. G. (1989) Aid to the evaluation of therapeutic studies. *Pediatrics*, **84**, 815–27. [16.4]
Richmond, R. L., Austin, A. and Webster, I. W. (1988) Predicting abstainers in a smoking cessation programme administered by general practitioners. *Int. J. Epidemiol.*, **17**, 530–4. [12.5.2]
Roberts, R. S., Spitzer, W. O., Delmore, T. and Sackett, D. L. (1978) An empirical demonstration of Berkson's bias. *J. Chron. Dis.*, **31**, 119–28. [5.10.1]
Rockwood, K., Stolee, P., Robertson, D. and Shillington, E. R. (1989) Response bias in a health status survey of elderly people. *Age Ageing*, **18**, 177–82. [5.12.2]
Rosenthal, F. S., Bakalian, A. E., Lou, C. and Taylor, H. R. (1988) The effect of sunglasses on ocular exposure to ultraviolet radiation. *Am. J. Public Health*, **78**, 72–4. [9.8.7]
Roth, J. A., Eilber, F. R., Nizze, J. A. and Morton, D. L. (1975) Lack of correlation between skin reactivity to dinitrochlorobenzene and croton oil in patients with cancer. *N. Engl. J. Med.*, **293**, 388–9. [Ex 10.1]
Royston, J. P. (1983) A simple method for evaluating the Shapiro-Francia $W'$ test for non-Normality. *Statistician*, **32**, 297–300. [11.6, App B]
Royston, J. P., Flecknell, P. A. and Wootton, R. (1982) New evidence that the intra-uterine growth-retarded piglet is a member of a discrete subpopulation. *Biol. Neonate*, **42**, 100–4. [7.5.3]
Sackett, D. L. (1979) Bias in analytic research. *J. Chron. Dis.*, **32**, 51–63. [5.10]
Sackett, D. L. (1986) Rational therapy in the neurosciences: the role of the randomized trial. *Stroke*, **17**, 1323–9. [5.]
Sackett, D. L. and Gent, M. (1979) Controversy in counting and attributing events in clinical trials. *N. Engl. J. Med.*, **301**, 1410–12. [15.4.5]
Sacks, H. S., Chalmers, T. C. and Smith, H. (1983) Sensitivity and specificity of clinical trials: randomized v historical controls. *Arch. Intern. Med.*, **143**, 753–5. [15.2.4]
Sankaranarayanan, R., Mohideen, M. N., Nair, M. K. and Padmanabhan, T. K. (1989) Aetiology of oral cancer in patients $\leq 30$ years of age. *Br. J. Cancer*, **59**,

439–40. [Ex 10.6]
Schiff, E., Peleg, E., Goldenberg, M., *et al.* (1989) The use of aspirin to prevent pregnancy-induced hypertension and lower the ratio of thromboxane $A_2$ to prostacyclin in relatively high risk pregnancies. *N. Engl. J. Med.*, **321**, 351–6. [Ex 10.7, Ex 15.5]
Schlesselman, J. J. (1982) *Case-control Studies. Design, conduct, analysis*, Oxford: University Press. [5.10.6, 5.14]
Schoenfeld, D. A. and Richter, J. R. (1982) Nomograms for calculating the number of patients needed for a clinical trial with survival as an endpoint. *Biometrics*, **38**, 163–70. [13.7]
Schoolman, H. M., Becktel, J. M., Best, W. R. and Johnson, A. F. (1968) Statistics in medical research: principles versus practices. *J. Lab. Clin. Med.*, **71**, 357–67. [1.3, 9.]
Schor, S. and Karten, I. (1966) Statistical evaluation of medical journal manuscripts. *J. Am. Med. Ass.*, **195**, 1123–8. [16.3.1]
Seddon, H. J. (1937) Clinical evidence and statistical proof. *Lancet*, **ii**, 412. [1.5]
Seely, S. (1985) Relation between pork consumption and cirrhosis. *Lancet*, **i**, 925. [11.8]
Shaper, A. G., Pocock, S. J., Phillips, A. N. and Walker, M. (1986) Identifying men at high risk of heart attacks: strategy for use in general practice. *Br. Med. J.*, **293**, 474–9. [1.4.1, 12.5.2]
Shapiro, C. M., Beckmann, E., Christiansen, N., *et al.* (1986) Immunologic status of patients in remission from Hodgkin's disease and disseminated malignancies. *Am. J. Med. Sci.*, **293**, 366–70. [7.3, 9.7, 9.7.1]
Sheps, S. B. and Schechter, M. T. (1984) The assessment of diagnostic tests. A survey of current medical research. *J. Am. Med. Ass.*, **252**, 2418–22. [14.4.8, 16.3.2, 16.4]
Silman, A. J. (1985) Failure of random zero sphygmomanometer in general practice. *Br. Med. J.*, **290**, 1781–2. [7.7.1]
Silverman, W. A. (1985) *Human Experimentation: a guided step into the unknown*, Oxford: University Press. [15.2.1, 15.2.9]
Simon, R. (1986) Confidence intervals for reporting results of clinical trials. *Ann. Intern. Med.*, **105**, 429–35. [13.4.5, 13.4.7]
Simon, R. and Makuch, R. W. (1984) A non-parametric graphical representation of the relationship between survival and the occurrence of an event: application to responder versus non-responder bias. *Stat. Med.*, **3**, 35–44. [13.5.3]
Simon, R. and Wittes, R. E. (1985) Methodologic guidelines for reports of clinical trials. *Cancer Treat. Rep.*, **69**, 1–3. [15.6.1, 16.4]
Sivell, L. M. and Wenlock, R. W. (1983) The nutritional composition of British bread: London area study. *Hum. Nut.: Appl. Nut.*, **37A**, 459–69. [3.7.3]
Smith, D. G., Clemens, J., Crede, W., *et al.* (1987) Impact of multiple comparisons in randomized clinical trials. *Am. J. Med.*, **83**, 545–50. [15.4.7]
Smith, R. (1981) The relation between consumption and damage. *Br. Med. J.*, **283**, 895–8. [11.8]
Smithells, R. W., Sheppard, S., Schorah, C. J., *et al.* (1980) Possible prevention of neural-tube defects by periconceptional vitamin supplementation. *Lancet*, **i**, 339–40. [15.2.4, 15.2.9]
Snedecor, G. W. (1950) The statistical part of the scientific method. *Ann. N.Y. Acad. Sci.*, **52**, 792–9. [8.]
Solberg, H. E. (1987) Approved recommendation (1986) on the theory of reference values. Part 1. The concept of reference values. *J. Clin. Chem. Clin. Biochem.*, **25**, 337–42. [14.5]

Sprent, P. (1989) *Applied Nonparametric Statistical Methods*, London: Chapman and Hall, 142–55. [11.14]
Stacpoole, P. W., Lorenz, A. C., Thomas, R. G. and Harman, E. M. (1988) Dichloroacetate in the treatment of lactic acidosis. *Ann. Intern. Med.*, **108**, 58–63. [Ex 11.1]
Storr, J., Barrell, E., Barry, W., *et al.* (1987) Effect of a single oral dose of prednisolone in acute childhood asthma. *Lancet*, **i**, 879–82. [Ex 10.3]
Stuart, J., Stone, P. C. W., Freyburger, G., *et al.* (1989) Instrument precision and biological variability determine the number of patients required for rheological studies. *Clin. Hemorheol.*, **9**, 181–97. [16.3.2]
Thakur, C. P. and Sharma, D. (1984) Full moon and crime. *Br. Med. J.*, **289**, 1789–91. [4.8]
Thomas, E. J. and Cooke, I. D. (1987) Impact of gestrinone on the course of asymptomatic endometriosis. *Br. Med. J.*, **294**, 272–4. [Ex 9.7]
Thompson, E. M., Price, A. B., Altman, D. G., *et al.* (1985) Quantitation in inflammatory bowel disease using computerised interactive image analysis. *J. Clin. Pathol.*, **38**, 631–8. [12.6]
Thuesen, L., Christiansen, J. S., Falstie-Jensen, N., *et al.* (1985) Increased myocardial contractility in short-term Type 1 diabetic patients: an echocardiographic study. *Diabetologia*, **28**, 822–6. [8.6, 11.6, 11.10]
Tibshirani, R. (1982) A plain man's guide to the proportional hazards model. *Clin. Invest. Med.*, **5**, 63–8. [13.6.3]
Toulon, P., Jacquot, C., Capron, L., *et al.* (1987) Antithrombin III and heparin cofactor II in patients with chronic renal failure undergoing regular haemodialysis. *Thromb. Haemostas.*, **57**, 263–8. [7.3, Ex 9.6]
Tufte, E. R. (1983) *The Visual Display of Quantitative Information*, Cheshire, Conn.: Graphics Press. [3.7.3, 16.3.5]
Tukey, J. W. (1977) *Exploratory Data Analysis*, Reading, Mass.: Addison-Wesley. [3.7.3]
Tyson, J. E., Furzan, J. A., Reisch, J. S. and Mize, S. G. (1983) An evaluation of the quality of therapeutic studies in perinatal medicine. *J. Pediatr.*, **102**, 10–13. [16.3.1]
Ueshima, H., Ogihara, T., Baba, S., *et al.* (1987) The effect of reduced alcohol consumption on blood pressure: a randomised, controlled, single blind study. *J. Hum. Hypertension*, **1**, 113–19. [15.4.1, 15.4.10]
Wainer, H. (1984) How to display data badly. *Am. Stat.*, **38**, 137–47. [16.3.5]
Wald, N. and Cuckle, H. (1989) Reporting the assessment of screening and diagnostic tests. *Br. J. Obstet. Gynaecol.*, **96**, 389–96. [16.4]
Weindling, A. M., Bamford, F. N. and Whittall, R. A. (1986) Health of juvenile delinquents. *Br. Med. J.*, **292**, 447. [10.7.2]
Weiss, S. H., Goedert, J. J., Sarngadharan, M. G., *et al.* (1985) Screening test for HTLV-III (AIDS agent) antibodies. *J. Am. Med. Ass.*, **253**, 221–5. [14.4.4, 14.4.8]
Welle, S. L., Seaton, T. B. and Campbell, R. G. (1986) Some metabolic effects of overeating in man. *Am. J. Clin. Nutr.*, **44**, 718–24. [Ex 12.1]
Weller, M. P. I. and Weller, B. (1986) Crime and psychopathology. *Br. Med. J.*, **292**, 55–6. [5.13]
Williams, C. J., Davies, C., Raval, M., *et al.* (1989) Comparison of starting antiemetic treatment 24 hours before or concurrently with cytotoxic chemotherapy. *Br. Med. J.*, **298**, 430–1. [Ex 9.4]
Woods, J. R., Williams, J. G. and Tavel, M. (1989) The two-period crossover design in medical research. *Ann. Intern. Med.*, **110**, 560–6. [15.2.5]

Yusuf, S., Collins, R., Peto, R., *et al.* (1985) Intravenous and intracoronary fibrinolytic therapy in acute myocardial infarction: overview of results on mortality, reinfarction and side-effects from 33 randomized controlled trials. *Eur. Heart J.*, **6**, 556–85. [15.5.2]

Zelen, M. (1979) A new design for randomized clinical trials. *N. Engl. J. Med.*, **300**, 1242–5. [15.2.5]

Zhang, Y., Nitter-Hauge, S., Ihlen, H., *et al.* (1986) Measurement of aortic regurgitation by Doppler echocardiography. *Br. Heart J.*, **55**, 32–8. [14.2.1]

Zweig, J. P. and Csank, J. Z. (1978) The application of a Poisson model to the annual distribution of daily mortality at six Montreal hospitals. *J. Epidem. Comm. Hlth.*, **32**, 206–11. [4.8]

# Index

The prefix N refers to an entry in Appendix A on mathematical notation